PRACTICAL GUIDE TO MAMMOGRAPHY INTERPRETATION AND REPORTING

REMON M. HANA

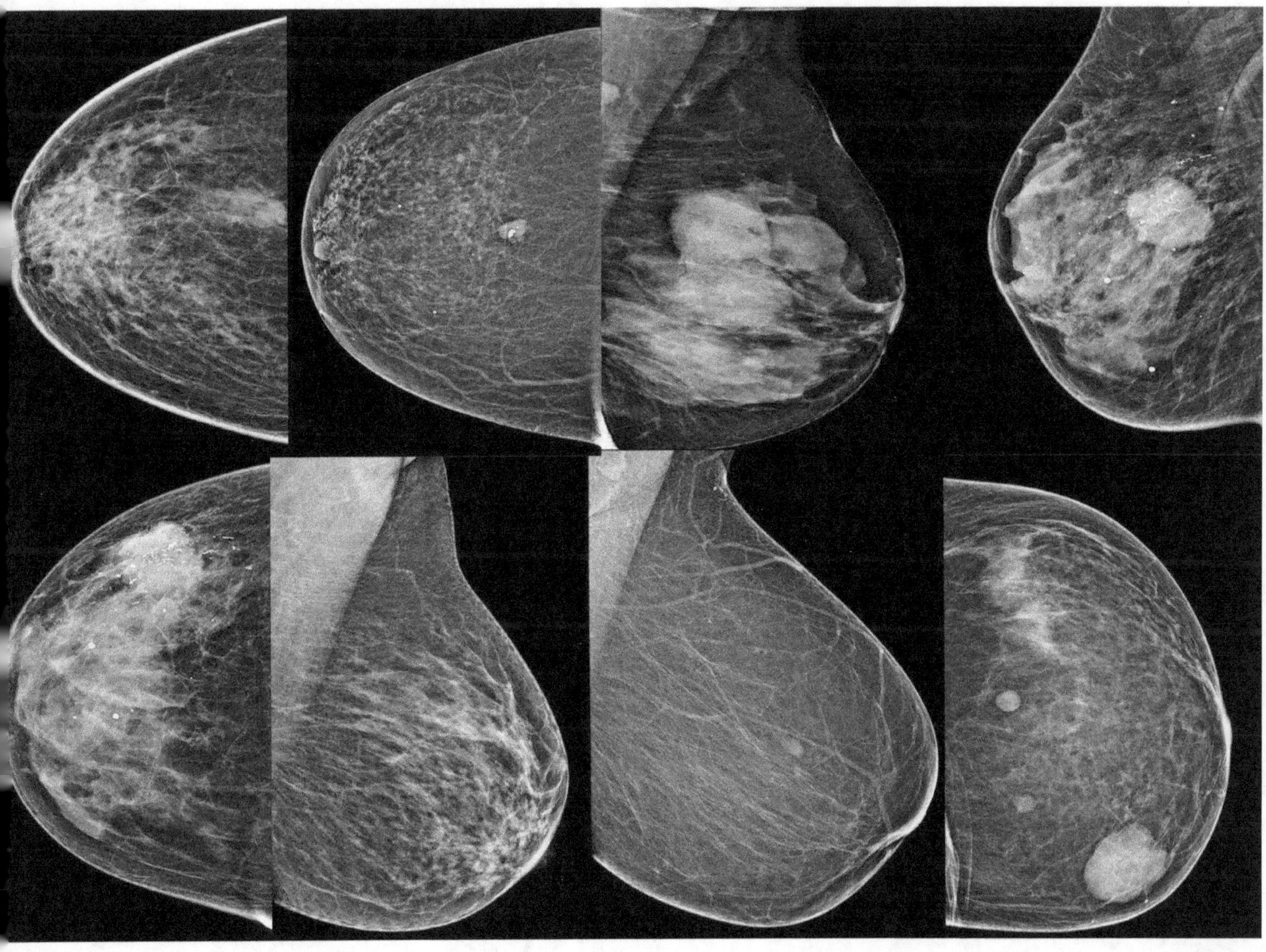

PRACTICAL GUIDE TO MAMMOGRAPHY INTERPRETATION AND REPORTING

ALL CASES PRESENTED IN THIS BOOK ARE FROM OUR CLINIC

First Edition

Remon M. Hana

AUTHOR NAME
COPYRIGHT AND DISCLAIMER

Notice to the Reader:
Medicine is an ever-changing science. As new research and clinical experience broaden our knowledge, changes in treatment and drug therapy are required. The authors and the publisher of this work have checked with sources believed to be reliable in their efforts to provide information that is complete and generally in accord with the standards accepted at the time of publication. However, in view of the possibility of human error or changes in medical sciences, neither the authors nor the publisher nor any other party who has been involved in the preparation or publication of this work warrants that the information contained herein is in every respect accurate or complete, and they disclaim all responsibility for any errors or omissions or for the results obtained from the use of the information contained in this work.

Contact **Dr. Remon M. Hana**: remonotawa@gmail.com

WhatsApp: +201142412106

ACKNOWLEDGMENTS

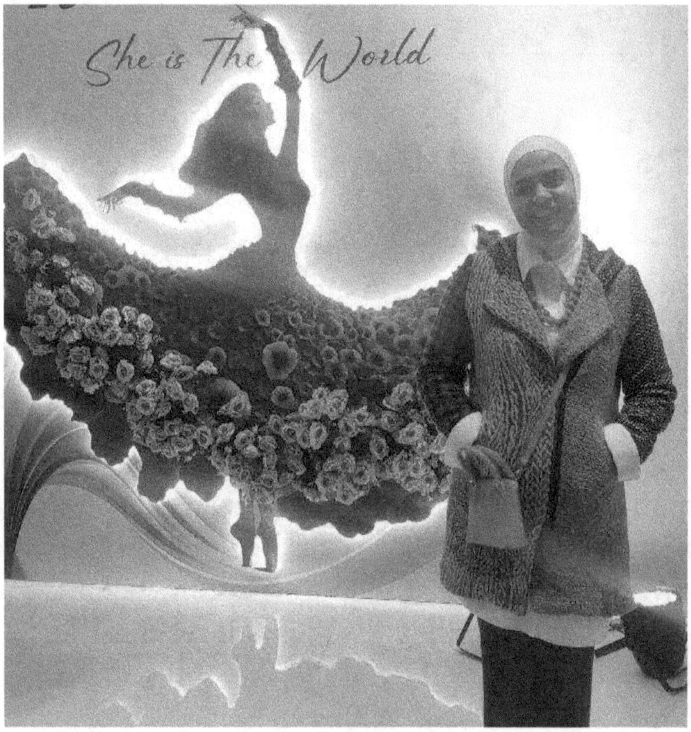

I would like to express my deepest gratitude and appreciation to **Dr. Heba Nabil, MD — *Consultant of Radiology and Women's Imaging*** — for all your support, invaluable guidance, mentorship, kindness, and mindfulness. Thank you for being a brilliant example of breast imaging leadership.

Contact **Dr. Heba Nabil:** dr.heba_nabil@hotmail.com

PREFACE

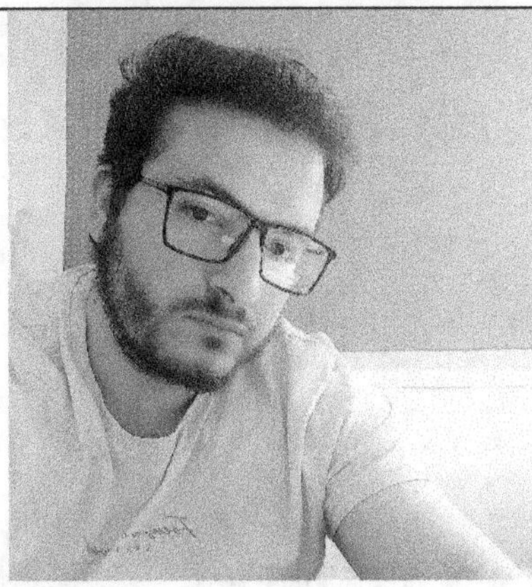

Breast cancer is the leading cause of cancer-related death among women worldwide. For both screening and diagnostic purposes, mammography and ultrasound are the primary imaging modalities used to evaluate breast lesions. Early diagnosis of breast cancer during asymptomatic stages is crucial for a favorable prognosis and improved quality of life. Diagnostic errors can cause delays in detection, which may result in poor consequences. Therefore, the role of the radiologist is critical.

The aim of this book is to provide radiologists and radiology residents specializing in breast imaging with simple, evidence-based methods to interpret and report mammograms confidently.

Feel free to contact me: remonotawa@gmail.com

WhatsApp: +201142412106

Remon M. Hana
March 2026

TABLE OF CONTENTS

CHAPTER 1: BREAST ANATOMY

- The breast overlies the **second to sixth ribs**. Typically, a breast contains **15 – 20 lobes**.
- Lobes can be broken down into lobules that contain milk-producing bulbs
- Bulbs and lobules are connected by ducts
- Mammary lobes coalesce into one lactiferous duct that extends to the nipple.

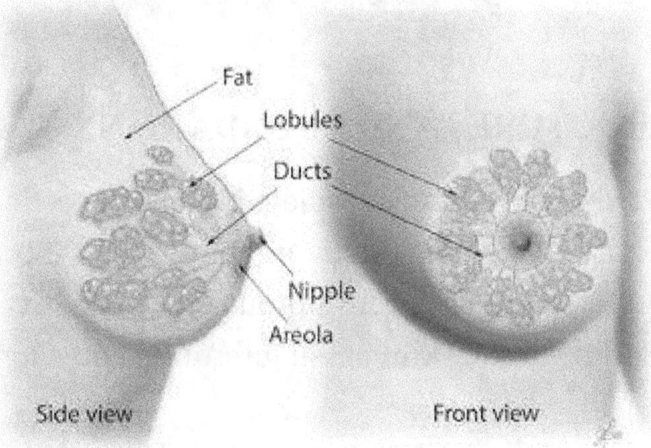

THE TERMINAL DUCTAL LOBULAR UNIT (TDLU)

- **The functional unit of the breast** is the Terminal Ductal Lobular Unit (TDLU). This microscopic structure is **the Holy Grail of breast pathology** because nearly all breast malignancies (ductal and lobular carcinomas) and many benign processes (cysts, fibroadenomas, adenosis) originate here. The TDLU consists of the extralobular terminal duct and the lobule itself, which contains the acini (ductules) responsible for milk production. These units drain into larger collecting ducts, which converge toward the nipple. On a mammogram, we cannot resolve individual TDLUs, but we visualize their aggregation as the fibroglandular density.

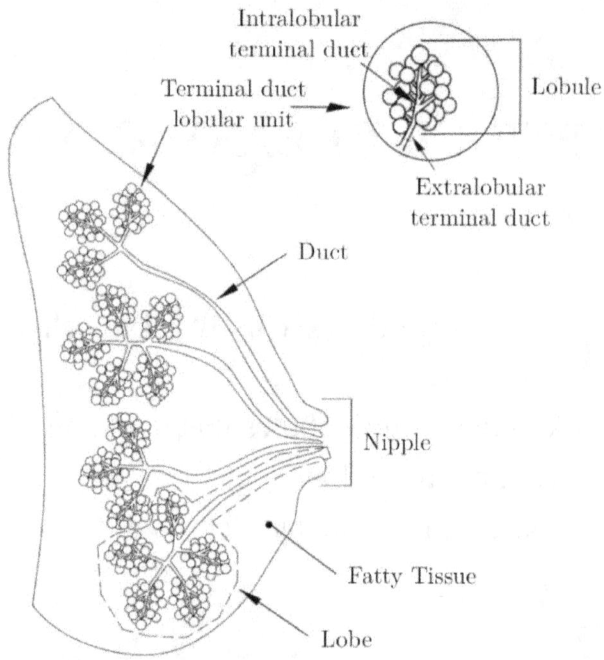

SUPPORTIVE STRUCTURES AND BOUNDARIES

- **The breast parenchyma** is encapsulated by the superficial and deep layers of the superficial fascia. The structural integrity of the breast is maintained by Cooper's Ligaments. These are fibrous bands that extend from the deep fascia to the dermis of the skin, passing through and supporting the breast parenchyma.
- **Radiological Significance:** Pathological processes that infiltrate these ligaments cause them to shorten and retract. This traction on the skin creates the "**dimpling**" or **skin retraction** often seen clinically with invasive carcinomas. On mammography, **thickening or straightening of Cooper's ligaments is a subtle sign of malignancy or edema.**

THE RETROMAMMARY SPACE

- Posterior to the breast tissue and anterior to the pectoralis muscle fascia lies a layer of **adipose tissue** called the retromammary space. Preserving the visualization of this fat line on a mammogram is critical for exclusion of deep chest wall invasion.

PHYSIOLOGICAL CHANGES

- The breast is **a dynamic organ** subject to hormonal regulation, primarily by estrogen and progesterone.
- **Proliferative Phase**: During puberty and pregnancy, hormonal stimulation causes ductal elongation and lobular proliferation. This increases radiographic density.
- **Lactation**: The lobules become hypertrophic and secretory. The breast becomes extremely dense radiographically, which significantly lowers the sensitivity of mammography. This is why ultrasound is often the first line of investigation in lactating women.
- **Involution**: With the cessation of ovarian function at menopause, the glandular elements atrophy and are **replaced by adipose tissue**. This process, termed involution, typically progresses from the posterior to the anterior breast. This fatty replacement is advantageous for the radiologist, as cancers (which appear white) are easily detected against the dark background of fat.

CHAPTER 2: BREAST CANCER ESSENTIAL

EPIDEMIOLOGY

- Breast cancer is the most common cancer in women worldwide according to the WHO reports, and its incidence is increasing particularly in developing countries where most cases are diagnosed in late stages.
- 1 in 8 lifetime probability of developing breast cancer among women; 1 in 1,000 lifetime probability among men.
- In 2016: 246,660 new invasive and 61,000 in situ breast cancers are expected among women in the United States and 2,600 new breast cancers among men
- Second leading cause of cancer mortality (15% of all cancer deaths) in women, (lung cancer is the leading cause of cancer-related deaths among women).

RISK FACTORS

- higher incidence among women// incidence increases with advancing age substantially higher for women age 50 and older //Personal history of breast cancer//Prior breast biopsy with certain benign diagnoses: atypical ductal hyperplasia, lobular neoplasia (atypical lobular hyperplasia and lobular carcinoma in situ), juvenile papillomatosis//Family history of breast cancer involving first degree relative particularly if the cancer is bilateral or diagnosed in premenopausal relative//BRCA1 and BRCA2 gene mutations//History of chest wall exposure to high-dose radiation (prior treatment of lymphoma)//Early menarche //Late menopause/Bilateral oophorectomy before age 40 may decrease breast cancer risk by 50%//Women with natural menopause before age 45 have half the risk of breast cancer compared to women who undergo menopause after age 55//

Late first term pregnancy// Nulliparity //Postmenopausal obesity//Hormone replacement therapy.

SCREENING MAMMOGRAPHY

- An annual screening mammogram should be obtained in women at the age of 40. Baseline mammography begins at age 35.
- Screening begins earlier if there is a history' of premenopausal cancer in a first degree relative (mother or sister), at 10 years minus the age of breast cancer onset. Example: if patient's mother developed breast cancer at the age of 40, the annual screening mammogram in the daughter would begin at the age of 30.

DIAGNOSTIC MAMMOGRAPHY

- The diagnostic mammogram involves performing additional views (such as coned/compression, magnification, and rolled views); 10 to 15% of breast cancers are not detected by mammography (not seen by mammography). Approximately 10% of breast cancers are clinically palpable, but evade mammographic detection, emphasizing the important role of monthly self-breast examination. Indications for ordering a diagnostic mammogram –
- Any patient with a personal history' of breast cancer.
- Active clinical symptoms (such as a breast lump, pain, or discharge).
- An abnormal screening mammogram.

HISTOPATHOLOGY

- **DUCTAL CARCINOMA IN-SITU (DCIS)** - type of early breast cancer confined to the inside of the ductal system.
- **INFILTRATING DUCTAL CARCINOMA (IDC)** - the most common type of breast cancer; accounts for 78% of all breast cancers. Common appearance - stellate (star like) or well-circumscribed (rounded) areas on mammograms; stellate lesions generally have a poorer prognosis; spiculated mass is the most common mammographic finding; associated with malignant pleomorphic type micro-calcifications. Clinical presentation - hard, fixed, palpable mass with or without skin dimpling and retraction.

- **MEDULLARY CARCINOMA** - accounts for 15% of breast cancers; most frequently occurs in women in their late 40s and 50s; on pathology, cells resemble the gray matter of the brain.
- **INFILTRATING LOBULAR CARCINOMA (ILC)** - accounts for 5% of breast cancers; a type of breast cancer that usually appears as a subtle thickening in the upper outer quadrant of the breast; with or without breast asymmetry or architectural distortion. Often positive for estrogen and progesterone receptors; tumors respond well to hormone therapy.
- **TUBULAR CARCINOMA** - accounts for 2% of breast cancers; tubular carcinoma cels have a distinctive tubular structure on histopathology; prevalent in women aged 50 and above; excellent 10-year survival rate of 95%.
- **MUCINOUS (COLLOID) CARCINOMA** - accounts for 1% to 2% of breast cancers; main differentiating features are mucus production and cells that are poorly defined; favorable prognosis in most cases.
- **INFLAMMATORY BREAST CANCER (IBC)** - accounts for 1% to 5% of breast cancers; rare and very aggressive type of breast cancer that obstructs lymphatics, resulting in characteristic inflammatory' appearance of the breast.
- **PHYLLOIDES TUMOR**- accounts <0.5% of breast cancers; uncommon fibroepithelial breast tumors which can re-grow; like fibroadenoma but has increased cellularity in the stroma, typically benign but has malignant potential, when malignant 25% metastasize. Imaging findings - smooth and solid lobular mass, occasionally with cystic components.
- **PAGET DISEASE** - uncommon peri-areolar malignancy presenting as inflammation or rash resembling eczema; occurs in women over age 50; underlying malignancy present in 95% of patients. Diagnosis - punch skin biopsy; followed by work-up for occult breast cancer.

CHAPTER 3:X-RAY MAMMOGRAPHY

CONVENTIONAL X-RAY MAMMOGRAPHY (SCREENING, DIAGNOSTIC)

- The corner stone of breast imaging.
- The most widely used screening modality.
- Should meet the Mammography Quality Standards Act (MQSA) legislation and regulations published by the Food and Drug Administration (FDA).
- Needs expertise technician and radiology specialist.
- High resolution (at least 5MP dual head) display screens are mandatory.

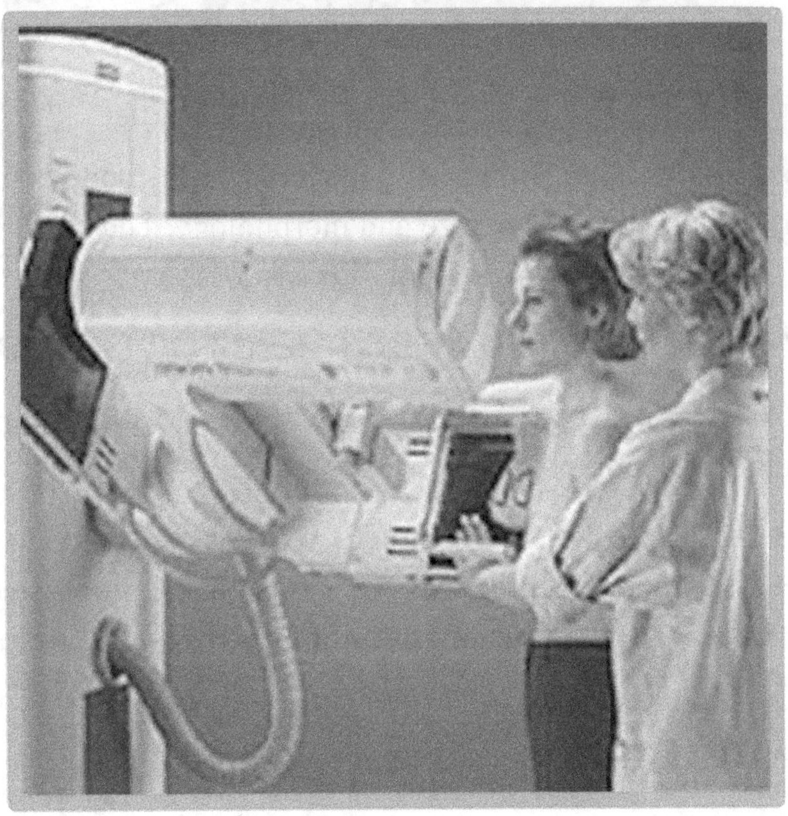

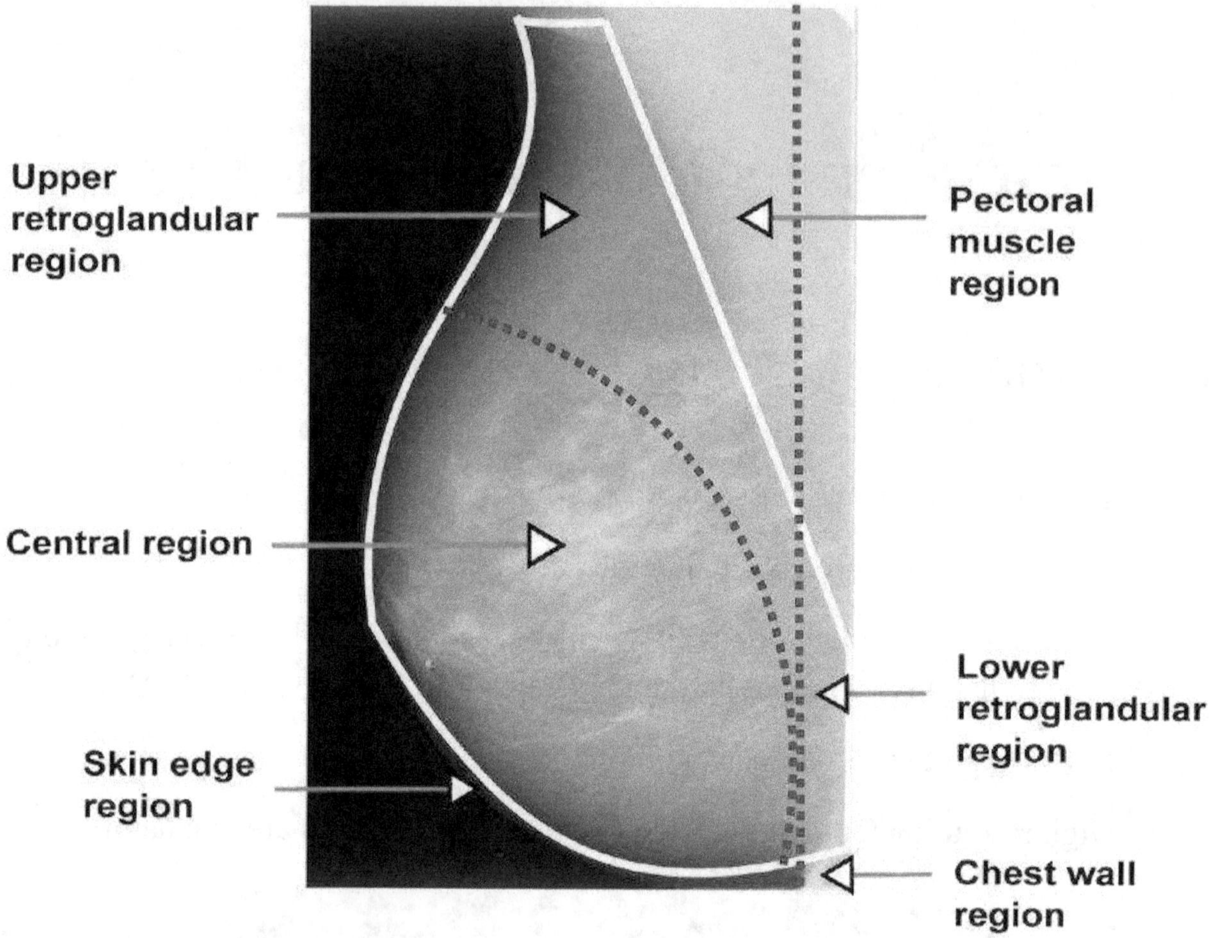

MAMMOGRAPHY VIEWS

- Breast is a mobile organ. However, depending on the body habitus of the patient, breast tissue varies in size and morphology. The goal of positioning is to visualize the maximum amount of breast tissue.

TWO STANDARD VIEWS MUST BE TAKEN FOR EACH BREAST:

1. **CC (CRANIO-CAUDAL) VIEW** is one of the two standard projections in a screening mammography.
2. **MLO (MEDIO-LATRAL OBLIQUE) VIEW** is the second standard projection in routine screening mammography. **MLO view is considered the most important view as maximum breast tissue is portrayed in this view.**

ROUTINE MAMMOGRAM

- Routine mammography: **MLO and CC views**. **RCC**, right craniocaudal; **LCC**, left craniocaudal; **RMLO**, right mediolateral oblique; **LMLO**, left mediolateral oblique views of a normal mammogram

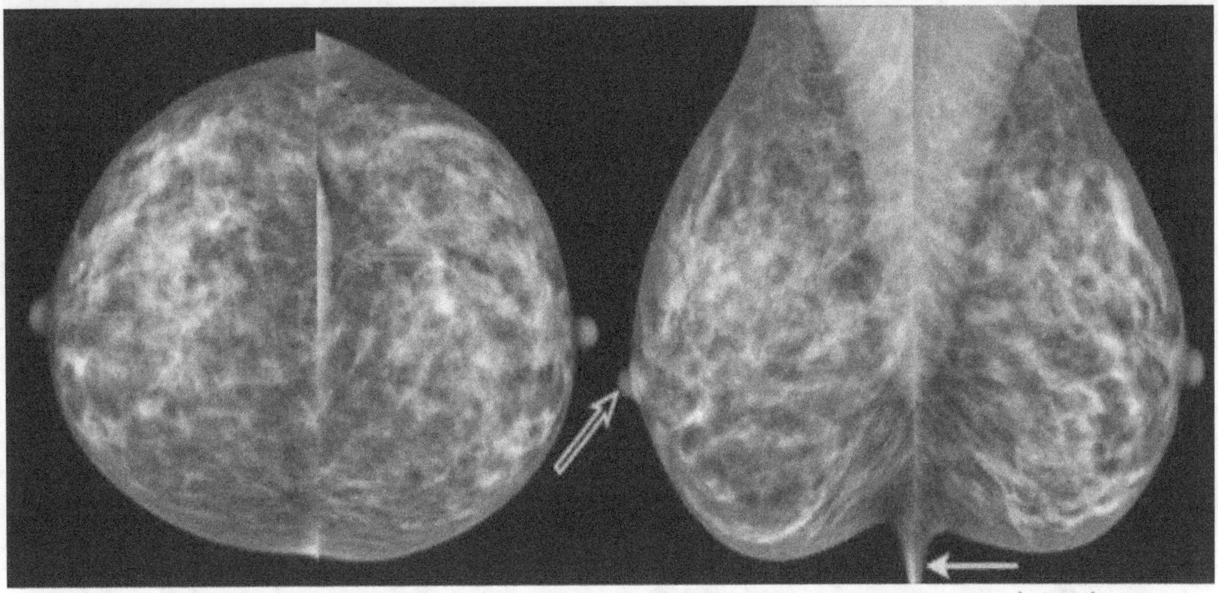

CC views: solid arrow (nipple in profile). Open arrow (pectoralis muscle)

MLO views: open arrow (nipple in profile). Closed arrow (inframammary fold)

ADDITIONAL VIEWS

- The patient's body habitus, anomalies, breast symptoms and other systemic diseases that can impact the mammogram should be and views should be added upon accordingly. Altering standard views or adding images may be necessary. This can help detect an otherwise occult cancer. ***Examples***: Lateral views /Cleavage view/Axillary view /Rolled views/Spot compression/cone views/Magnification views/Tangential views/

MALE MAMMOGRAPHY

- The most common indication is gynaecomastia, rarely breast cancer (1%–2%). The positioning method is similar to that of small female breast and both CC and MLO are taken.

AREAS THAT CAN BE MISSED IN MAMMOGRAPHY (BLIND OR FORBIDDEN AREAS)

- **THE MILKY WAY (RETROMAMMARY FAT)**: a 3-4 cm wide band parallel to the edge of the pectoral muscle
- **RETRO GLANDULAR CLEAR SPACE** between the posterior border of the breast parenchyma and the chest wall on any view, especially on the CC view.
- **INFRA-MAMMARY FOLD.**
- **MEDIAL HALF OF THE BREAST.**
- **RETROAREOLAR REGION.**

CONTRAST ENHANCED SPECTRAL MAMMOGRAPHY (CESM)

- Imaging of an iodinated contrast agent using mammographic x-ray imaging equipment which can be done using 2D imaging.

DIGITAL BREAST TOMOSYNTHESIS (DBT)

- In DBT, the compressed breast tissue is imaged in a three-dimensional manner by performing a series of low-dose radiographic exposures and using the resultant projection image dataset to reconstruct cross-sectional in-plane images in standard mammographic views.
- Improved visualization of breast detail at diagnostic DBT allows improved characterization of findings, including normal structures and breast cancer.

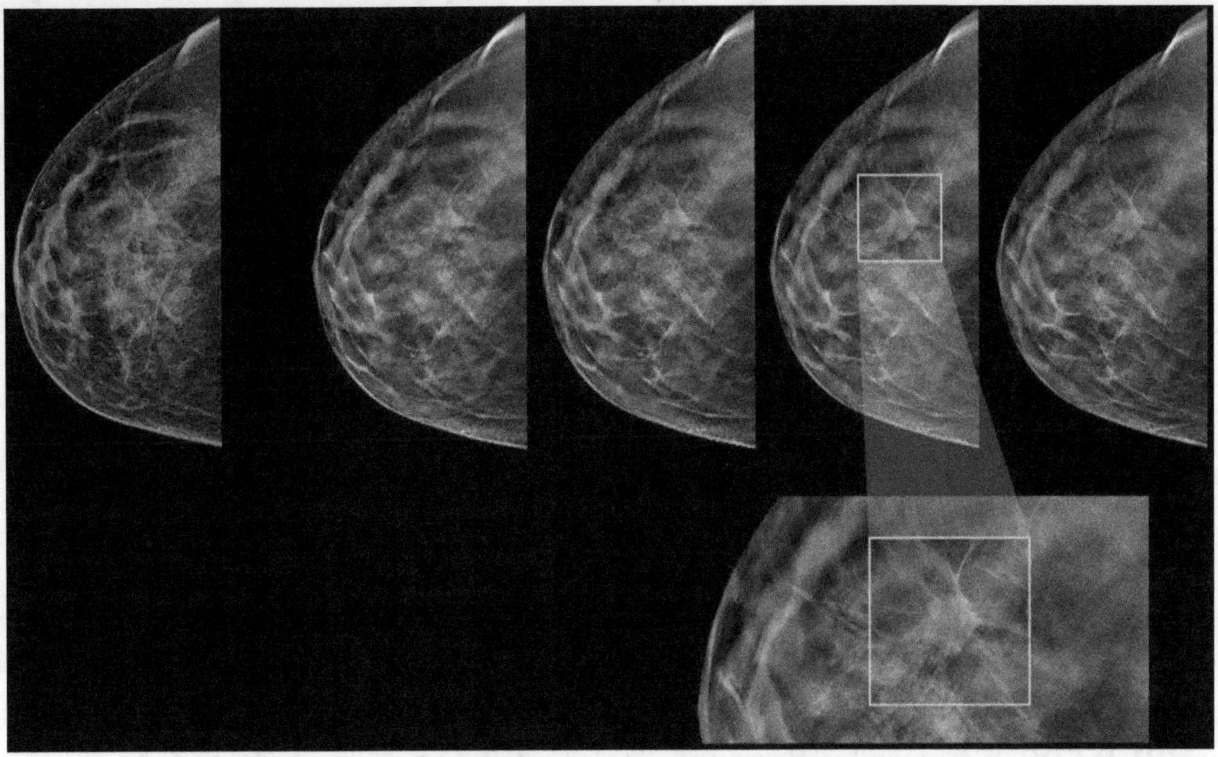

DIGITAL BREAST TOMOSYNTHESIS (DBT)

CHAPETR 4: MAMMOGRAM REPORTING AND BI-RADS LEXICON (BIRADS v2025)

American College of Radiology Breast Imaging Reporting and Data System (ACR BI-RADS®) according to latest edition (The ACR BI-RADS® v2025 Manual the 5th Edition)

— **BI-RADS 0:** Further imaging required

— **BI-RADS 1:** Normal, no suspicion of malignancy; usual screening recommended (as appropriate for the patient's age and risk)

— **BI-RADS 2:** Benign lesion (e.g., **cyst, internal mammary lymph node or <u>Fibroadenoma, as proven by follow-up</u>**) **one or more simple cysts, intramammary lymph nodes, postsurgical fluid collections, breast implants, or complicated cysts/probable fibroadenomas that are <u>unchanged for at least 2 or 3 years</u>, while still concluding that there is no sonographic evidence of malignancy**

— **BI-RADS 3:** Probably benign; short-term follow-up (usually at 6 months) recommended (**solid lesion with typically benign features conglomeration of microcysts**)

For US solid mass with a circumscribed margin, oval shape, and parallel orientation (most commonly fibroadenoma) and an isolated complicated cyst & clustered microcysts

— **BI-RADS 4:** Suspicious finding (**all solid lesions without <u>typically benign features</u>**); histopathologic assessment recommended.

— **BI-RADS 5:** Highly suspicious of malignancy; histopathologic verification recommended.

— **BI-RADS 6:** Proven malignancy It is also used when imaging is performed to assess response to neoadjuvant chemotherapy.

Final Assessment Categories			
Category		Management	Likelihood of cancer
0	Need additional imaging or prior examinations	Recall for additional imaging and/or await prior examinations	n/a
1	Negative	Routine screening	Essentially 0%
2	Benign	Routine screening	Essentially 0%
3	Probably Benign	Short interval-follow-up (6 month) or continued	>0 % but ≤ 2%
4	Suspicious	Tissue diagnosis	4a. low suspicion for malignancy (>2% to ≤ 10%) 4b. moderate suspicion for malignancy (>10% to ≤ 50%) 4c. high suspicion for malignancy (>50% to <95%)
5	Highly suggestive of malignancy	Tissue diagnosis	≥95%
6	Known biopsy-proven	Surgical excision when clinical appropriate	n/a

<table>
<tr><th colspan="4">MAMMOGRAPHY LEXICON</th></tr>
<tr><td>Breast composition</td><td colspan="3">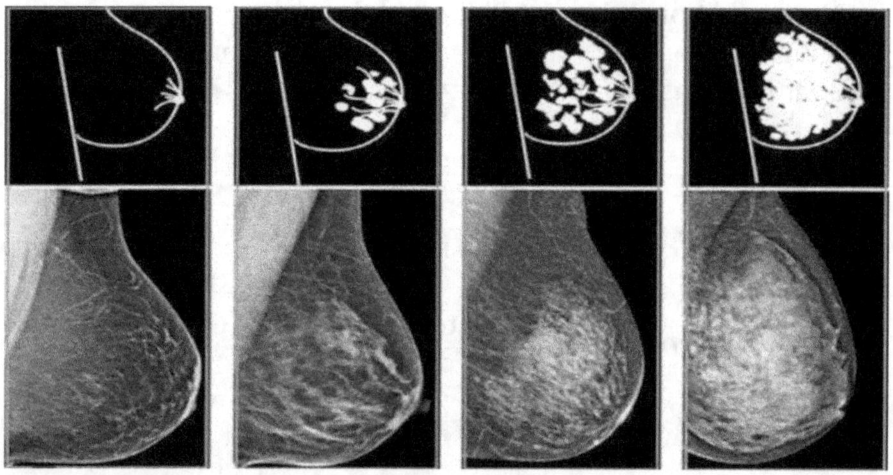
ACR-A. Entirely fatty.
ACR-B. Scattered areas of fibro glandular density.
ACR-C. Heterogeneously dense, which may obscure masses.
ACR-D. Extremely dense, which lowers sensitivity</td></tr>
<tr><td rowspan="3">Mass</td><td>Shape</td><td colspan="2">Oval// Lobulated/ Round// Irregular</td></tr>
<tr><td>Margin</td><td colspan="2">Circumscribed//Obscured// Indistinct// Spiculated</td></tr>
<tr><td>Density</td><td colspan="2">Fat//Low//Equal// High Density (compared to fibroglandular breast tissue)</td></tr>
<tr><td>Asymmetry</td><td colspan="3">Asymmetry (seen only in one projection) //Global// Focal //Developing (=that was not visible on a previous mammogram)</td></tr>
<tr><td>Architectural /Parenchymal distortion</td><td colspan="3">Distorted parenchyma with no visible mass</td></tr>
<tr><td>Calcification</td><td>Morphology</td><td>Benign</td><td>Skin/ Vascular/ Coarse or popcorn like/ Large rod like/ Round or punctate /Rim calcification/ Dystrophic /Fat</td></tr>
</table>

			necrosis /Milk of calcium /Suture
		Suspicious	*1. Amorphous (4B)* *2. Coarse heterogeneous(4B)* *3. Fine pleomorphic(4C)* *4. Fine linear or fine linear branching(4C)*
	Distribution	*Diffuse// regional// grouped// linear// segmental*	
Associated Features	*Skin / nipple retraction, skin thickening (>2 mm), trabecular thickening, axillary adenopathy, architectural distortion, calcification*		

SHAPE			
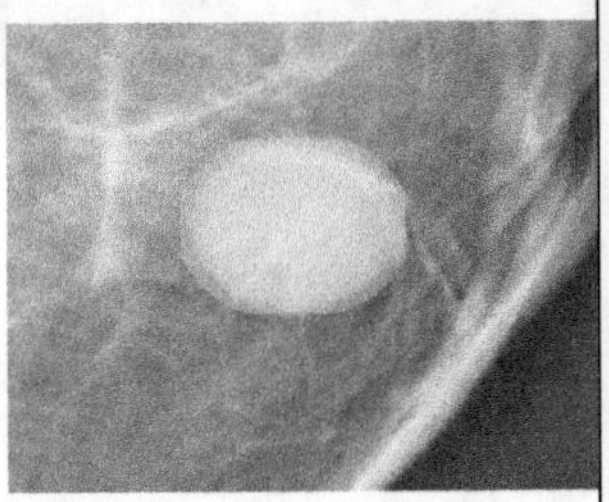	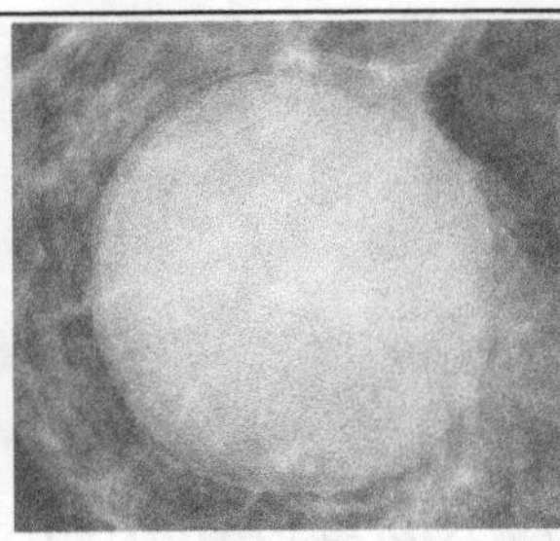	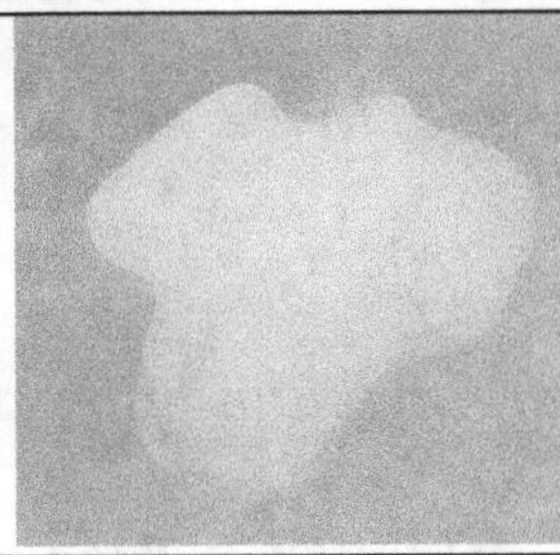	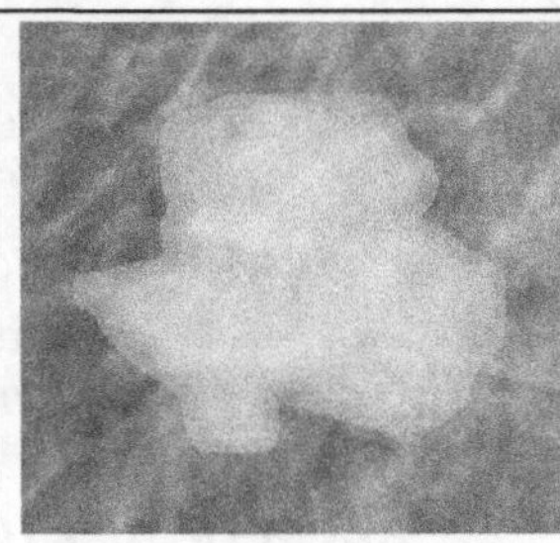
Oval	**Round**	**Lobulated**	**Irregular**
MARGIN			
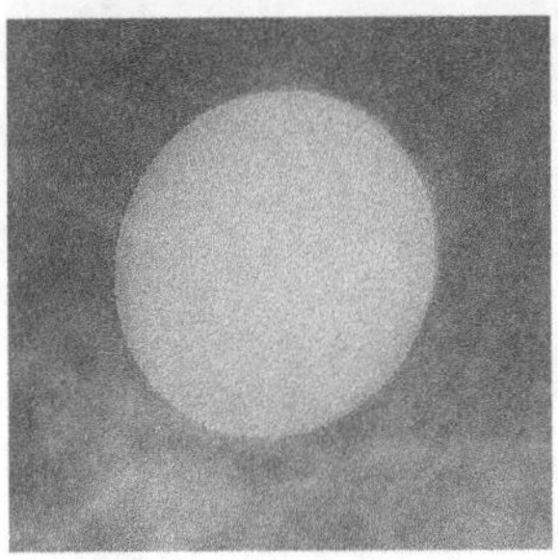	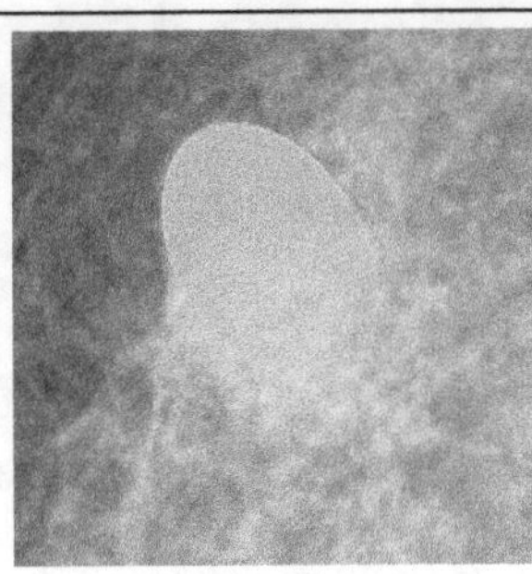	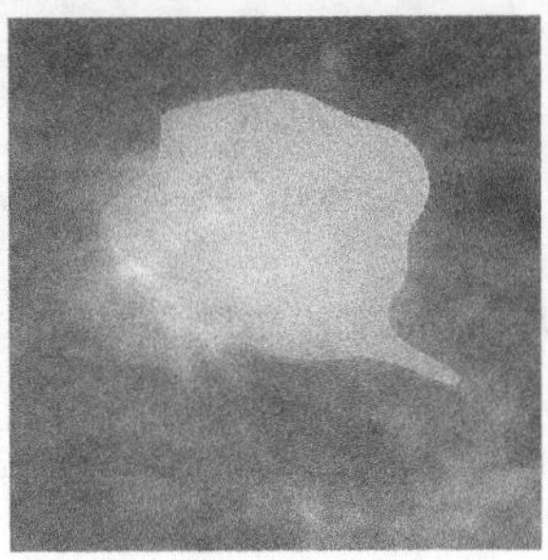	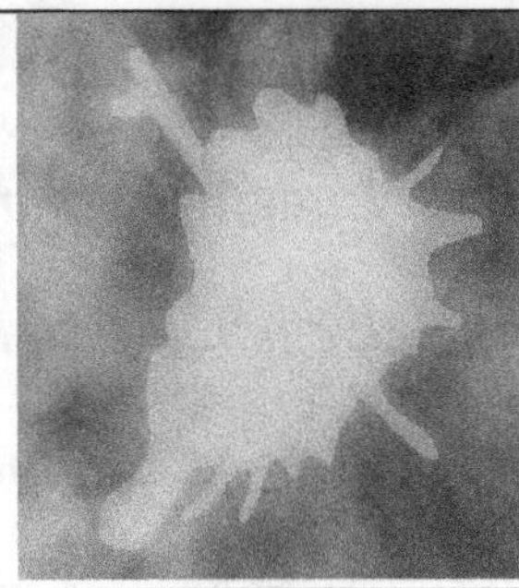
Circumscribed	**Obscured**	**Indistinct**	**Spiculated**
DENSITY			
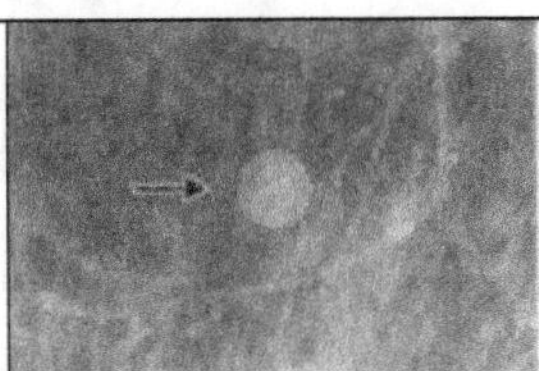	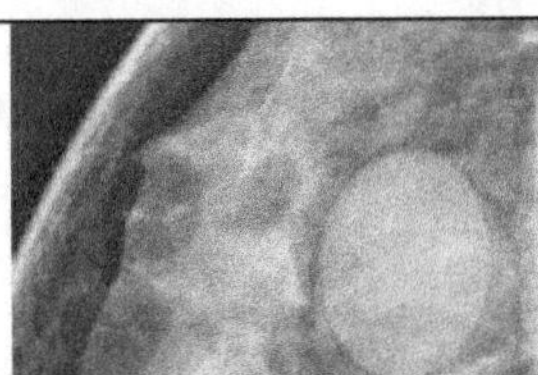	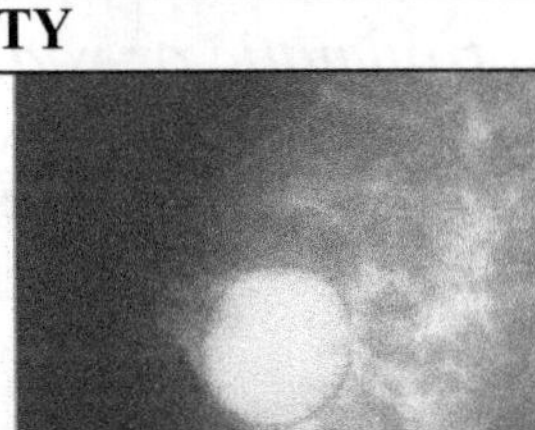	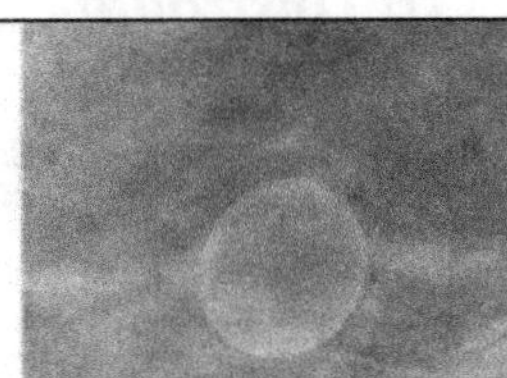
Low density	Equal density	High density	Fat-containing

DISTRIBUTION OF CALCIFICATION

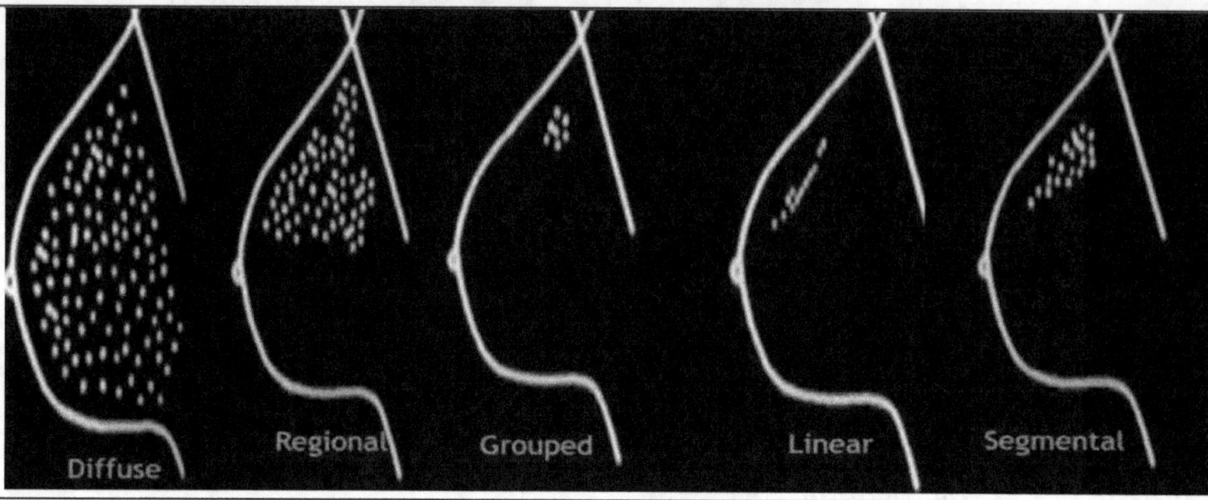

BENIGN CALCIFICATIONS = BI-RADS 2

1. ***Skin:*** *lucent centered, tangential views.*
2. ***Vascular:*** *Parallel tracks.*
3. ***Coarse (popcorn)****: involuting fibroadenoma.*
4. ***Large Rod-Like****: secretory disease, "plasma cell mastitis", duct ectasia (versus linear DCIS calcs).*
5. ***Round****: pearl shaped, formed in acini of Lobules.*
6. ***Lucent-Centered****: fat necrosis and fibroadenoma.*
7. ***Eggshell or rim****: under 1mm in thickness, cyst walls.*
8. ***Milk of calcium****: sedimented calcifications in cysts.*
9. ***suture****: post-irradiated breast (rare today).*
10. ***Dystrophic****: post traumatic or radiation.*
11. ***Punctate****: less than 0.5 mm (subset of "round")*

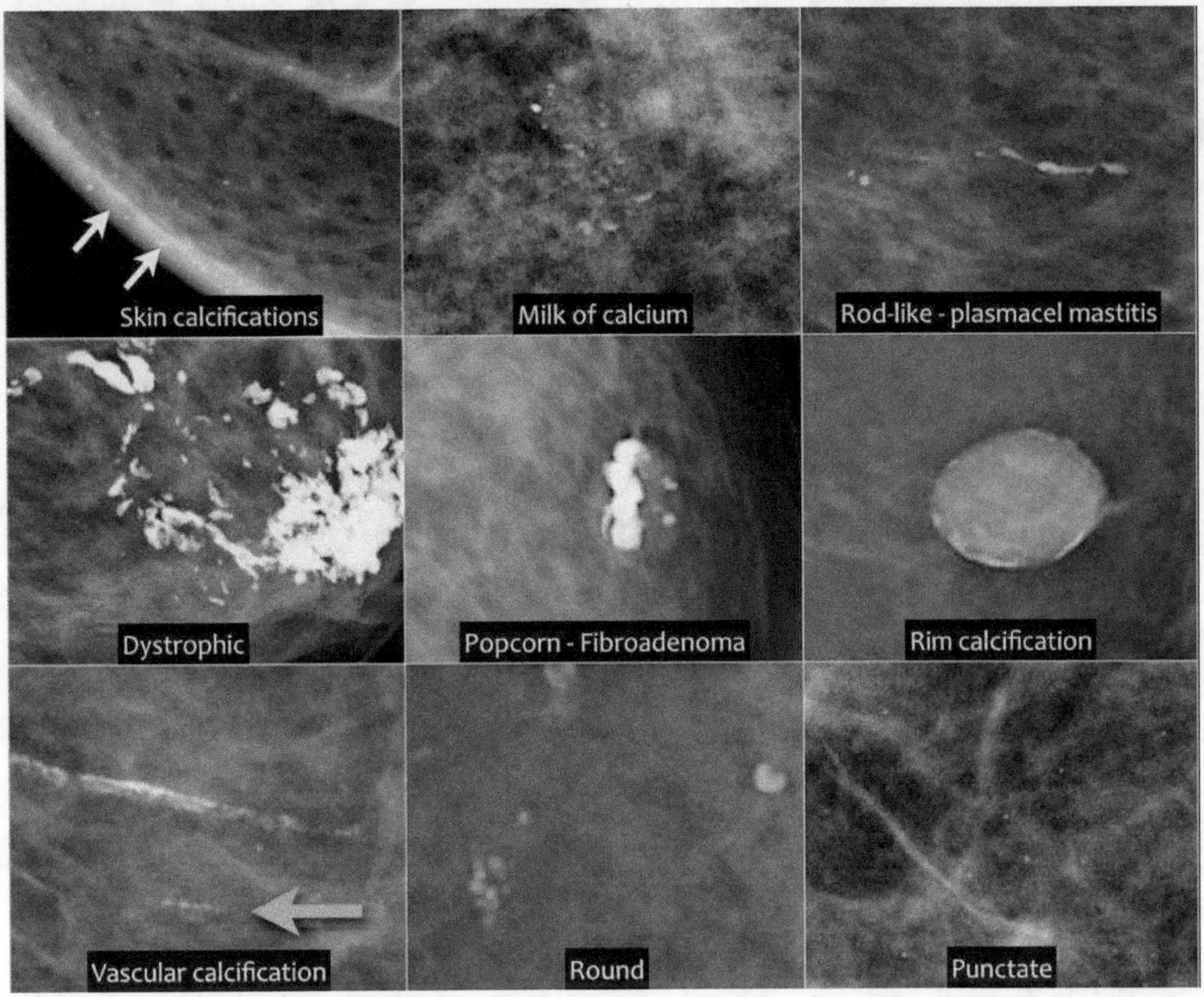

MALIGNANT CALCIFICATIONS = BI-RADS 4

- Significant correlation between histological subtypes of DCIS and calcification patterns.

Morphology

1. Amorphous
2. Course Heterogeneous
3. Fine pleomorphic
4. Fine linear/fine linear branching

LIKELIHOOD OF MALIGNANCY FROM

- Amorphous (21%) =BI-RADS 4B

- Course Heterogeneous (13%) =BI-RADS 4B
- Fine pleomorphic (29%) =BI-RADS 4C
- Fine linear/fine linear branching (70%) = BI-RADS 4C

Note: None of these rises to BI-RADS 5

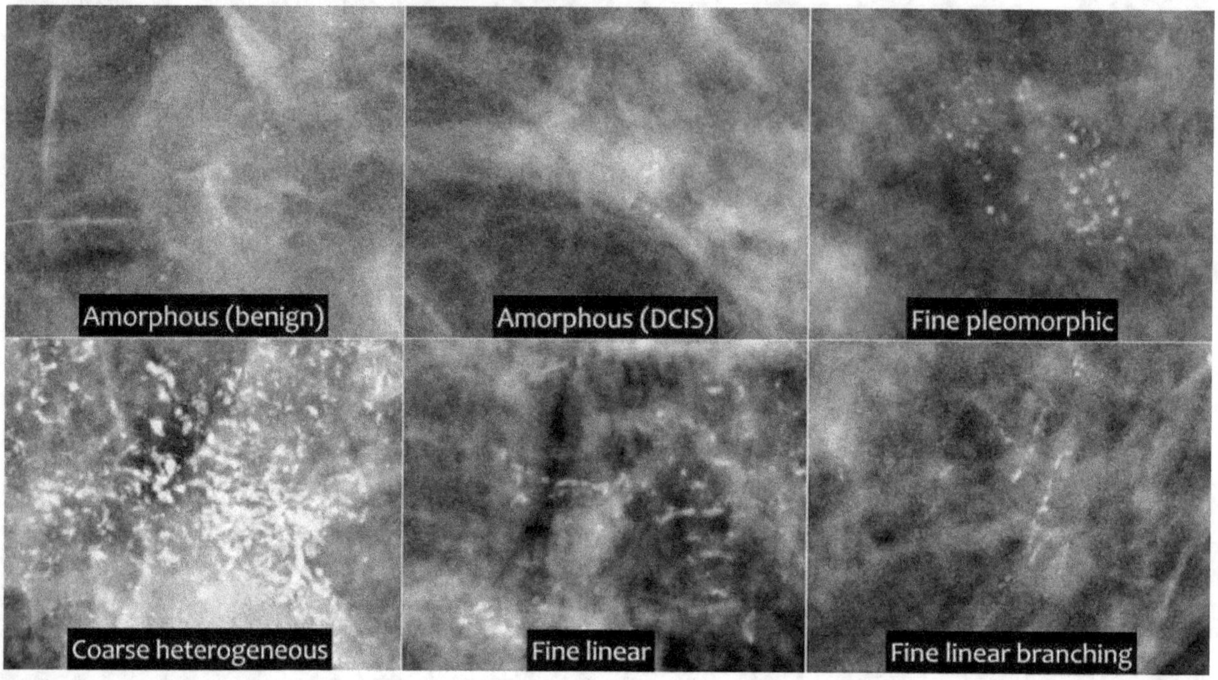

COARSE HETEROGENEOUS

- **Like aggregated pieces of broken glass**

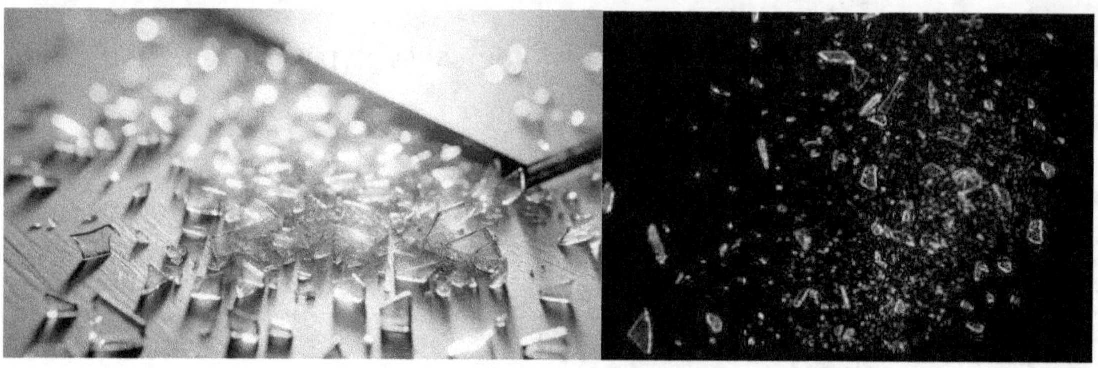

FINE PLEOMORPHIC

- **Different shapes and sizes no specific pattern**

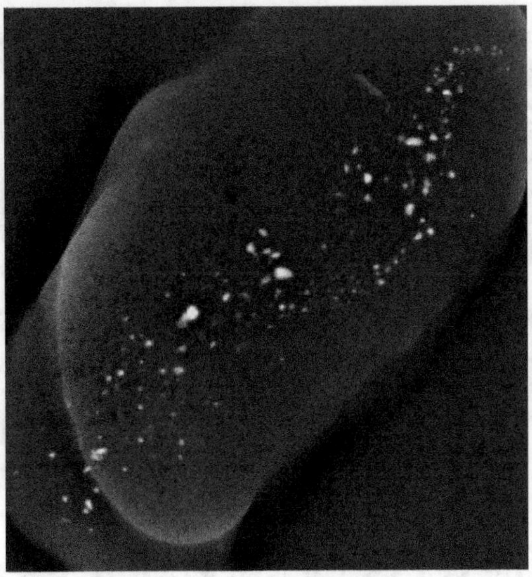

AMORPHOUS

- **Like powder hard to see**

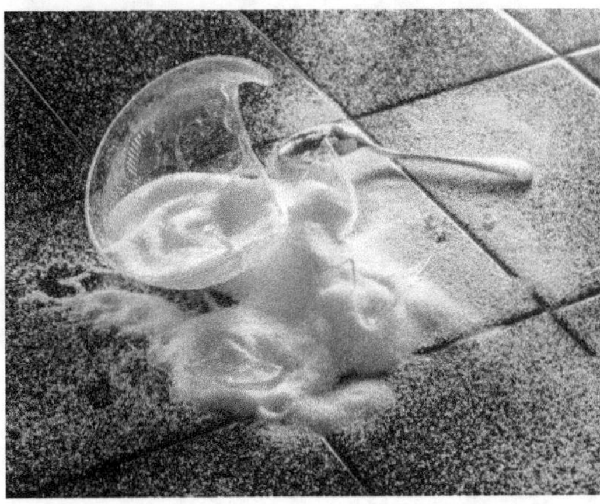

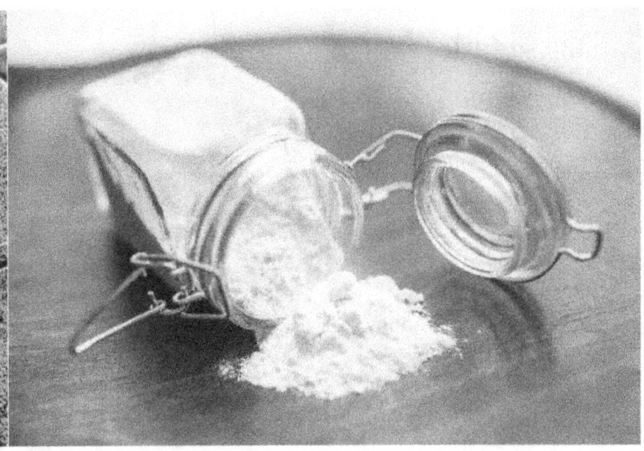

FINE LINEAR /FINE-LINEAR BRANCHING

- **Linear pattern along the duct/ with branching pattern**

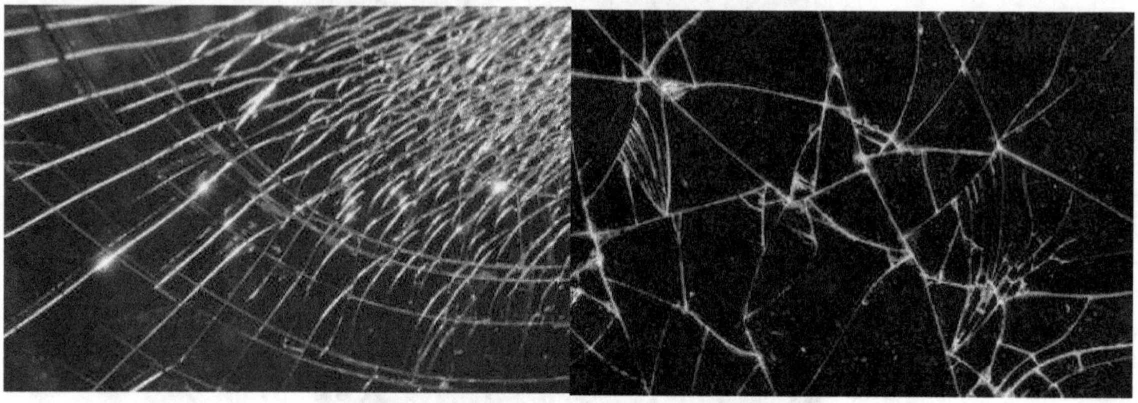

LOCALIZATION OF MASS IN MAMMOGRAPHY

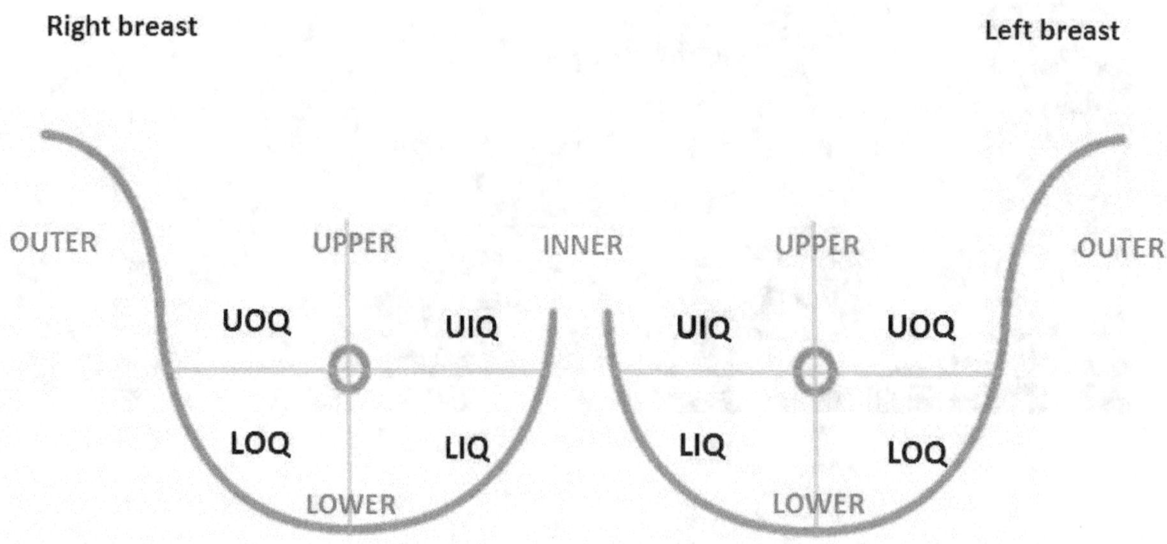

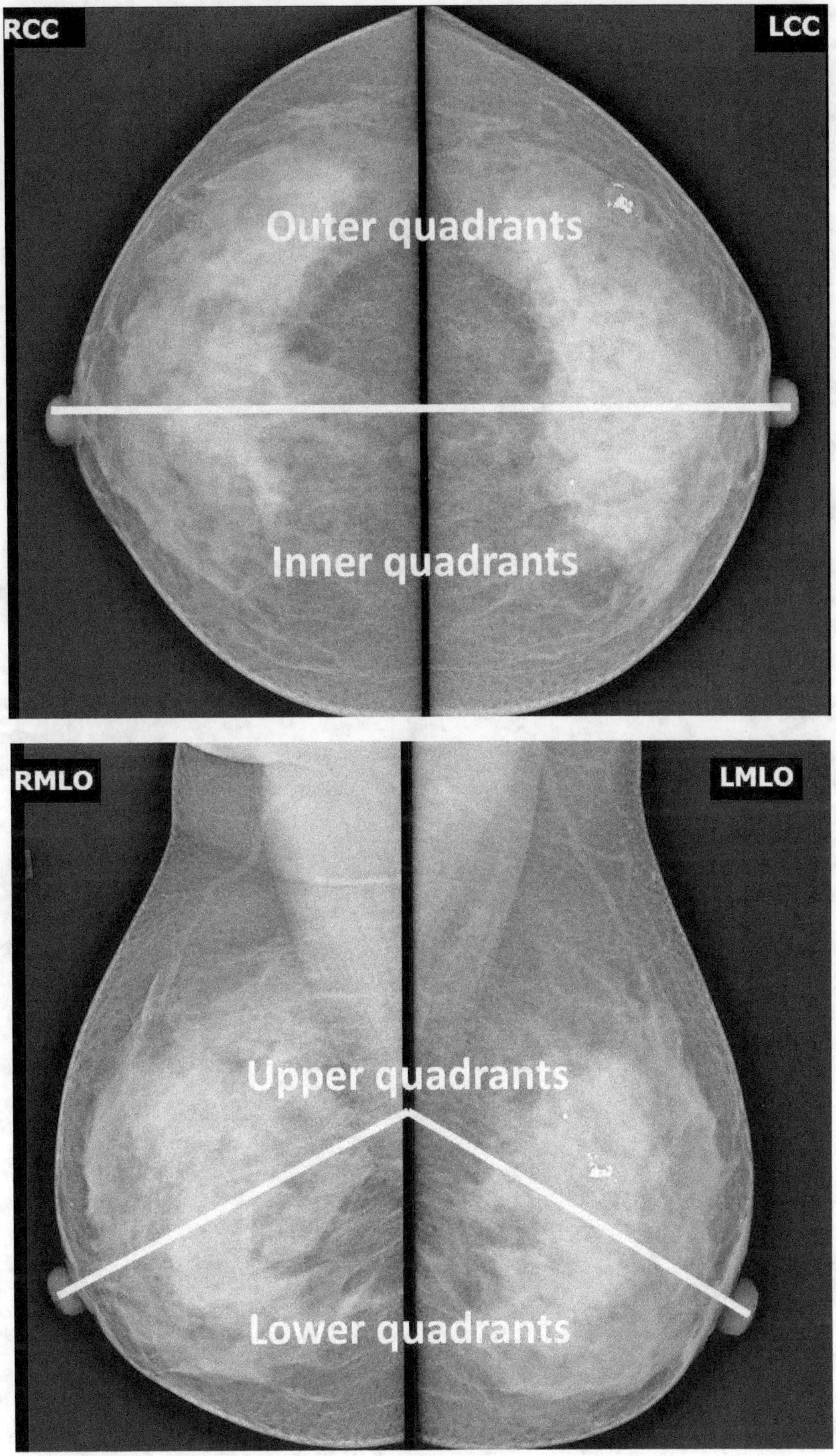
RCC
LCC
Outer quadrants
Inner quadrants
RMLO
LMLO
Upper quadrants
Lower quadrants

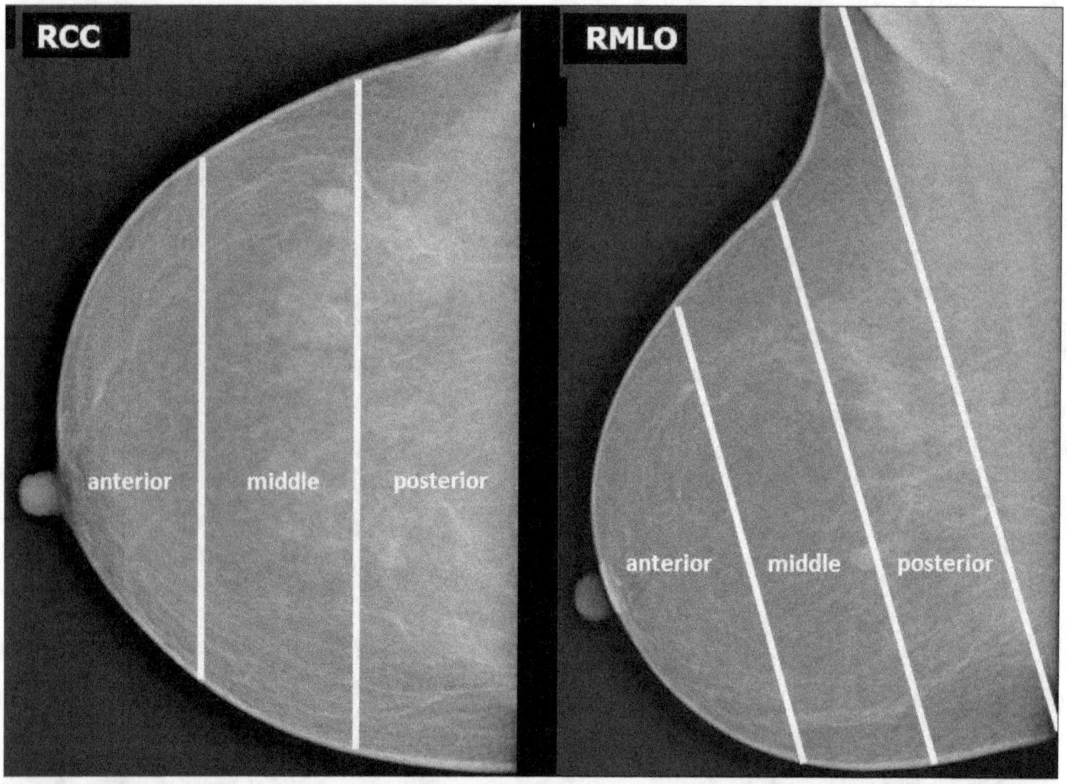

RCC
RMLO
anterior
middle
posterior
anterior
middle
posterior

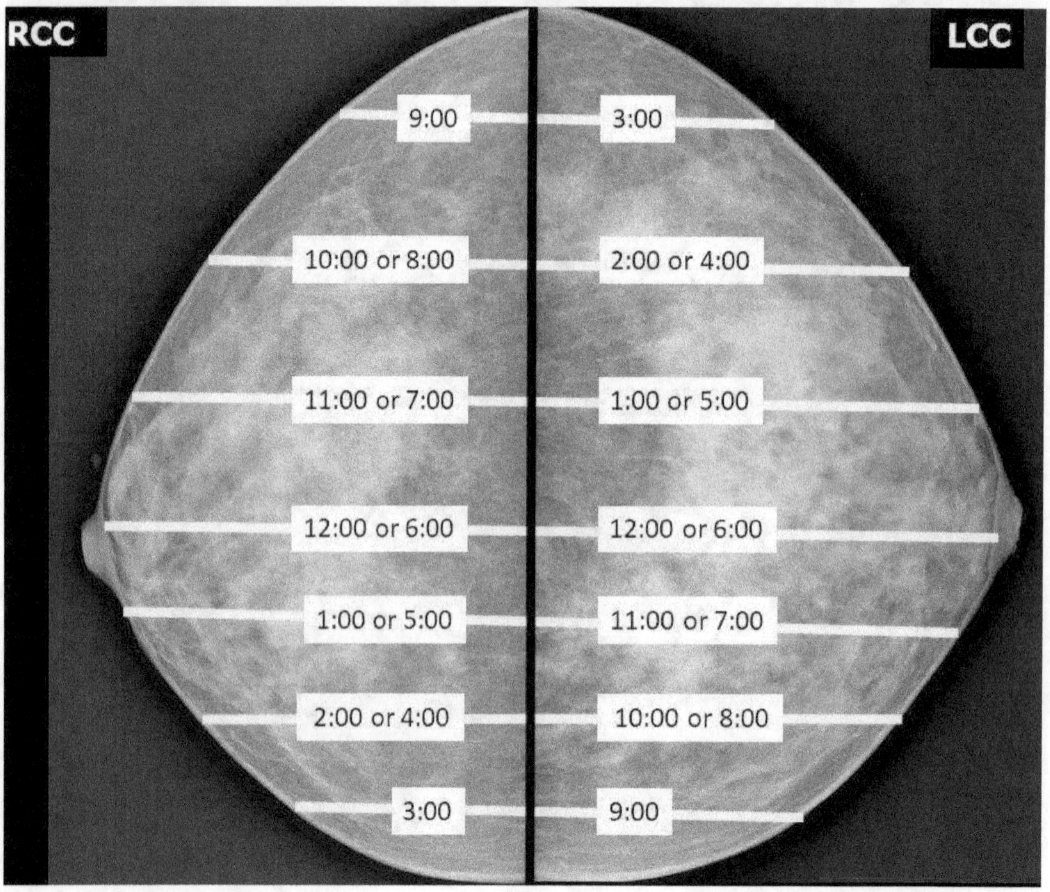

RCC
LCC
9:00
3:00
10:00 or 8:00
2:00 or 4:00
11:00 or 7:00
1:00 or 5:00
12:00 or 6:00
12:00 or 6:00
1:00 or 5:00
11:00 or 7:00
2:00 or 4:00
10:00 or 8:00
3:00
9:00

CHAPTER 5: REPORTING NOTES

-VE Findings
• No Focal mass lesion • No Focal parenchymal asymmetry /Global parenchymal asymmetry • No Parenchymal architectural distortion • No Suspicious Micro-Calcifications • No dermal changes/axillary lymphadenopathy
+VE Findings
A) <u>**If there is mass lesion**</u> 1. Right / Left UOQ LOQ UIQ LIQ (<u>**location**</u>) 2. Oval / Round / Irregular (<u>**shape**</u>) 3. Circumscribed /Obscured / Indistinct / Spiculated (<u>**margin**</u>) 4. of fat density / of low density/ of equal density/ of high density (<u>**density**</u>) 5. associated with or without suspicious micro-calcifications (<u>**micro-calcifications**</u>) **B)** Right / Left UOQ LOQ UIQ LIQ **Focal parenchymal asymmetry** **C)** Right / Left **Global parenchymal asymmetry** **D)** Right / Left UOQ LOQ UIQ LIQ Diffuse/Regional/Grouped of **suspicious micro-calcifications** **E)** UOQ LOQ UIQ LIQ Diffuse/Regional/Grouped **benign clarifications** (skin, vascular, rod like, rounded, Rim calcification, coarse popcorn)

F) Associated Features

1. **Retracted Nipple and areolar region**
2. **Mild marked focal Diffuse skin thickening**
3. **Single / Multiple axillary enlarged lymphadenopathies.**

REPORTING TIPS AND TRICKS

(BI-RADS 0) Further imaging required *(US Correlation / Dynamic Contrast-Enhanced Breast MRI Correlation)*

(BI-RADS 1) Normal *(Routine Annual Screening)*

(BI-RADS 2) Benign Finding *(Routine Annual Screening)*

- *Involuting calcified fibroadenomas (calcified circumscribed)*
- *Skin, Vascular calcifications*
- *Metallic foreign bodies (such as surgical clips)*
- *Fat-containing lesions (such as oil cysts, lipomas, galactoceles, and mixed-density hamartomas)*
- *Intra-mammary lymph nodes*
- *Breast Implants*
- *Global asymmetry* ***WITHOUT*** *clinical or sonographic correlate/ associated calcifications or parenchymal distortion, retracted nipple, No thickened skin…etc)*
- *Architectural distortion clearly related to prior surgery*

(BI-RADS 3) = Probably benign *(Short Term Follow Up = usually 6 months)*

- *Non-calcified **circumscribed** solid mass*
- *Focal asymmetry without (Clinical or sonographic correlate,*
    - *Associated calcifications or parenchymal distortion Suspicious associated findings as retracted nipple, thickened skin...etc)*
- *Solitary group of punctate calcifications with no previous examinations for comparison*

In follow up if the lesion increased in size or extent, biopsy will be recommended.
In screening mammograms, we only give BIRADS 0-1-2-4-5 not 3

(BI-RADS 4) = Histopathological Correlation

- *Irregular, new, or changing masses.*
- *Suspicious micro-calcifications*
- *Focal asymmetry Associated Suspicious micro-calcifications or parenchymal distortion Suspicious associated findings as retracted nipple, thickened skin...etc).*

(BI-RADS 5) = Histopathological Correlation

- *Typical Spiculated masses*
- *Irregular, new, or changing masses with Suspicious Micro-Calcifications / Lymphadenopathy/Retracted Nipple /Skin Changes*

(BI-RADS 6) *= Clinical Management = Tissue Proven Malignancy*

- *In case of tumoral marker clips and assessment response to neoadjuvant chemotherapy*

CHAPTER 6: CASES

CASE 1: 54-year-old female/Screening (=NO SYMPTOMS)

Right MLO	Left MLO

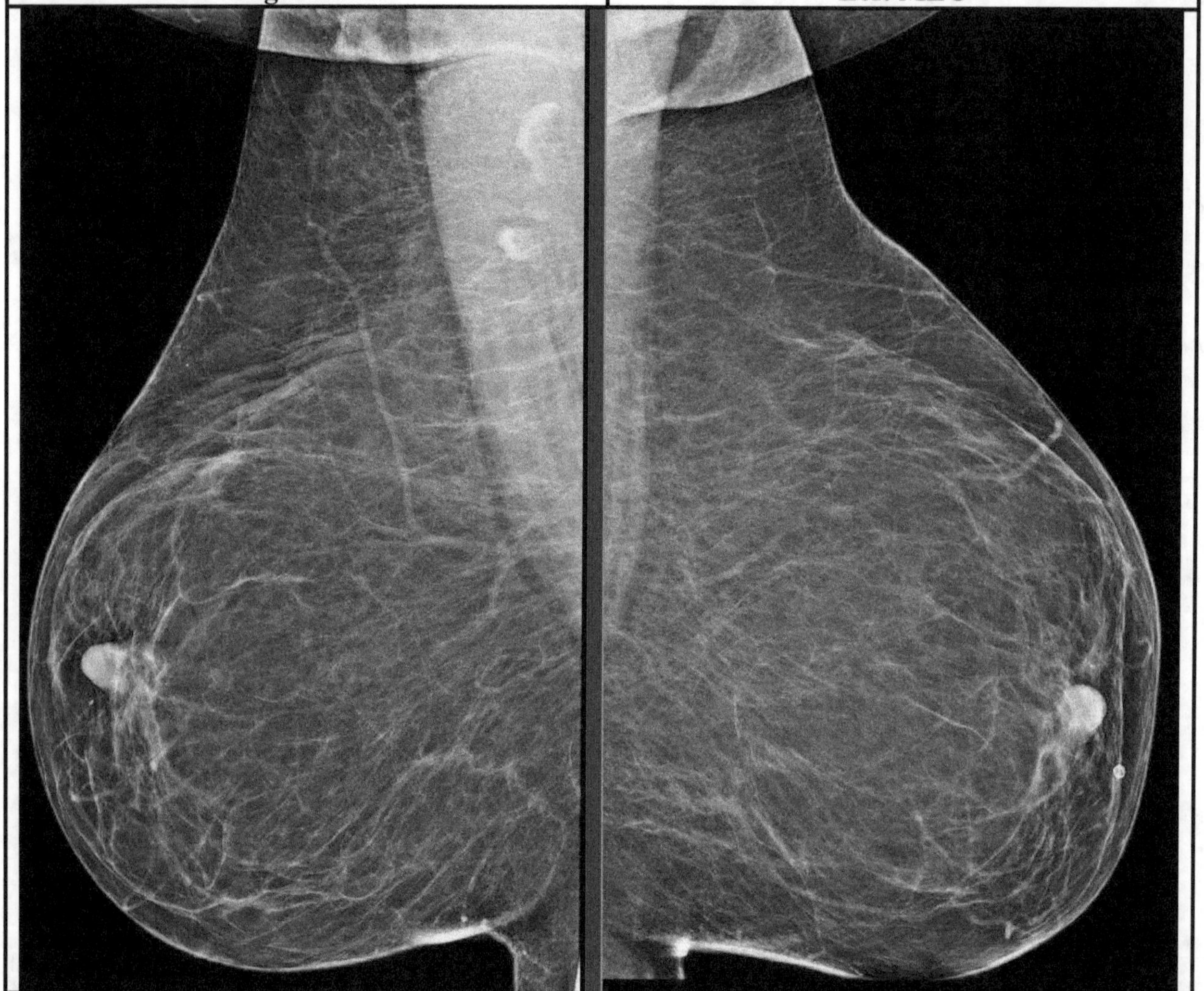

Right CC	Left CC

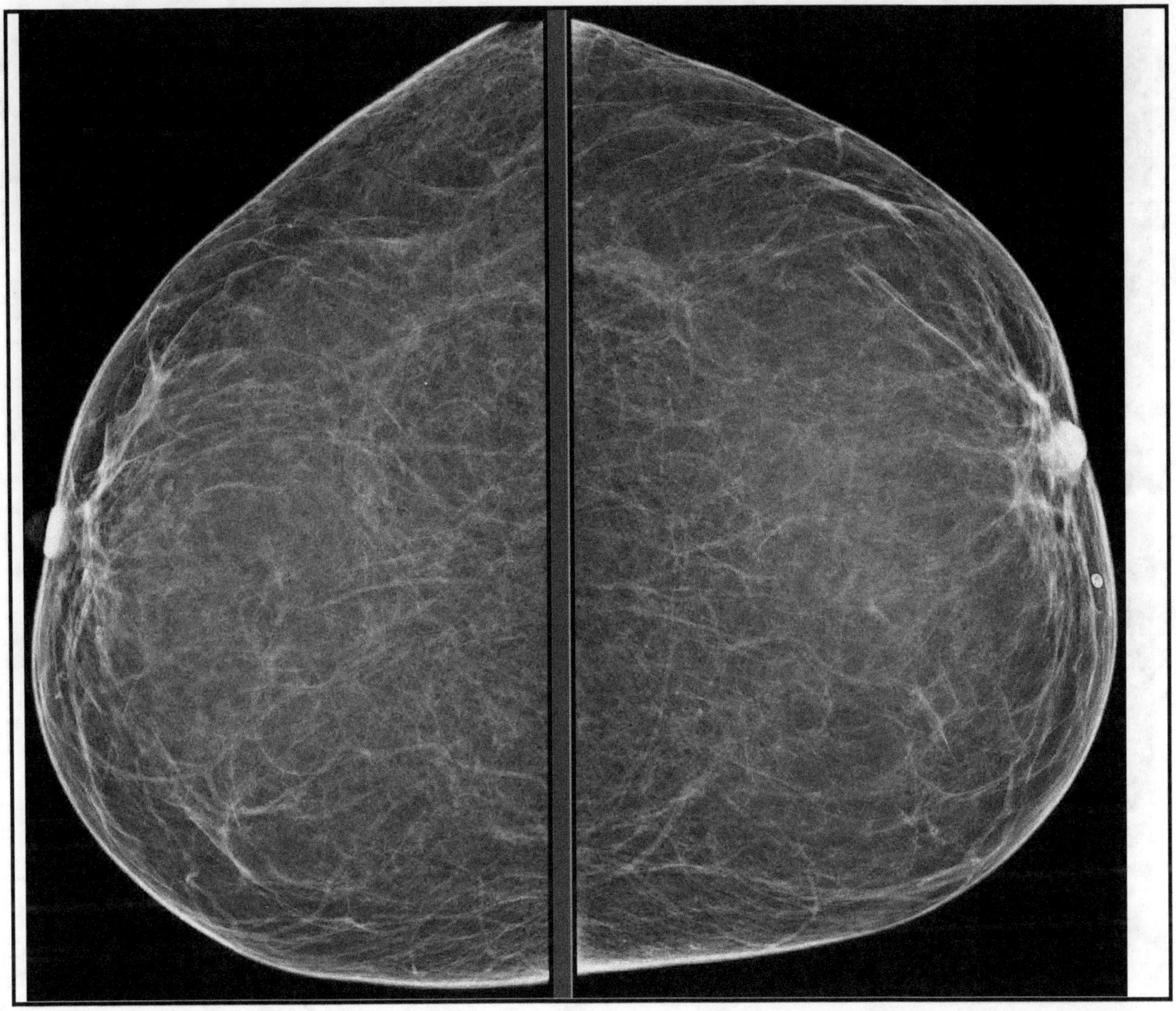

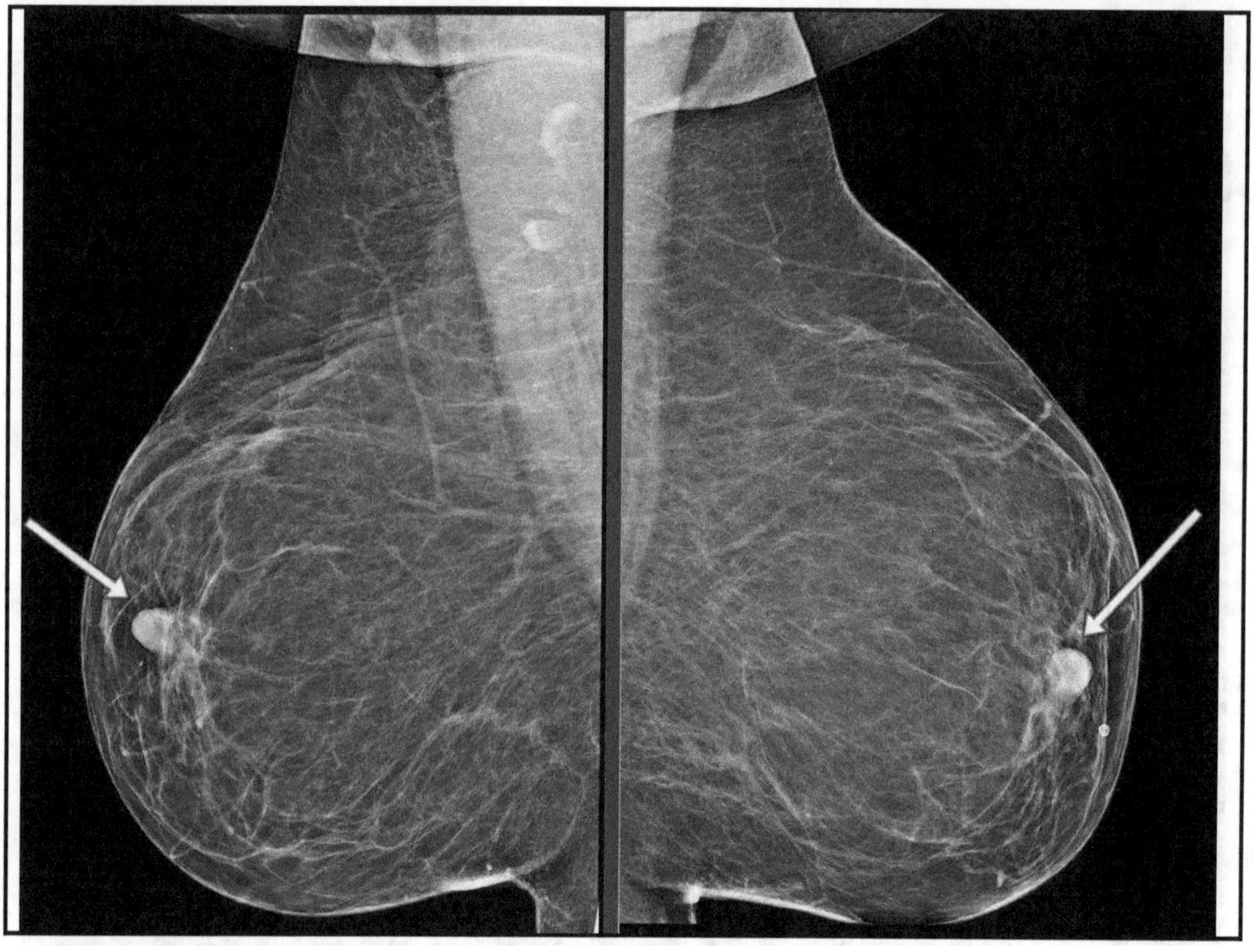

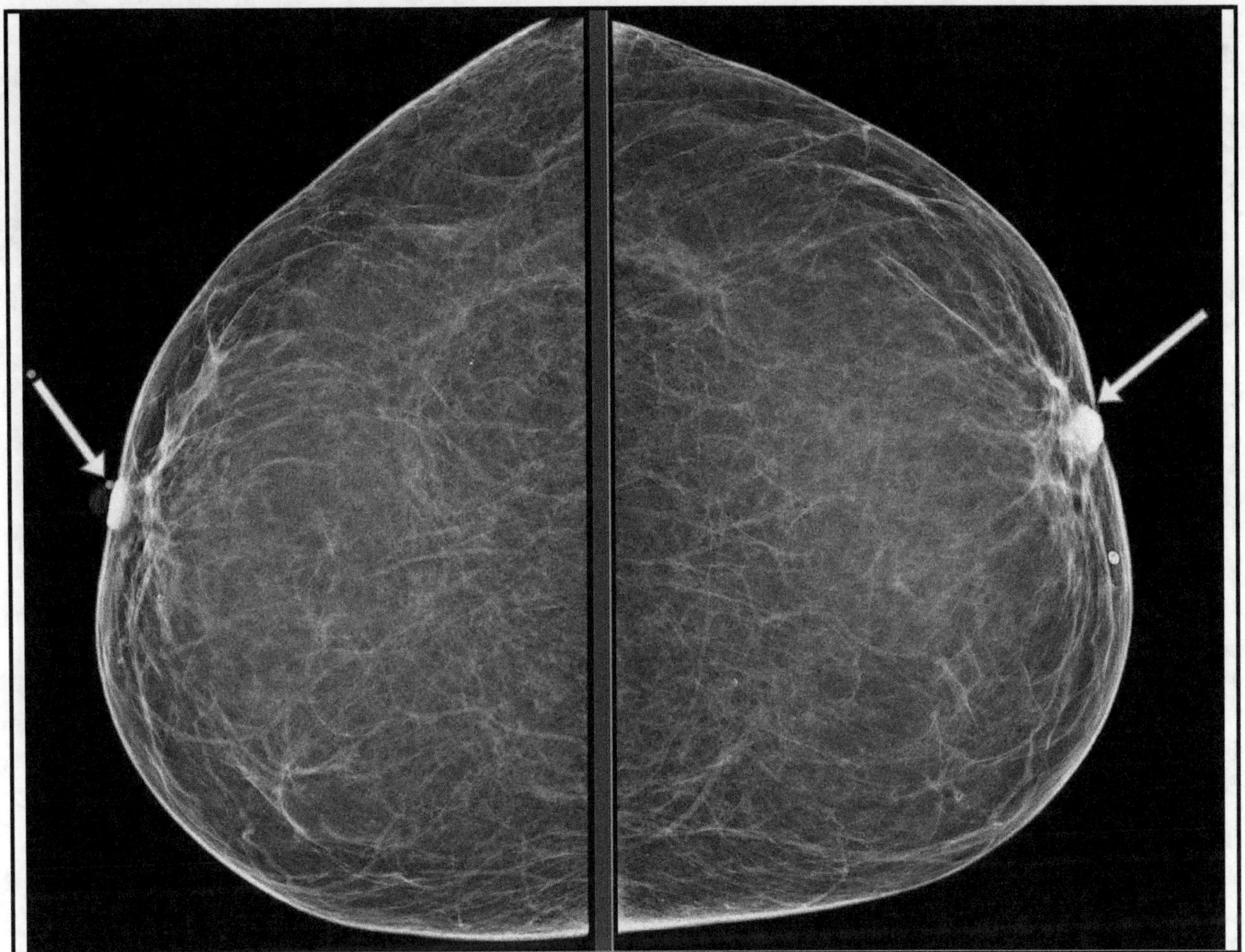

Technical error nipple not in profile mimic focal lesion

CASE 2: 53-year-old female/screening

Right MLO	Left MLO

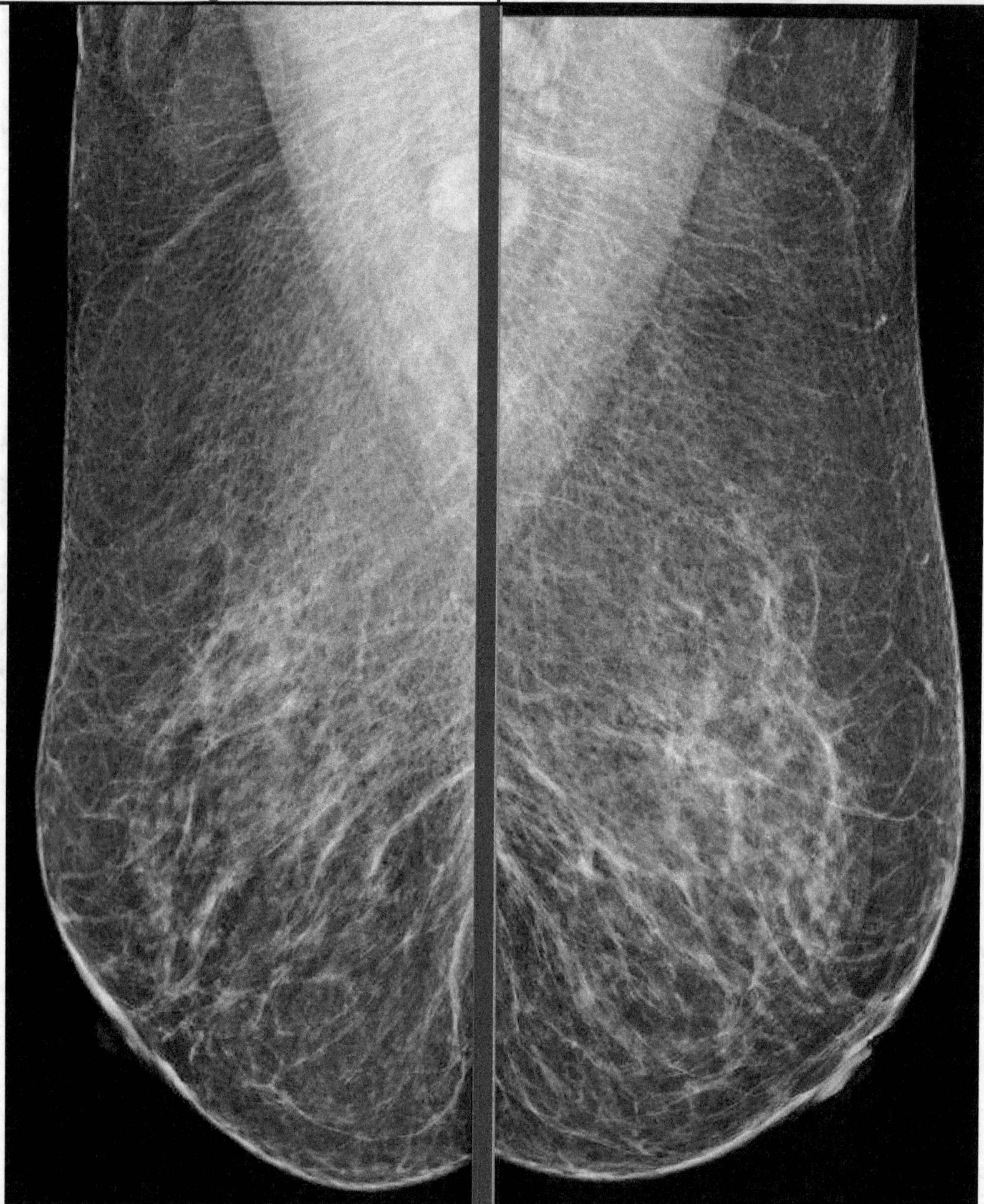

Right CC	Left CC

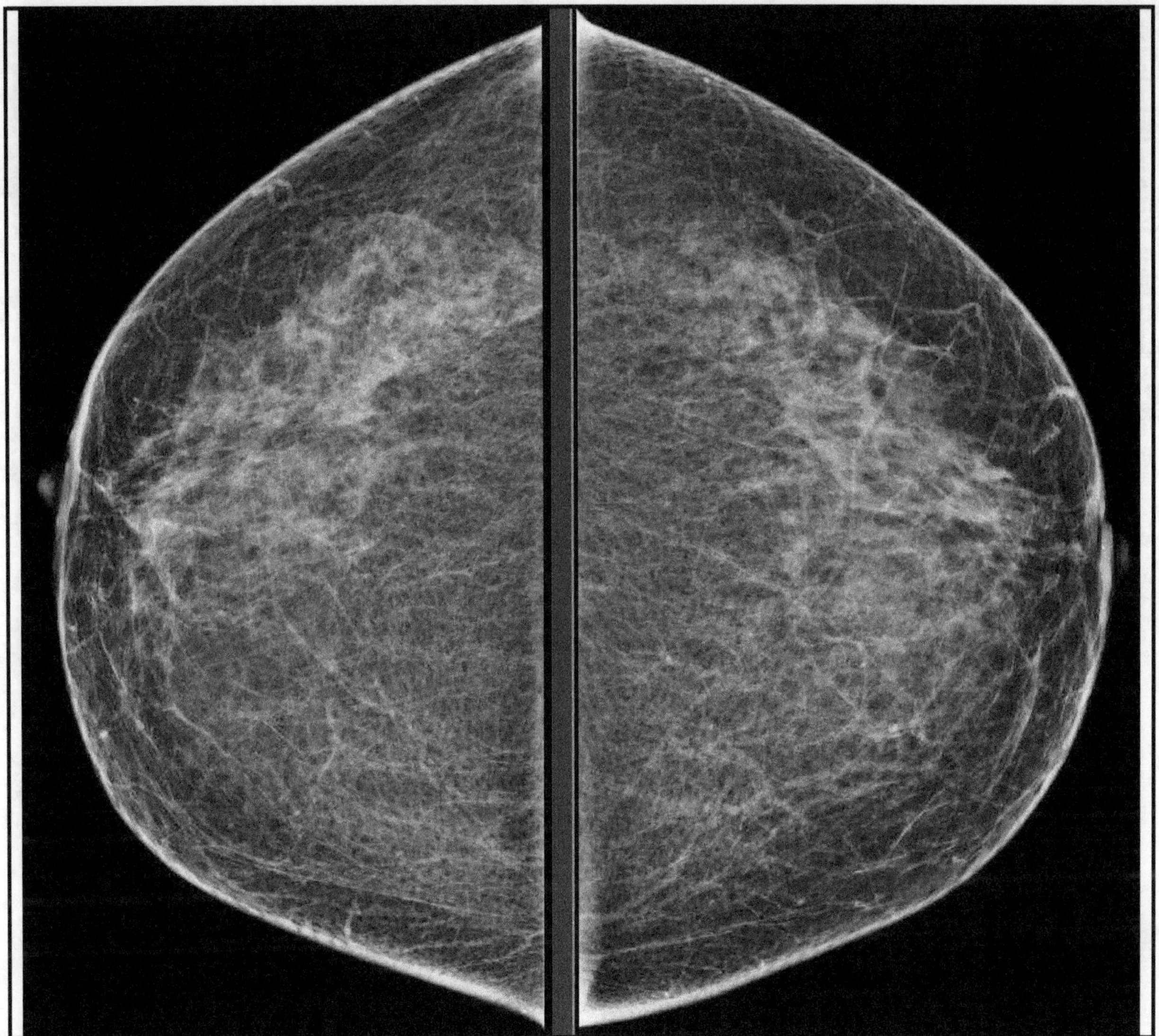

RIGHT BREAST	
Breast Parenchymal Density	***Scattered areas of fibroglandular density (ACR B)***
Focal Mass	None
Asymmetric Density	None
Parenchymal Distortion	None
Calcification	None
Skin Thickening	None
Axillary Nodes	None

LEFT BREAST	
Breast Parenchymal Density	***Scattered areas of fibroglandular density (ACR B)***
Focal Mass	None
Asymmetric Density	None
Parenchymal Distortion	None
Calcification	None
Skin Thickening	None
Axillary Nodes	None

IMPRESSION:

RIGHT BREAST: (BI-RADS 1)
LEFT BREAST: (BI-RADS 1)

RECOMMENDATION: Routine Annual screening

CASE 3: 57-year-old female/screening	
Right MLO	Left MLO

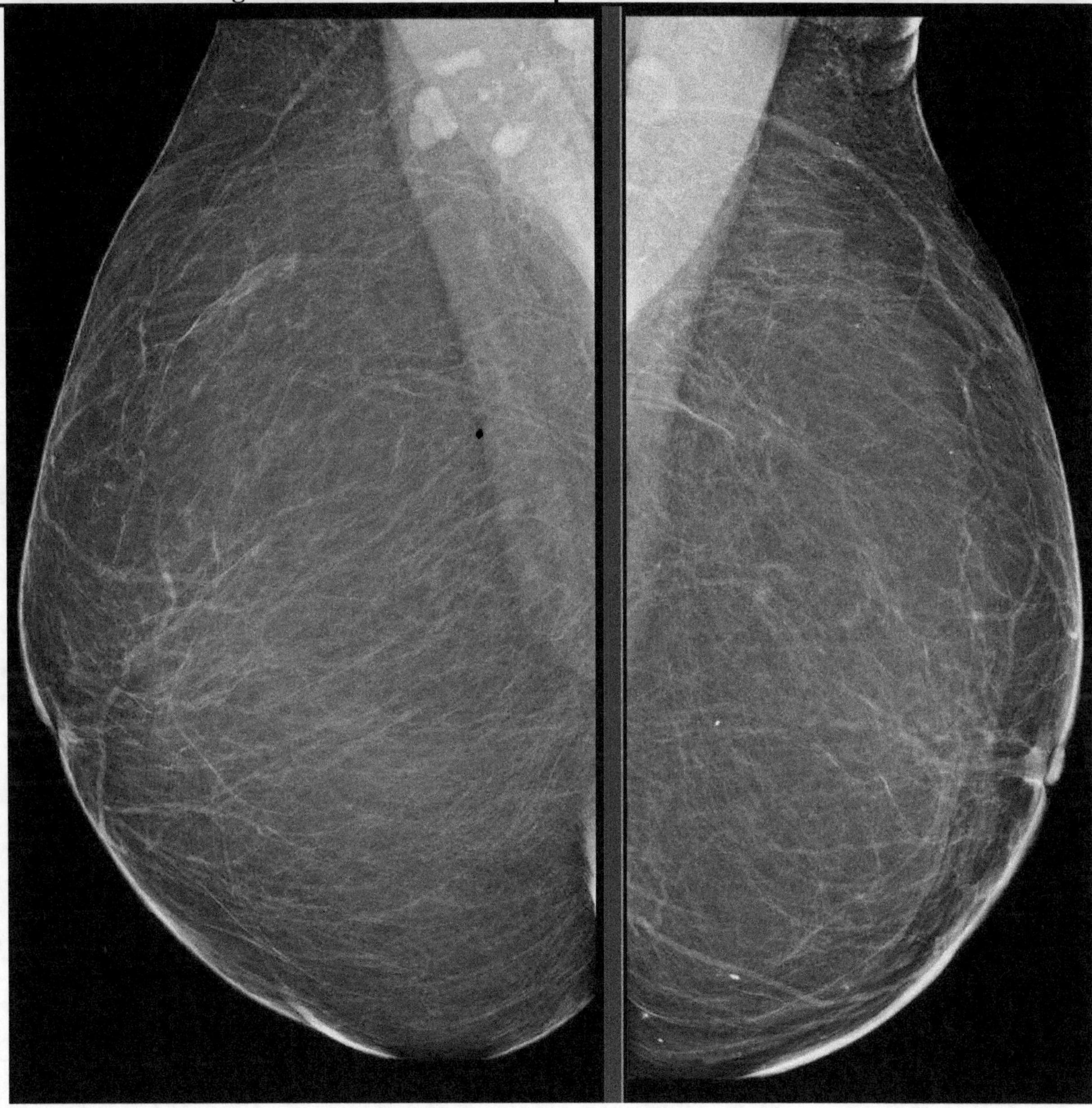

Right CC	Left CC

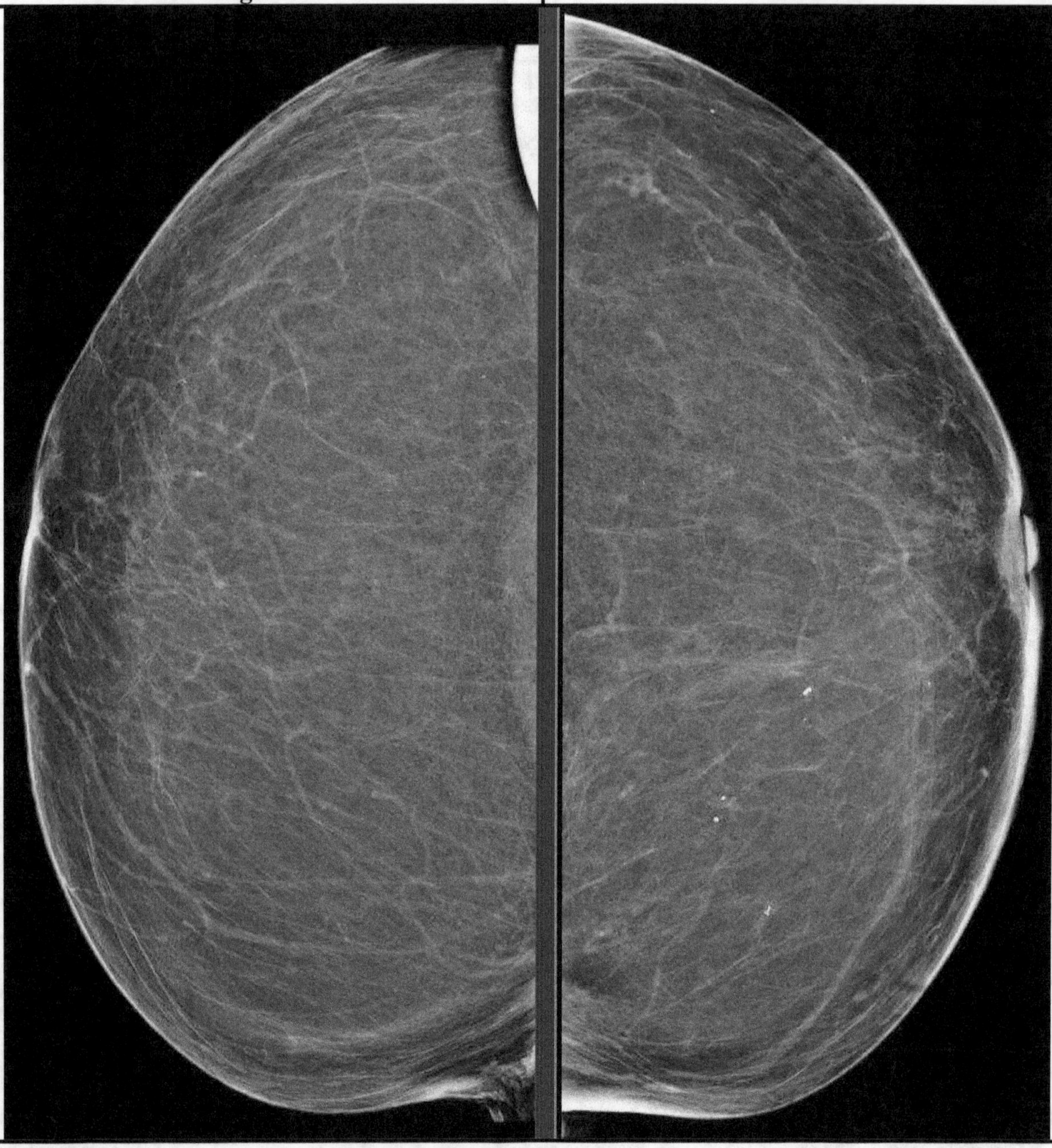

RIGHT BREAST	
Breast Parenchymal Density	***Almost entirely fatty (ACR A)***
Focal Mass	None
Asymmetric Density	None
Parenchymal Distortion	None
Calcification	None
Skin Thickening	None
Axillary Nodes	None

LEFT BREAST	
Breast Parenchymal Density	***Almost entirely fatty (ACR A)***
Focal Mass	None
Asymmetric Density	None
Parenchymal Distortion	None
Calcification	***skin calcifications***
Skin Thickening	None
Axillary Nodes	None

IMPRESSION:

RIGHT BREAST: (BI-RADS 1)
LEFT BREAST: (BI-RADS 2)

RECOMMENDATION: Routine Annual screening

CASE 4: 37-year-old female/screening

Right MLO	Left MLO

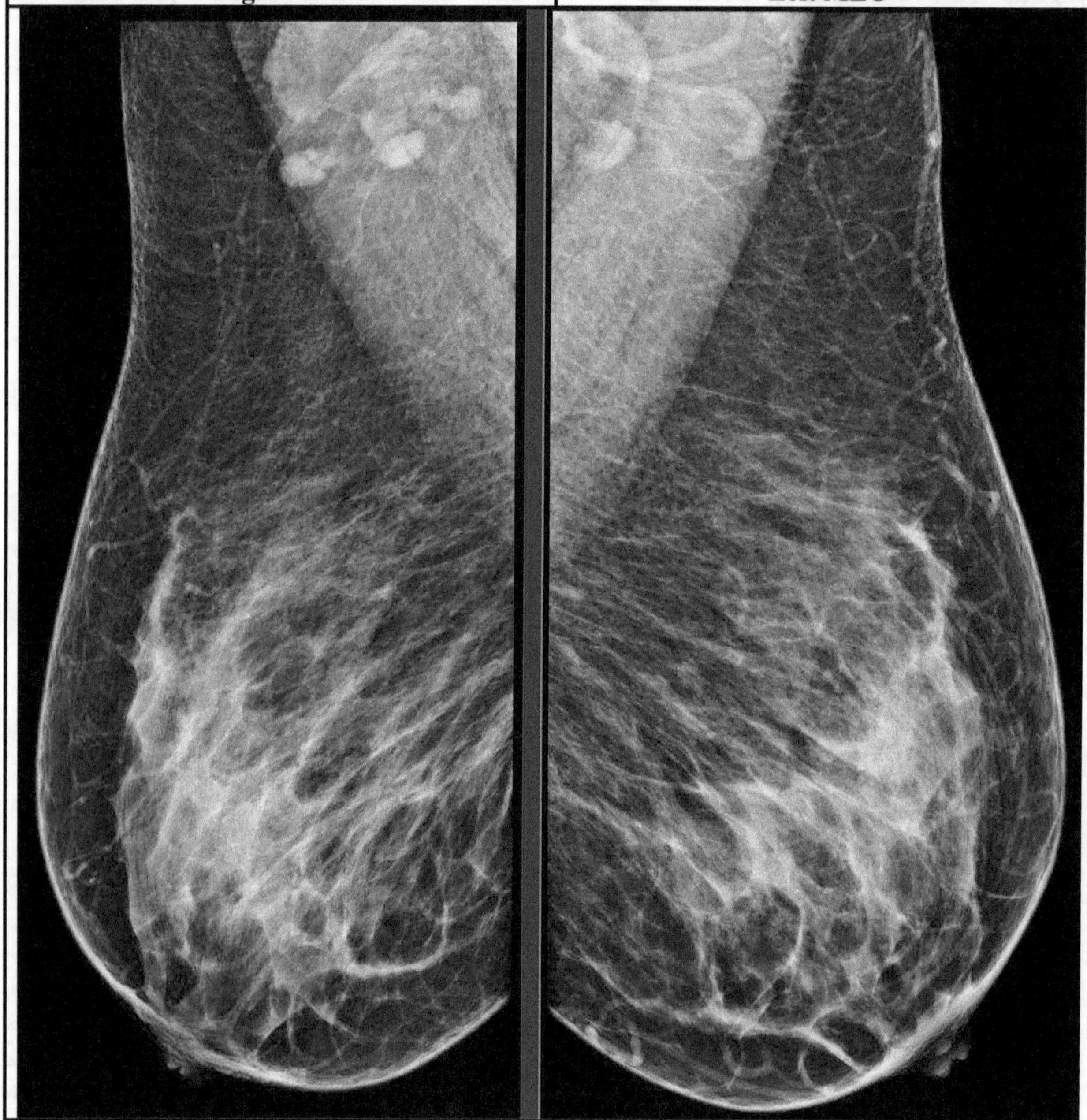

Right CC	Left CC

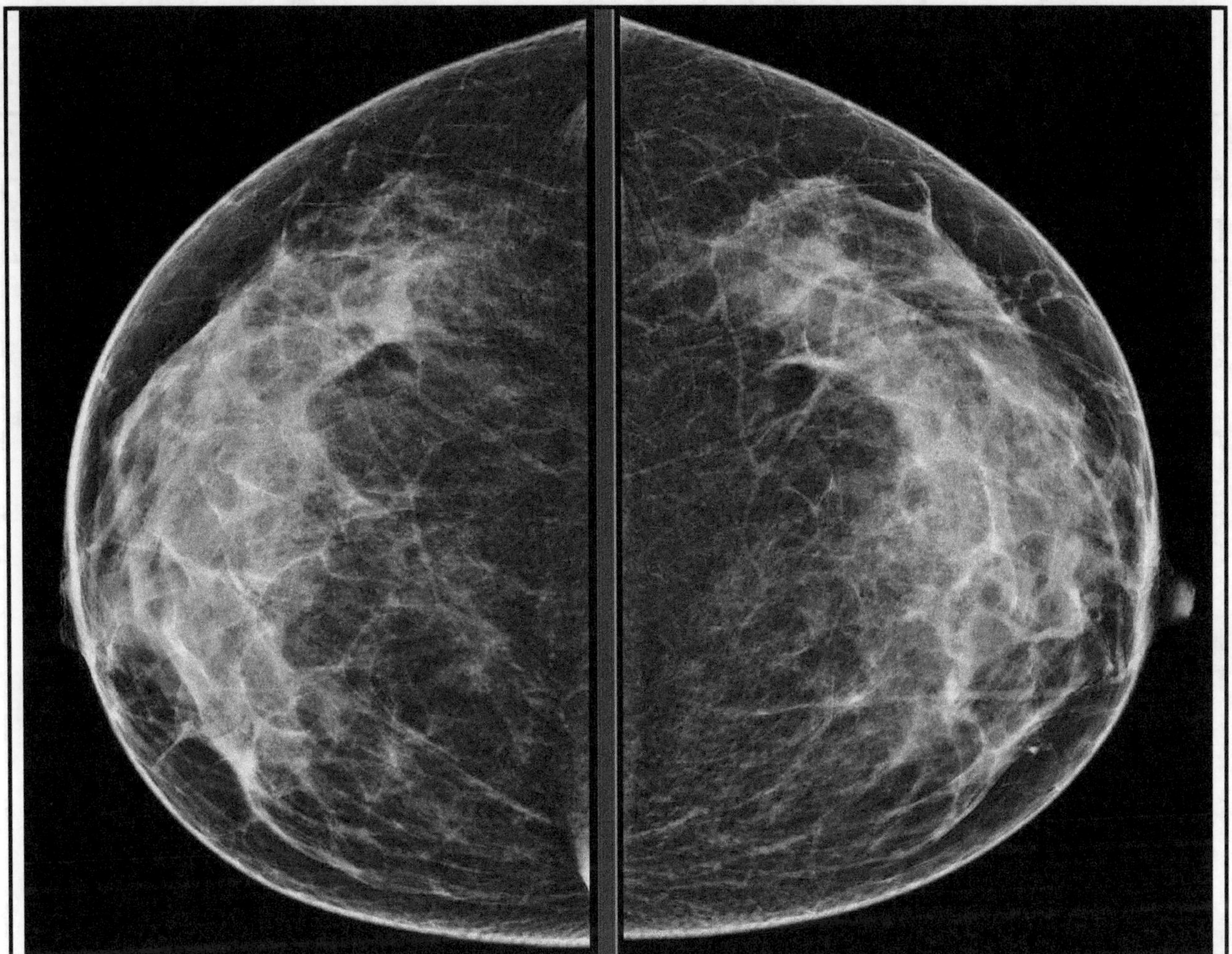

RIGHT BREAST	
Breast Parenchymal Density	***Heterogeneously dense, may obscure small masses (ACR C)***
Focal Mass	None
Asymmetric Density	None
Parenchymal Distortion	None
Calcification	None
Skin Thickening	None
Axillary Nodes	None

LEFT BREAST	
Breast Parenchymal Density	***Heterogeneously dense, may obscure small masses (ACR C)***
Focal Mass	None
Asymmetric Density	None
Parenchymal Distortion	None
Calcification	None
Skin Thickening	None
Axillary Nodes	None

IMPRESSION:

RIGHT BREAST: (BI-RADS 1)

LEFT BREAST: (BI-RADS 1)

RECOMMENDATION: Routine Annual screening

CASE 5: 26-year-old female/screening	
Right MLO	**Left MLO**
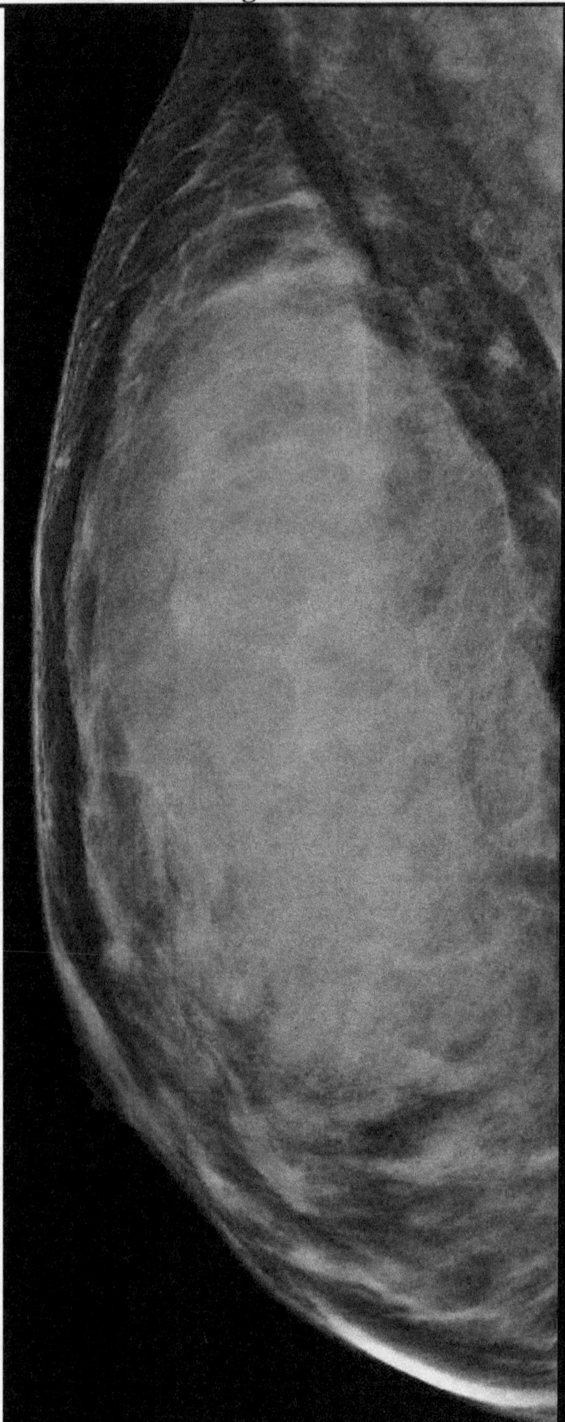	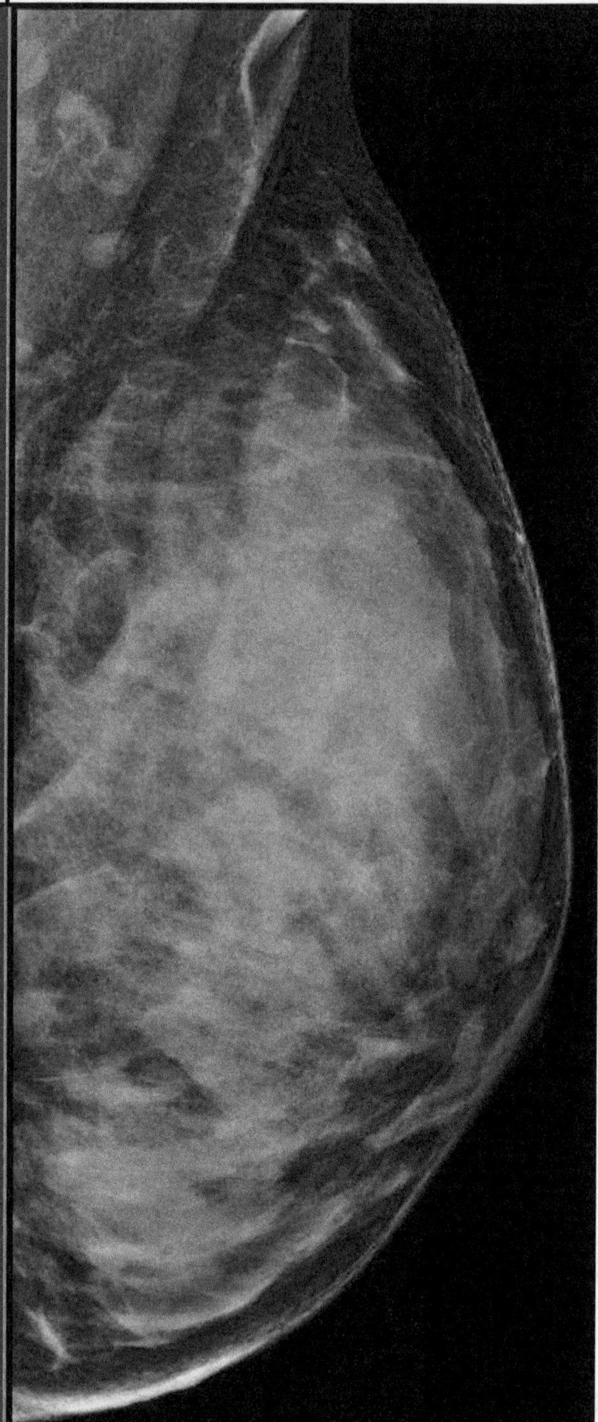

Right CC	Left CC

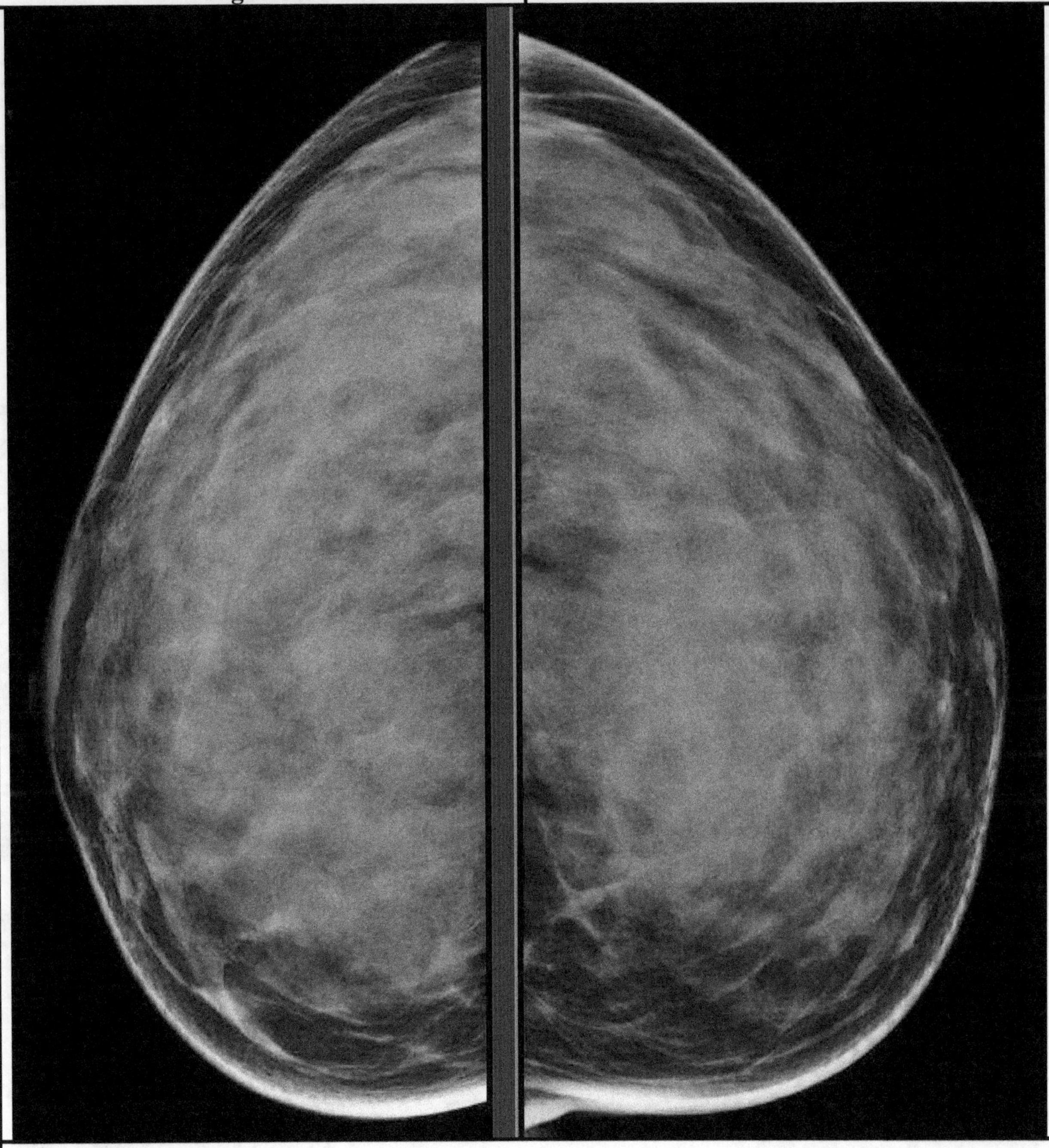

RIGHT BREAST	
Breast Parenchymal Density	***Extremely dense, which lowers the sensitivity of mammography (ACR D)***
Focal Mass	None
Asymmetric Density	None
Parenchymal Distortion	None
Calcification	None
Skin Thickening	None
Axillary Nodes	None

LEFT BREAST	
Breast Parenchymal Density	***Extremely dense, which lowers the sensitivity of mammography (ACR D)***
Focal Mass	None
Asymmetric Density	None
Parenchymal Distortion	None
Calcification	None
Skin Thickening	None
Axillary Nodes	None

IMPRESSION:

RIGHT BREAST: (BI-RADS 0)
LEFT BREAST: (BI-RADS 0)

RECOMMENDATION: US Correlation

CASE 6: 38-year-old female/screening	
Right MLO	Left MLO

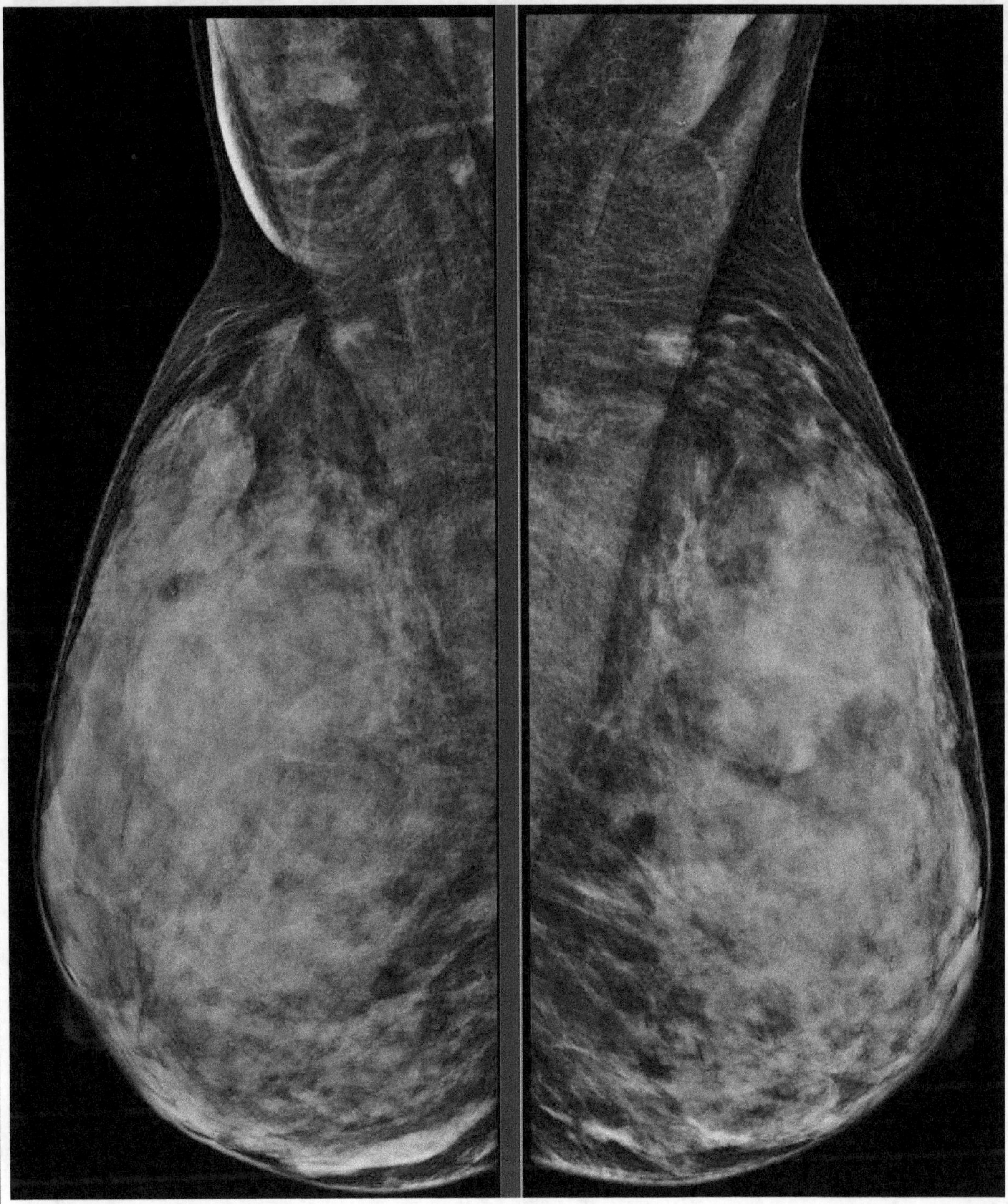

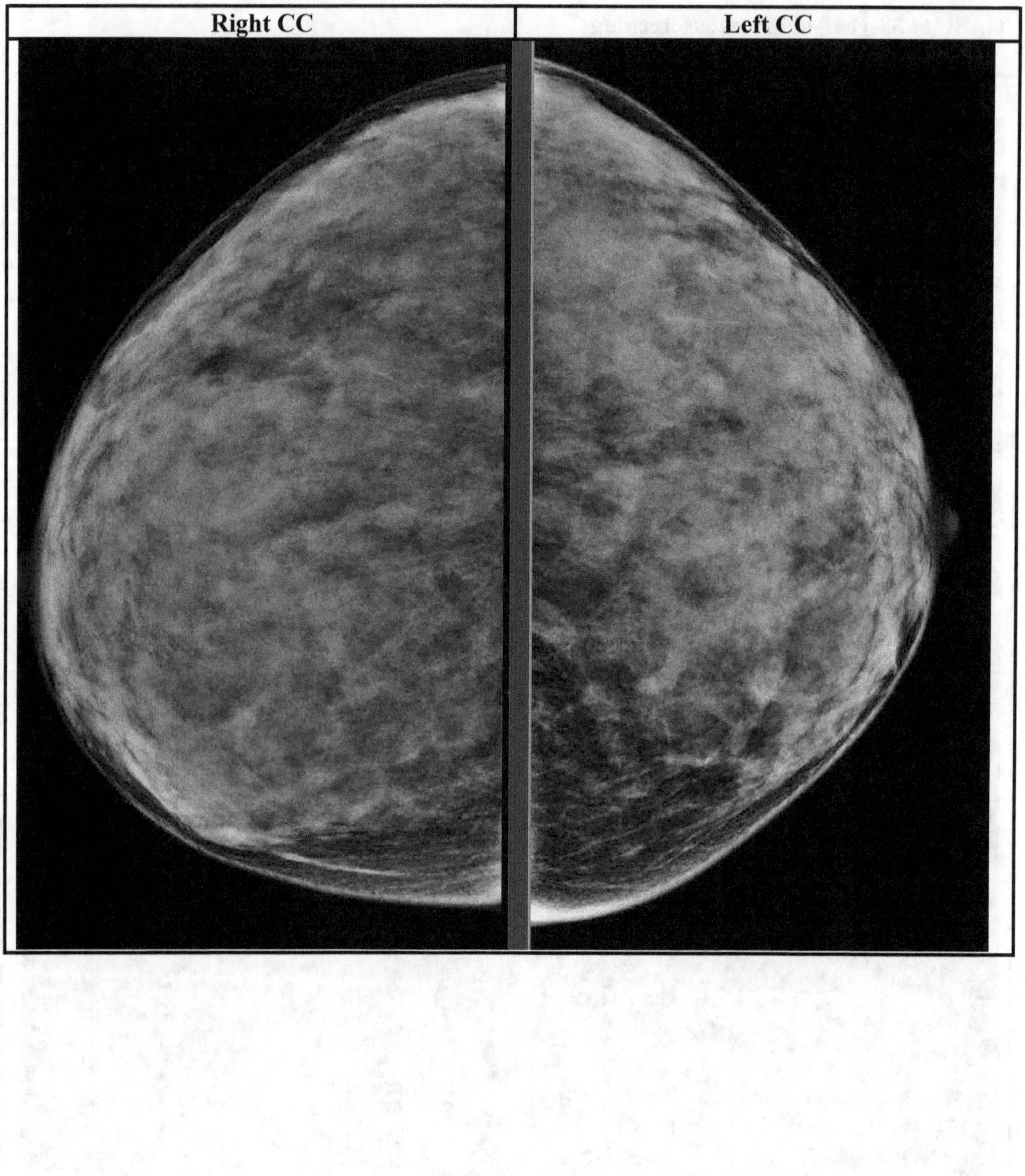
Right CC
Left CC

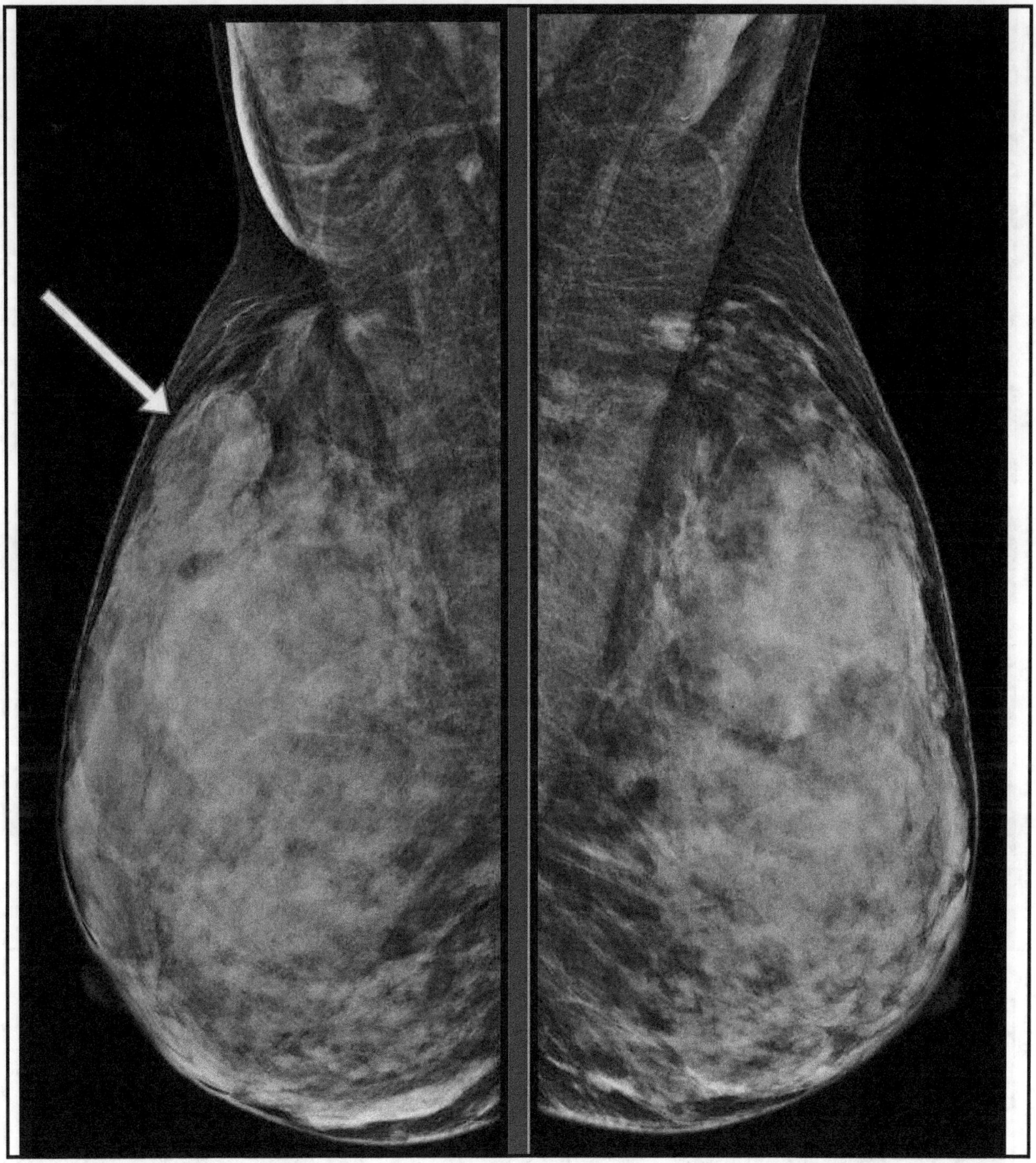

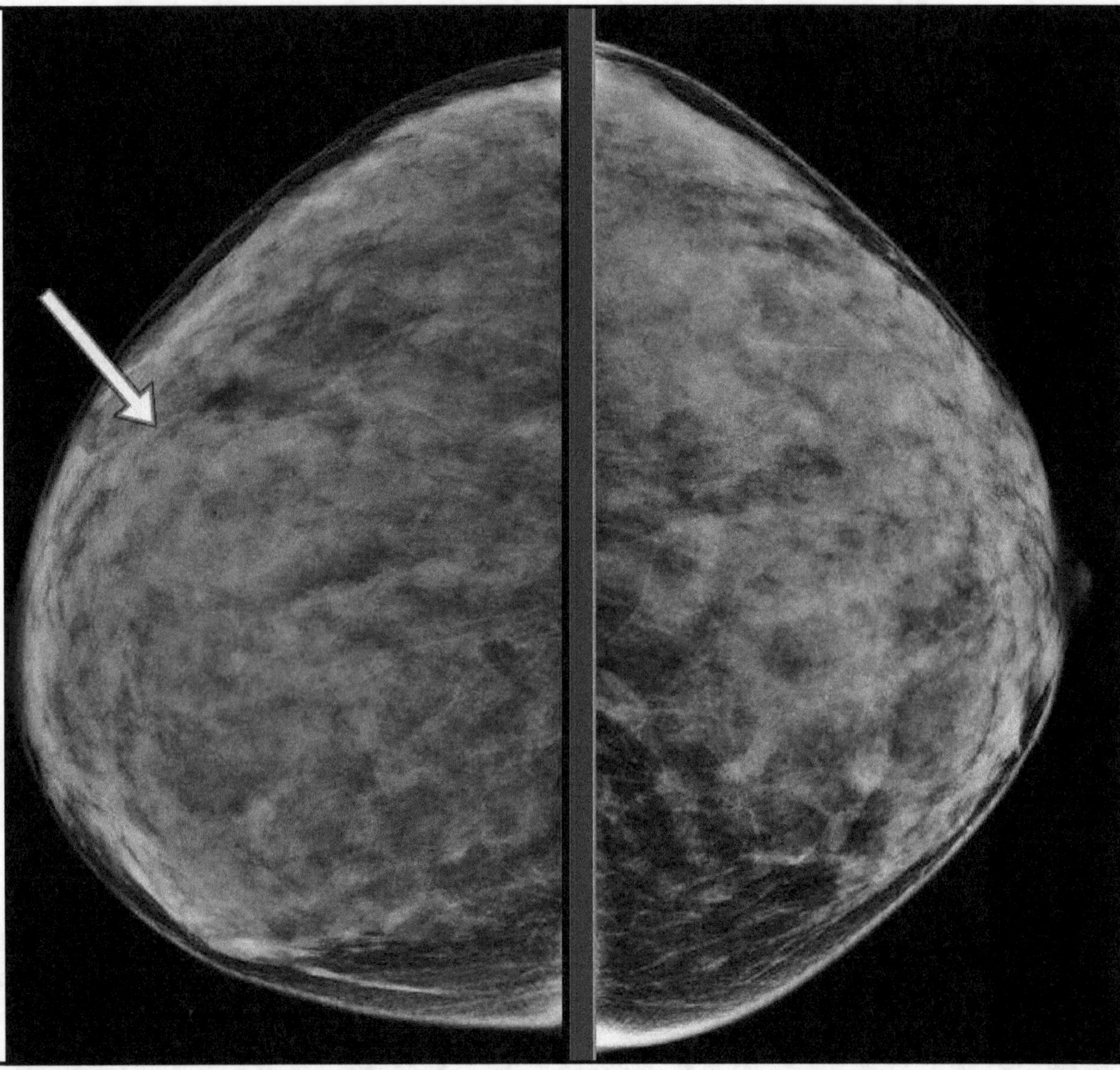

RIGHT BREAST	
Breast Parenchymal Density	***Extremely dense, which lowers the sensitivity of mammography (ACR D)/Axillary Accessory Breast***
Focal Mass	***UOQ Circumscribed Mass Lesion of Equal Density***
Asymmetric Density	None
Parenchymal Distortion	None
Calcification	None
Skin Thickening	None
Axillary Nodes	None

LEFT BREAST	
Breast Parenchymal Density	***Extremely dense, which lowers the sensitivity of mammography (ACR D)***
Focal Mass	None
Asymmetric Density	None
Parenchymal Distortion	None
Calcification	None
Skin Thickening	None
Axillary Nodes	None

IMPRESSION:

RIGHT BREAST: (BI-RADS 0)
LEFT BREAST: (BI-RADS 0)

RECOMMENDATION: US Correlation

CASE 7: 39-year-old female/screening

Right MLO	Left MLO

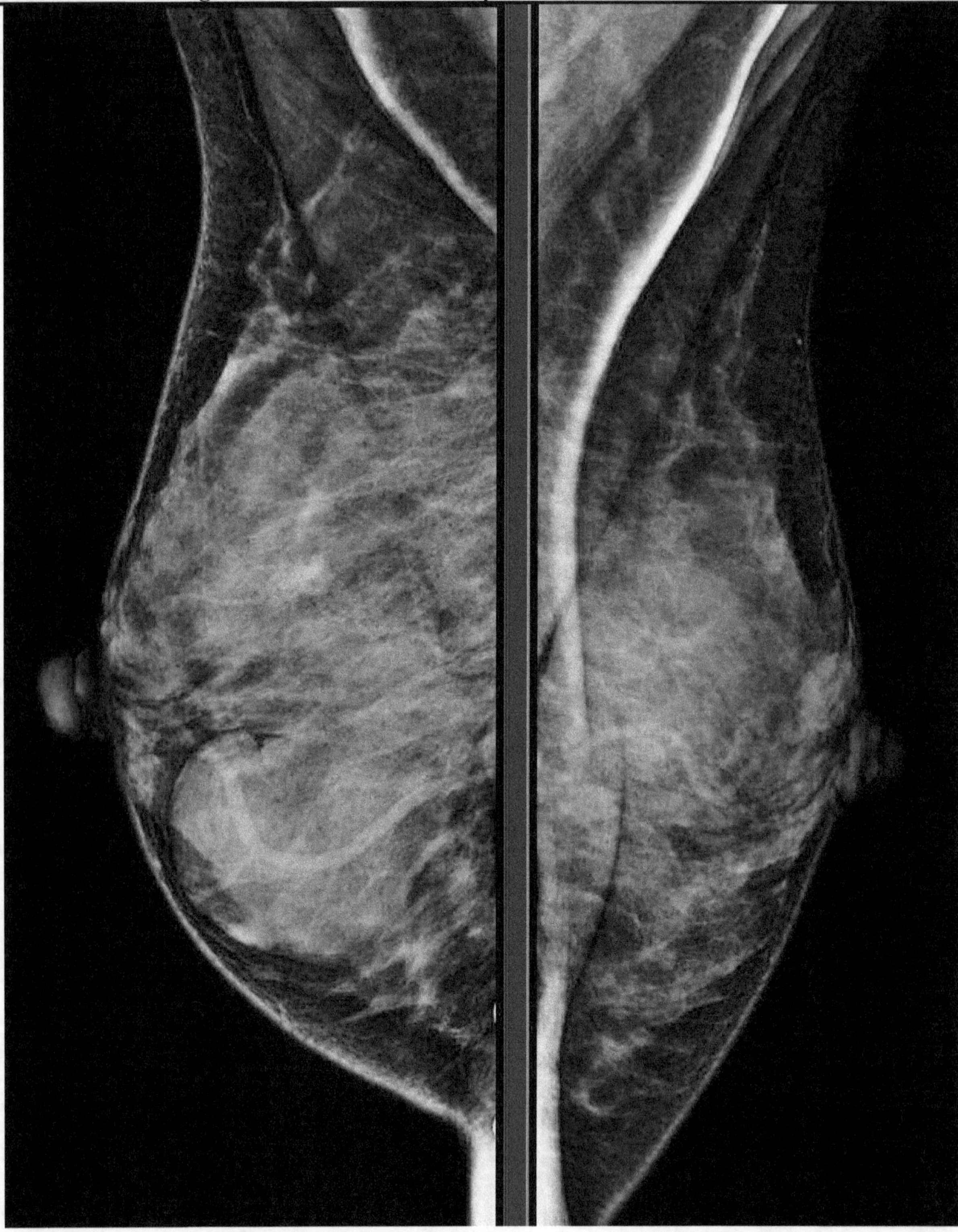

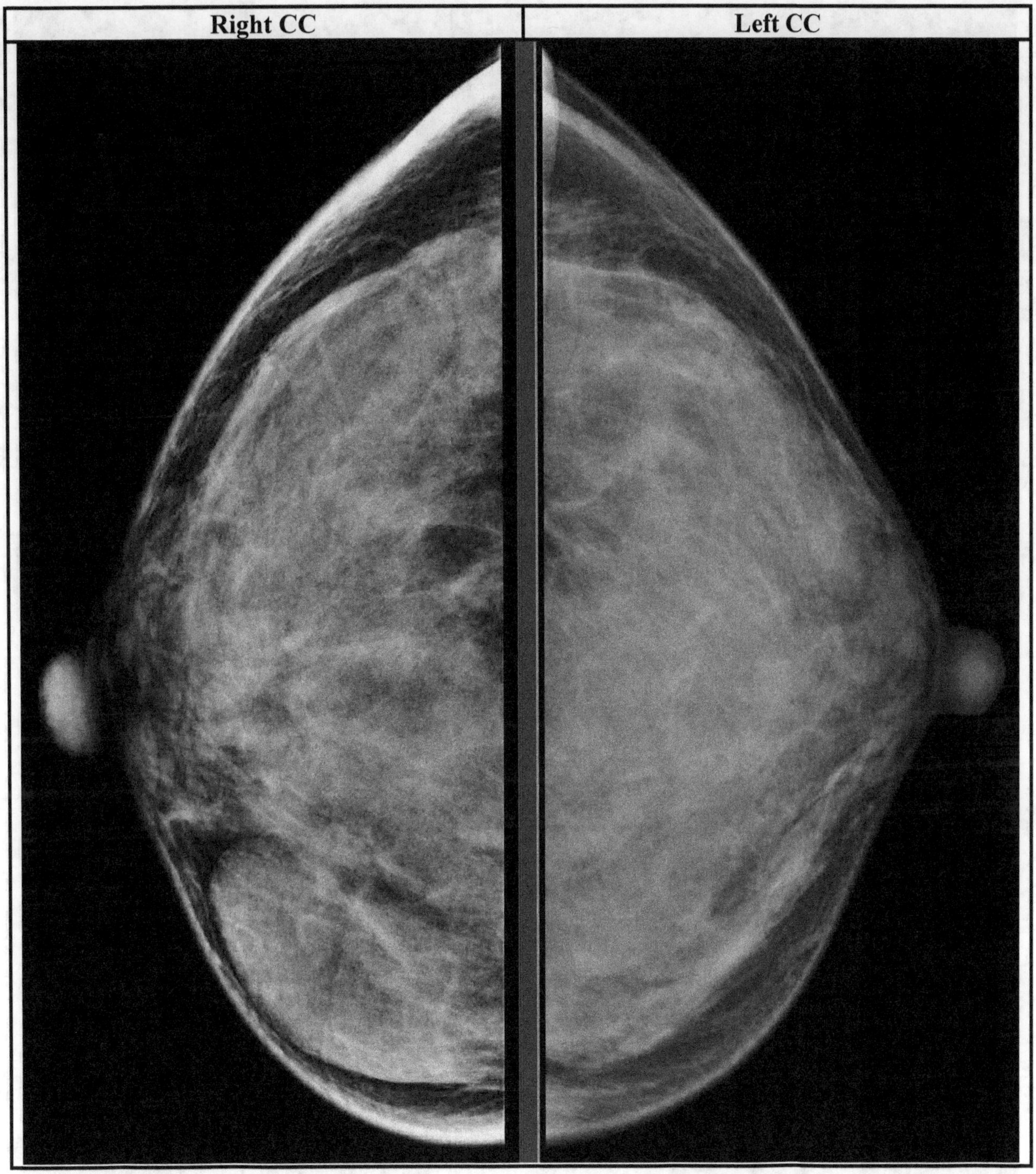
Right CC
Left CC

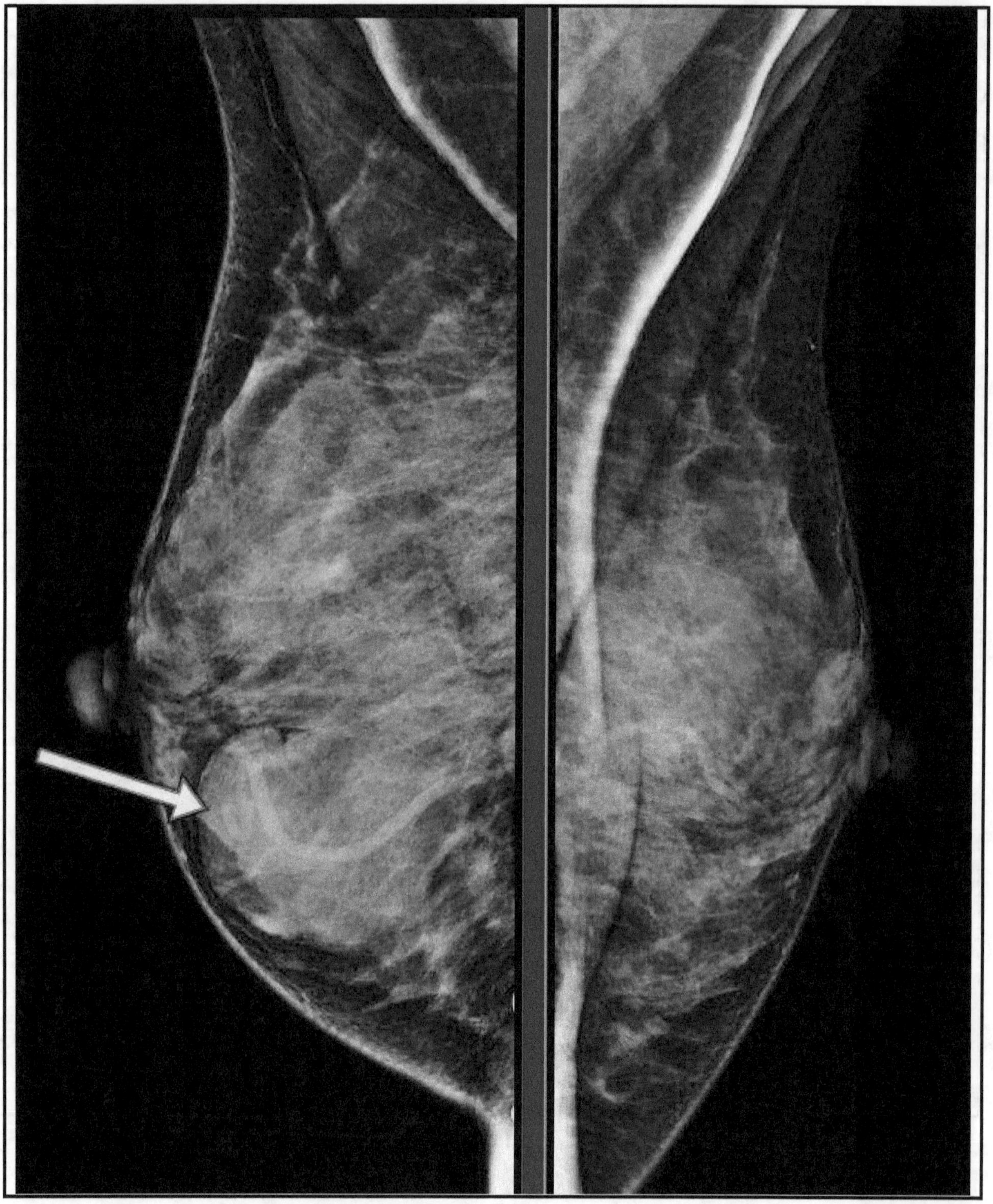

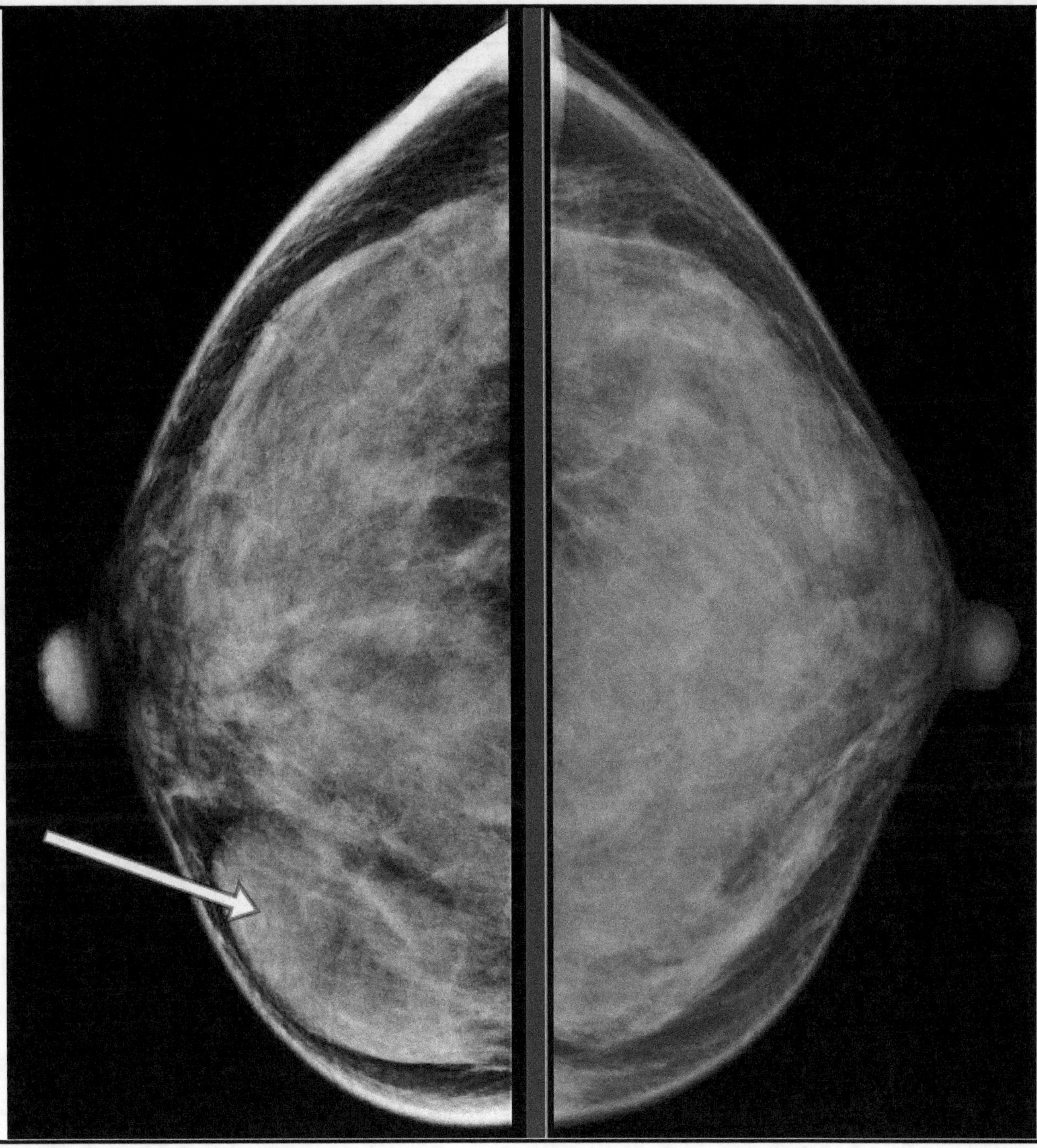

RIGHT BREAST	
Breast Parenchymal Density	***Extremely dense, which lowers the sensitivity of mammography (ACR D)***
Focal Mass	NONE
Asymmetric Density	***LIQ focal asymmetry***
Parenchymal Distortion	None
Calcification	None
Skin Thickening	None
Axillary Nodes	None

LEFT BREAST	
Breast Parenchymal Density	***Extremely dense, which lowers the sensitivity of mammography (ACR D)***
Focal Mass	None
Asymmetric Density	None
Parenchymal Distortion	None
Calcification	None
Skin Thickening	None
Axillary Nodes	None

IMPRESSION:

RIGHT BREAST: (BI-RADS 0)
LEFT BREAST: (BI-RADS 0)

RECOMMENDATION: US Correlation

CASE 8: 41-year-old female/screening

Right MLO	Left MLO
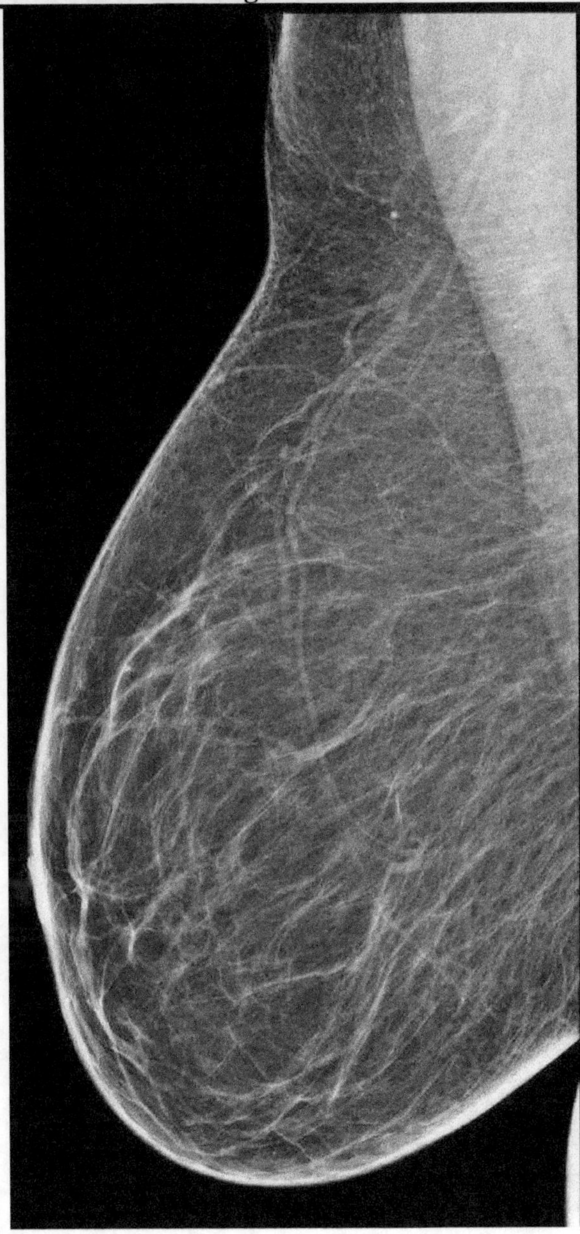	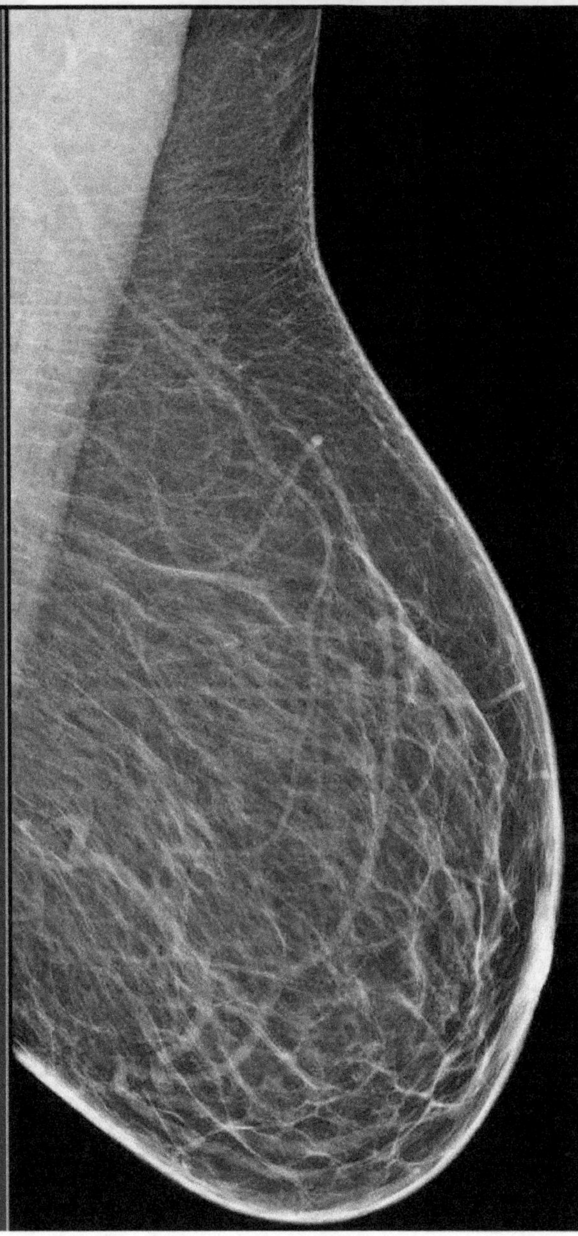

Right CC	Left CC

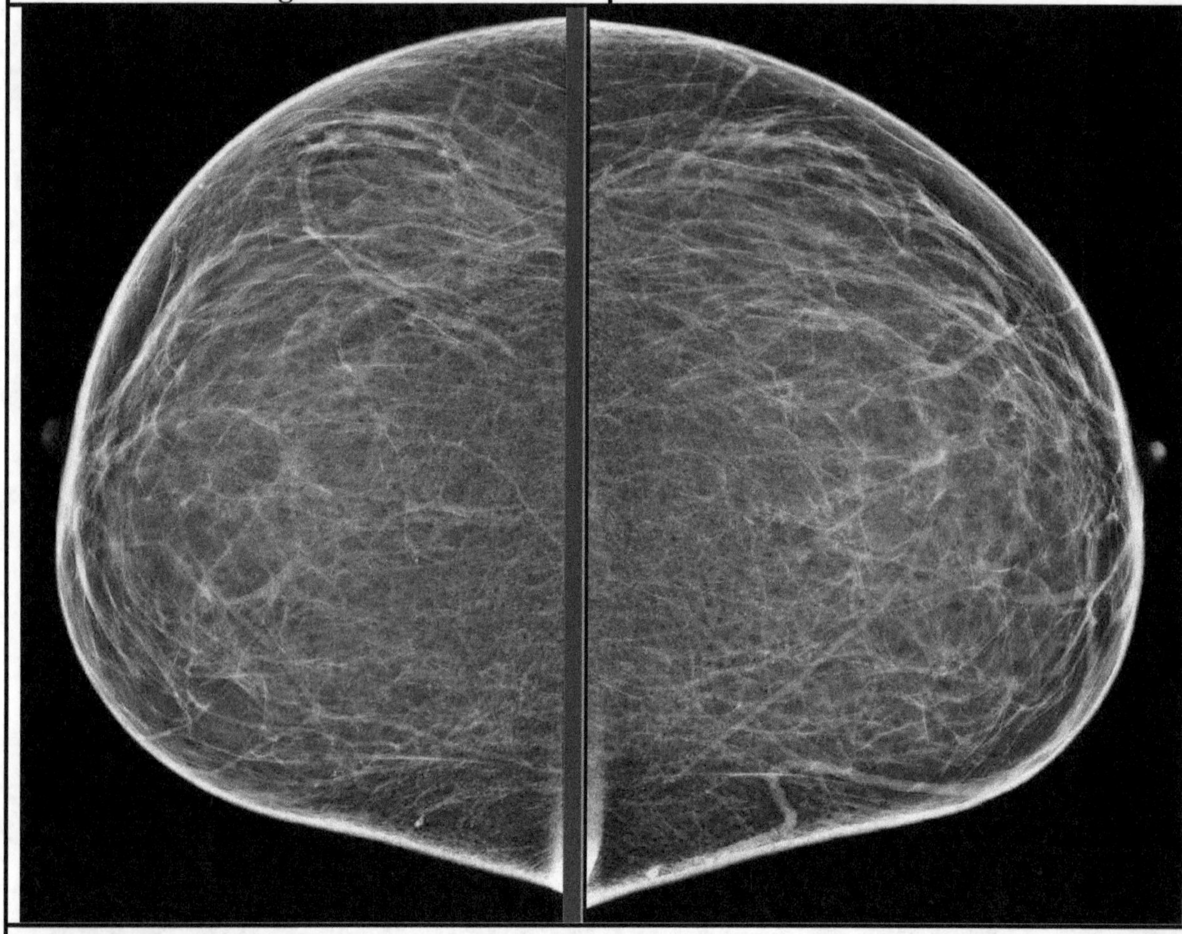

RIGHT BREAST	
Breast Parenchymal Density	***Scattered areas of fibroglandular density (ACR B)***
Focal Mass	None
Asymmetric Density	None
Parenchymal Distortion	None
Calcification	None
Skin Thickening	None
Axillary Nodes	None

LEFT BREAST	
Breast Parenchymal Density	***Scattered areas of fibroglandular density (ACR B)***
Focal Mass	None
Asymmetric Density	None
Parenchymal Distortion	None
Calcification	None
Skin Thickening	None
Axillary Nodes	None

IMPRESSION:

RIGHT BREAST: (BI-RADS 1)

LEFT BREAST: (BI-RADS 1)

RECOMMENDATION: Routine Annual screening

CASE 9: 36-year-old female/screening

Right MLO	**Left MLO**
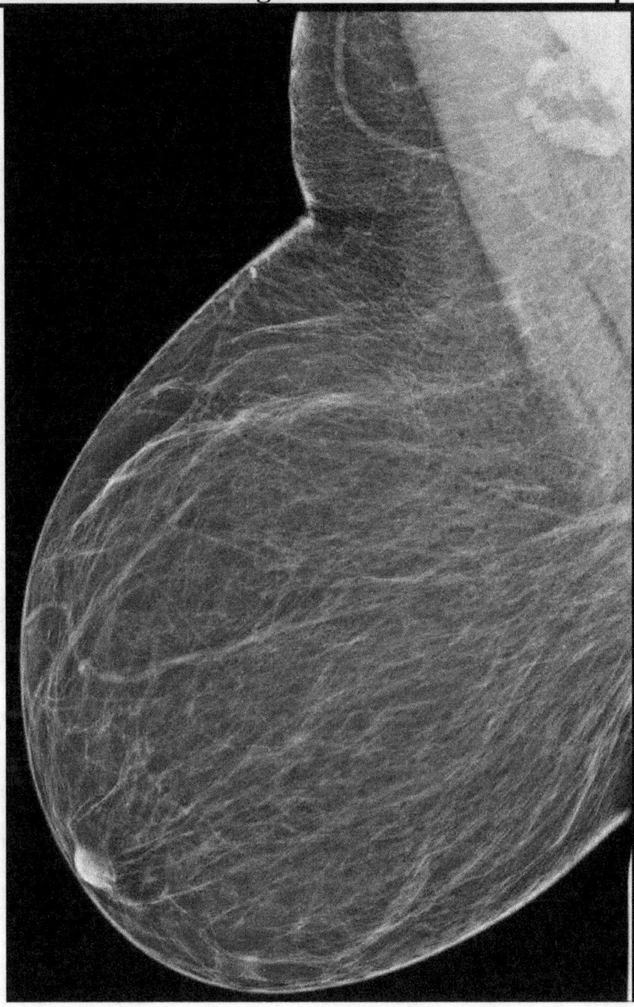	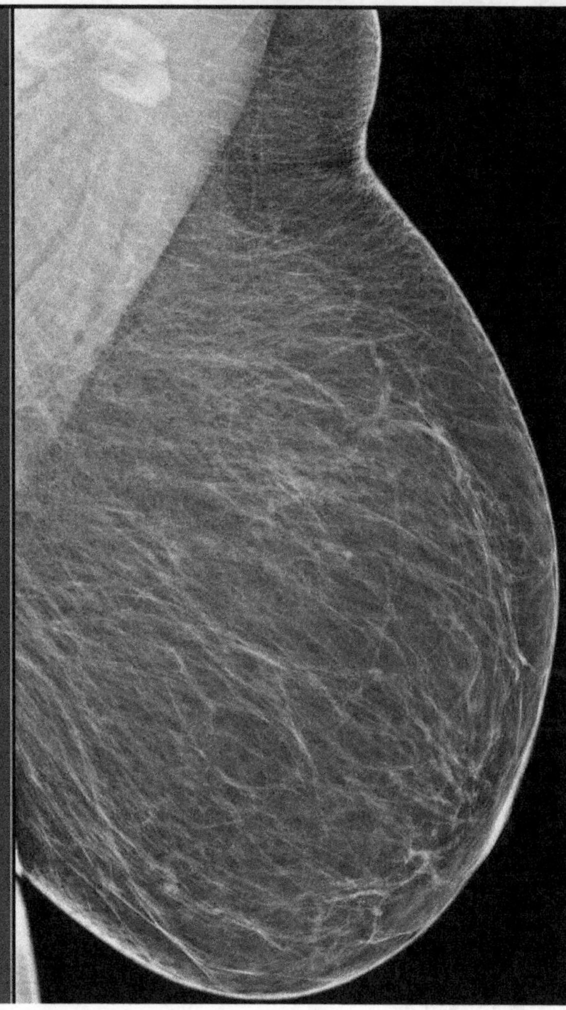

Right CC	Left CC

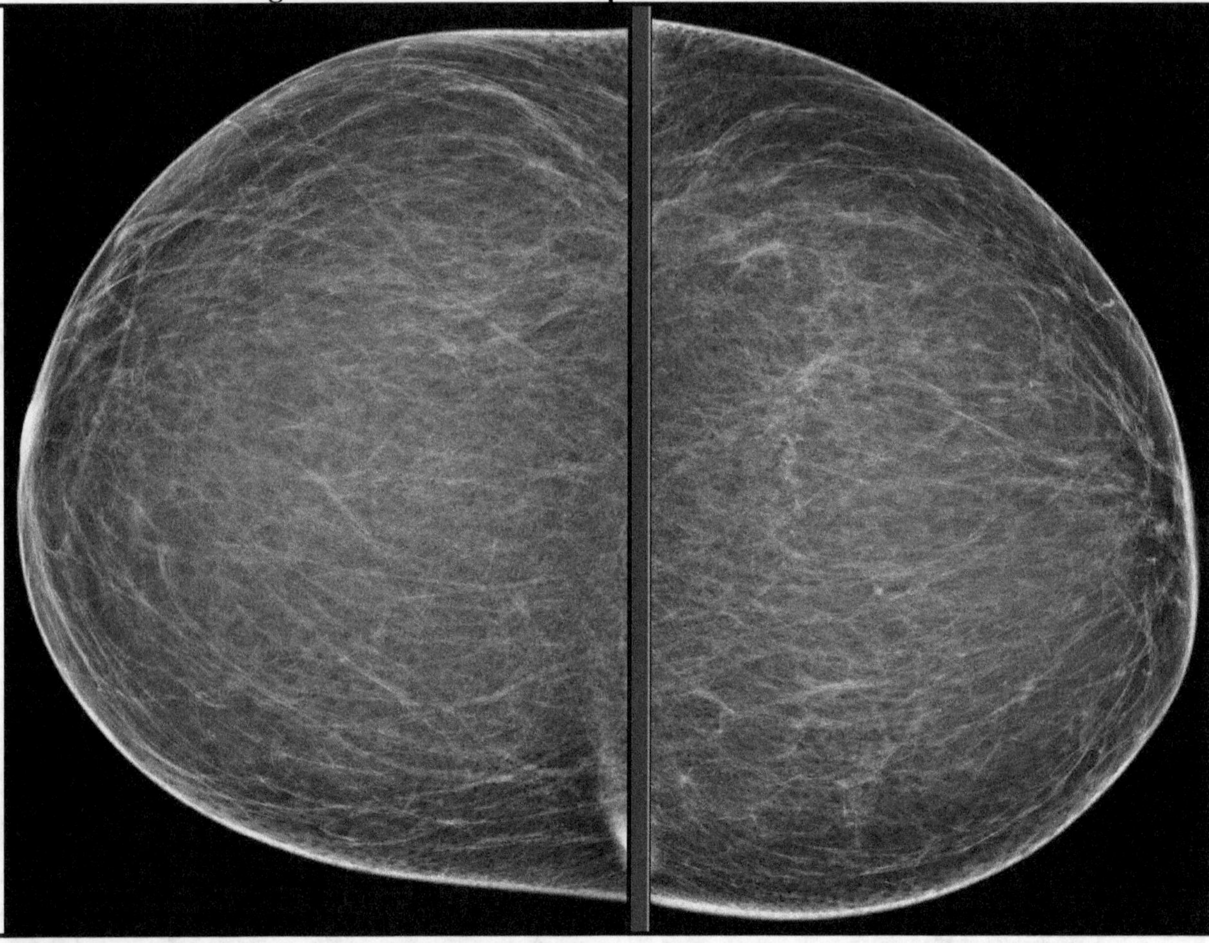

RIGHT BREAST	
Breast Parenchymal Density	***Almost entirely fatty (ACR A)***
Focal Mass	None
Asymmetric Density	None
Parenchymal Distortion	None
Calcification	None
Skin Thickening	None
Axillary Nodes	None

LEFT BREAST	
Breast Parenchymal Density	***Almost entirely fatty (ACR A)***
Focal Mass	None
Asymmetric Density	None
Parenchymal Distortion	None
Calcification	None
Skin Thickening	None
Axillary Nodes	None

IMPRESSION:

RIGHT BREAST: (BI-RADS 1)

LEFT BREAST: (BI-RADS 1)

RECOMMENDATION: Routine Annual screening

CASE 10: 47-year-old female/screening

Right MLO	**Left MLO**

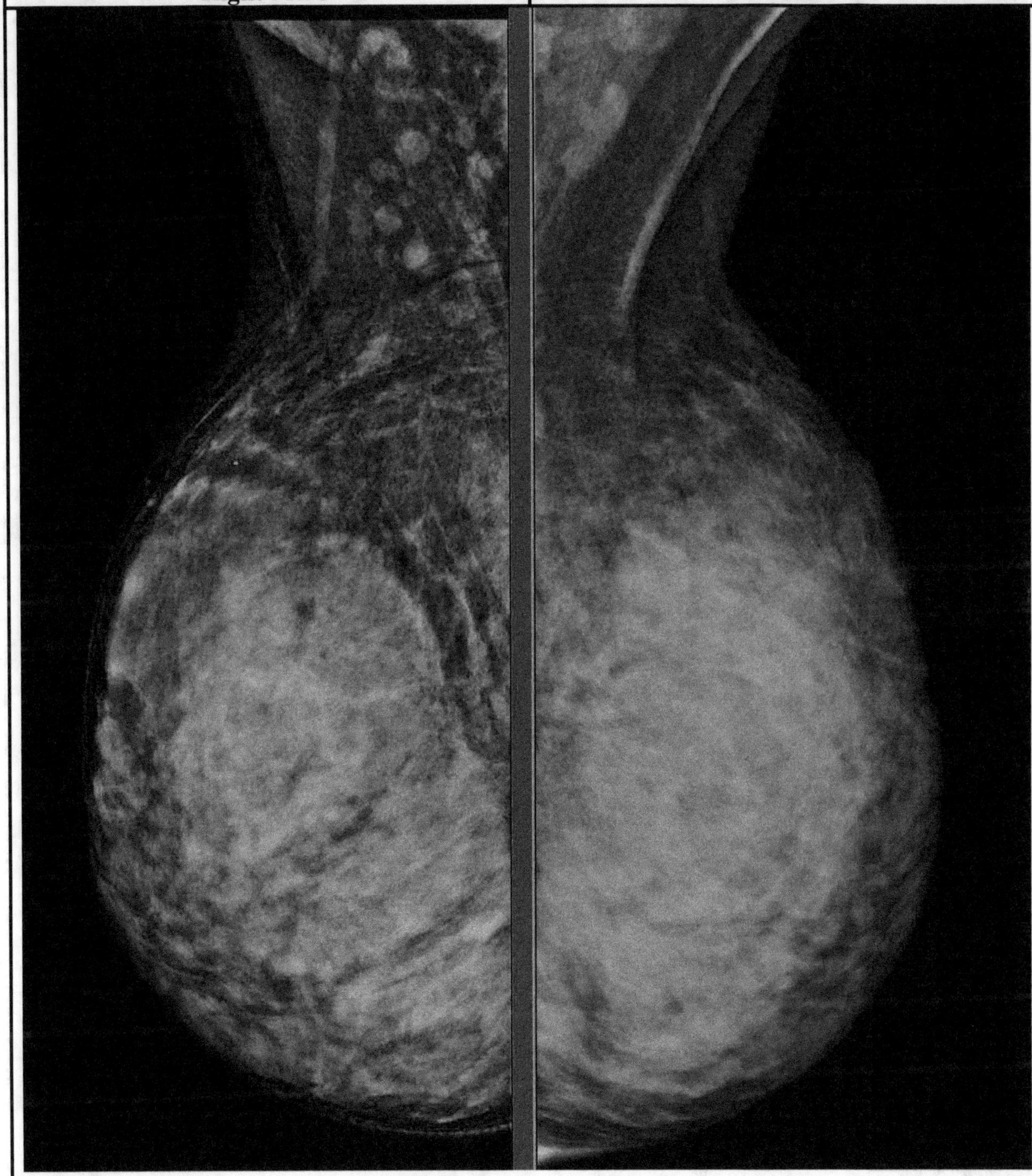

Right CC	Left CC

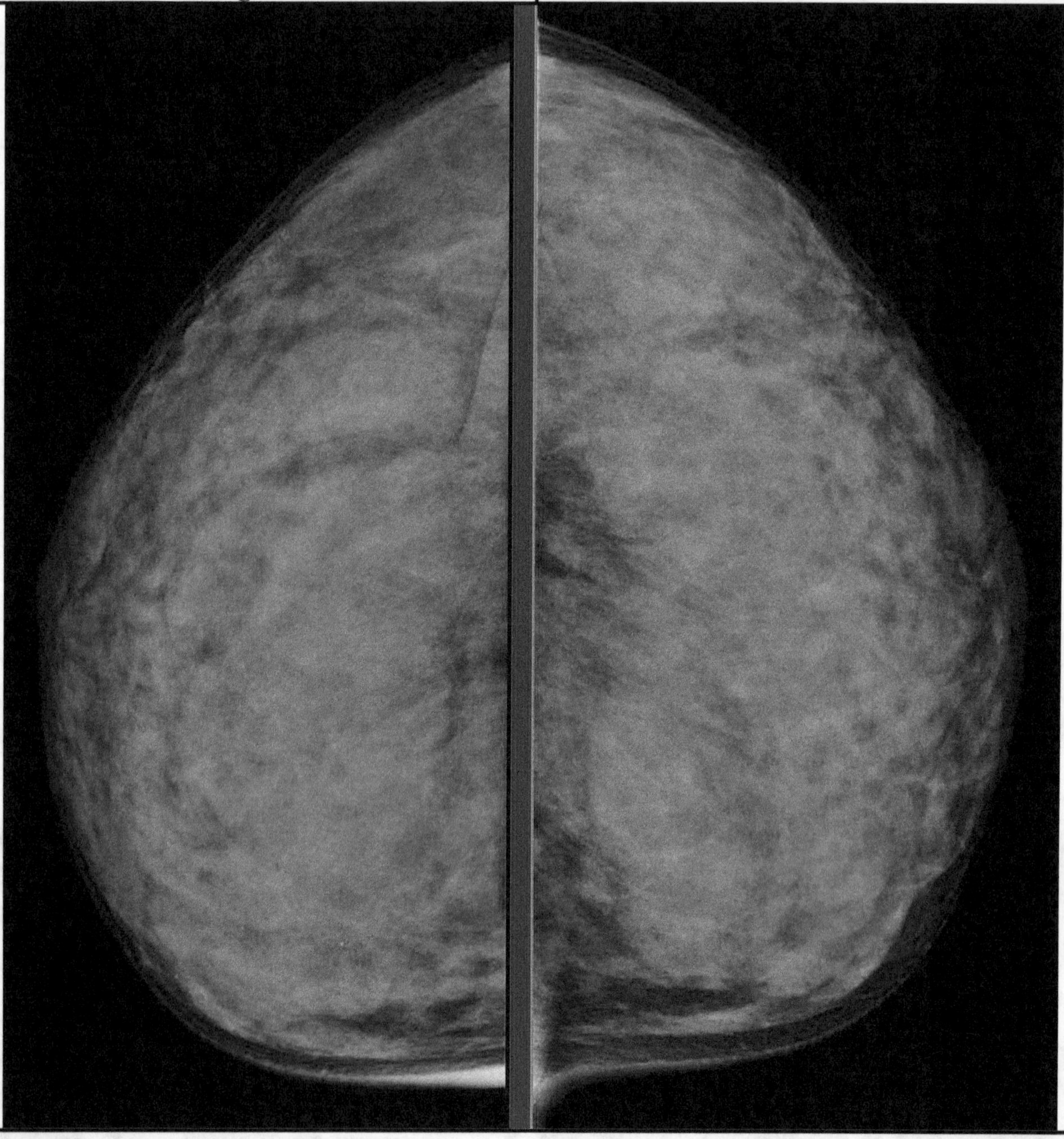

RIGHT BREAST	
Breast Parenchymal Density	*Extremely dense, which lowers the sensitivity of mammography (ACR D)*
Focal Mass	None
Asymmetric Density	None
Parenchymal Distortion	None
Calcification	None
Skin Thickening	None
Axillary Nodes	None

LEFT BREAST	
Breast Parenchymal Density	***Extremely dense, which lowers the sensitivity of mammography (ACR D)***
Focal Mass	None
Asymmetric Density	None
Parenchymal Distortion	None
Calcification	None
Skin Thickening	None
Axillary Nodes	None

IMPRESSION:

RIGHT BREAST: (BI-RADS 0)
LEFT BREAST: (BI-RADS 0)

RECOMMENDATION: US Correlation

CASE 11: 36-year-old female/screening

Right MLO	Left MLO

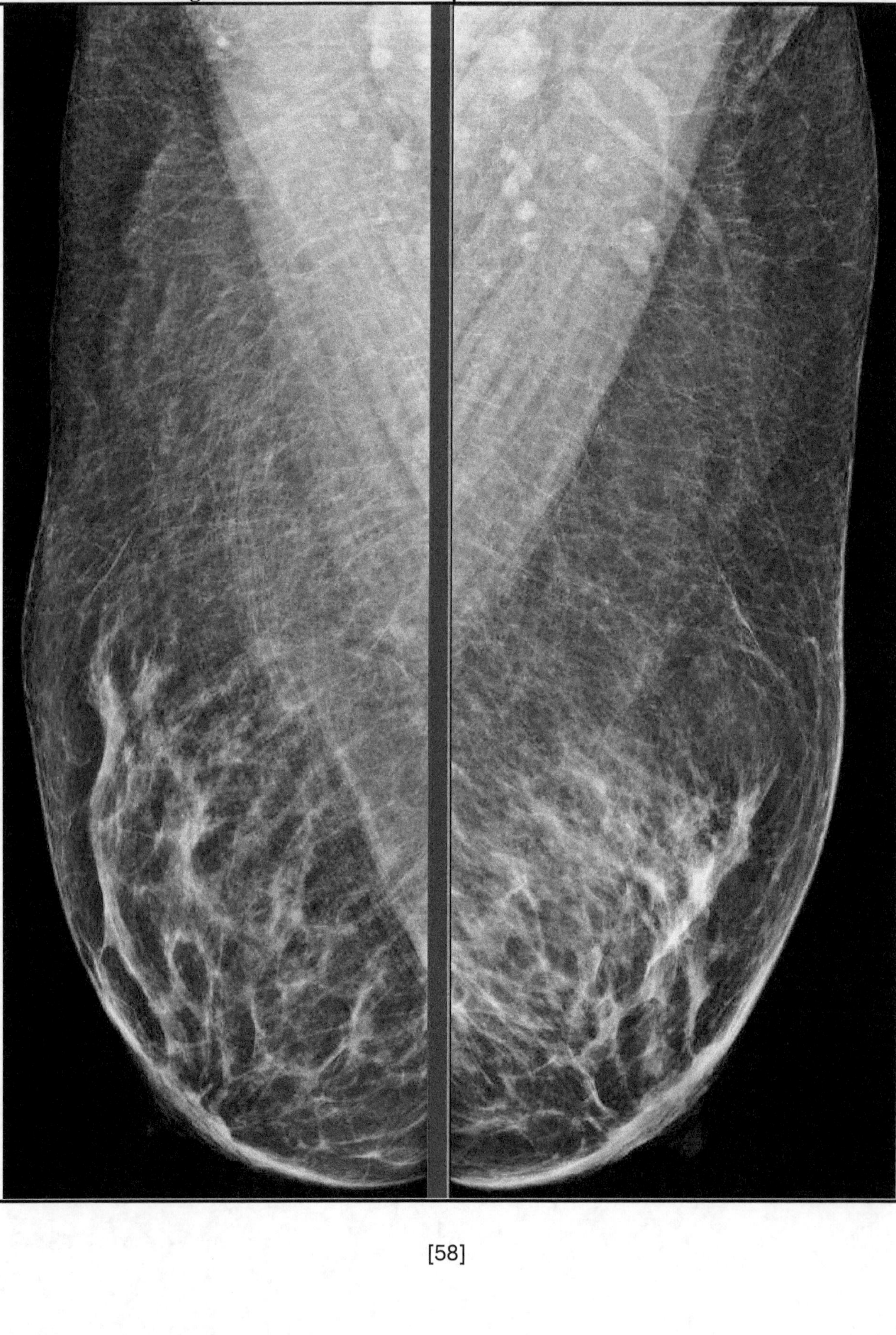

Right CC	Left CC

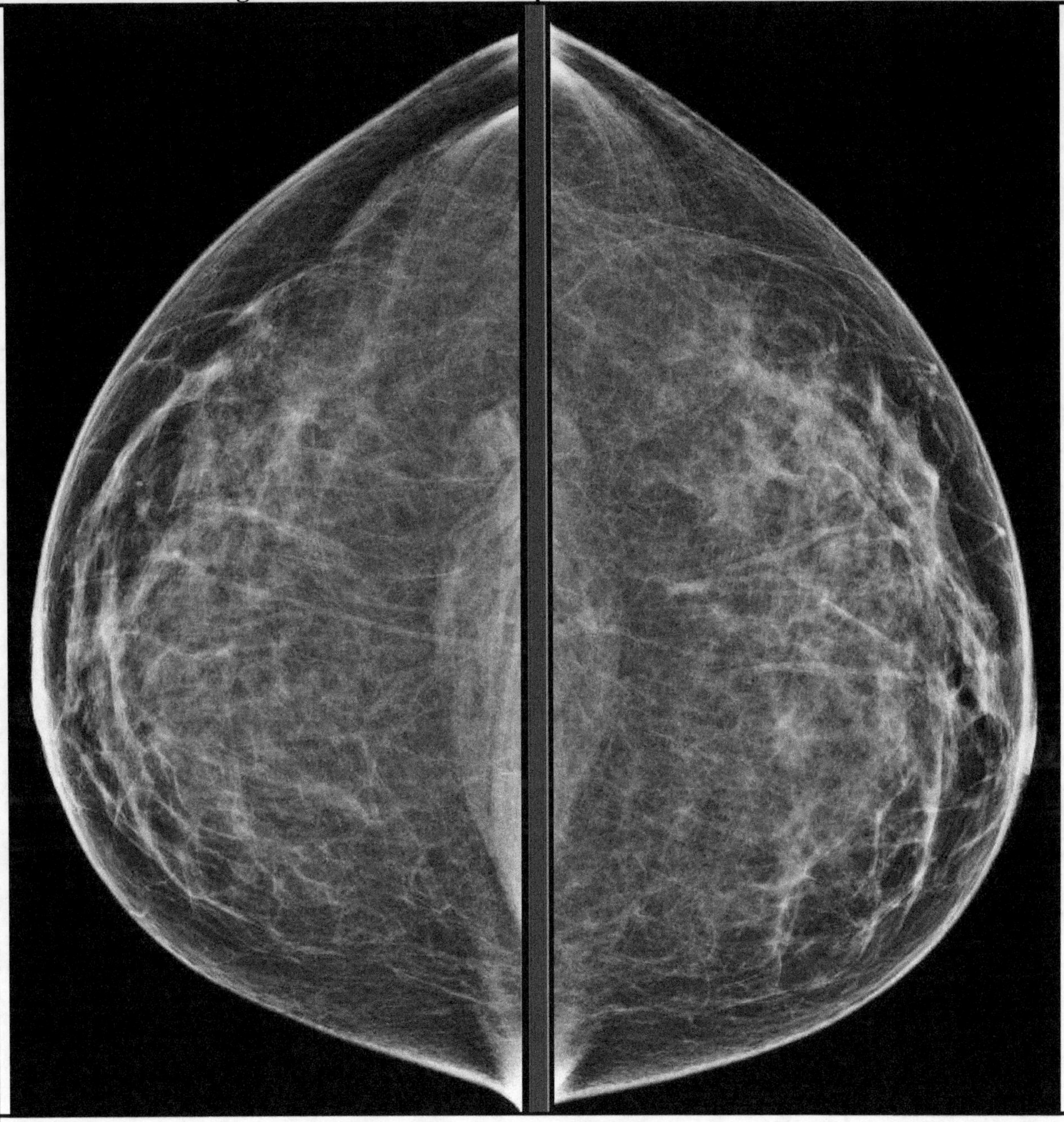

RIGHT BREAST	
Breast Parenchymal Density	***Scattered areas of fibroglandular density (ACR B)***
Focal Mass	None
Asymmetric Density	None
Parenchymal Distortion	None
Calcification	None
Skin Thickening	None
Axillary Nodes	None

LEFT BREAST	
Breast Parenchymal Density	***Scattered areas of fibroglandular density (ACR B)***
Focal Mass	None
Asymmetric Density	None
Parenchymal Distortion	None
Calcification	None
Skin Thickening	None
Axillary Nodes	None

IMPRESSION:

RIGHT BREAST: (BI-RADS 1)
LEFT BREAST: (BI-RADS 1)

RECOMMENDATION: Routine Annual screening

CASE 12: 44-year-old female/screening	
Right MLO	Left MLO

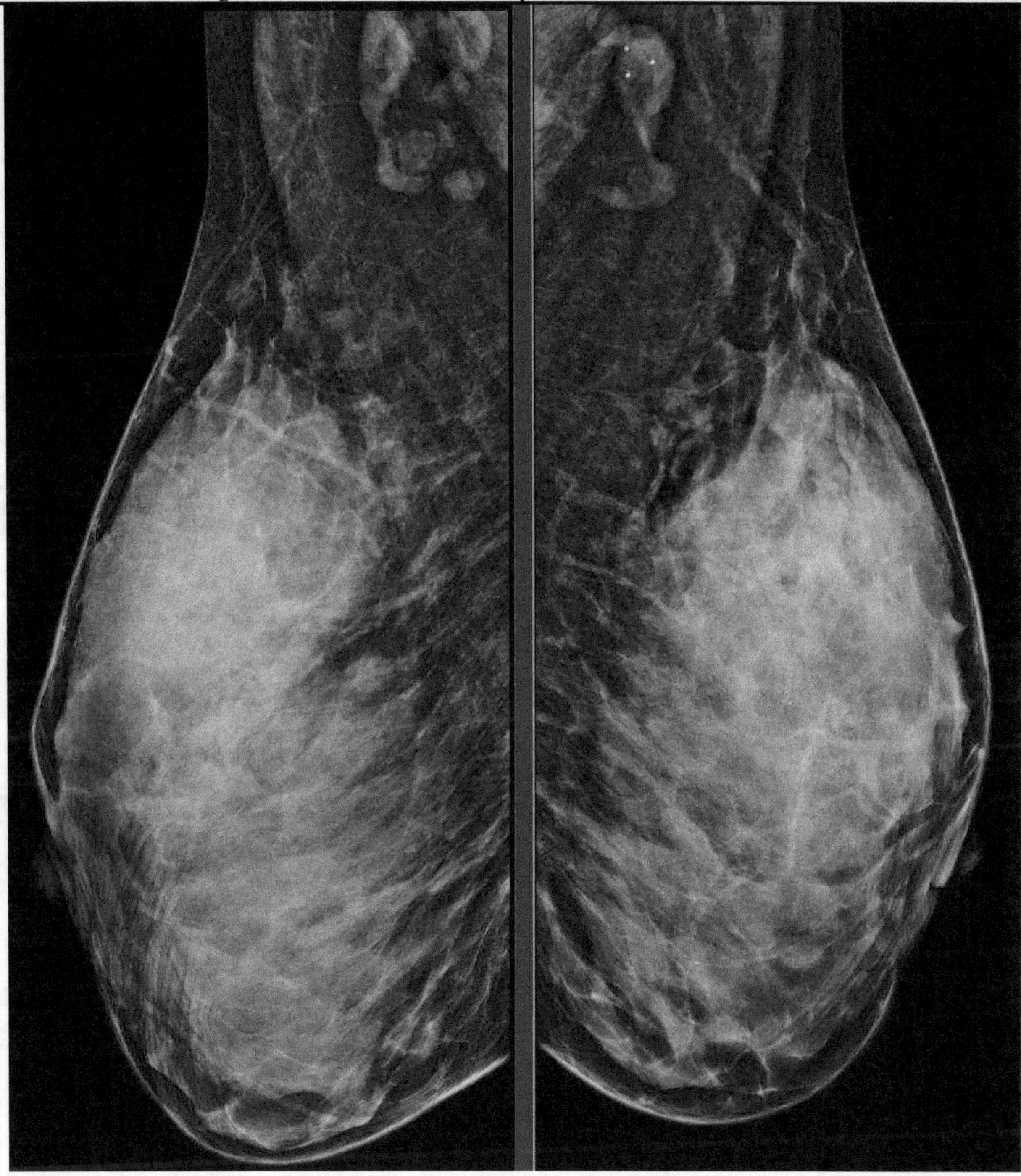

Right CC	Left CC

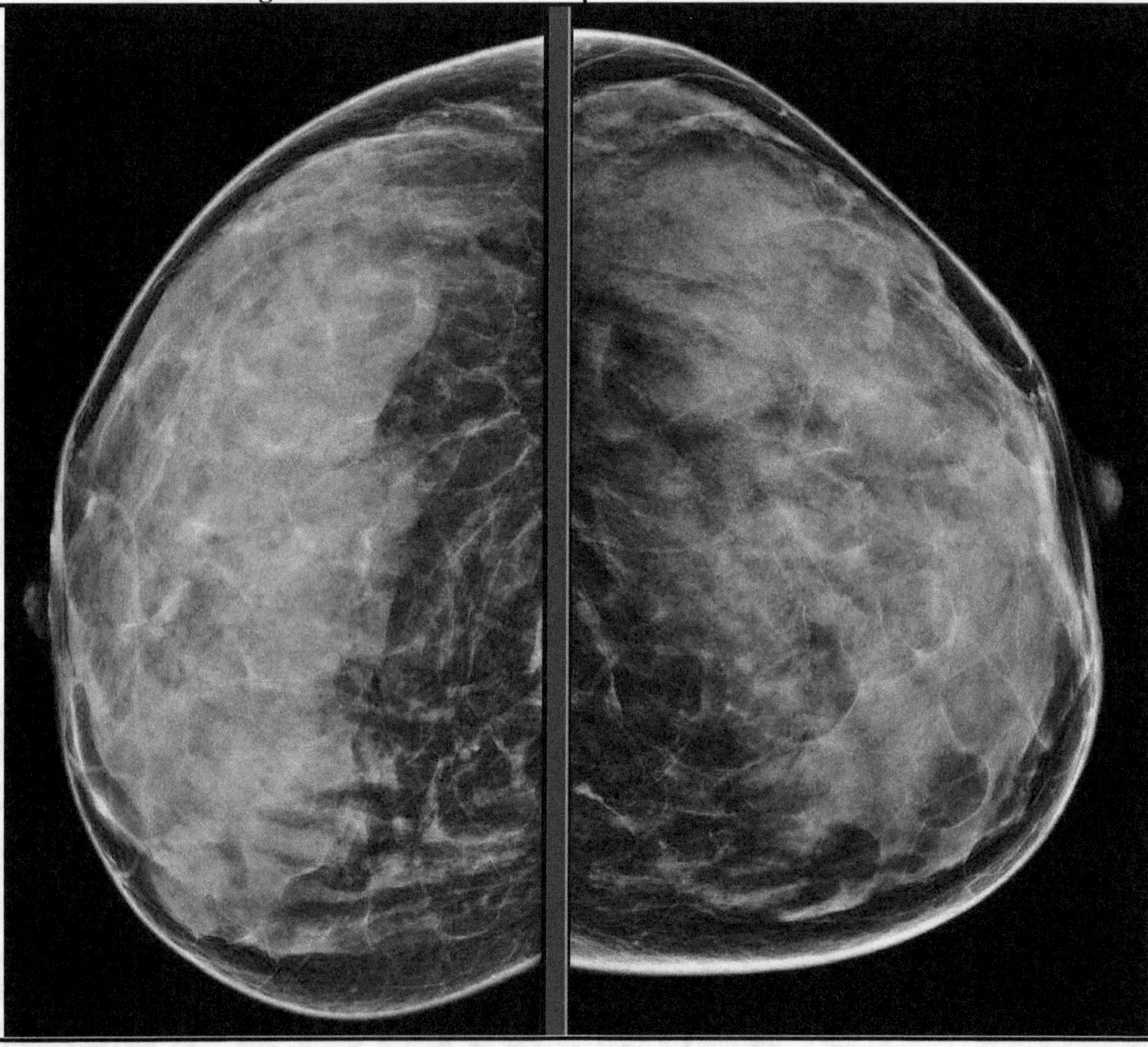

RIGHT BREAST	
Breast Parenchymal Density	***Extremely dense, which lowers the sensitivity of mammography (ACR D)***
Focal Mass	None
Asymmetric Density	None
Parenchymal Distortion	None
Calcification	None
Skin Thickening	None
Axillary Nodes	None

LEFT BREAST	
Breast Parenchymal Density	***Extremely dense, which lowers the sensitivity of mammography (ACR D)***
Focal Mass	None
Asymmetric Density	None
Parenchymal Distortion	None
Calcification	None
Skin Thickening	None
Axillary Nodes	None

IMPRESSION:

RIGHT BREAST: (BI-RADS 0)
LEFT BREAST: (BI-RADS 0)

RECOMMENDATION: US Correlation

CASE 13: 40-year-old female/screening

Right MLO	Left MLO

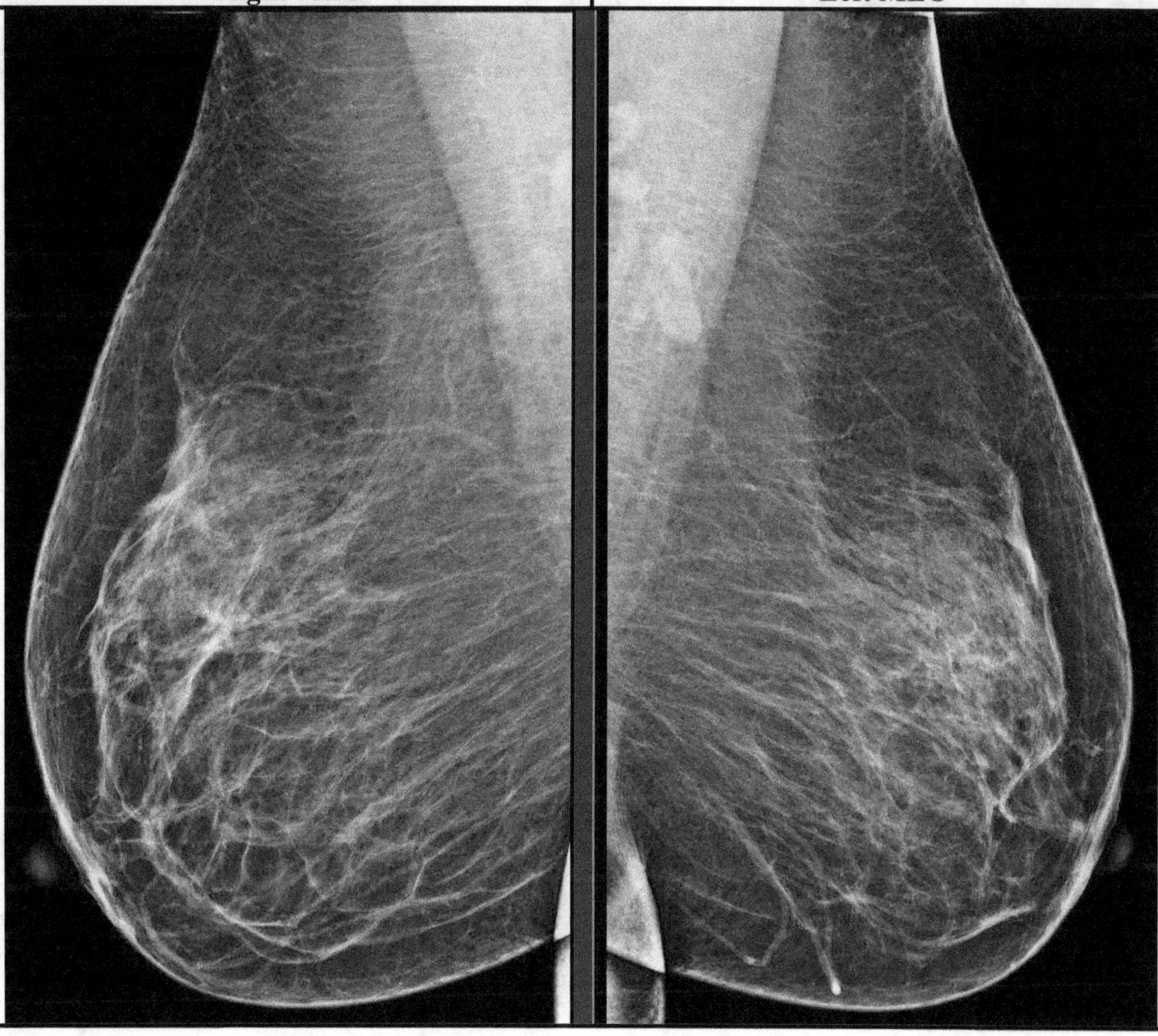

Right CC	Left CC

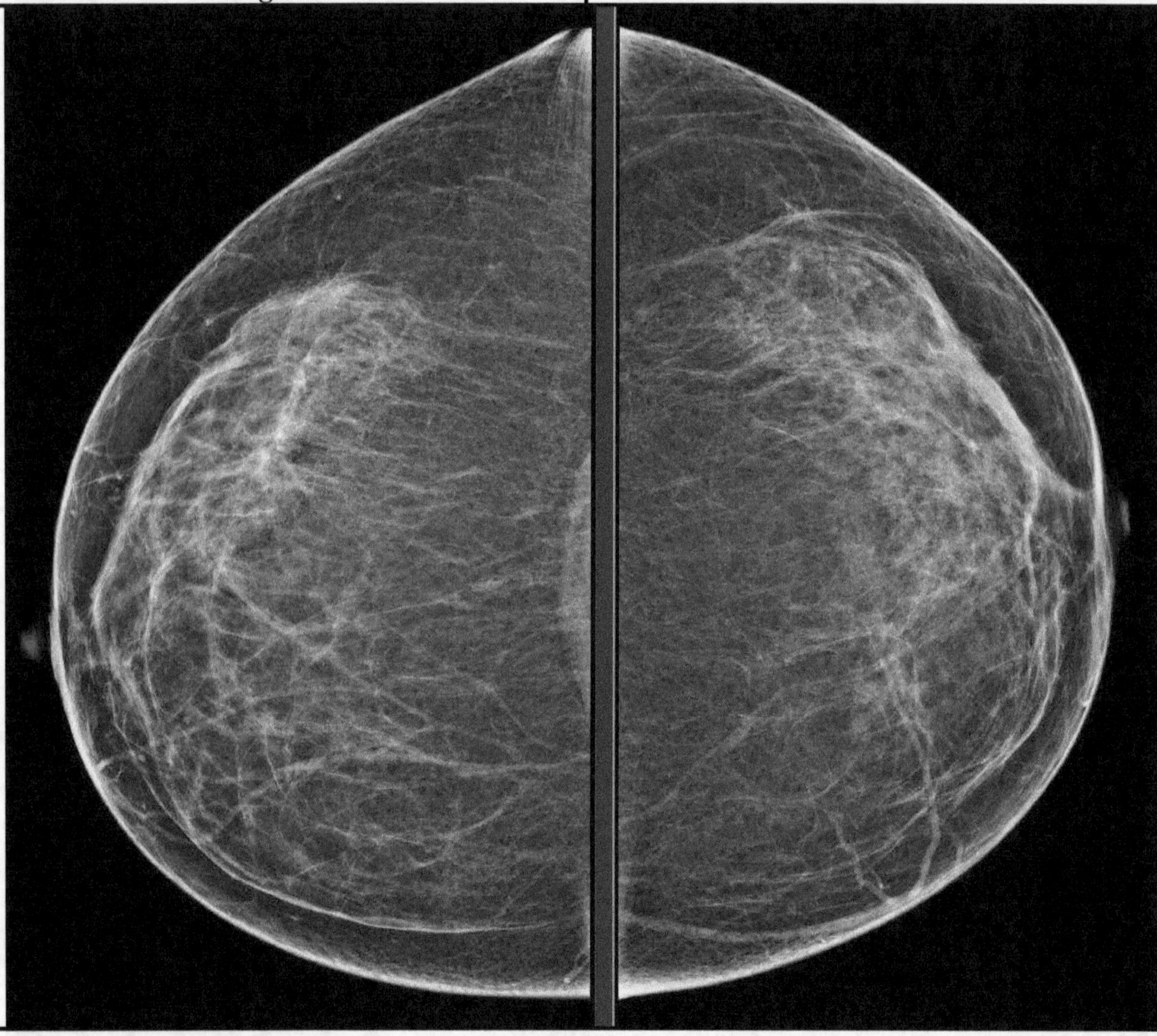

RIGHT BREAST	
Breast Parenchymal Density	***Scattered areas of fibroglandular density (ACR B)***
Focal Mass	None
Asymmetric Density	None
Parenchymal Distortion	None
Calcification	None
Skin Thickening	None
Axillary Nodes	None

LEFT BREAST	
Breast Parenchymal Density	***Scattered areas of fibroglandular density (ACR B)***
Focal Mass	None
Asymmetric Density	None
Parenchymal Distortion	None
Calcification	None
Skin Thickening	None
Axillary Nodes	None

IMPRESSION:

RIGHT BREAST: (BI-RADS 1)
LEFT BREAST: (BI-RADS 1)

RECOMMENDATION: Routine Annual screening

CASE 14: 38-year-old female/Diagnostic (=COME WITH SYMPTOMS LIKE LUMP /PAIN/ etc.…)

Right MLO	Left MLO

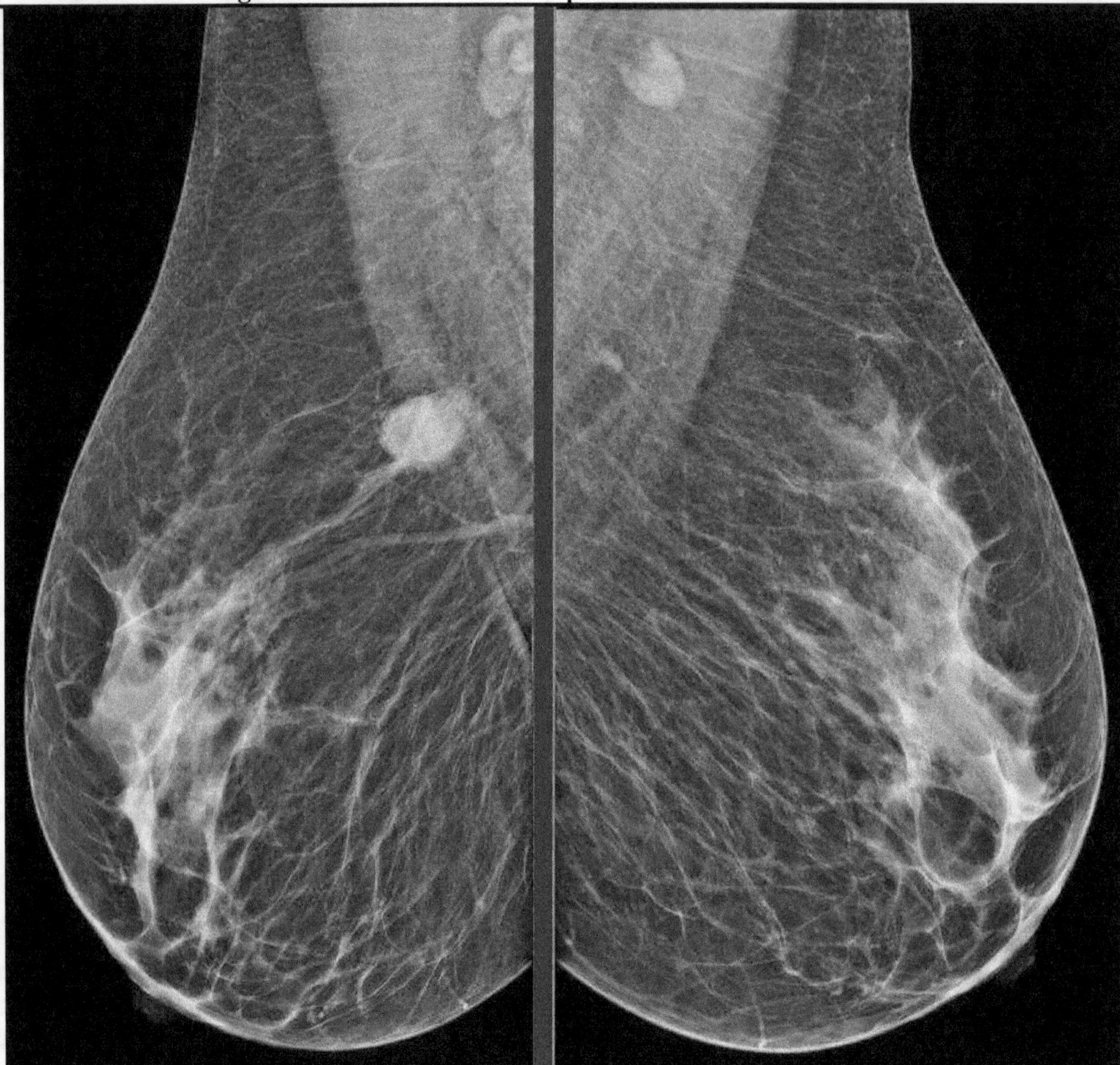

Right CC	Left CC

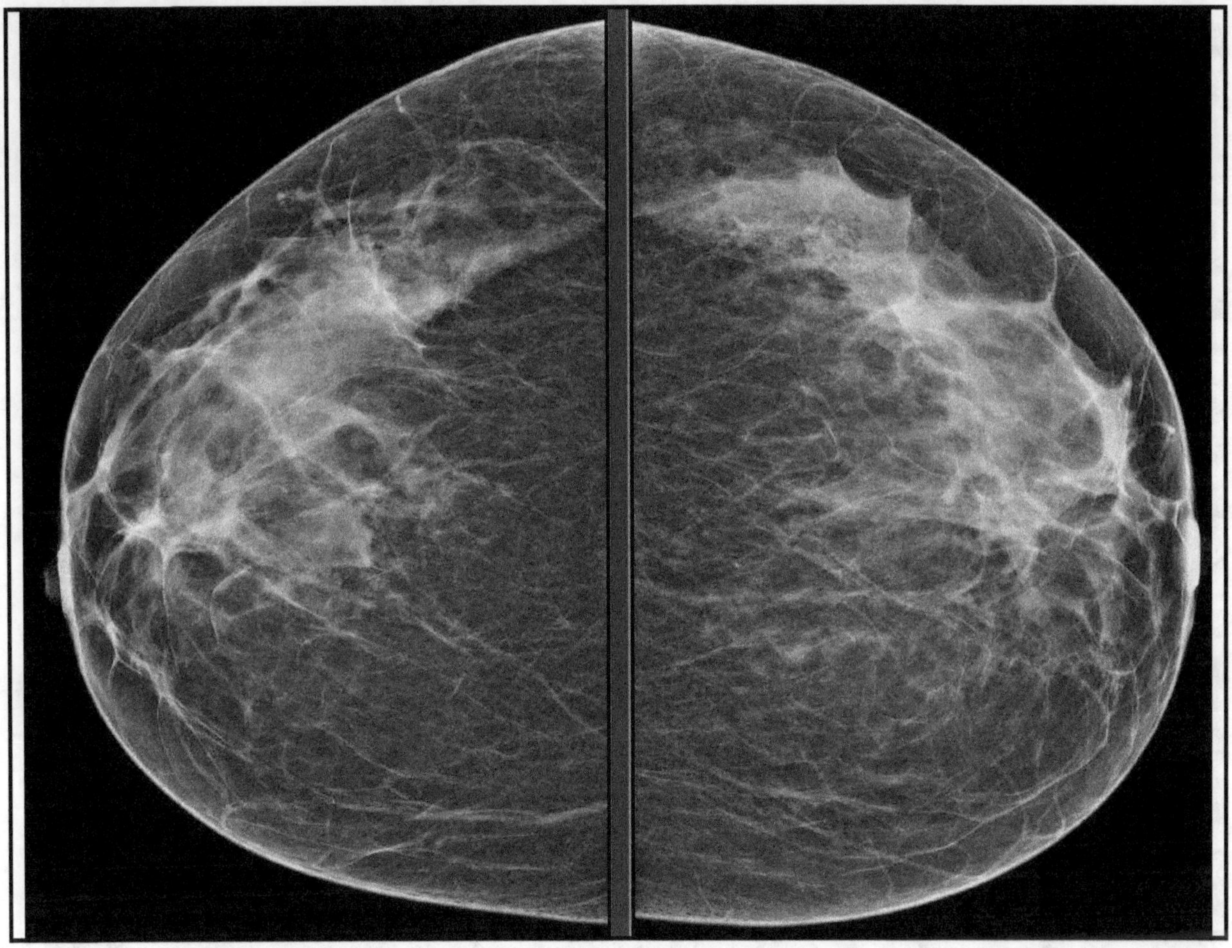

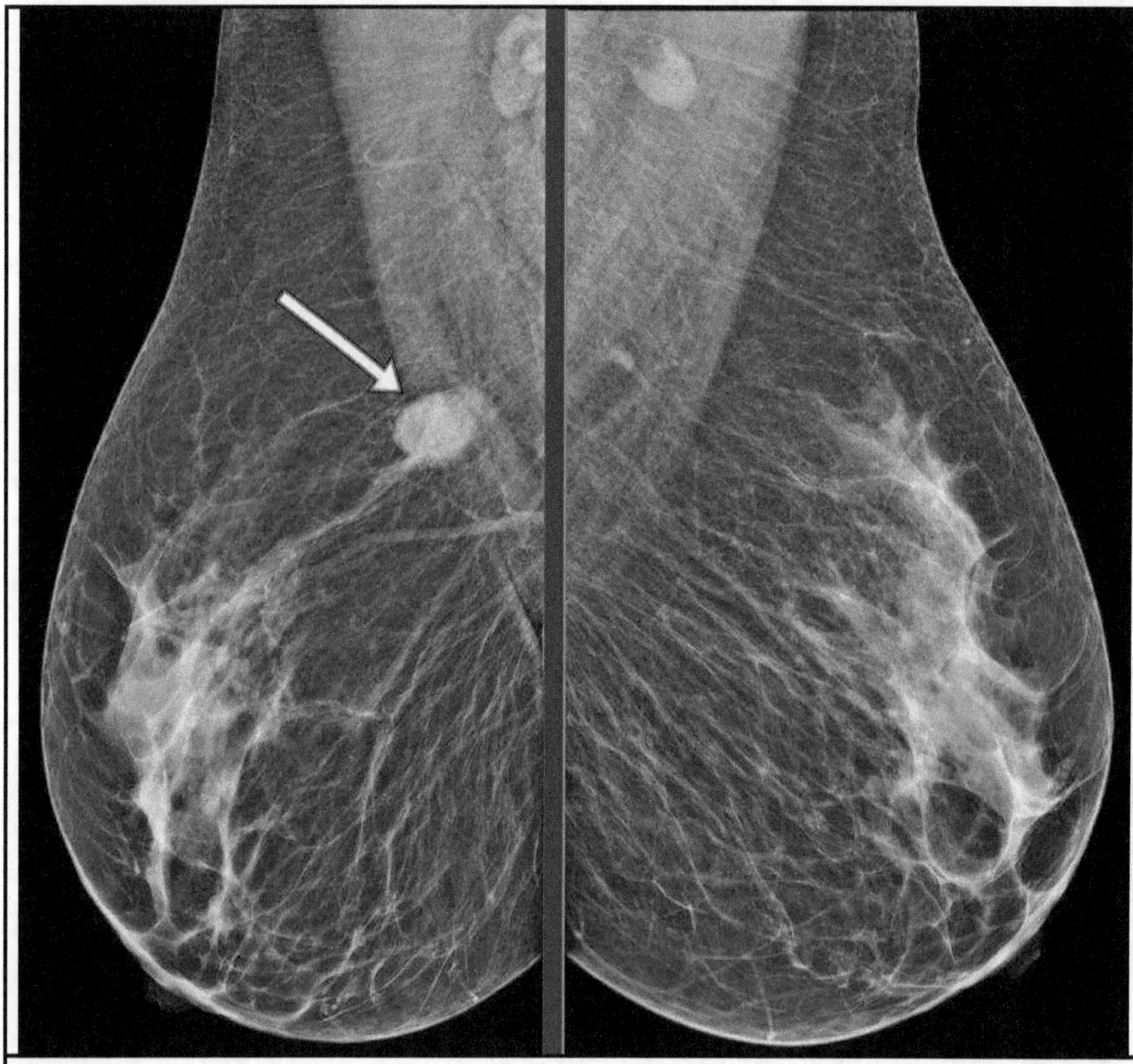

RIGHT BREAST	
Breast Parenchymal Density	***Heterogeneously dense, may obscure small masses (ACR C)***
Focal Mass	***UOQ Circumscribed Mass of equal-Density Measures (X)***
Asymmetric Density	None
Parenchymal Distortion	None
Calcification	None
Skin Thickening	None
Axillary Nodes	None

LEFT BREAST	
Breast Parenchymal Density	***Heterogeneously dense, may obscure small masses (ACR C)***
Focal Mass	None
Asymmetric Density	None
Parenchymal Distortion	None
Calcification	None
Skin Thickening	None
Axillary Nodes	None

IMPRESSION:

RIGHT BREAST: (BI-RADS 0)
LEFT BREAST: (BI-RADS 1)

RECOMMENDATION: US Correlation

CASE 15: 39-year-old female/screening

Right MLO	Left MLO
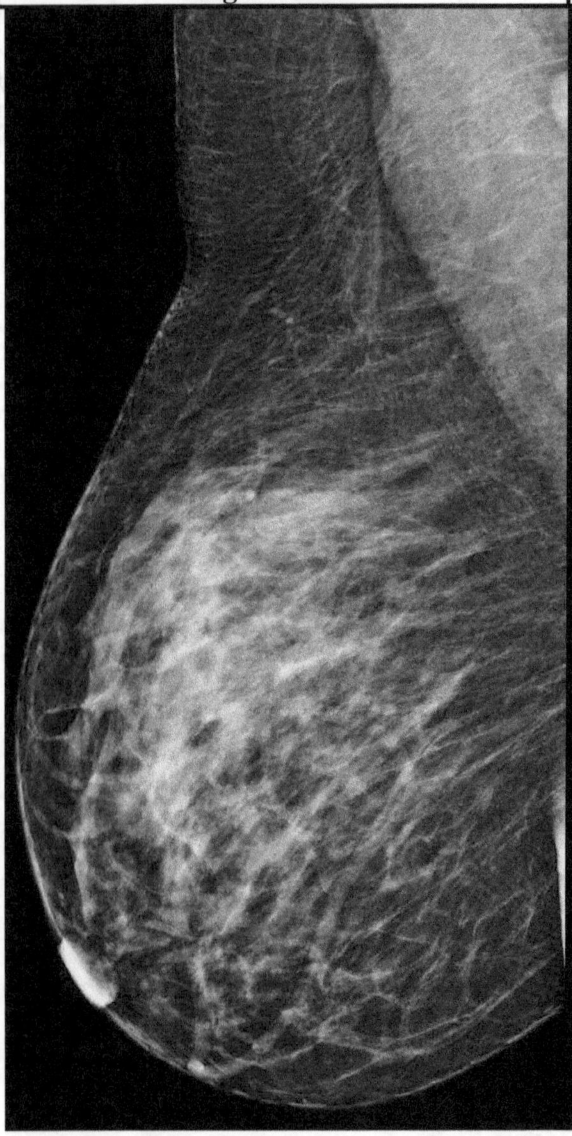	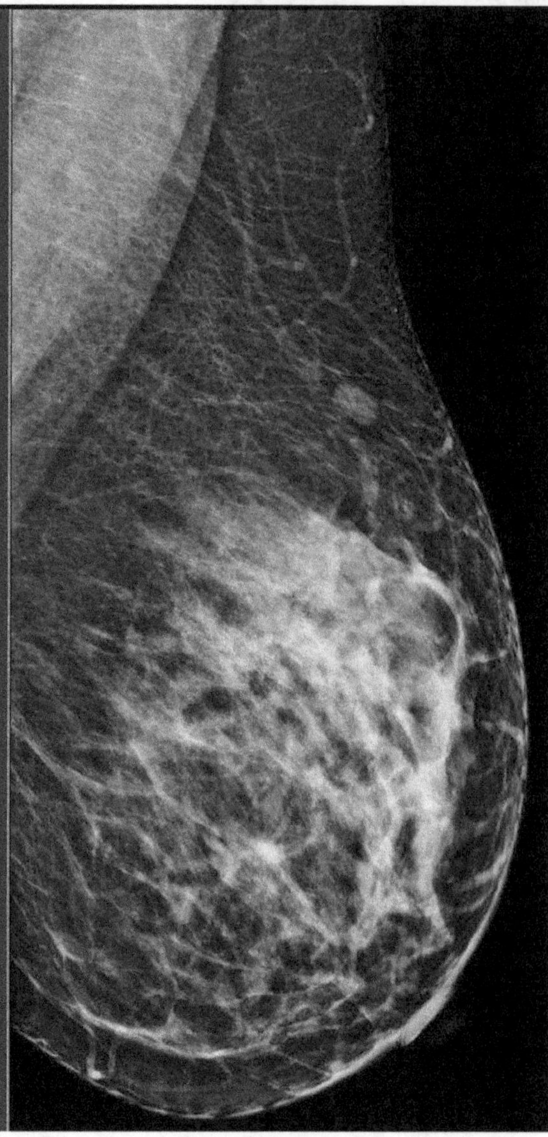

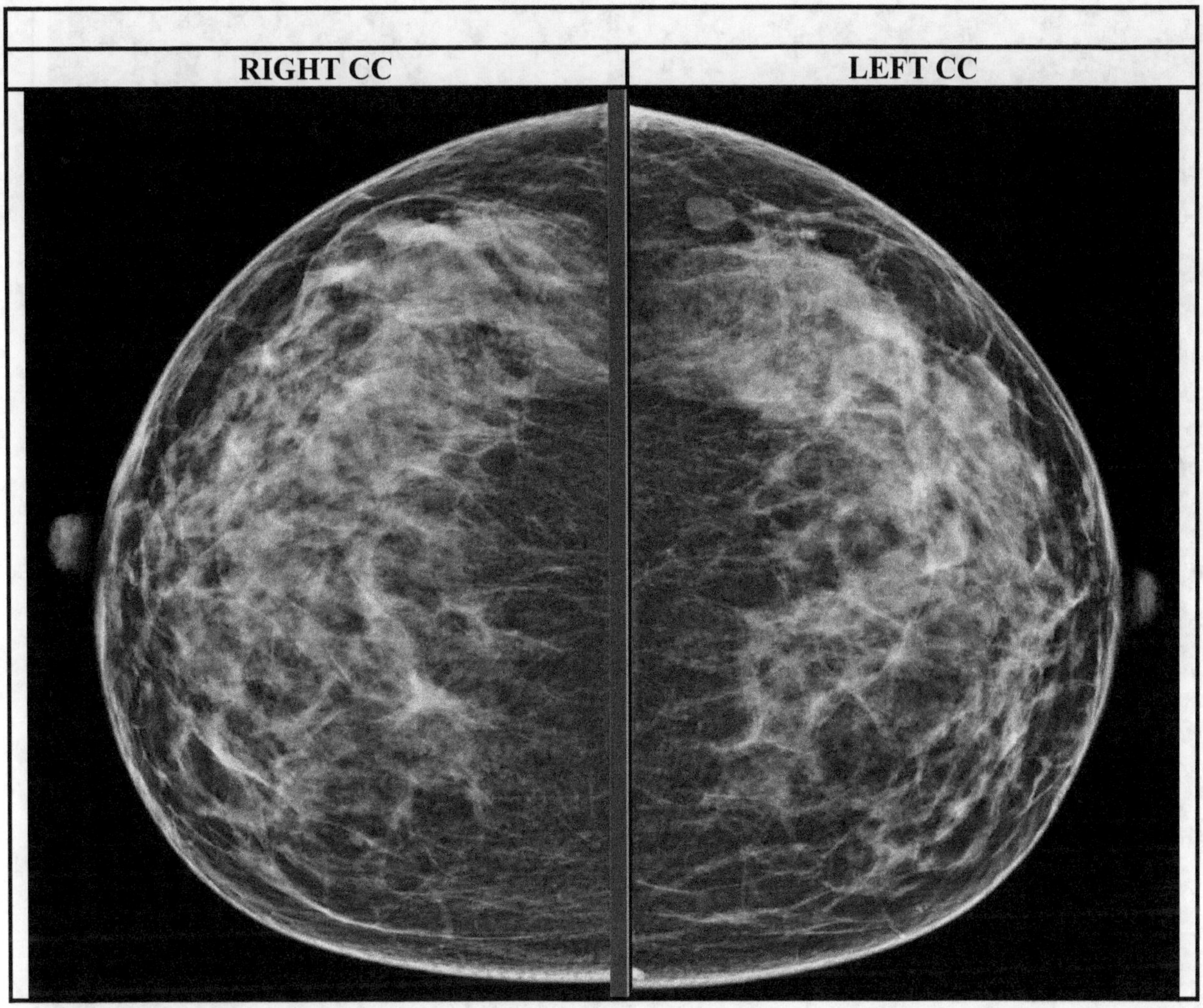
RIGHT CC
LEFT CC

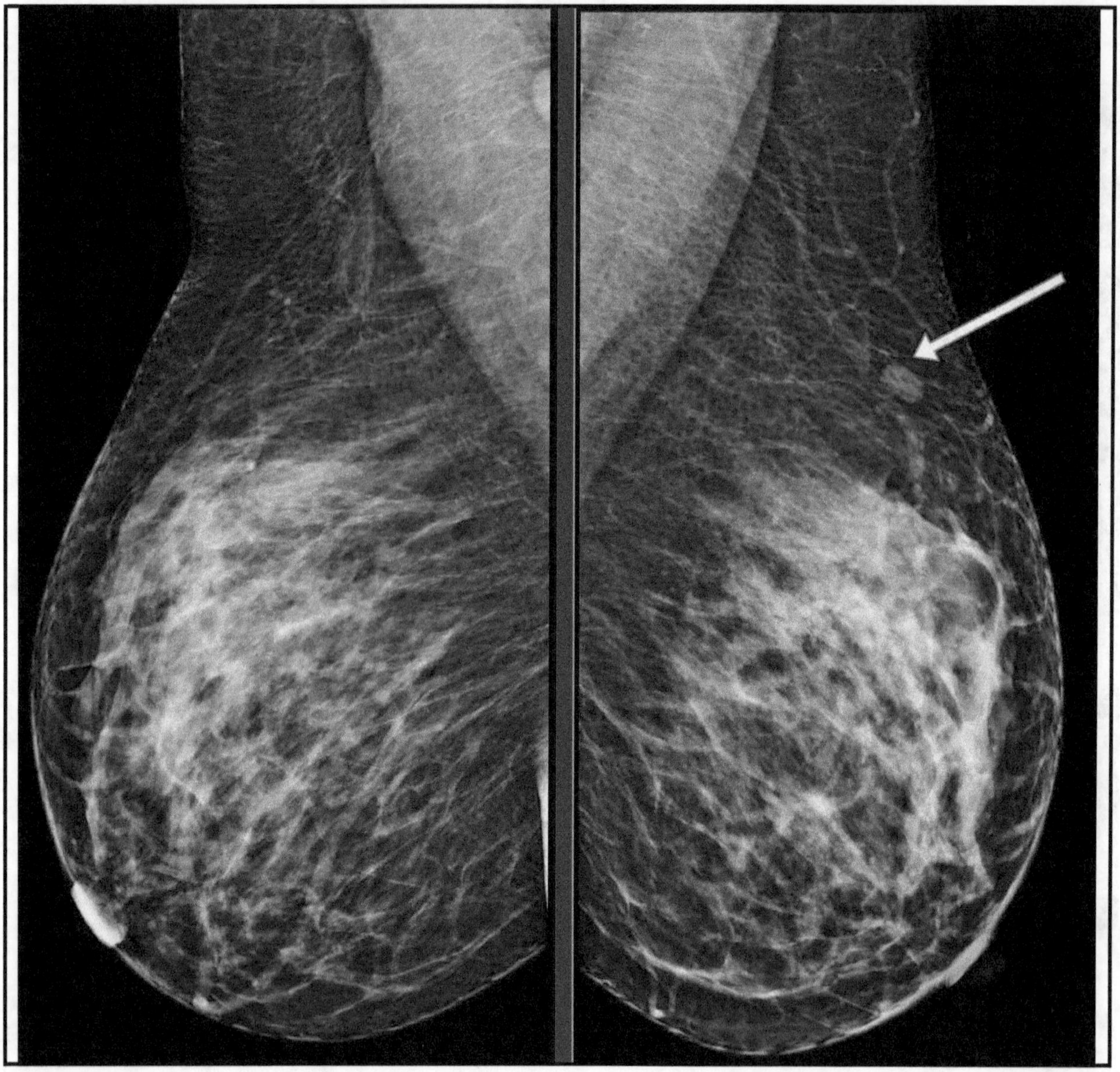

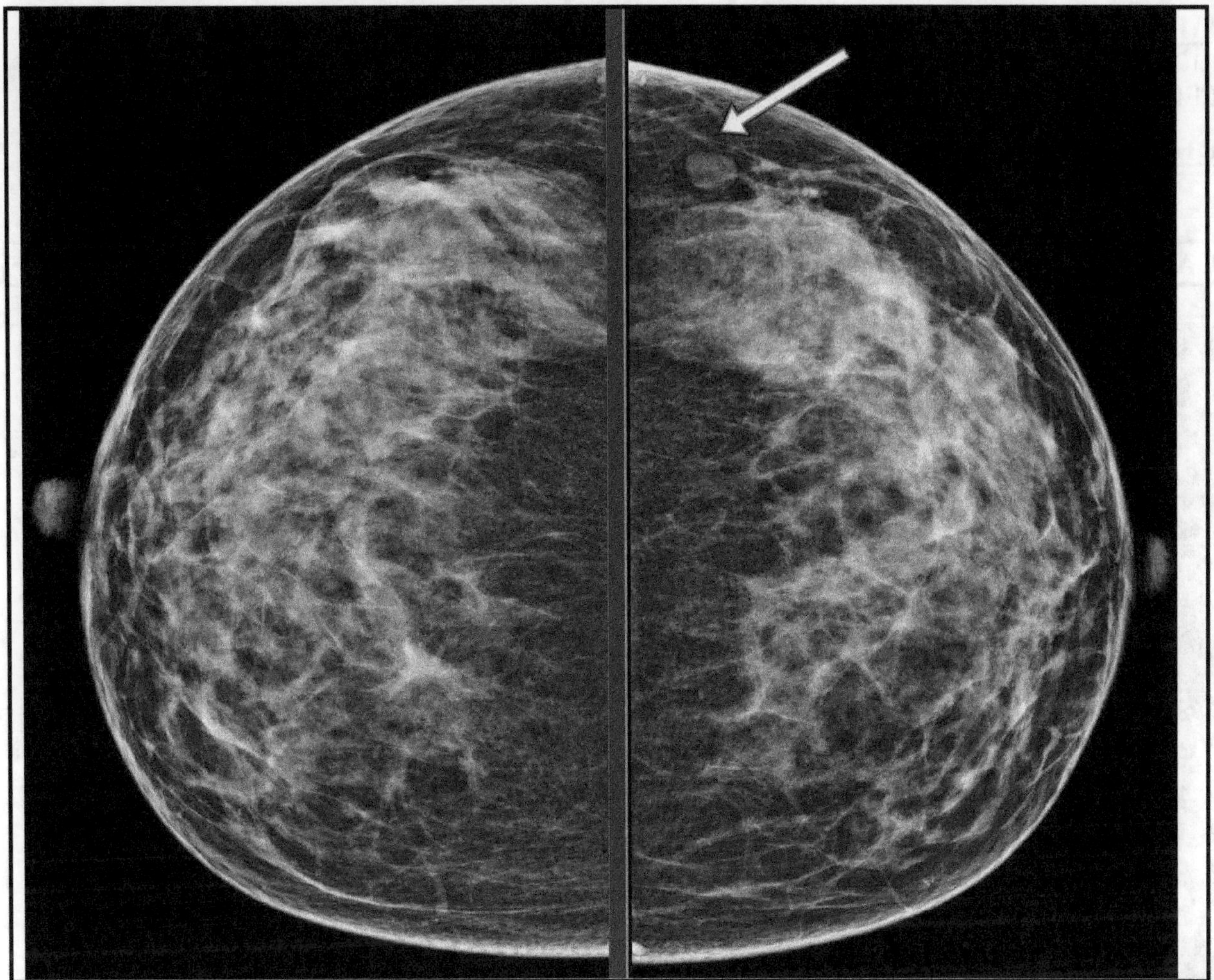

RIGHT BREAST	
Breast Parenchymal Density	***Heterogeneously dense, may obscure small masses (ACR C)***
Focal Mass	None
Asymmetric Density	None
Parenchymal Distortion	None
Calcification	None
Skin Thickening	None
Axillary Nodes	None

LEFT BREAST	
Breast Parenchymal Density	***Heterogeneously dense, may obscure small masses (ACR C)***
Focal Mass	None
Asymmetric Density	None
Parenchymal Distortion	None
Calcification	None
Skin Thickening	None
Axillary Nodes	None **N.B.** ***UOQ intramammary lymph node (IMLN)***

IMPRESSION:
RIGHT BREAST: (BI-RADS 1)
LEFT BREAST: (BI-RADS 1)

RECOMMENDATION: Routine Annual screening

CASE 16: 35-year-old female/Diagnostic

Right MLO	Left MLO

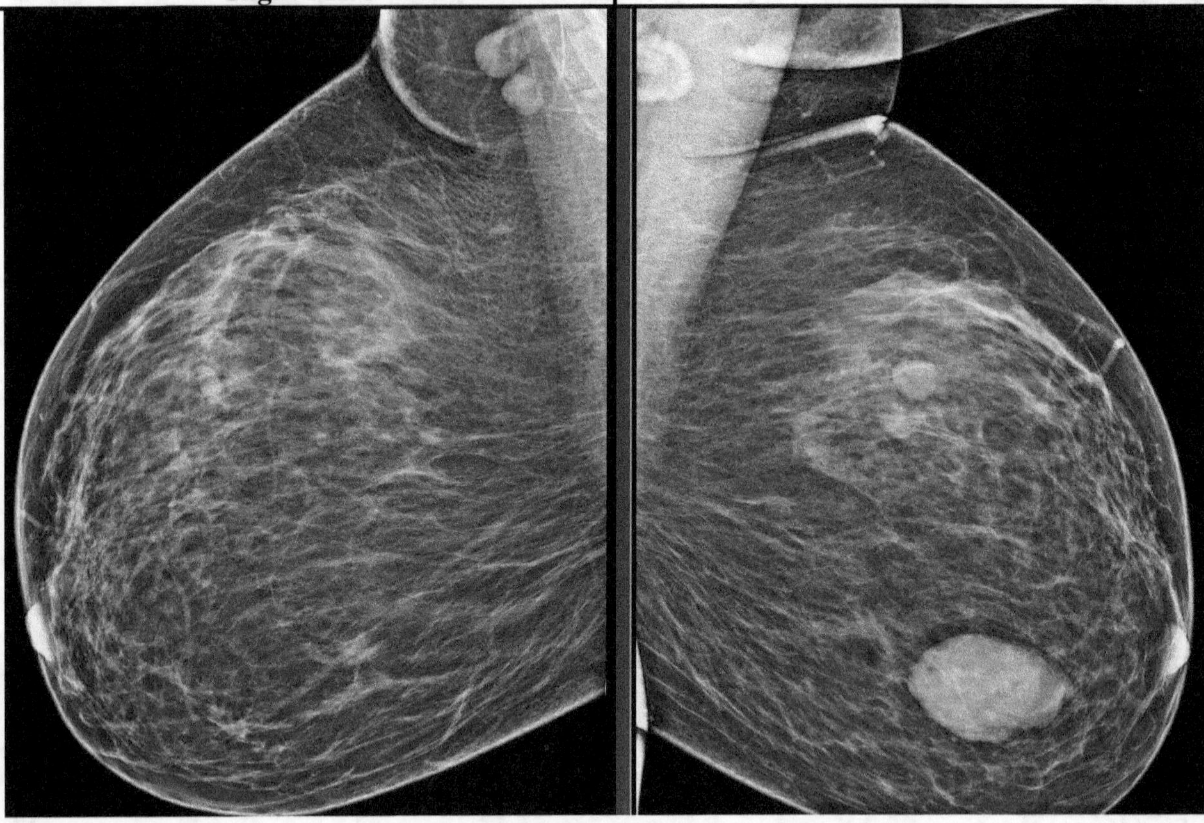

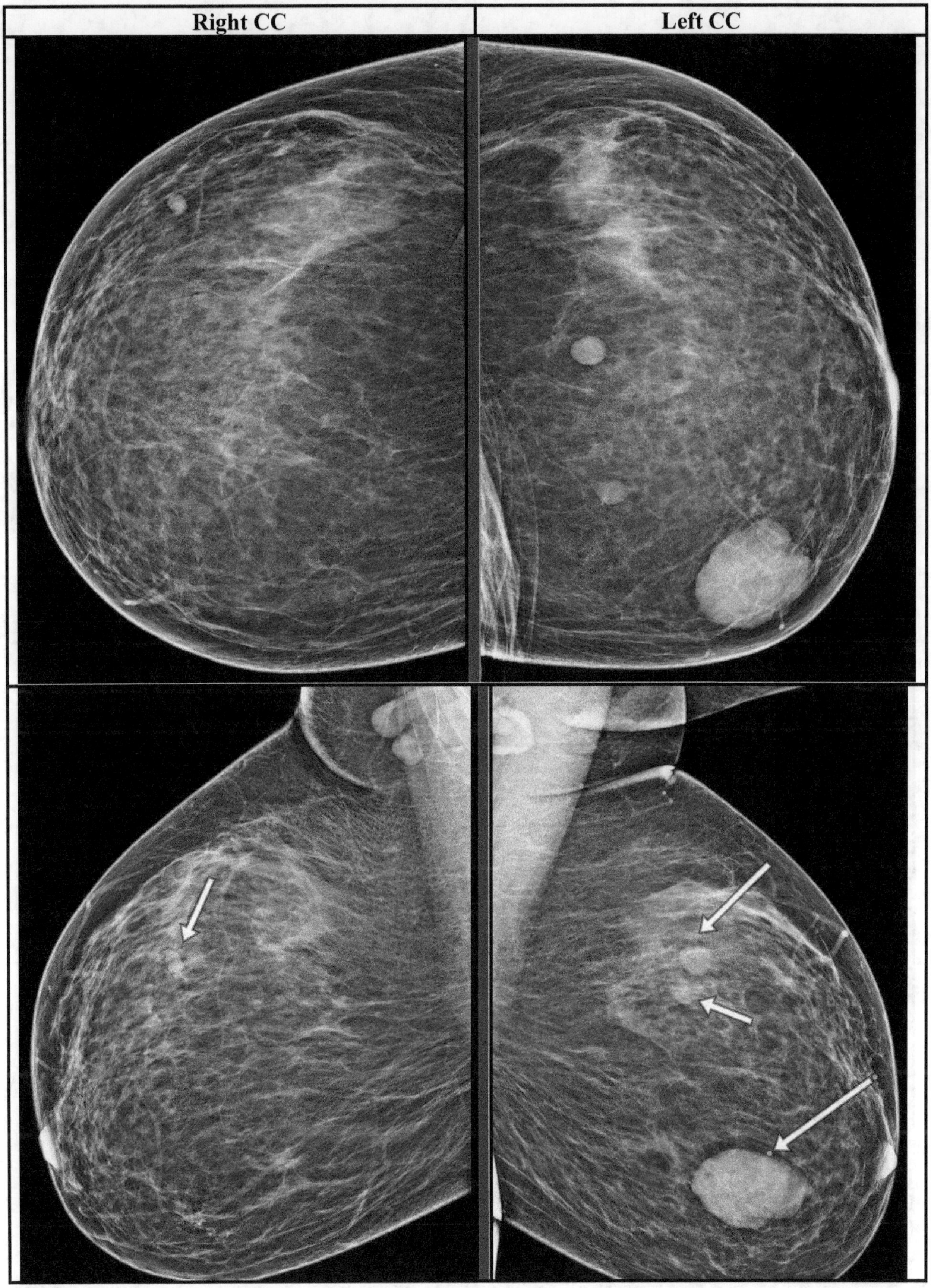
Right CC
Left CC

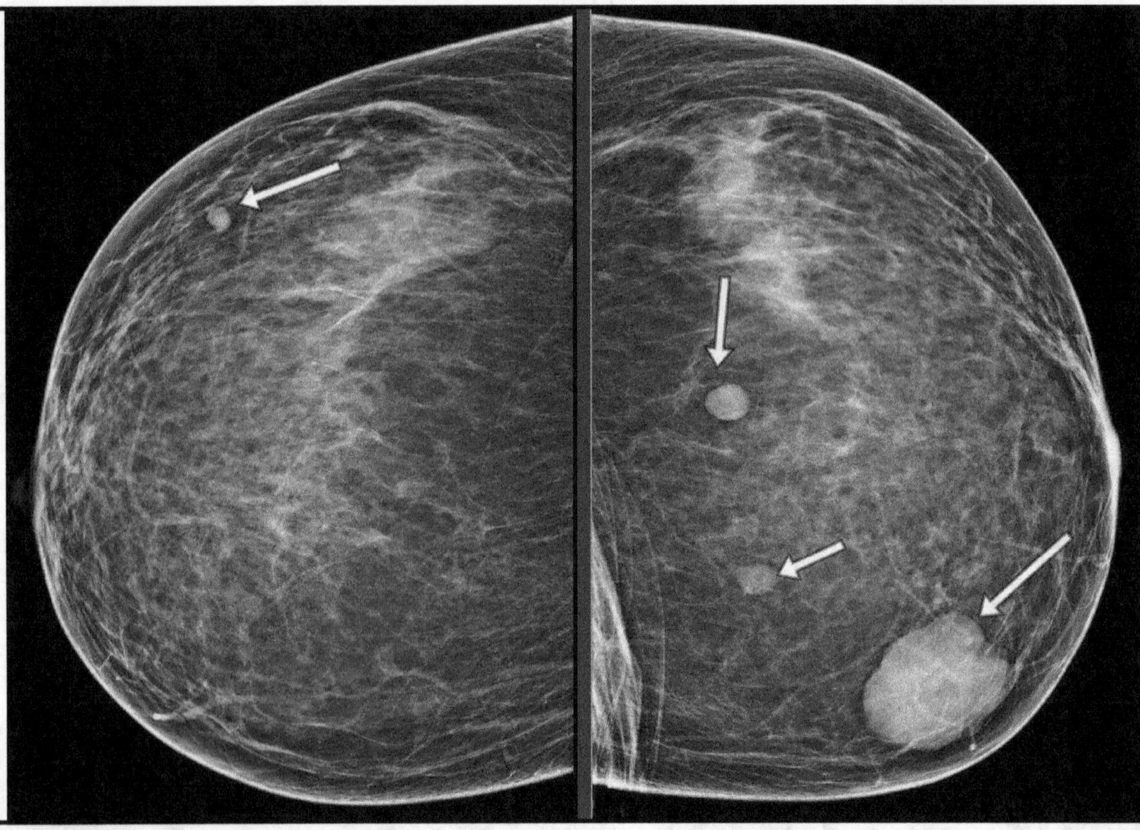

RIGHT BREAST	
Breast Parenchymal Density	***Scattered areas of fibroglandular density (ACR B)***
Focal Mass	None
Asymmetric Density	None
Parenchymal Distortion	None
Calcification	None
Skin Thickening	None
Axillary Nodes	None **IMLN**

LEFT BREAST	
Breast Parenchymal Density	***Scattered areas of fibroglandular density (ACR B)***
Focal Mass	***LIQ / Upper Central (12 O'clock) circumscribed mass lesions measures (x)***
Asymmetric Density	None
Parenchymal Distortion	None
Calcification	None
Skin Thickening	None
Axillary Nodes	None

IMPRESSION:
RIGHT BREAST: (BI-RADS 1)
LEFT BREAST: (BI-RADS 0)

RECOMMENDATION: US Correlation (***My Be Solid =Fibroadenoma Or Cystic***)

CASE 17: 54-year-old female/ Diagnostic	
Right MLO	**Left MLO**
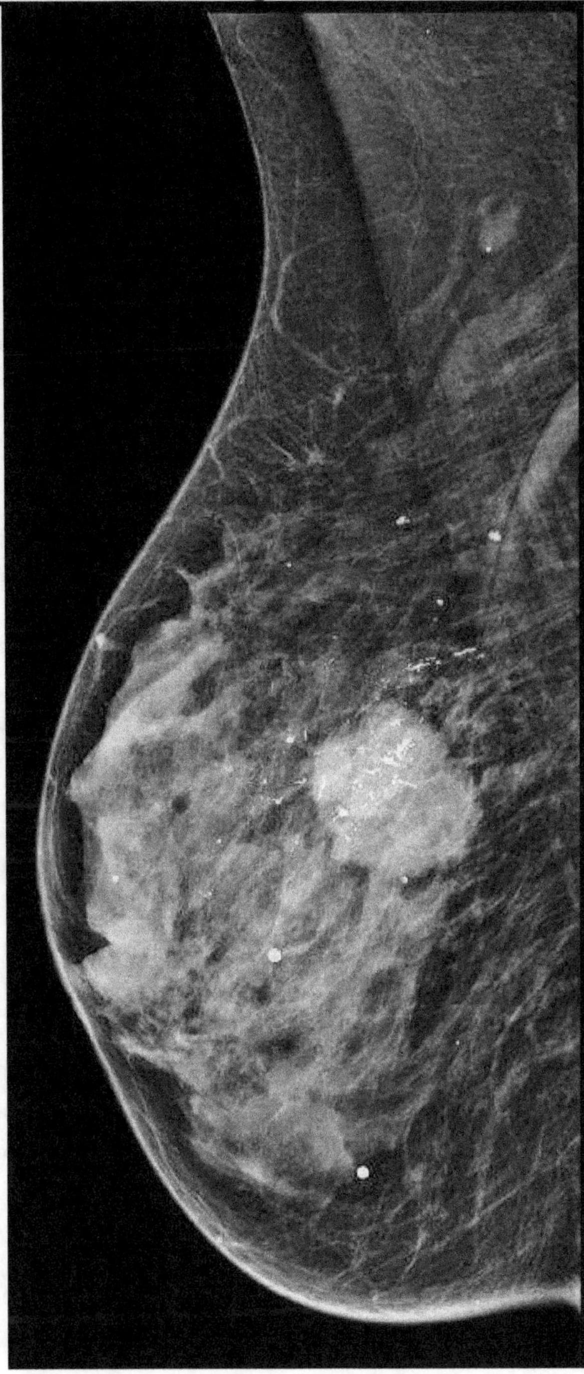	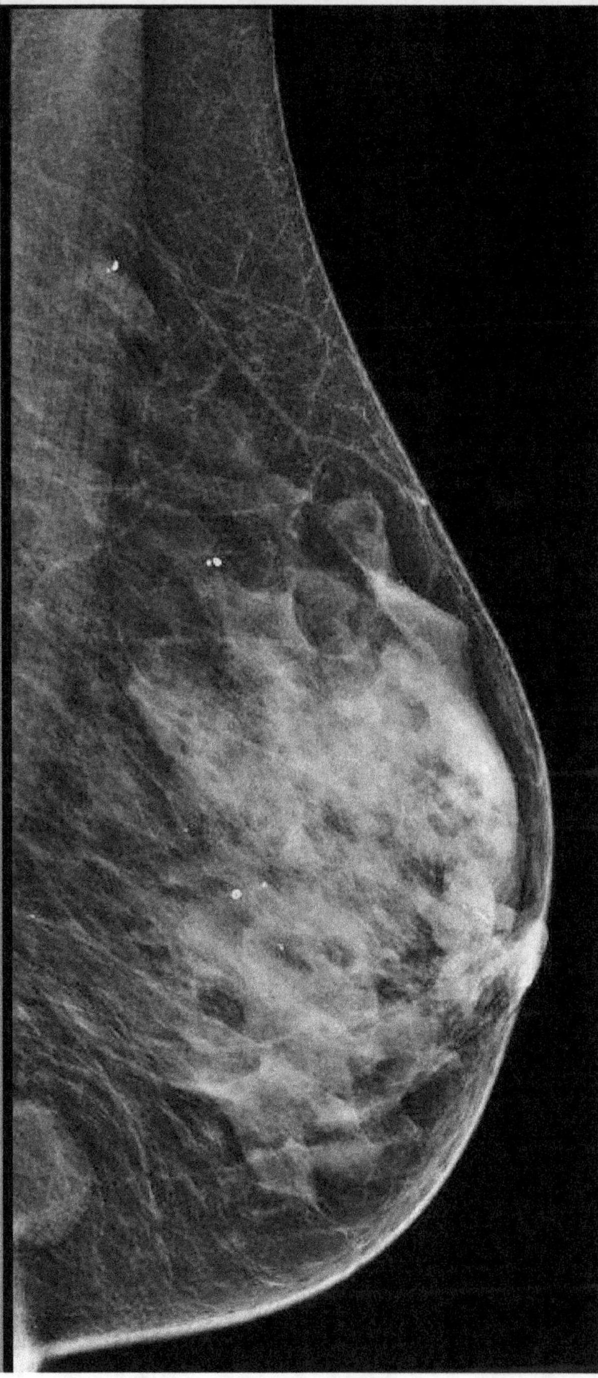

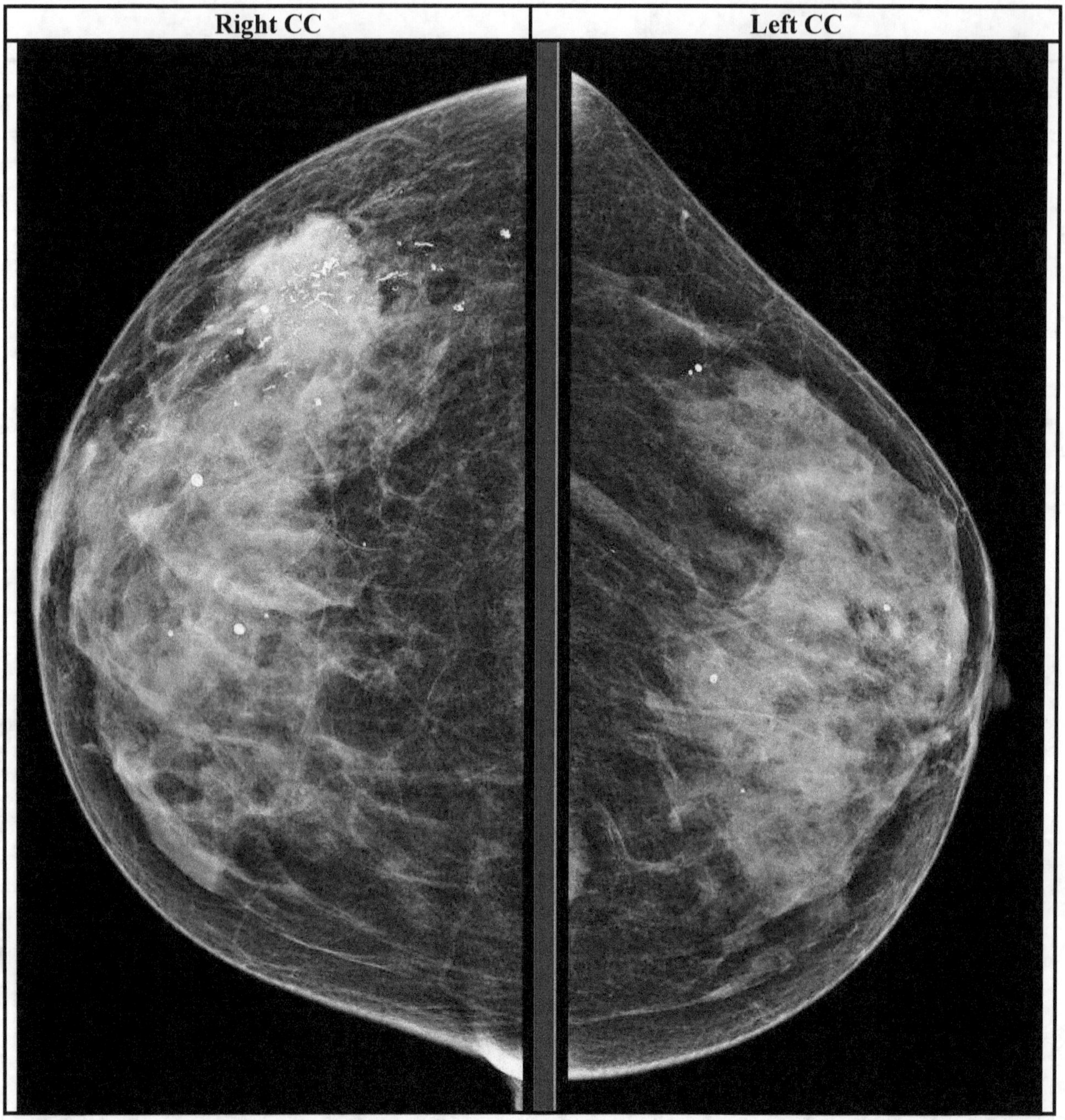
Right CC
Left CC

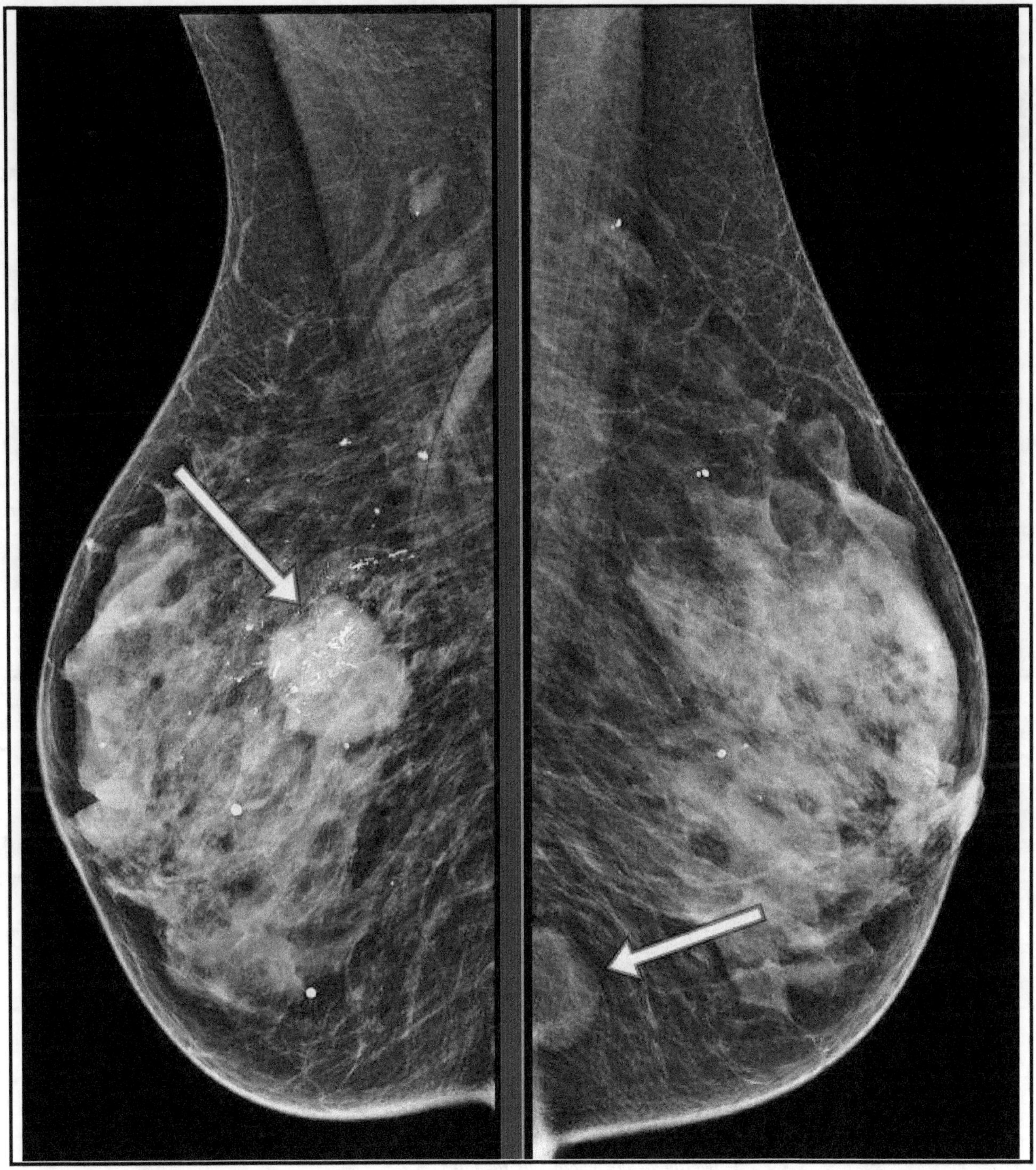

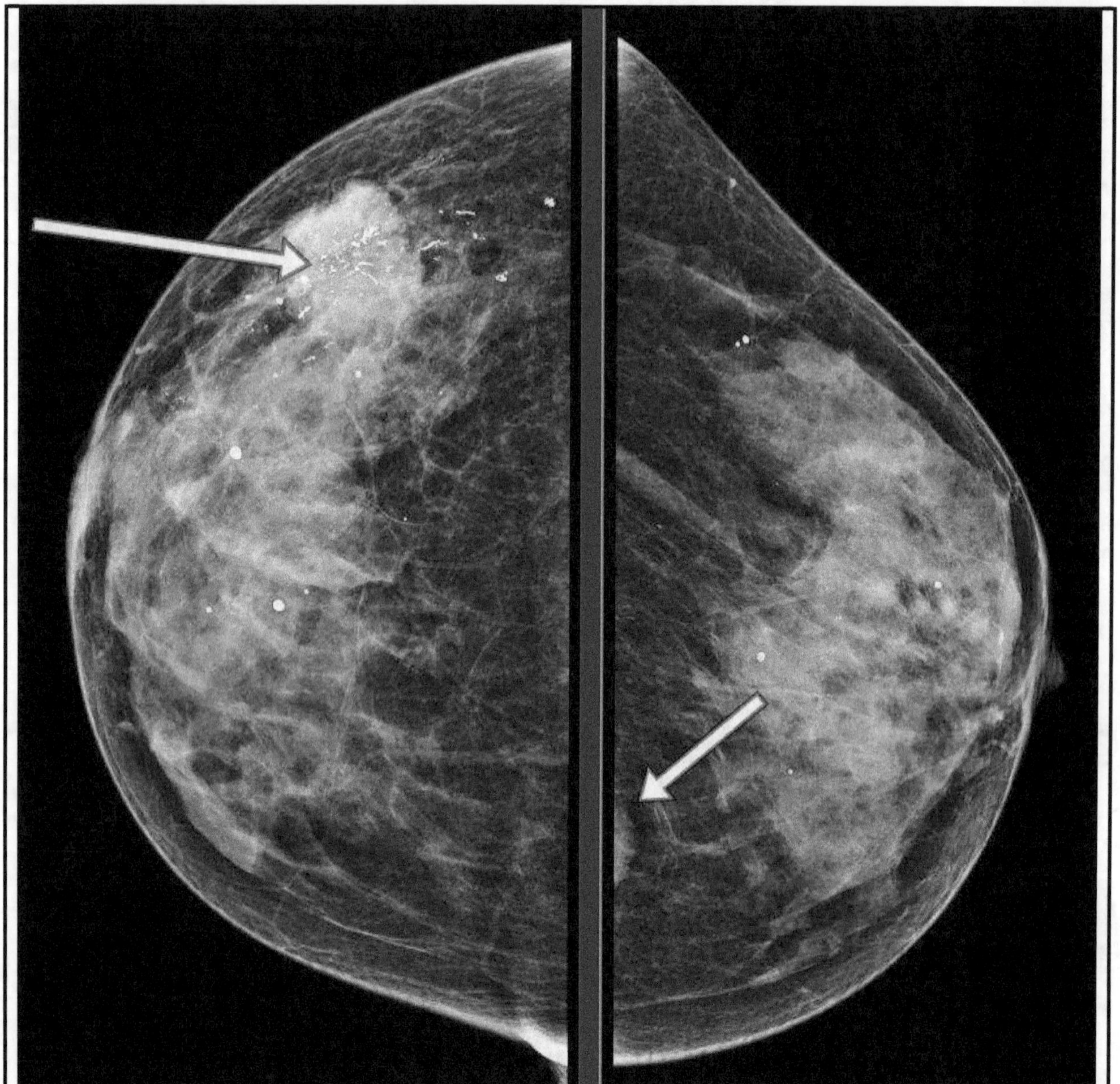

RIGHT BREAST	
Breast Parenchymal Density	***Heterogeneously dense, may obscure small masses (ACR C)***
Focal Mass	***UOQ Irregular lobulated mass lesion measures (x) associated with coarse heterogeneous micro-calcifications***
Asymmetric Density	None
Parenchymal Distortion	None
Calcification	***UOQ coarse heterogeneous micro-calcifications /benign skin calcifications***
Skin Thickening	None
Axillary Nodes	None

LEFT BREAST	
Breast Parenchymal Density	***Heterogeneously dense, may obscure small masses (ACR C)***
Focal Mass	***LIQ mass lesion measures (x)***
Asymmetric Density	None
Parenchymal Distortion	None
Calcification	***skin calcifications***
Skin Thickening	None
Axillary Nodes	None

IMPRESSION:

RIGHT BREAST: (BI-RADS 4C)
LEFT BREAST: (BI-RADS 0)

RECOMMENDATION: US Correlation/ Histopathological Correlation

CASE 18: 45-year-old female/ Diagnostic	
Right MLO	Left MLO

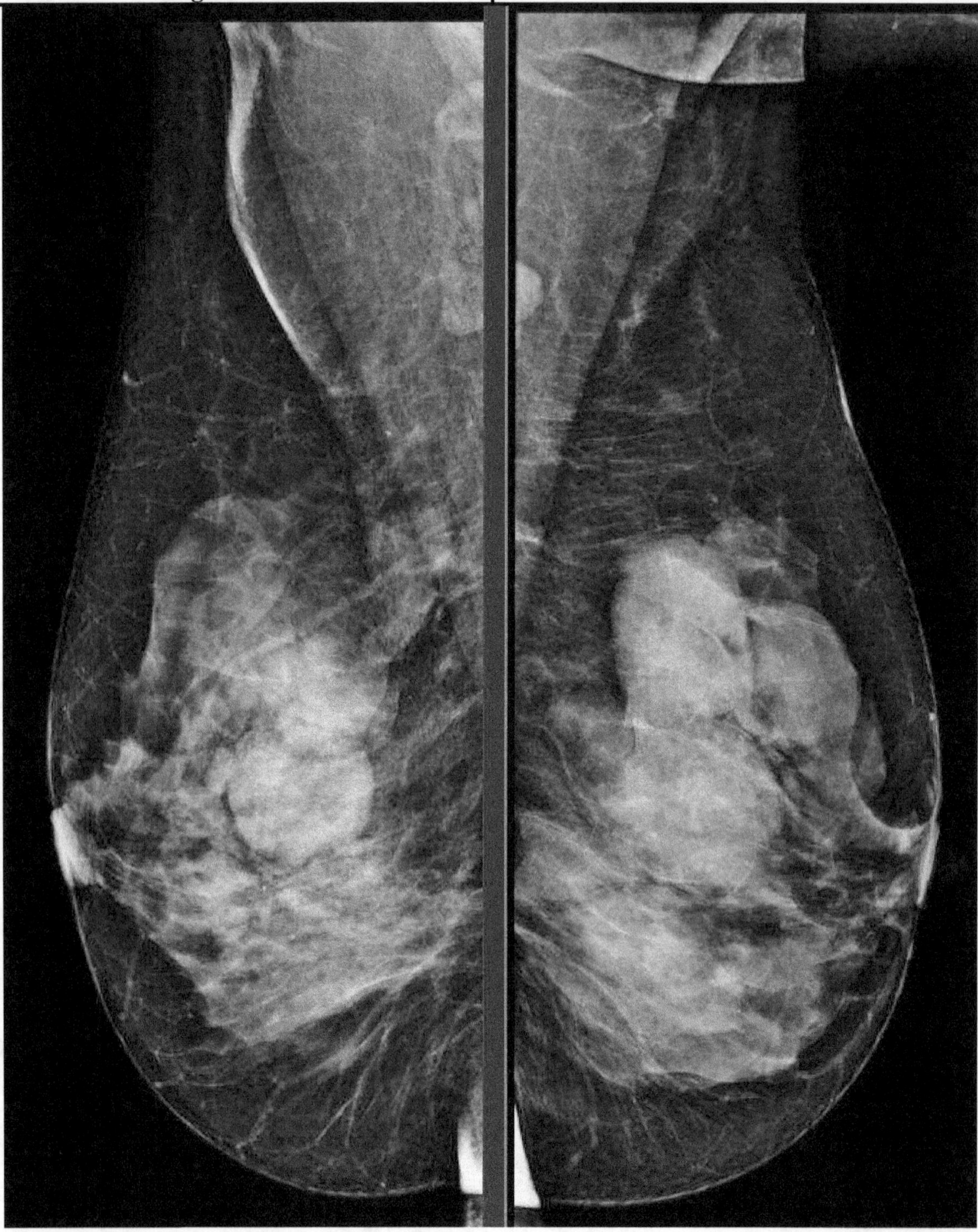

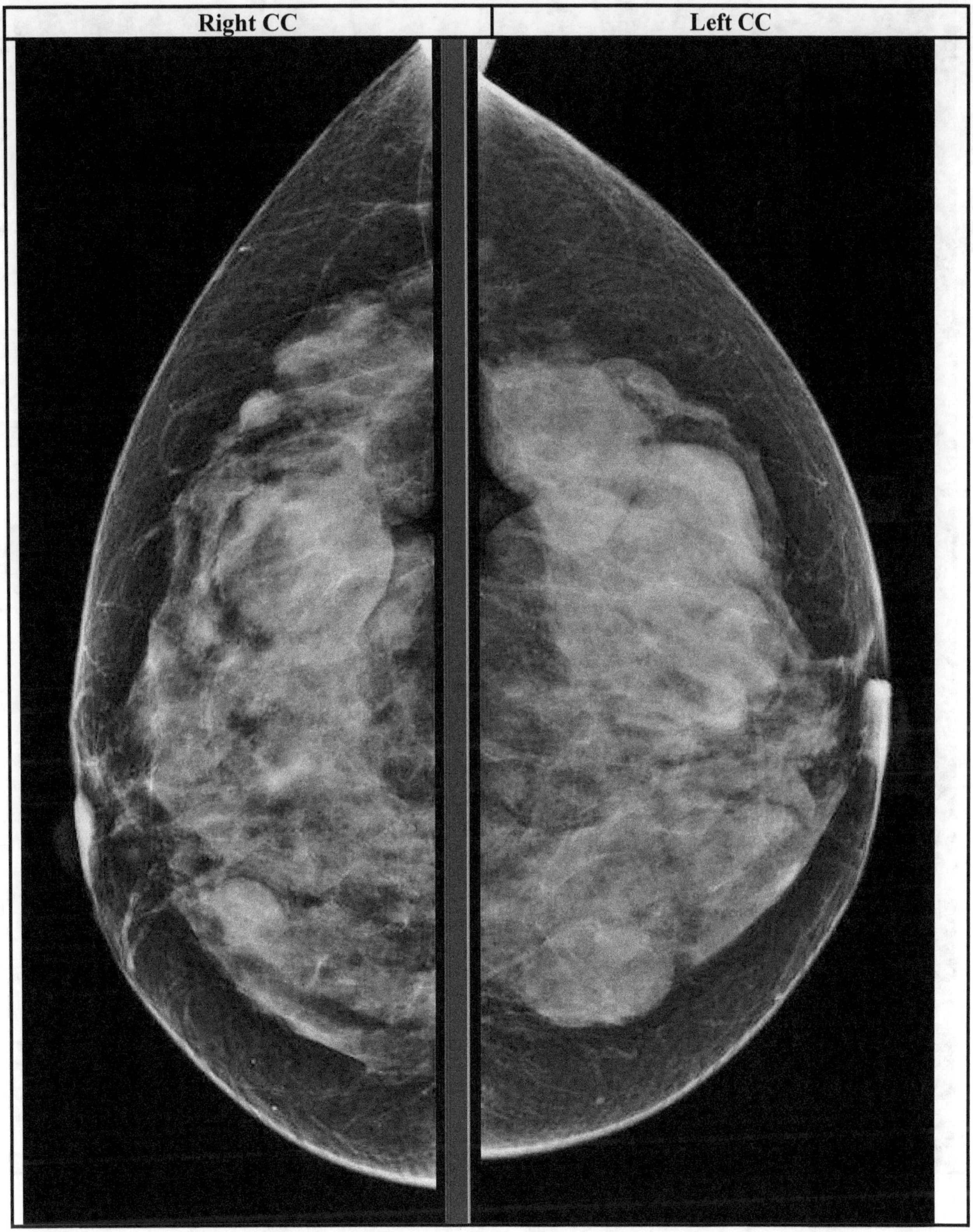
Right CC
Left CC

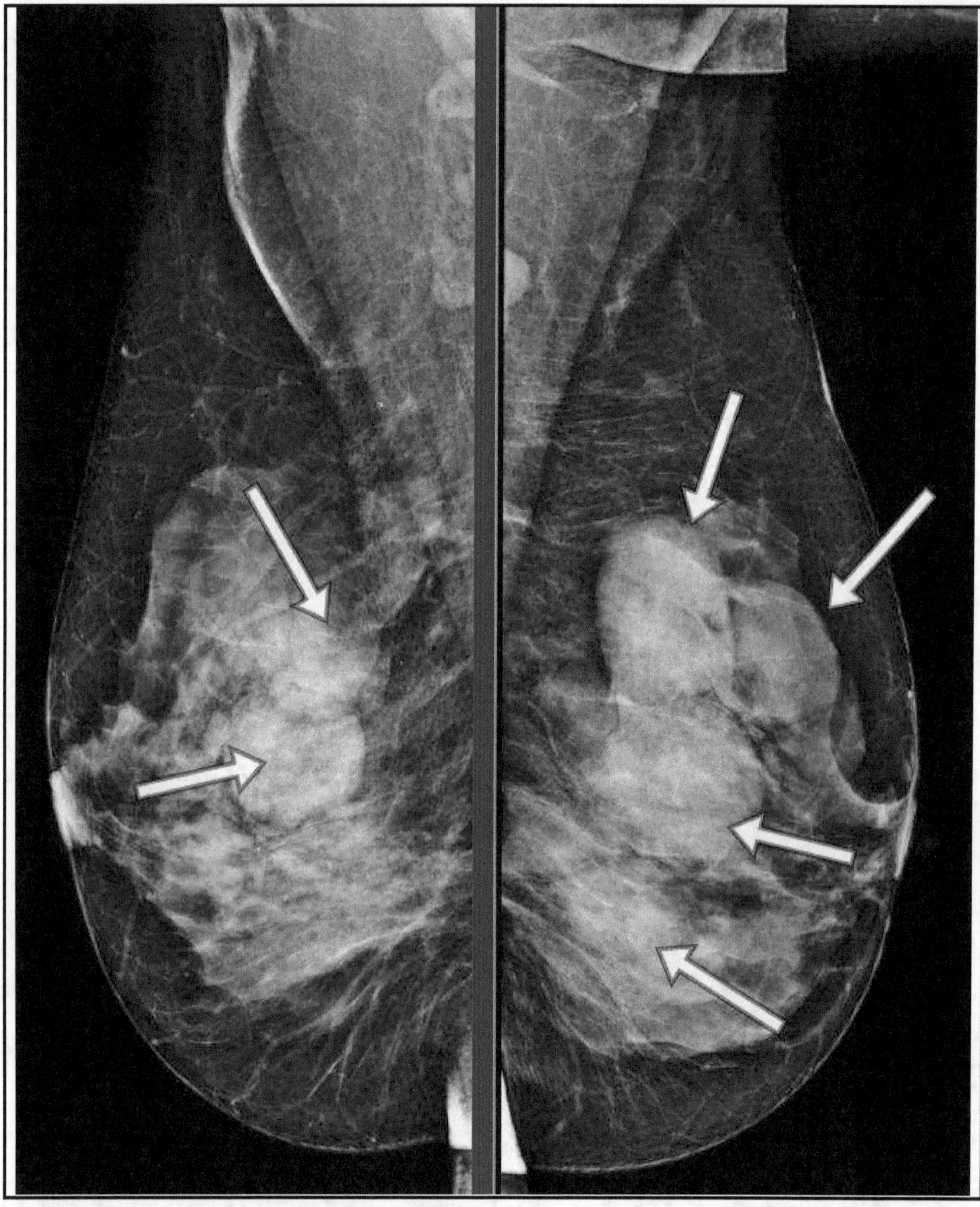

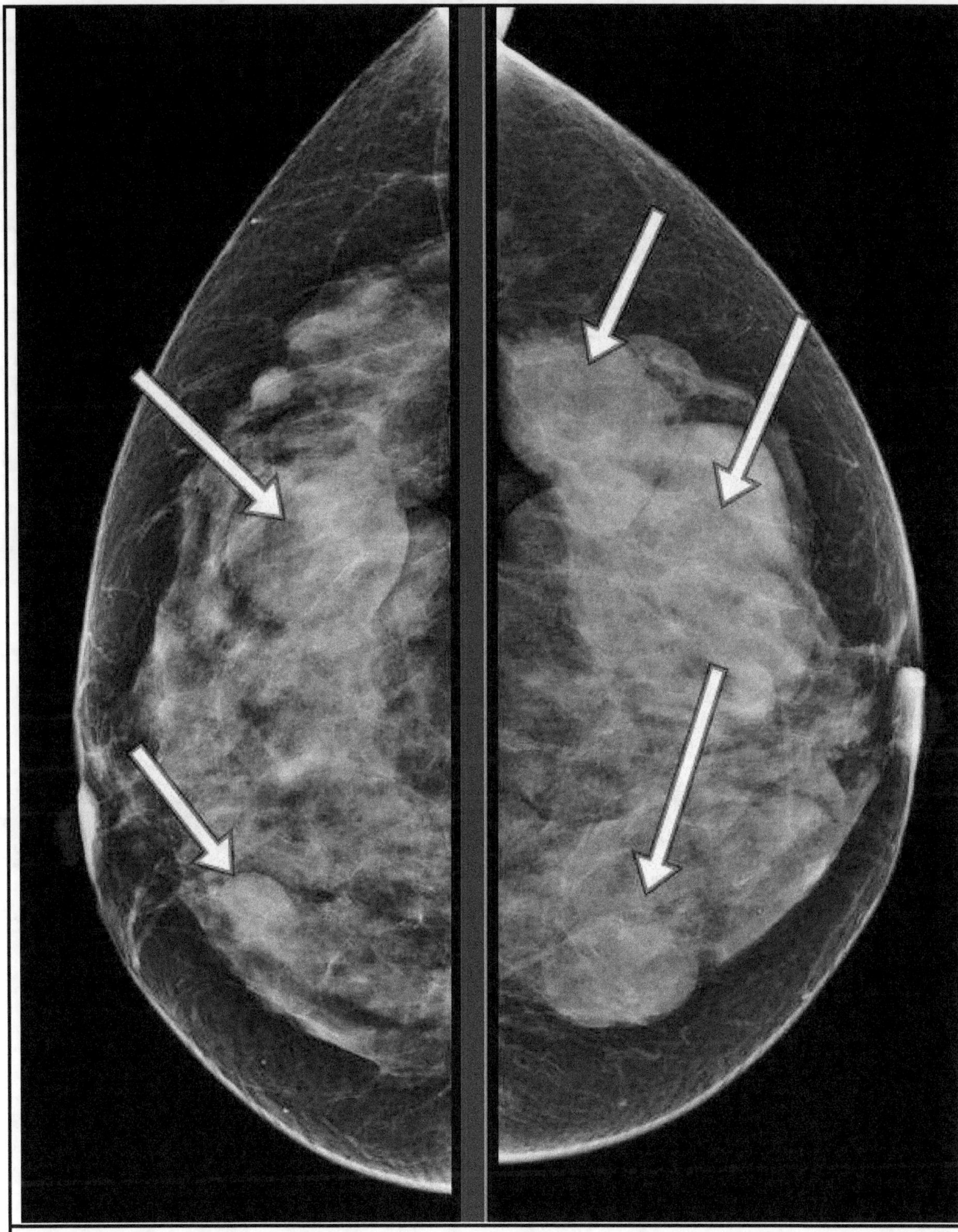

RIGHT BREAST	
Breast Parenchymal Density	*Extremely dense, which lowers the sensitivity of mammography (ACR D)*
Focal Mass	*Multiple oval circumscribed mass lesions*

Asymmetric Density	None
Parenchymal Distortion	None
Calcification	None
Skin Thickening	None
Axillary Nodes	None

LEFT BREAST	
Breast Parenchymal Density	***Extremely dense, which lowers the sensitivity of mammography (ACR D)***
Focal Mass	***Multiple oval circumscribed mass lesions***
Asymmetric Density	None
Parenchymal Distortion	None
Calcification	None
Skin Thickening	None
Axillary Nodes	None

IMPRESSION:

RIGHT BREAST: (BI-RADS 0)
LEFT BREAST: (BI-RADS 0)

RECOMMENDATION: US Correlation

US demonstrate (bilateral multiple cysts= fibrocystic changes)

CASE 19: 53-year-old female/screening	
Right MLO	Left MLO

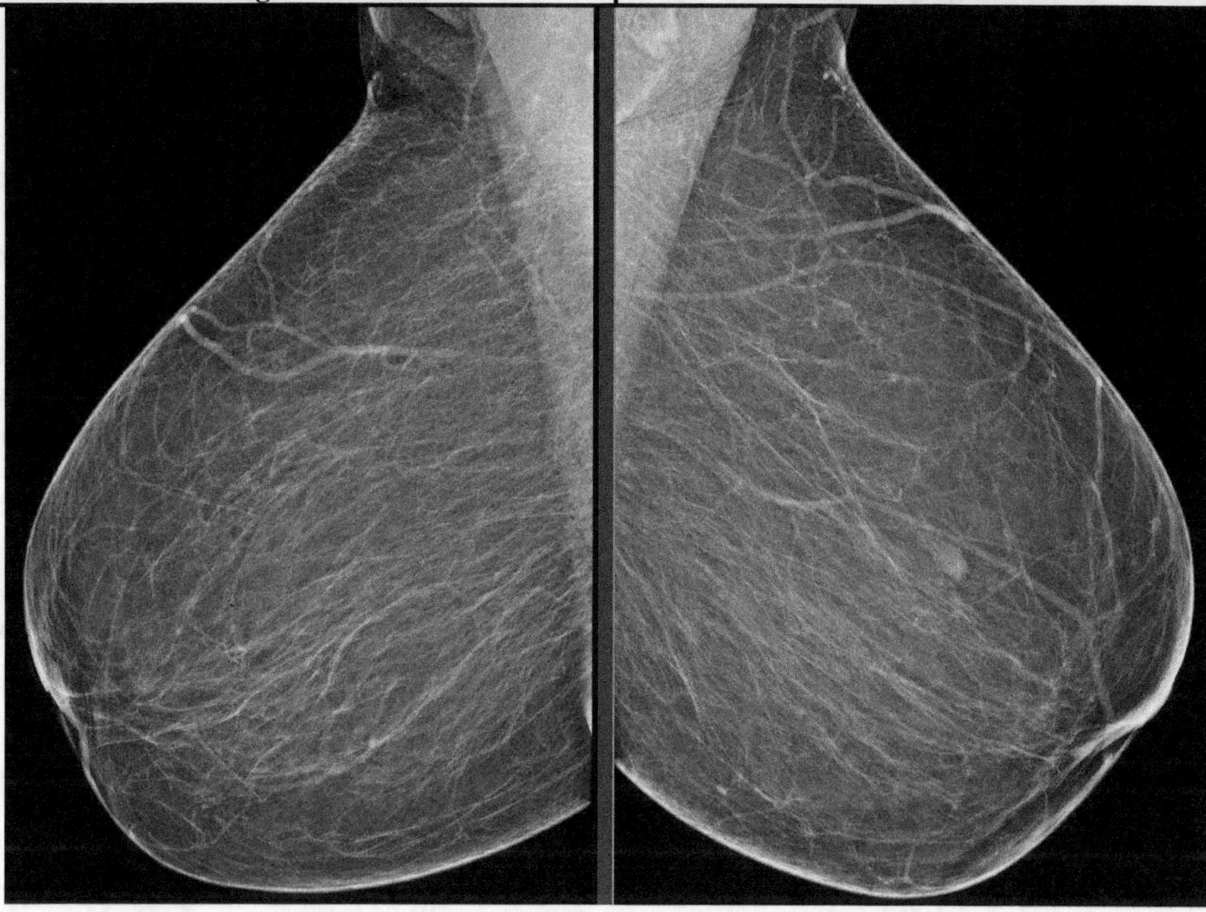

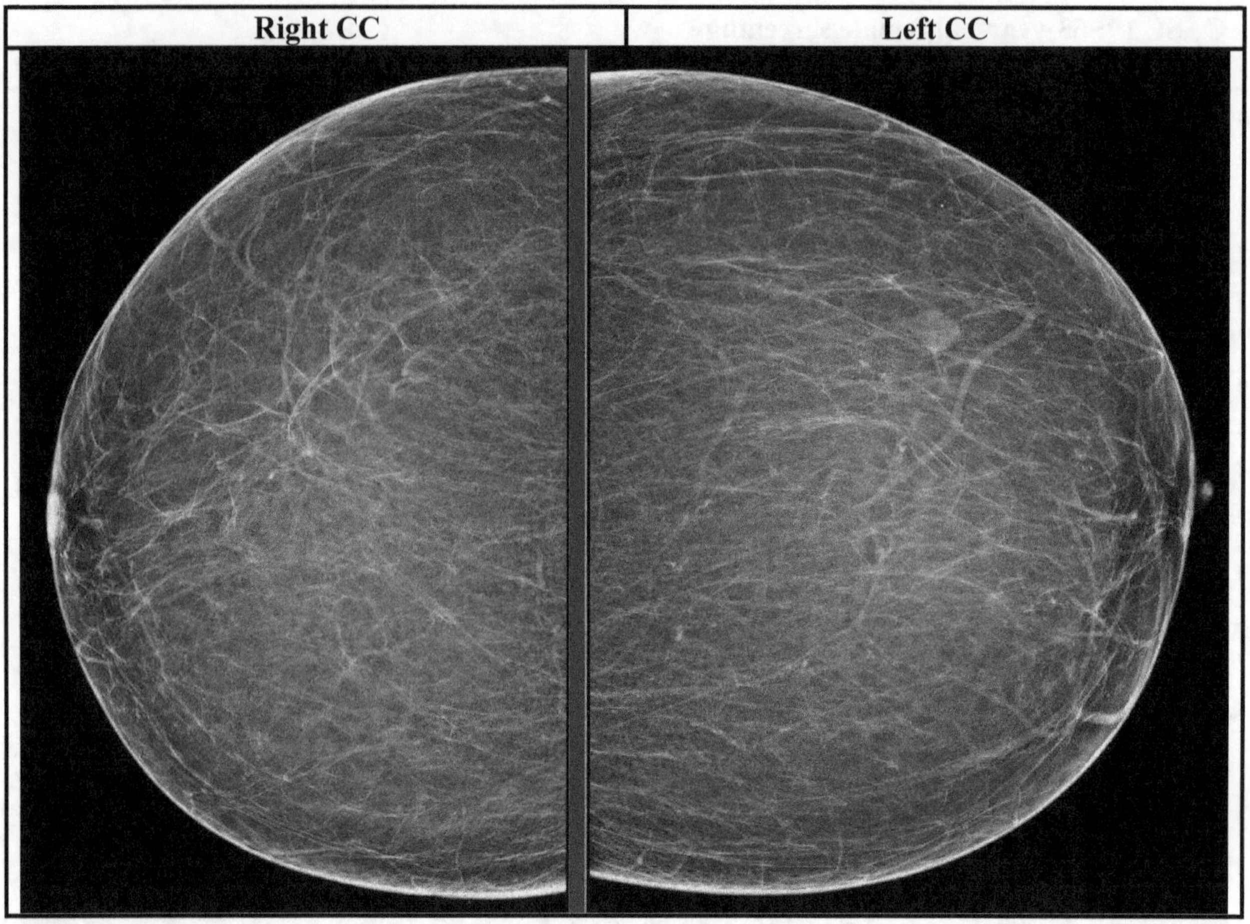
Right CC
Left CC

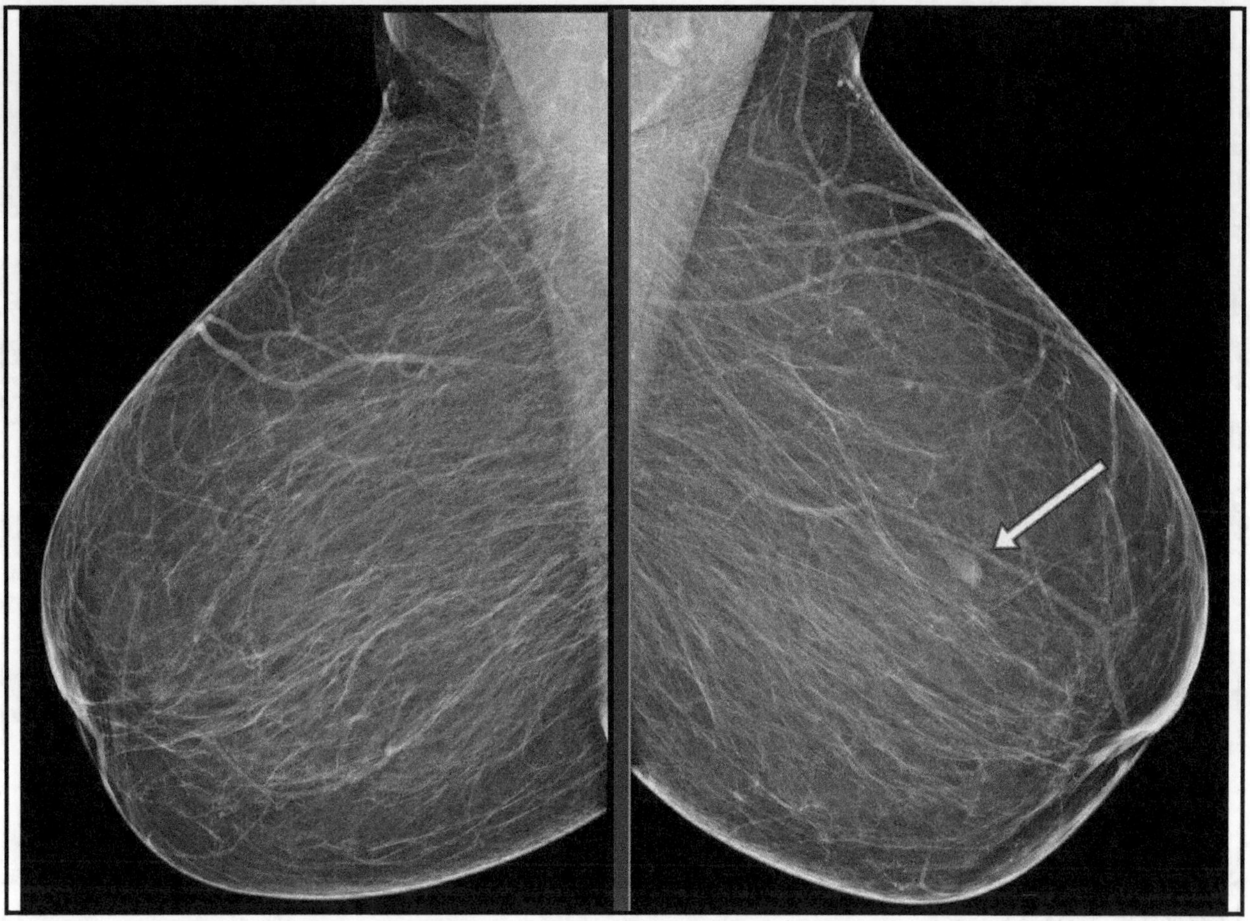

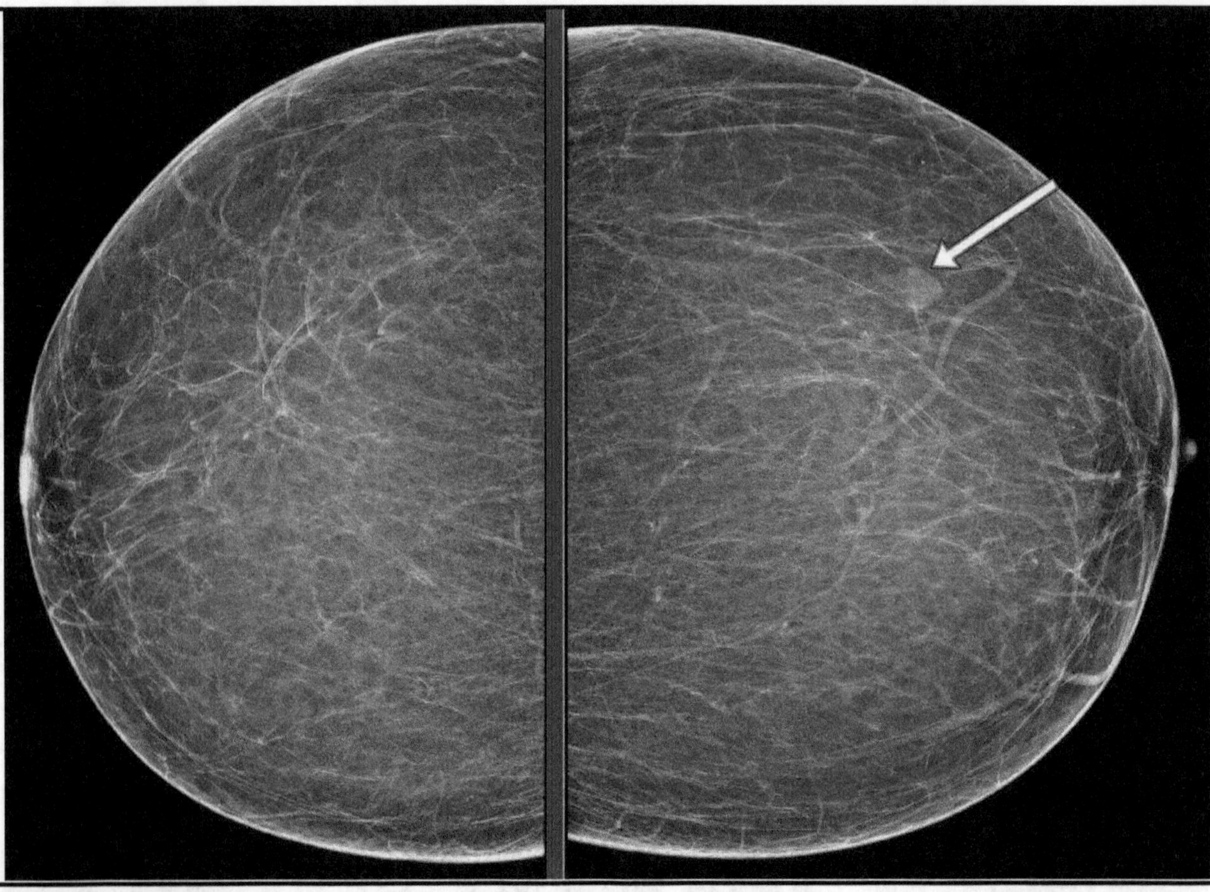

RIGHT BREAST	
Breast Parenchymal Density	***Almost entirely fatty (ACR A)***
Focal Mass	None
Asymmetric Density	None
Parenchymal Distortion	None
Calcification	None
Skin Thickening	None
Axillary Nodes	None

LEFT BREAST	
Breast Parenchymal Density	***Almost entirely fatty (ACR A)***
Focal Mass	None
Asymmetric Density	None
Parenchymal Distortion	None
Calcification	None
Skin Thickening	None
Axillary Nodes	None **IMLN**

IMPRESSION:
RIGHT BREAST: (BI-RADS 1)
LEFT BREAST: (BI-RADS 1)

RECOMMENDATION: Routine Annual screening

CASE 20: 59-year-old female/screening

Right MLO	Left MLO
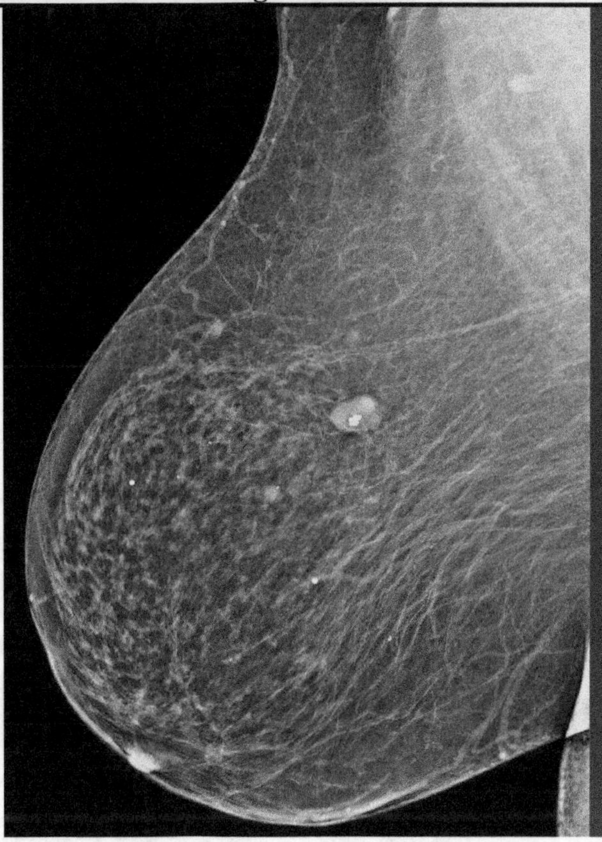	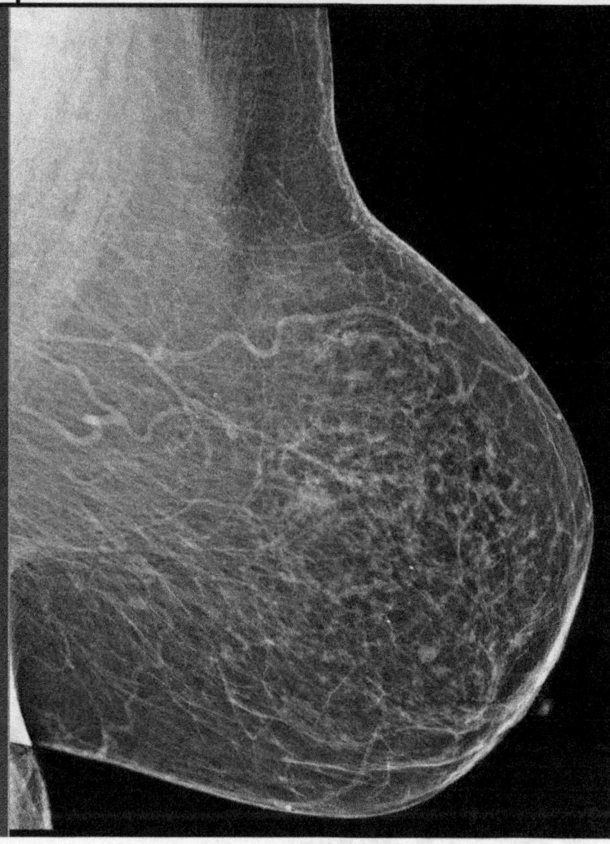

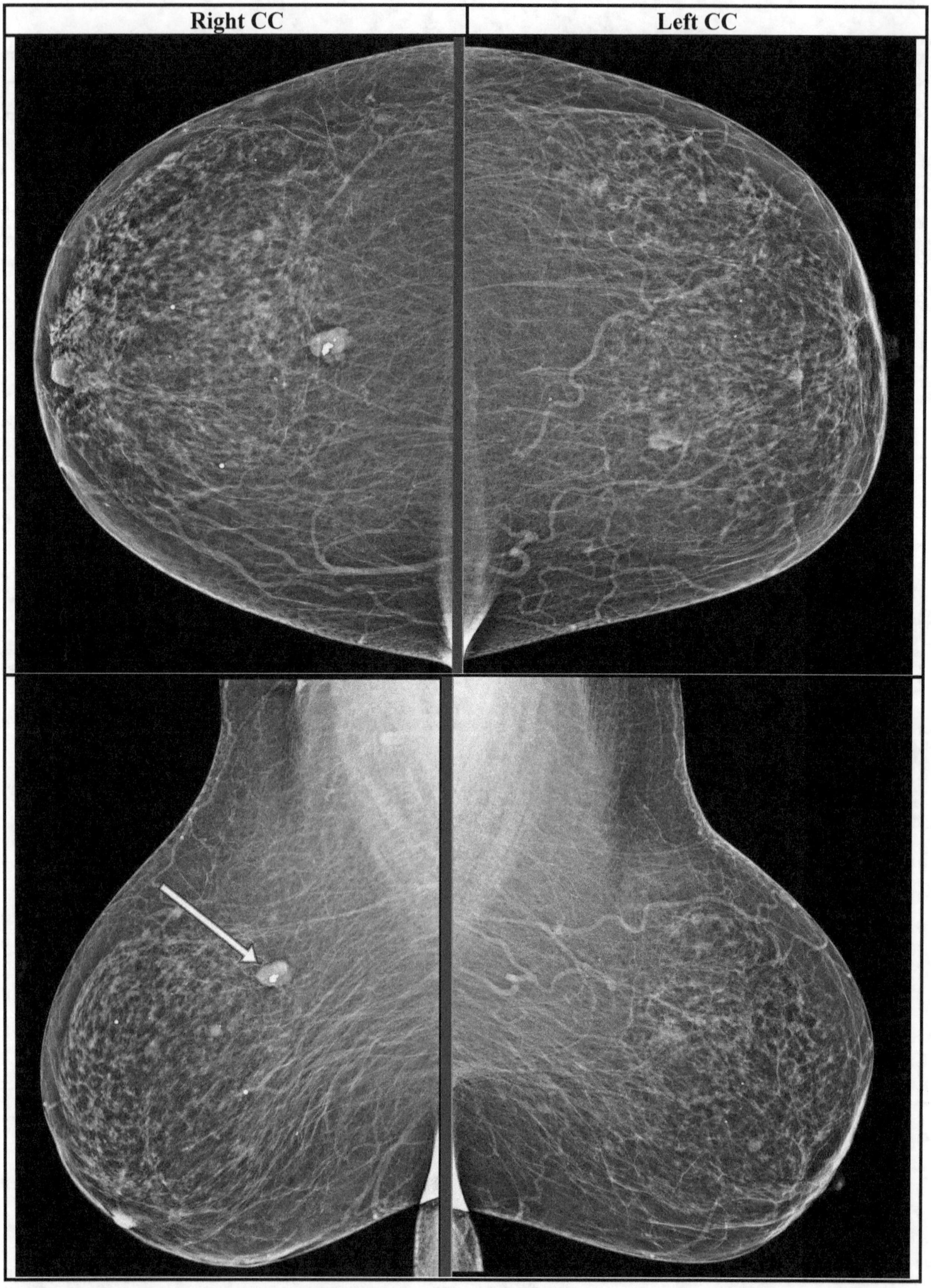
Right CC
Left CC

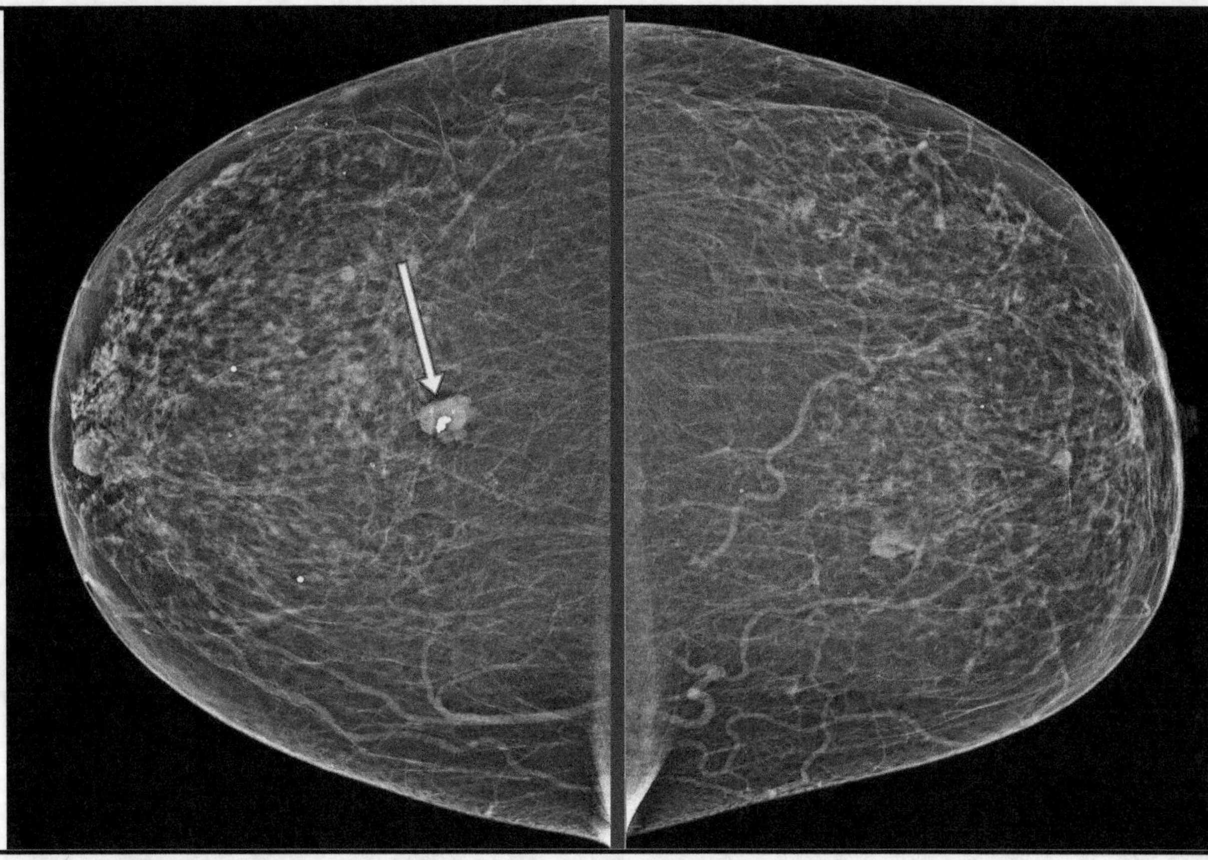

RIGHT BREAST	
Breast Parenchymal Density	***Scattered areas of fibroglandular density (ACR B)***
Focal Mass	***Upper central (12 o'clock) involuted fibroadenoma***
Asymmetric Density	None
Parenchymal Distortion	None
Calcification	None
Skin Thickening	None
Axillary Nodes	None

LEFT BREAST	
Breast Parenchymal Density	***Scattered areas of fibroglandular density (ACR B)***
Focal Mass	None
Asymmetric Density	None
Parenchymal Distortion	None
Calcification	None
Skin Thickening	None
Axillary Nodes	None

IMPRESSION:
RIGHT BREAST: (BI-RADS 2)
LEFT BREAST: (BI-RADS 1)

RECOMMENDATION: Routine Annual screening

CASE 21: 59-year-old female/ Diagnostic

Right MLO	Left MLO
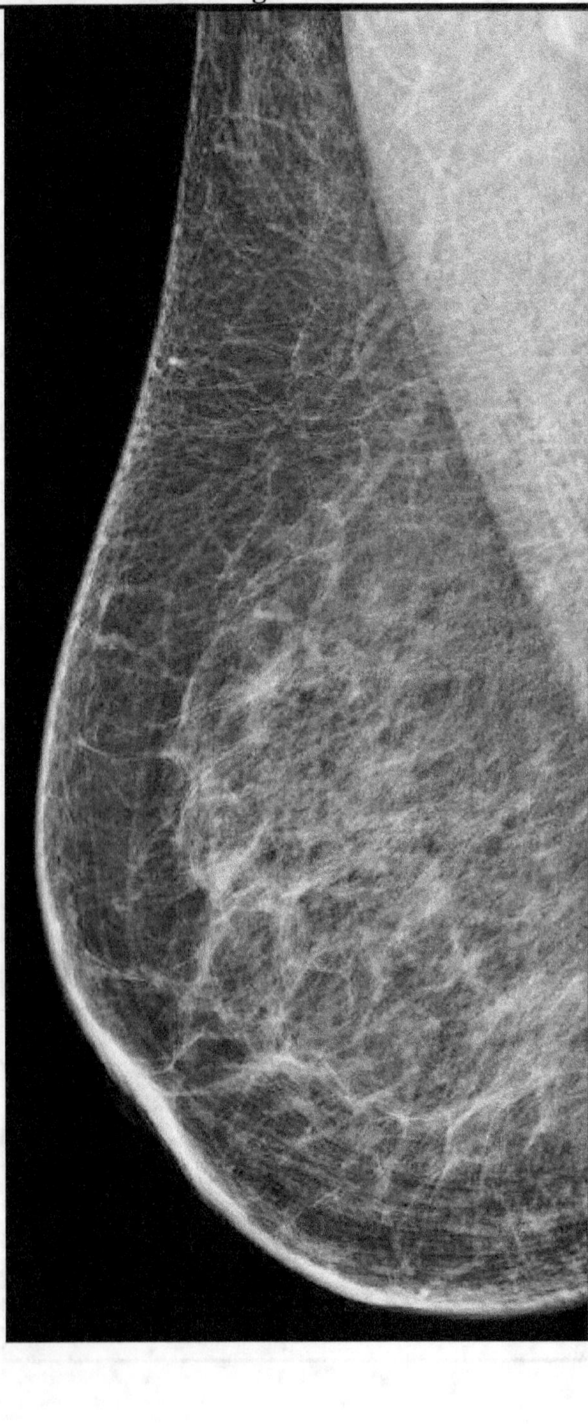	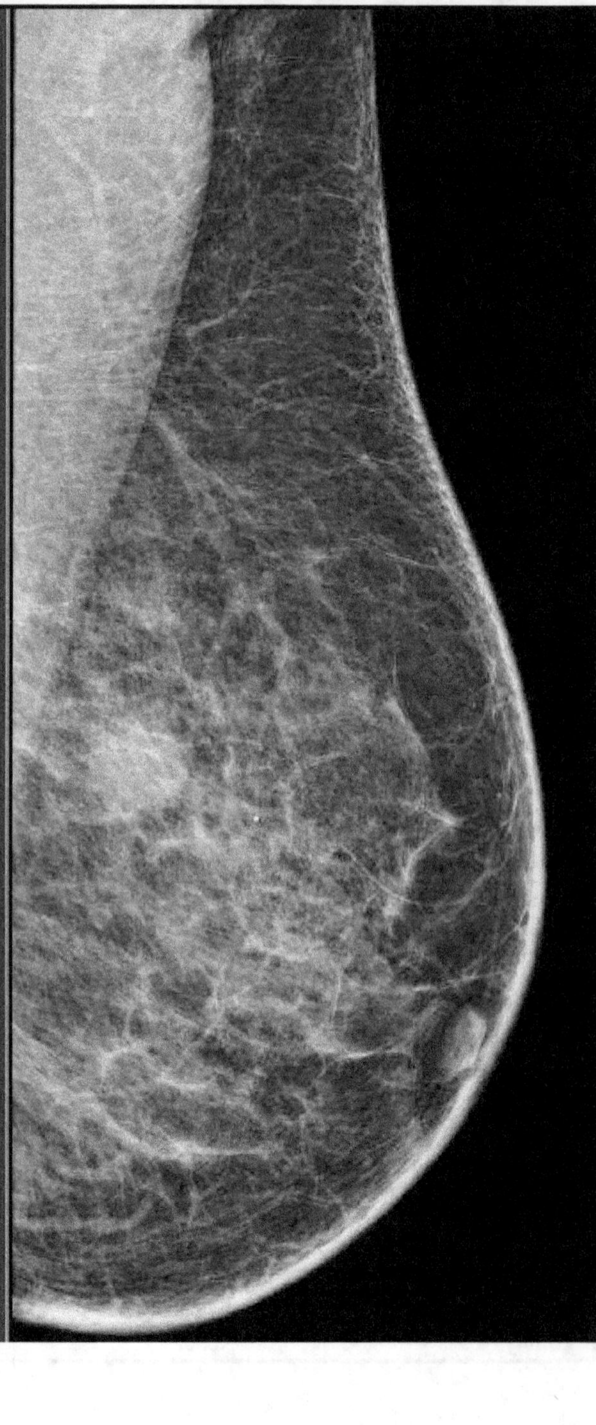

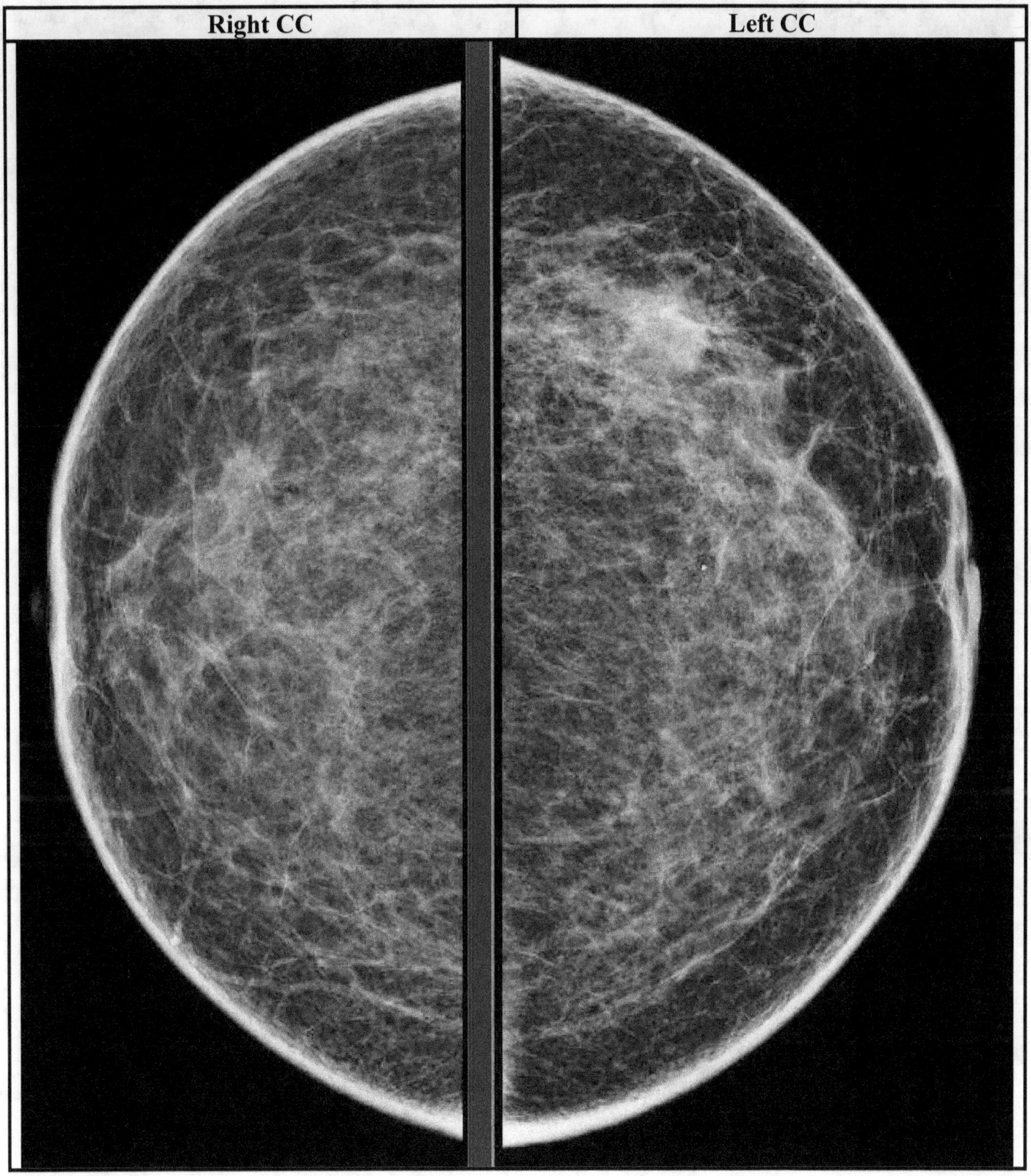
Right CC
Left CC

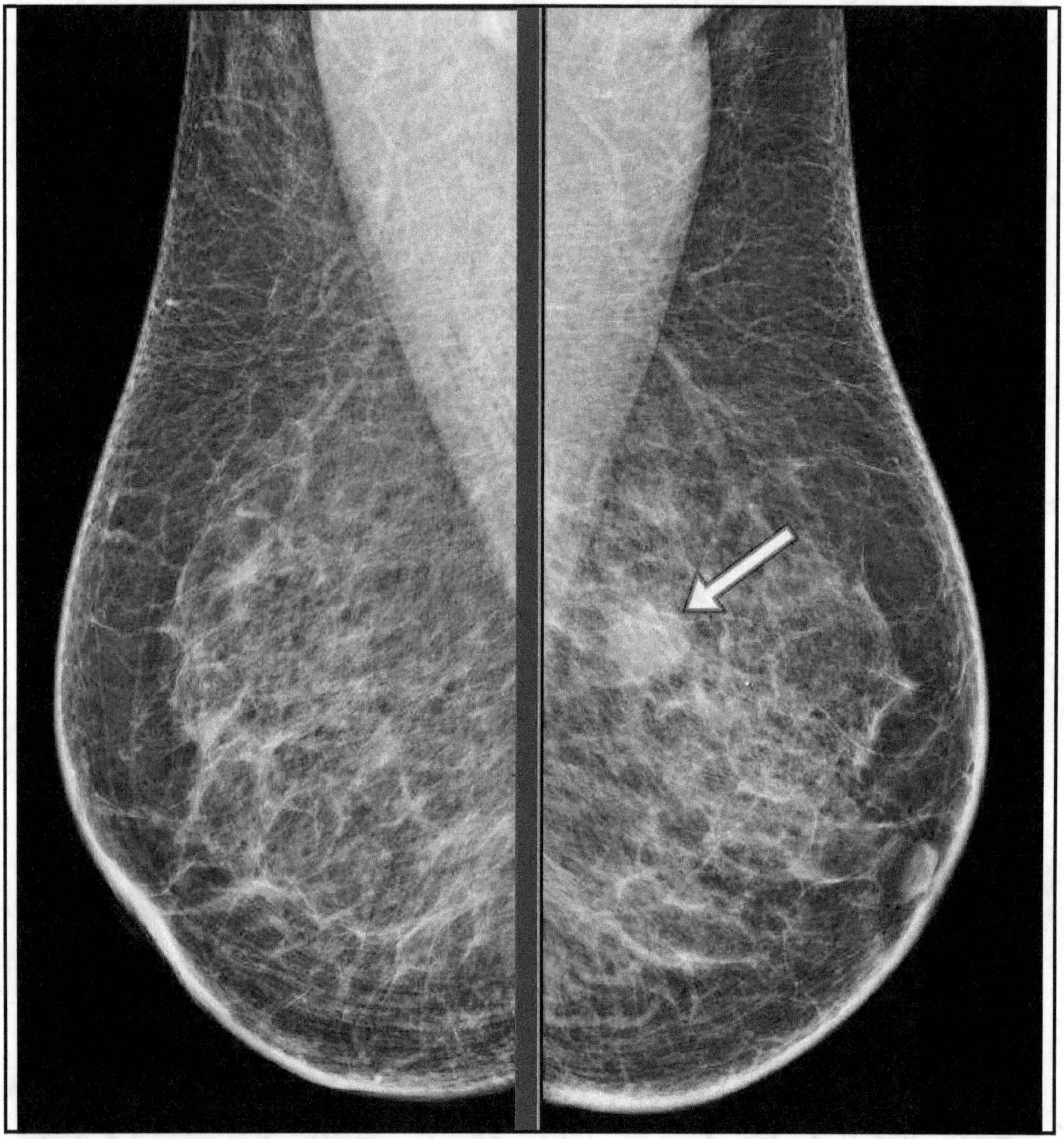

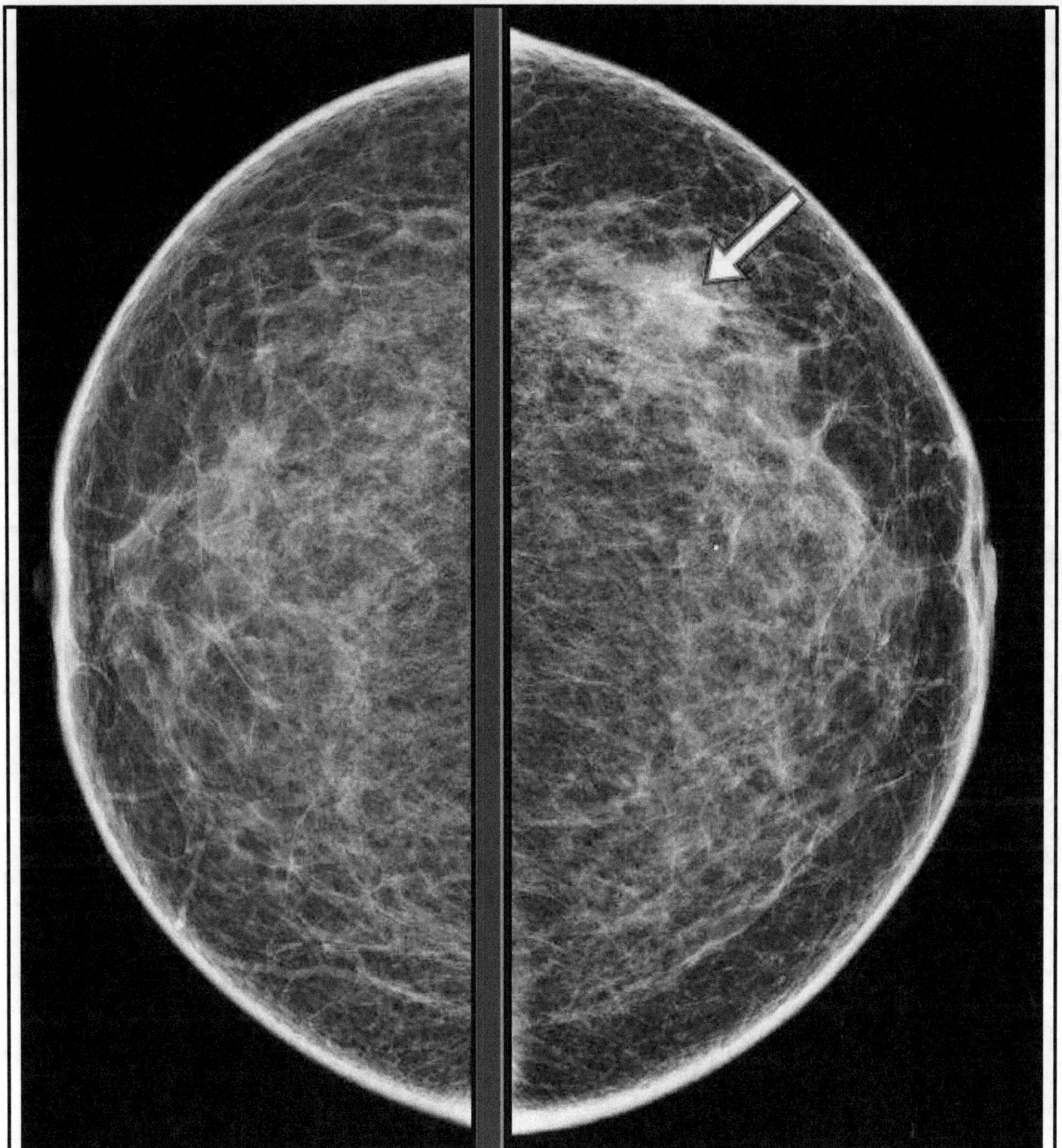

RIGHT BREAST	
Breast Parenchymal Density	***Scattered areas of fibroglandular density (ACR B)***
Focal Mass	None
Asymmetric Density	None
Parenchymal Distortion	None
Calcification	None
Skin Thickening	None
Axillary Nodes	None

LEFT BREAST	
Breast Parenchymal Density	***Scattered areas of fibroglandular density (ACR B)***
Focal Mass	***UOQ oval obscured mass lesion***
Asymmetric Density	None
Parenchymal Distortion	None
Calcification	None
Skin Thickening	None
Axillary Nodes	None

IMPRESSION:
RIGHT BREAST: (BI-RADS 1)
LEFT BREAST: (BI-RADS 4B)

RECOMMENDATION: Histopathological Correlation

CASE 22: 47-year-old female/ Diagnostic	
Right MLO	**Left MLO**

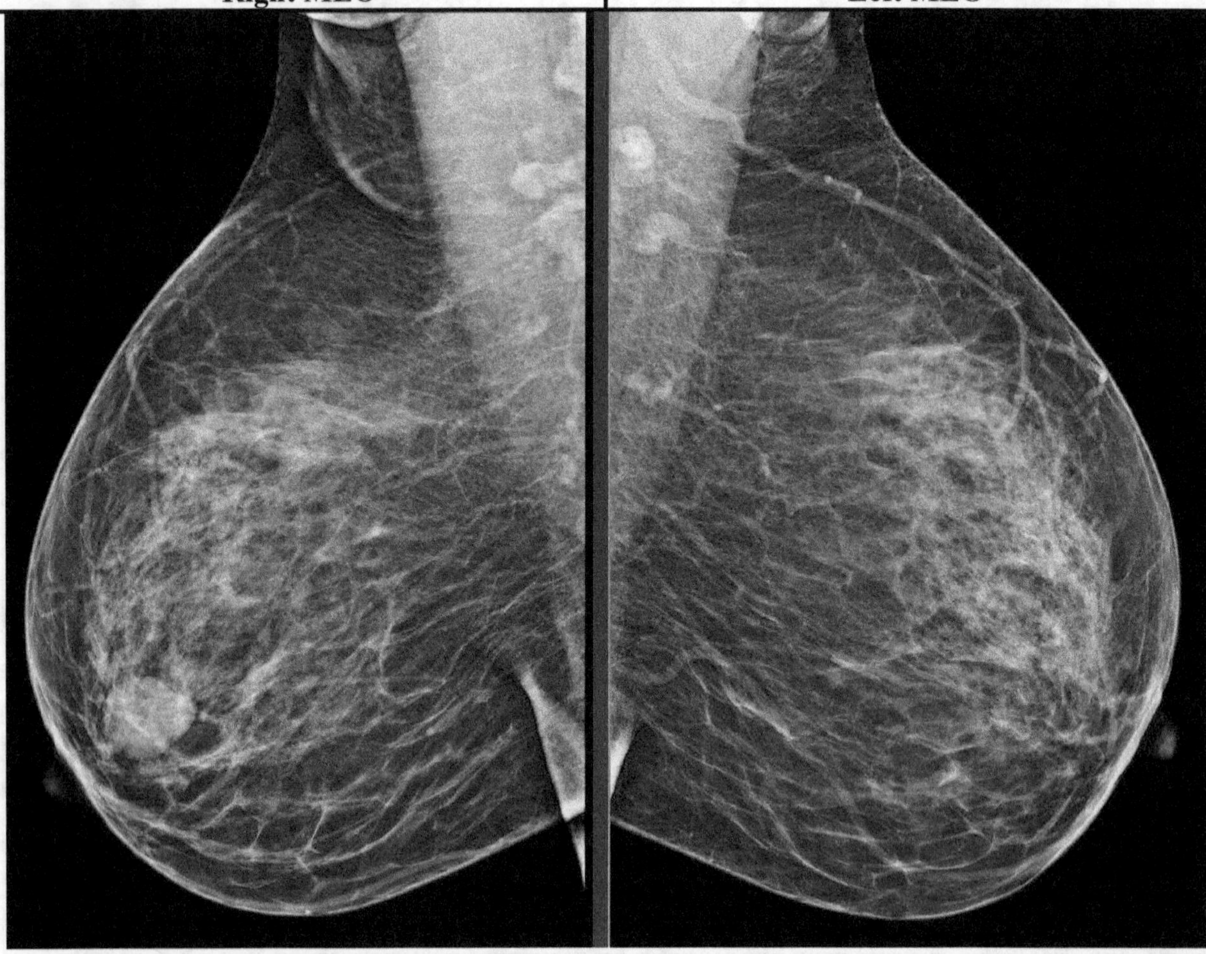

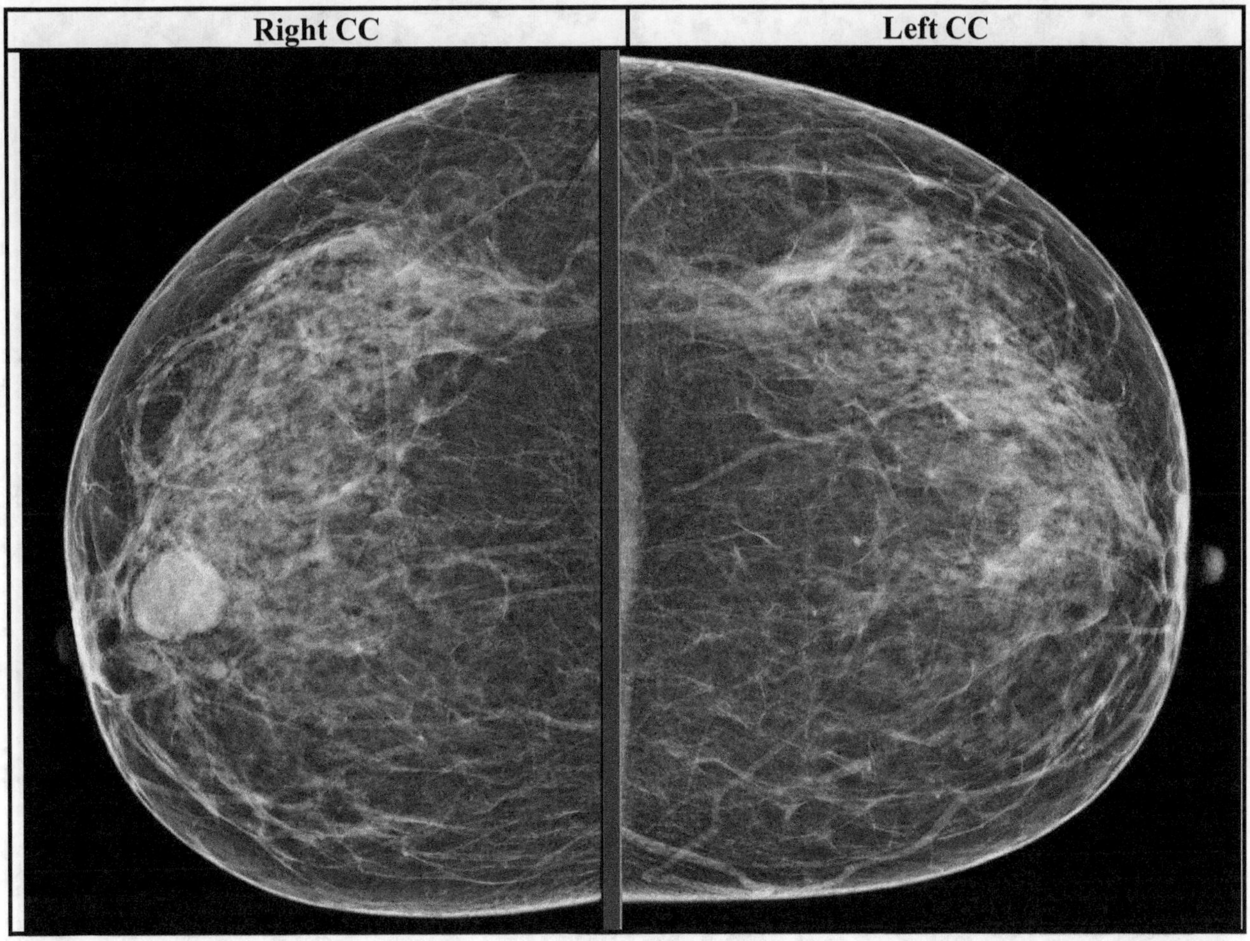
Right CC
Left CC

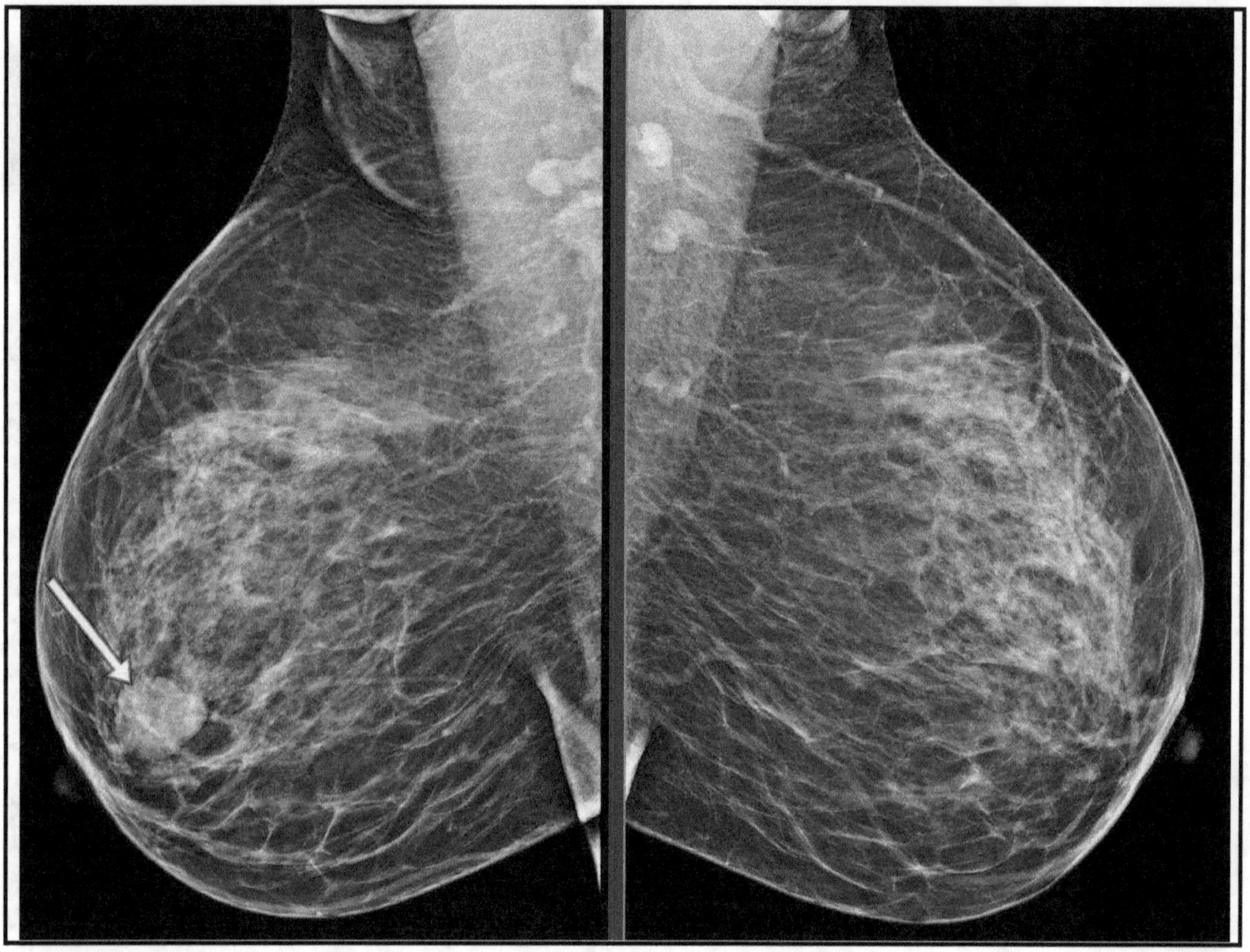

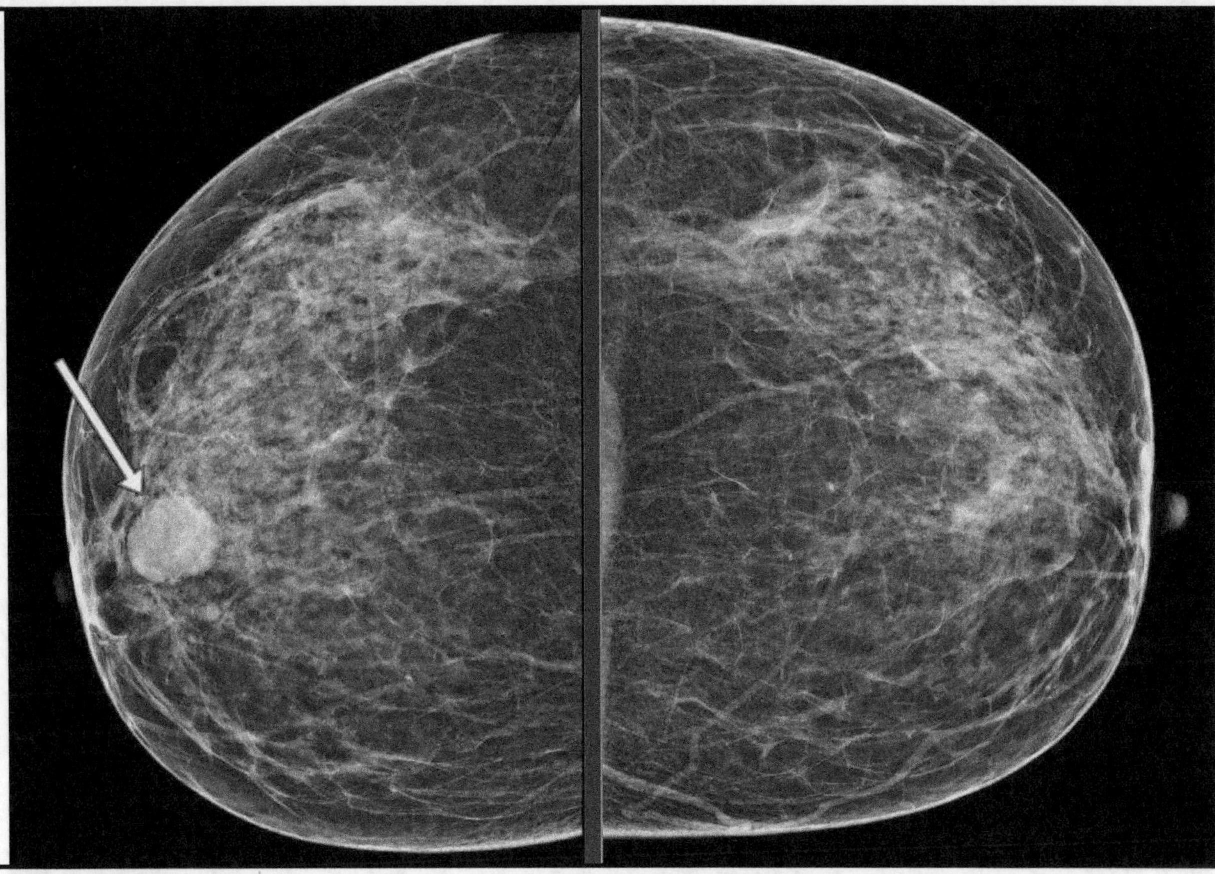

RIGHT BREAST	
Breast Parenchymal Density	***Scattered areas of fibroglandular density (ACR B)***
Focal Mass	***Upper central (12 o'clock) circumscribed mass lesion***
Asymmetric Density	None
Parenchymal Distortion	None
Calcification	None
Skin Thickening	None
Axillary Nodes	None

LEFT BREAST	
Breast Parenchymal Density	***Scattered areas of fibroglandular density (ACR B)***
Focal Mass	None
Asymmetric Density	None
Parenchymal Distortion	None
Calcification	None
Skin Thickening	None
Axillary Nodes	None

IMPRESSION:

RIGHT BREAST: (BI-RADS 0)
LEFT BREAST: (BI-RADS 1)

RECOMMENDATION: US Correlation

CASE 23: 64-year-old female/ Diagnostic

Right MLO	Left MLO

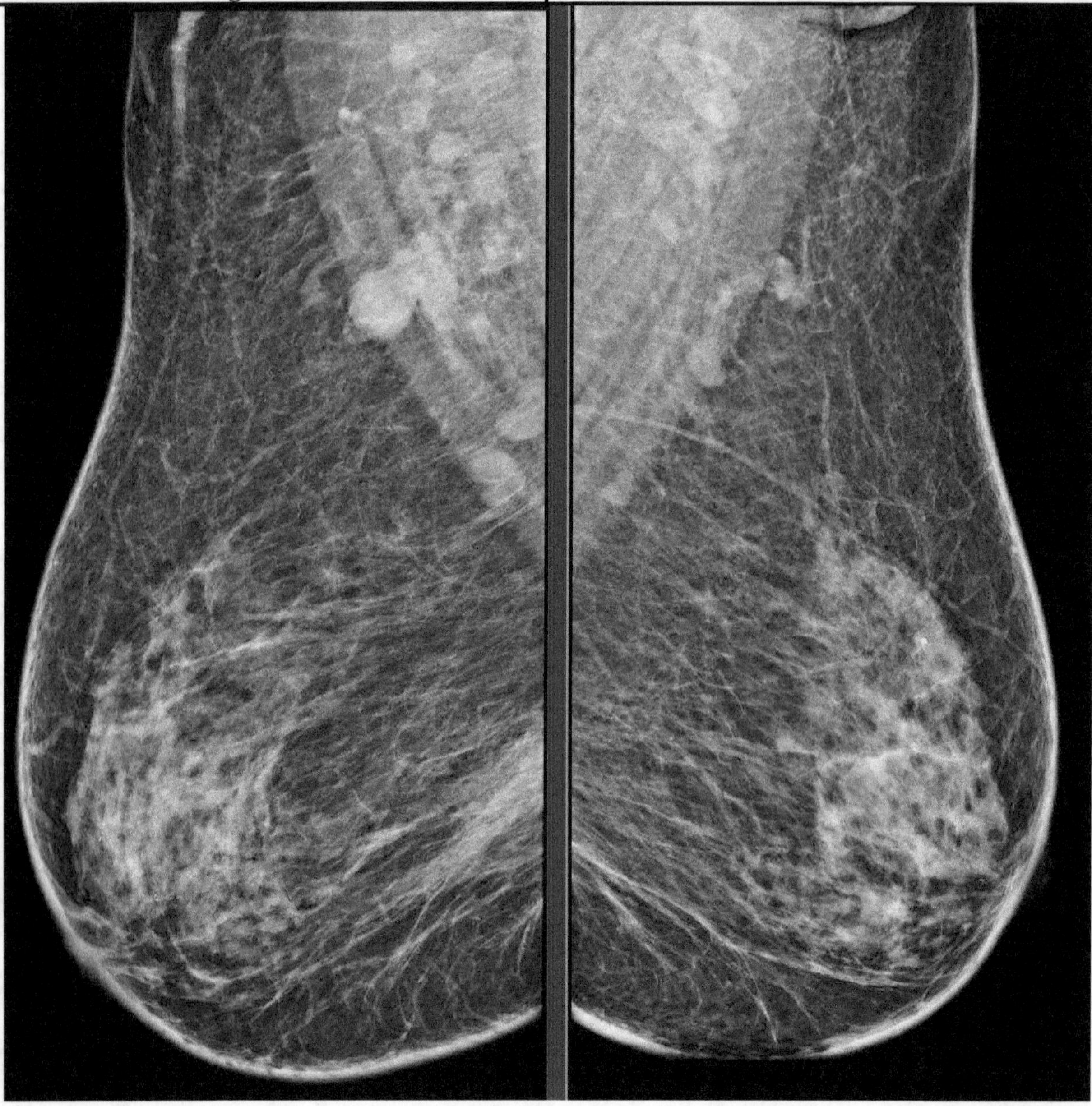

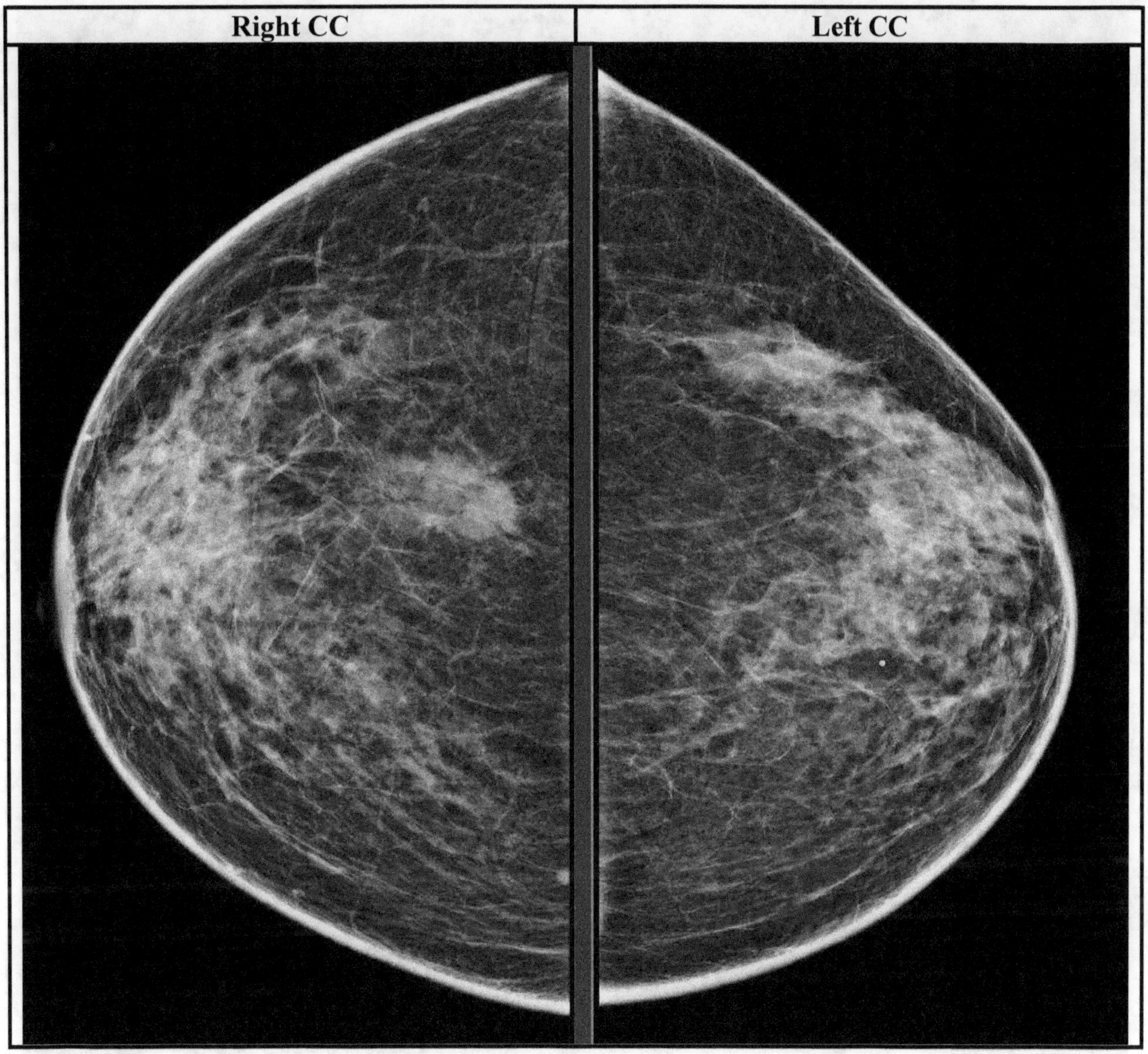
Right CC
Left CC

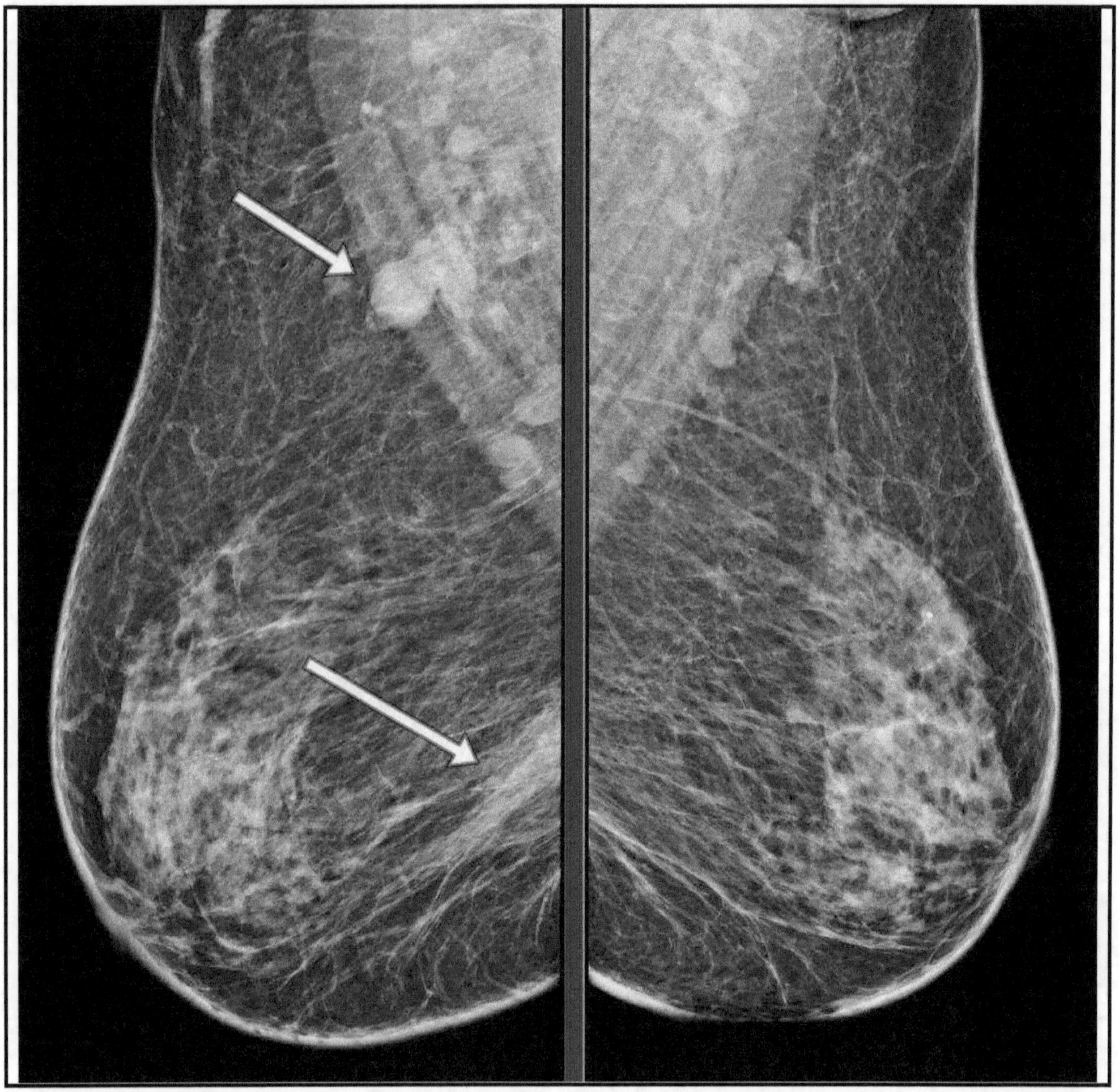

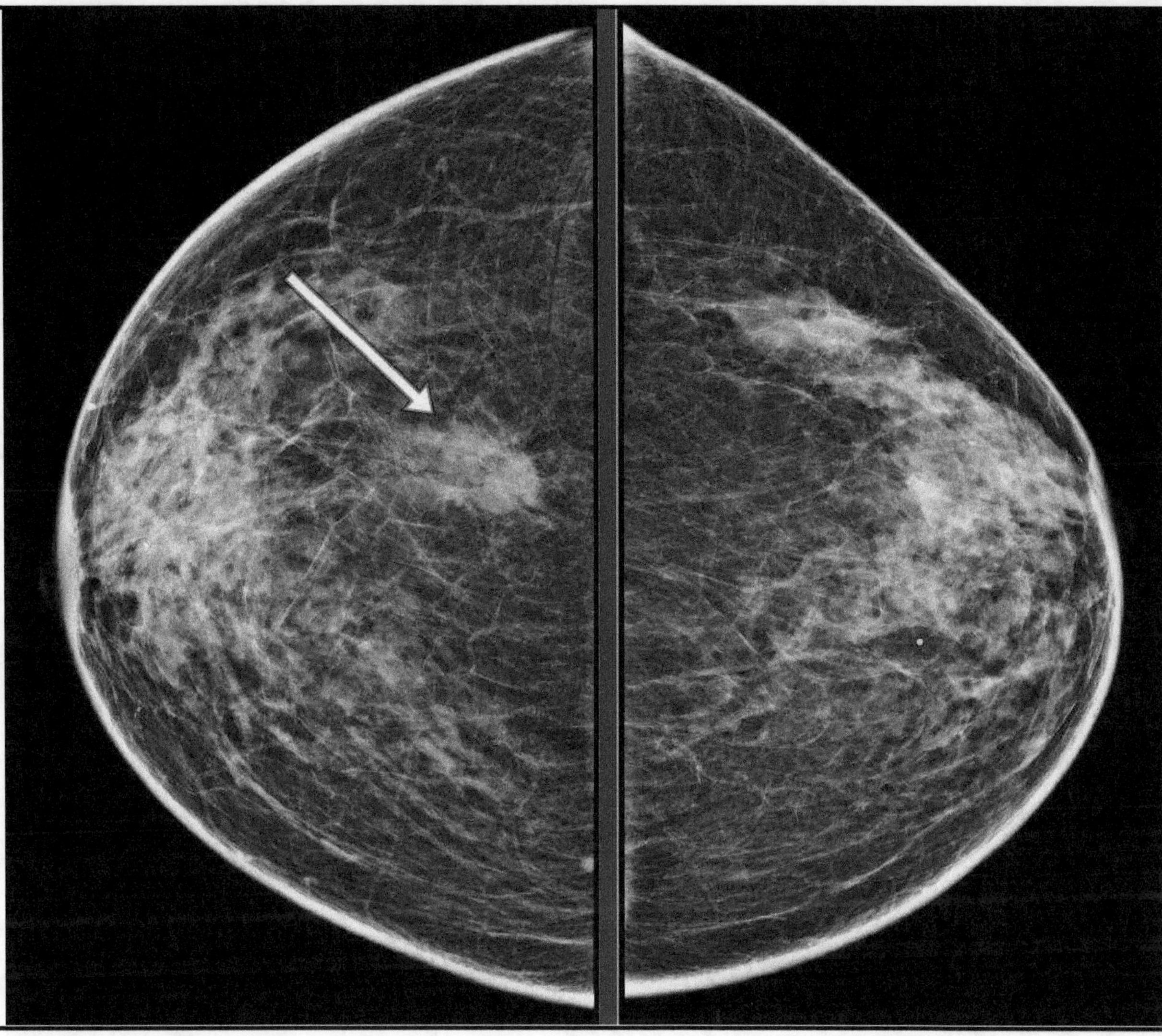

RIGHT BREAST	
Breast Parenchymal Density	***Heterogeneously dense, may obscure small masses (ACR C)***
Focal Mass	None
Asymmetric Density	***LOQ focal asymmetry***
Parenchymal Distortion	None
Calcification	None
Skin Thickening	None
Axillary Nodes	***Lymphadenopathy***

LEFT BREAST	
Breast Parenchymal Density	***Heterogeneously dense, may obscure small masses (ACR C)***
Focal Mass	None
Asymmetric Density	None
Parenchymal Distortion	None
Calcification	None
Skin Thickening	None
Axillary Nodes	None

IMPRESSION:

RIGHT BREAST: (BI-RADS 4C)
LEFT BREAST: (BI-RADS 1)

RECOMMENDATION: Histopathological Correlation

CASE 24: 43-year-old female/ Diagnostic	
Right MLO	**Left MLO**
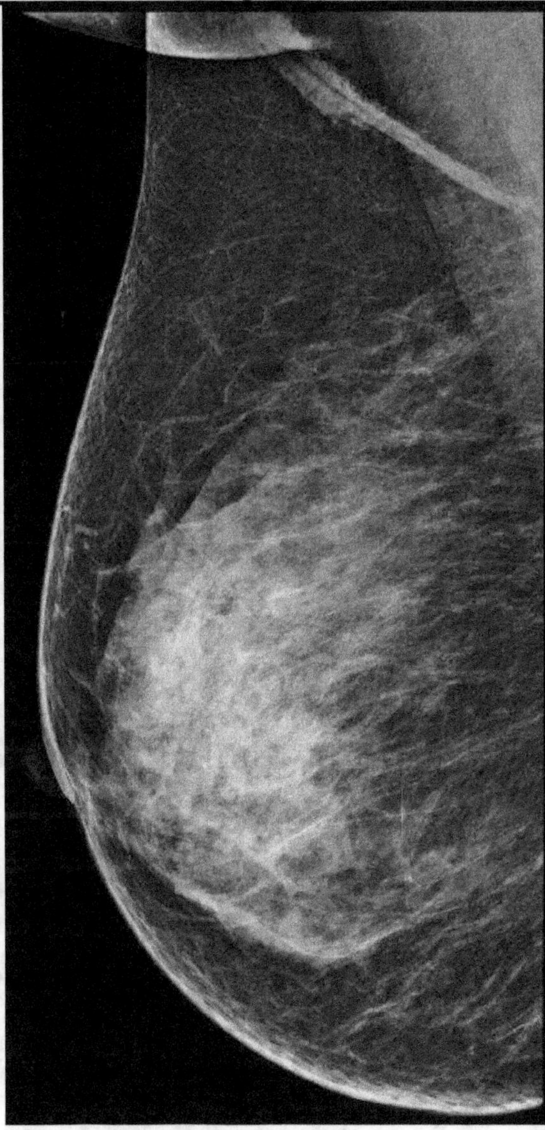	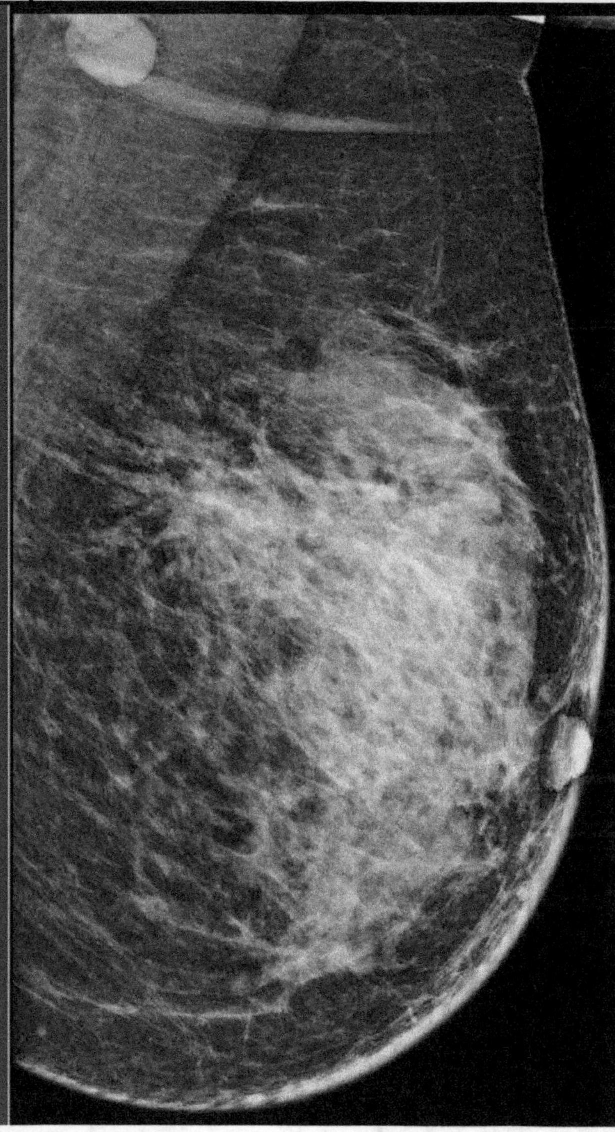

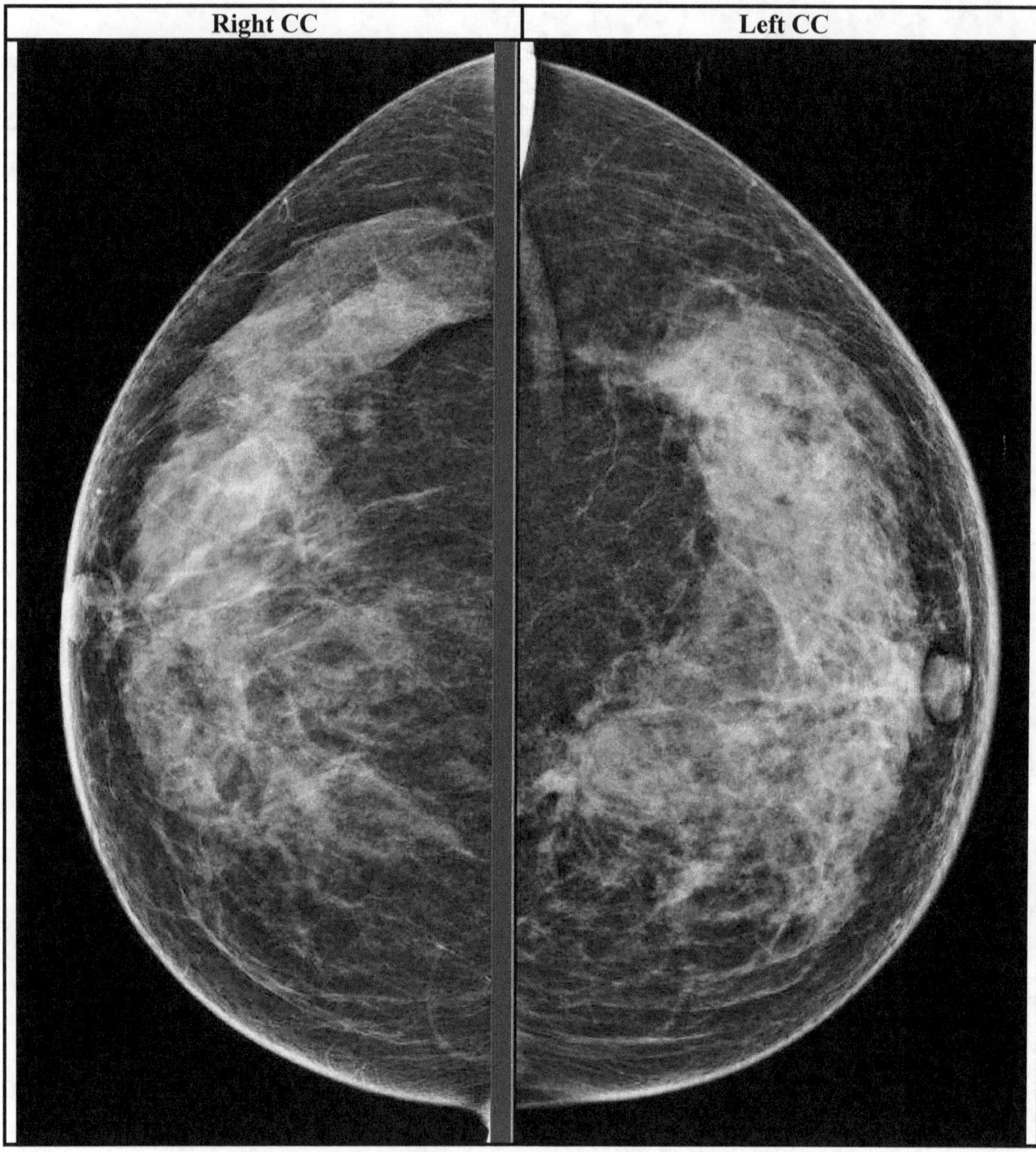
Right CC
Left CC

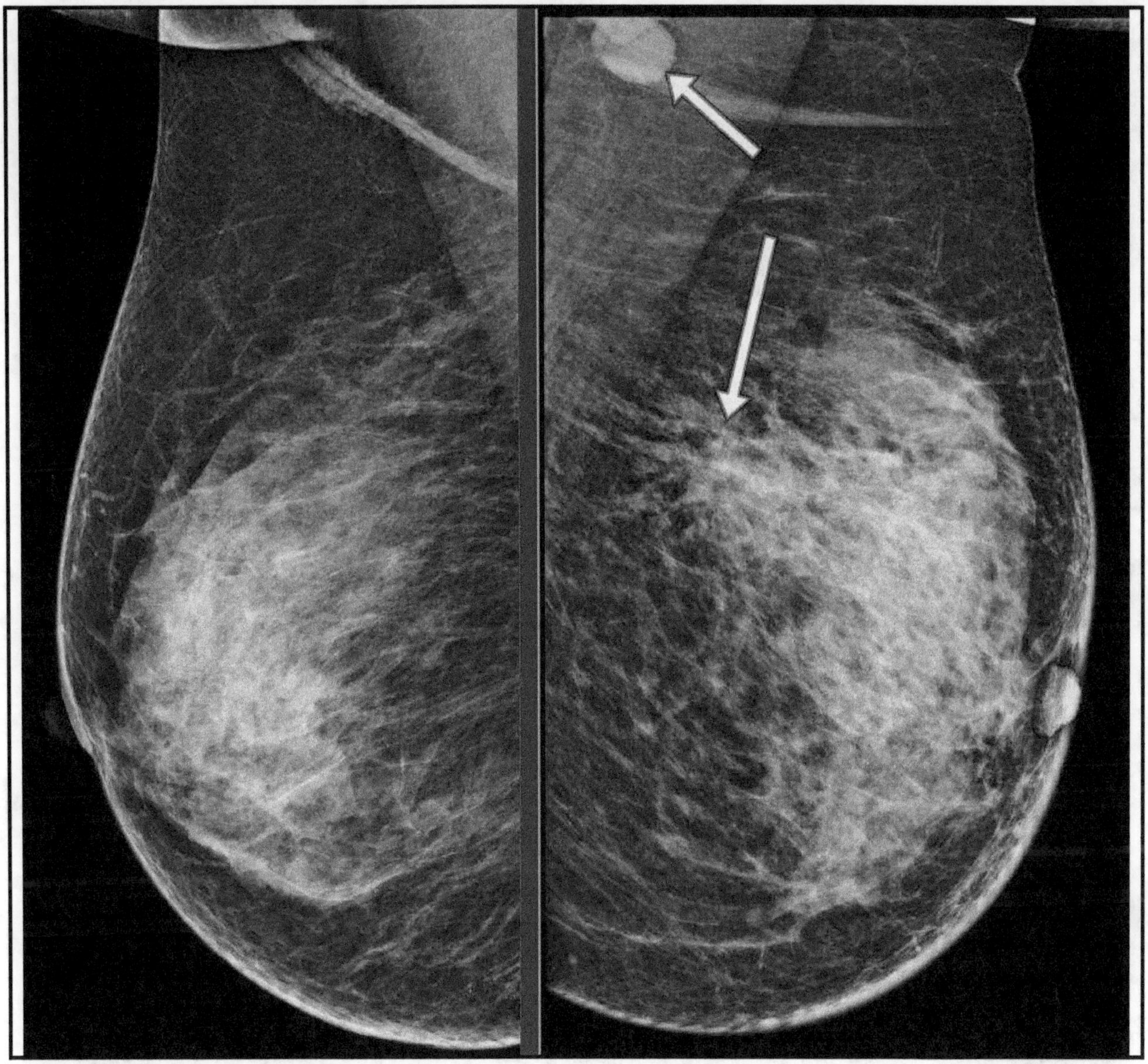

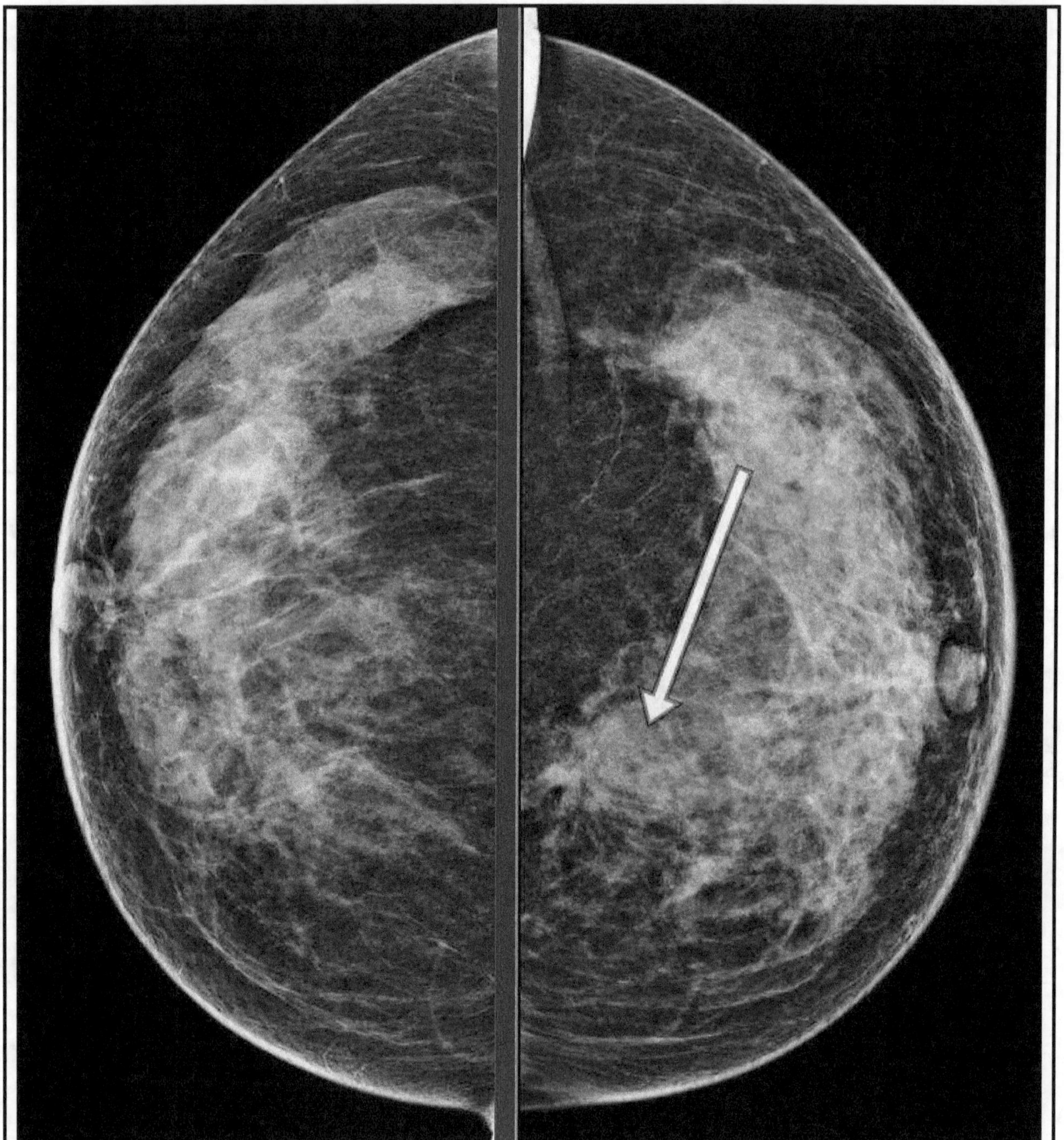

RIGHT BREAST	
Breast Parenchymal Density	***Heterogeneously dense, may obscure small masses (ACR C)***
Focal Mass	None
Asymmetric Density	None
Parenchymal Distortion	None
Calcification	None
Skin Thickening	None
Axillary Nodes	None

LEFT BREAST	
Breast Parenchymal Density	***Heterogeneously dense, may obscure small masses (ACR C)***
Focal Mass	None
Asymmetric Density	***UIQ focal asymmetry associated suspicious amorphous calcifications***
Parenchymal Distortion	None
Calcification	***UIQ suspicious amorphous calcifications***
Skin Thickening	None
Axillary Nodes	***Lymphadenopathy***

IMPRESSION:
RIGHT BREAST: (BI-RADS 1)
LEFT BREAST: (BI-RADS 4B)

RECOMMENDATION: Histopathological Correlation

CASE 25: 64-year-old female/ Diagnostic

Right MLO	Left MLO
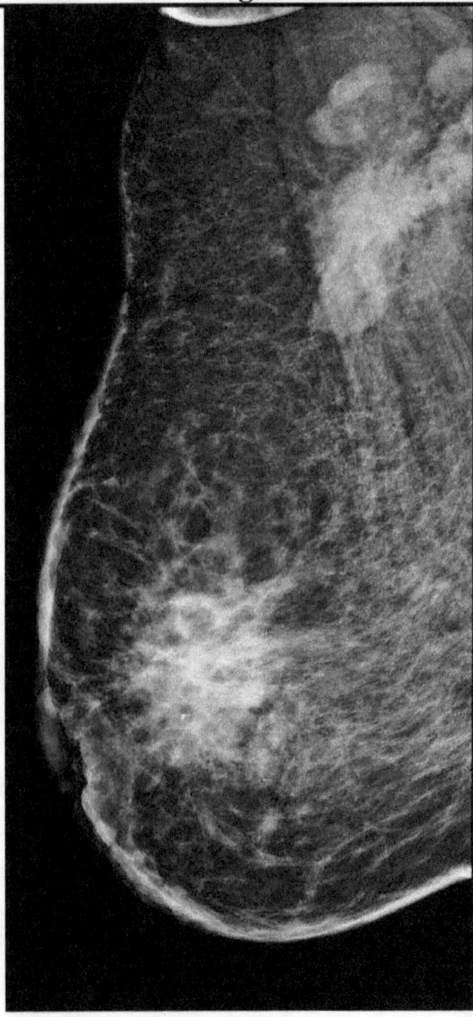	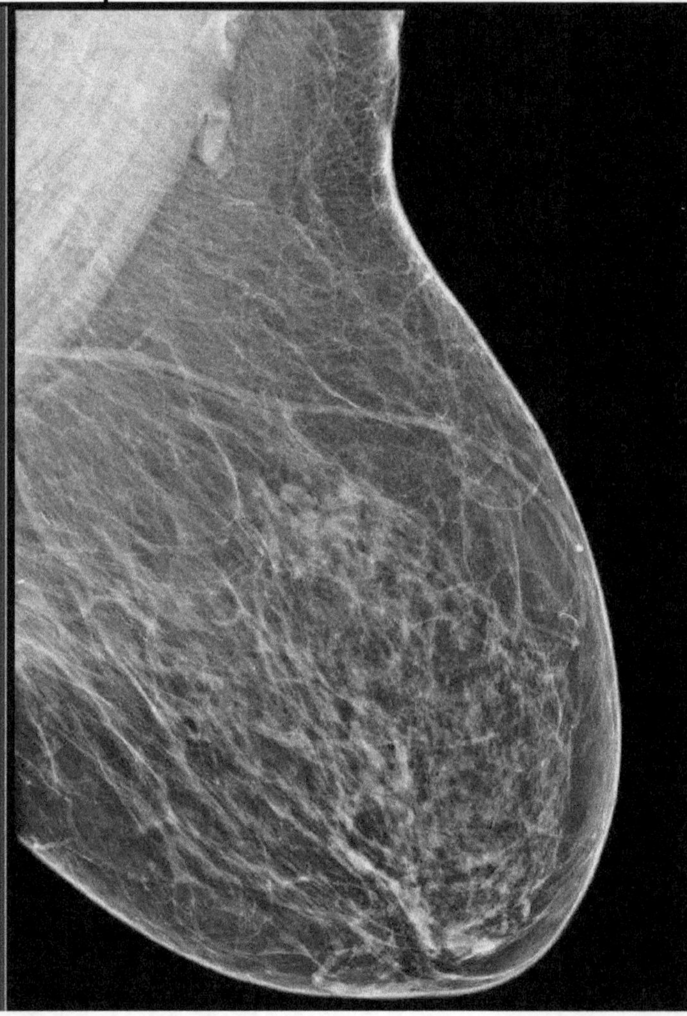

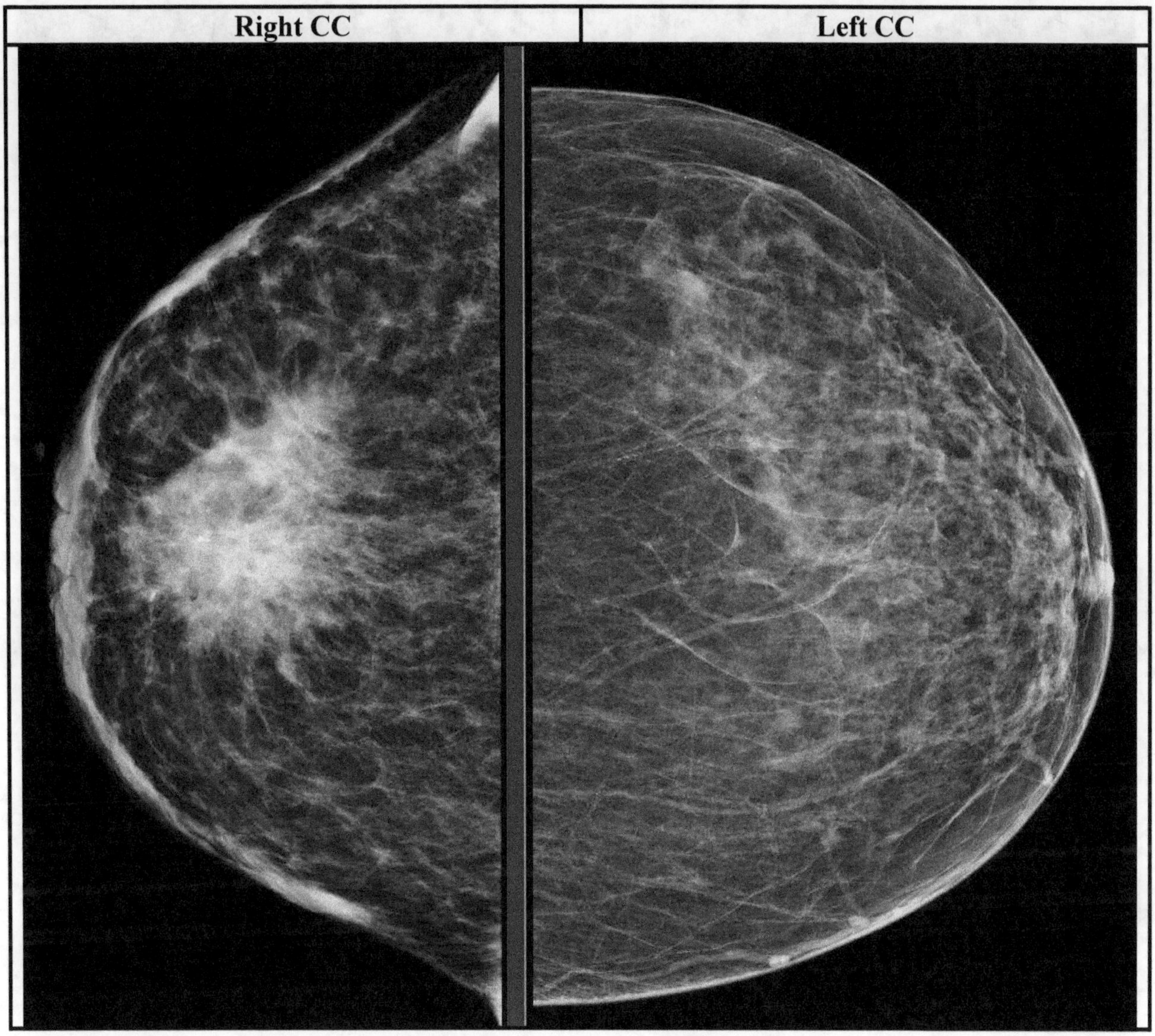
Right CC
Left CC

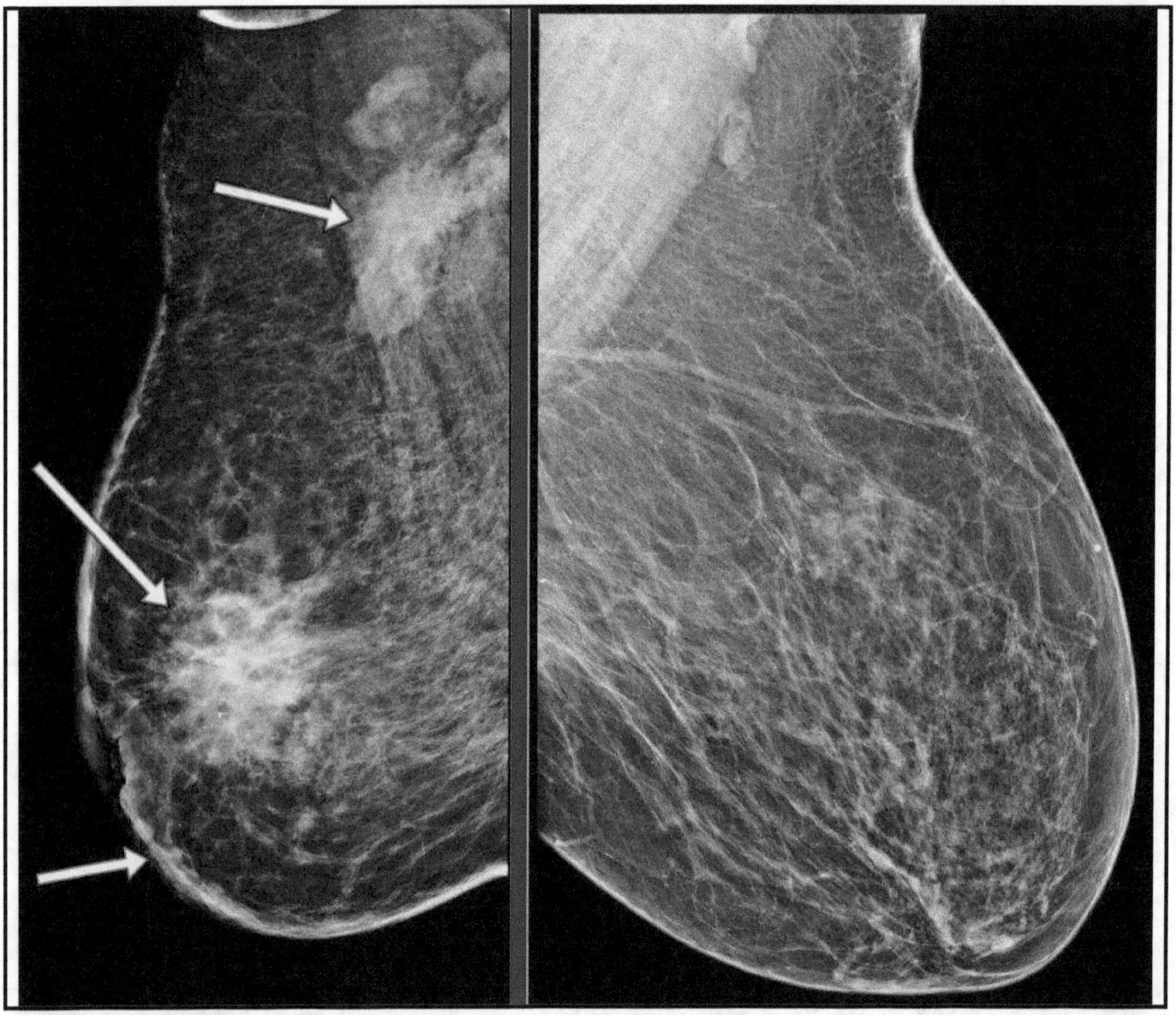

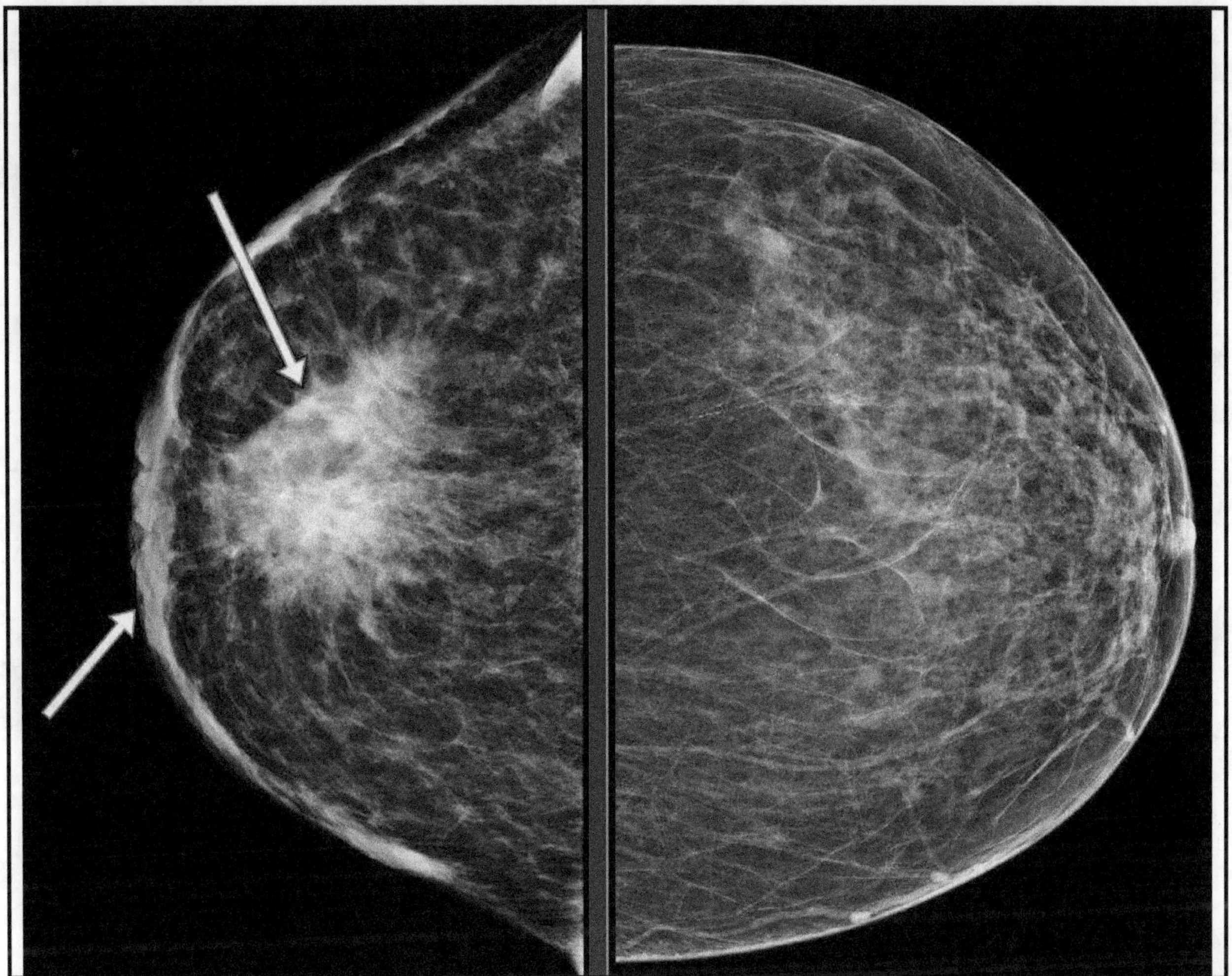

RIGHT BREAST	
Breast Parenchymal Density	***Scattered areas of fibroglandular density (ACR B)***
Focal Mass	***Retro-areolar spiculated mass lesion***
Asymmetric Density	None
Parenchymal Distortion	None
Calcification	None
Skin Thickening	***Positive***
Axillary Nodes	***lymphadenopathy***

LEFT BREAST	
Breast Parenchymal Density	***Scattered areas of fibroglandular density (ACR B)***
Focal Mass	None
Asymmetric Density	None
Parenchymal Distortion	None
Calcification	None
Skin Thickening	None
Axillary Nodes	None

IMPRESSION:

RIGHT BREAST: (BI-RADS 5)
LEFT BREAST: (BI-RADS 1)

RECOMMENDATION: Histopathological Correlation

CASE 26: 65-year-old female/ Diagnostic	
Right MLO	Left MLO
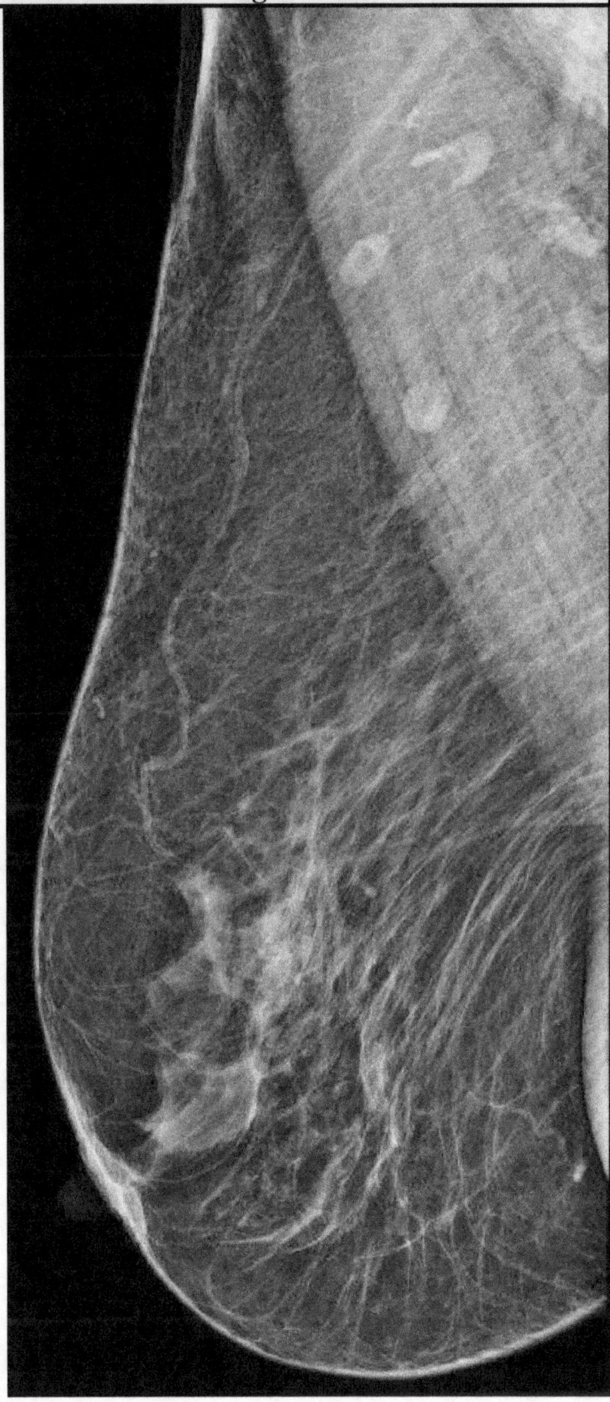	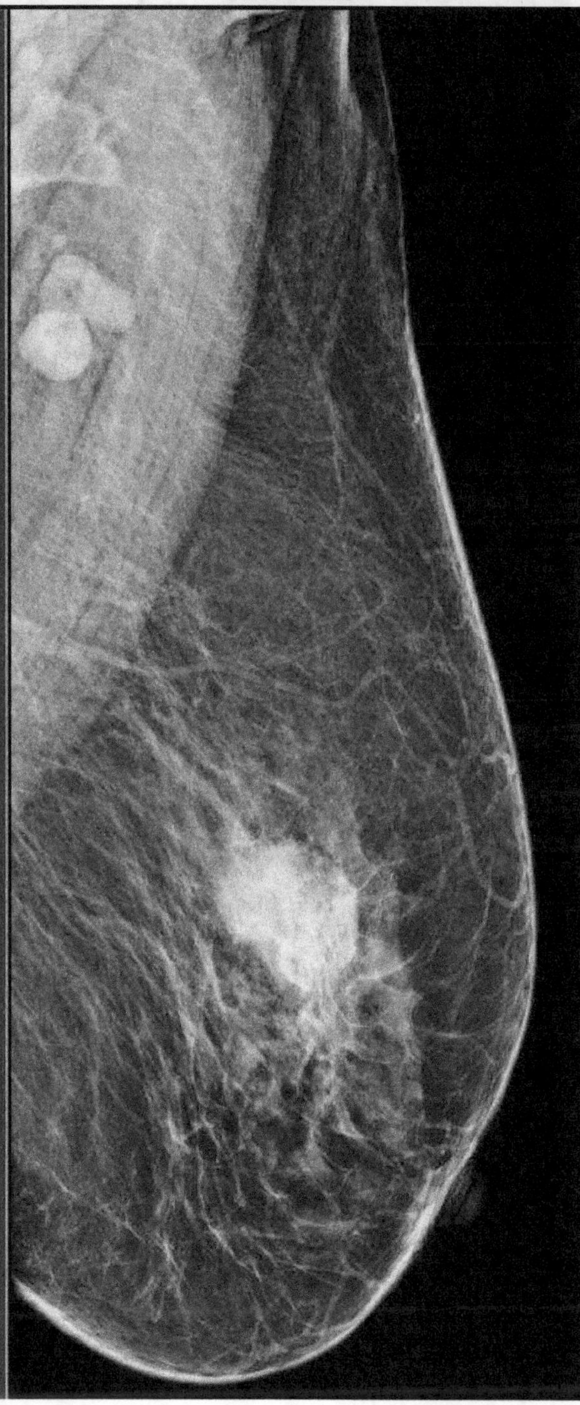

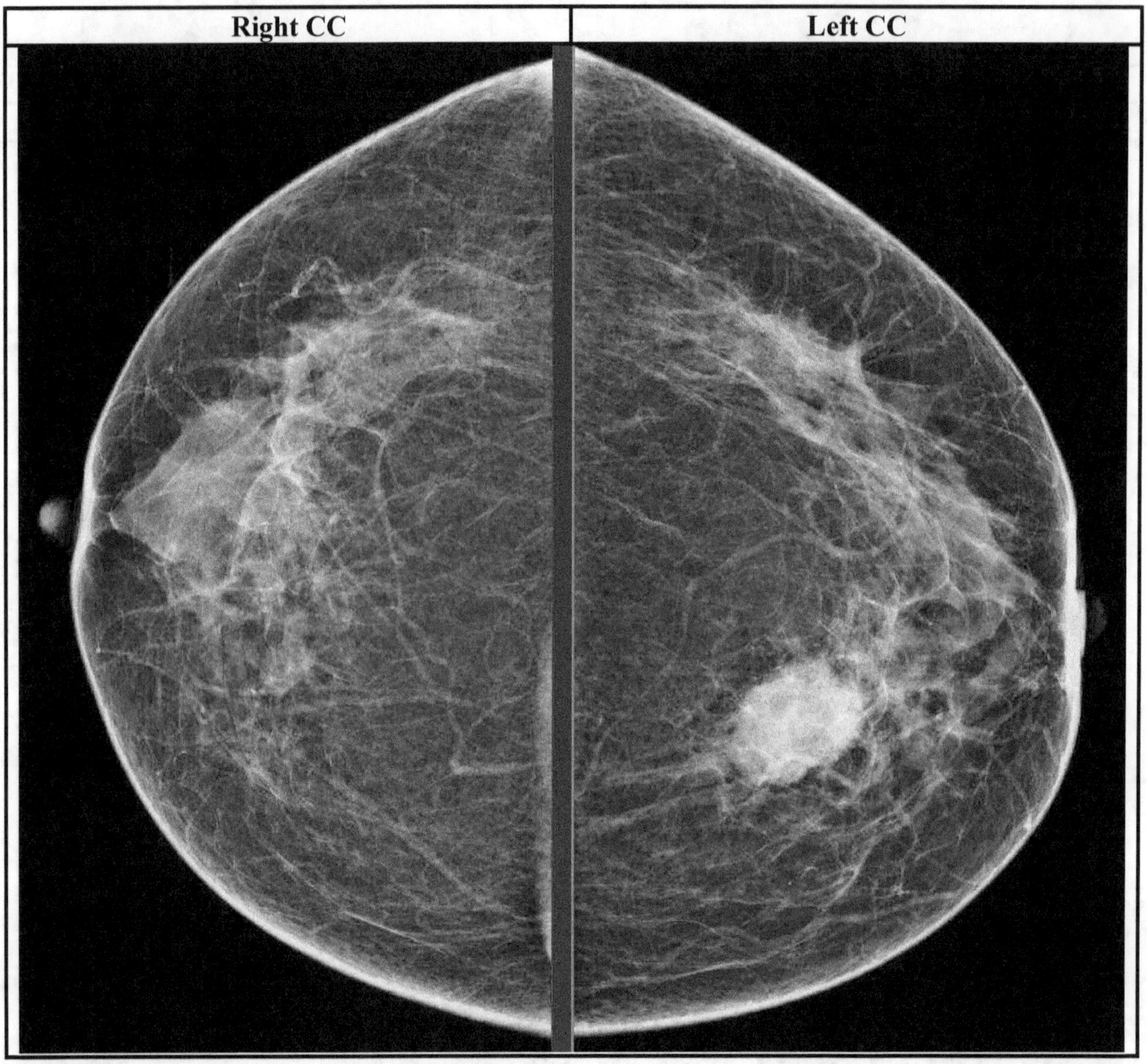
Right CC
Left CC

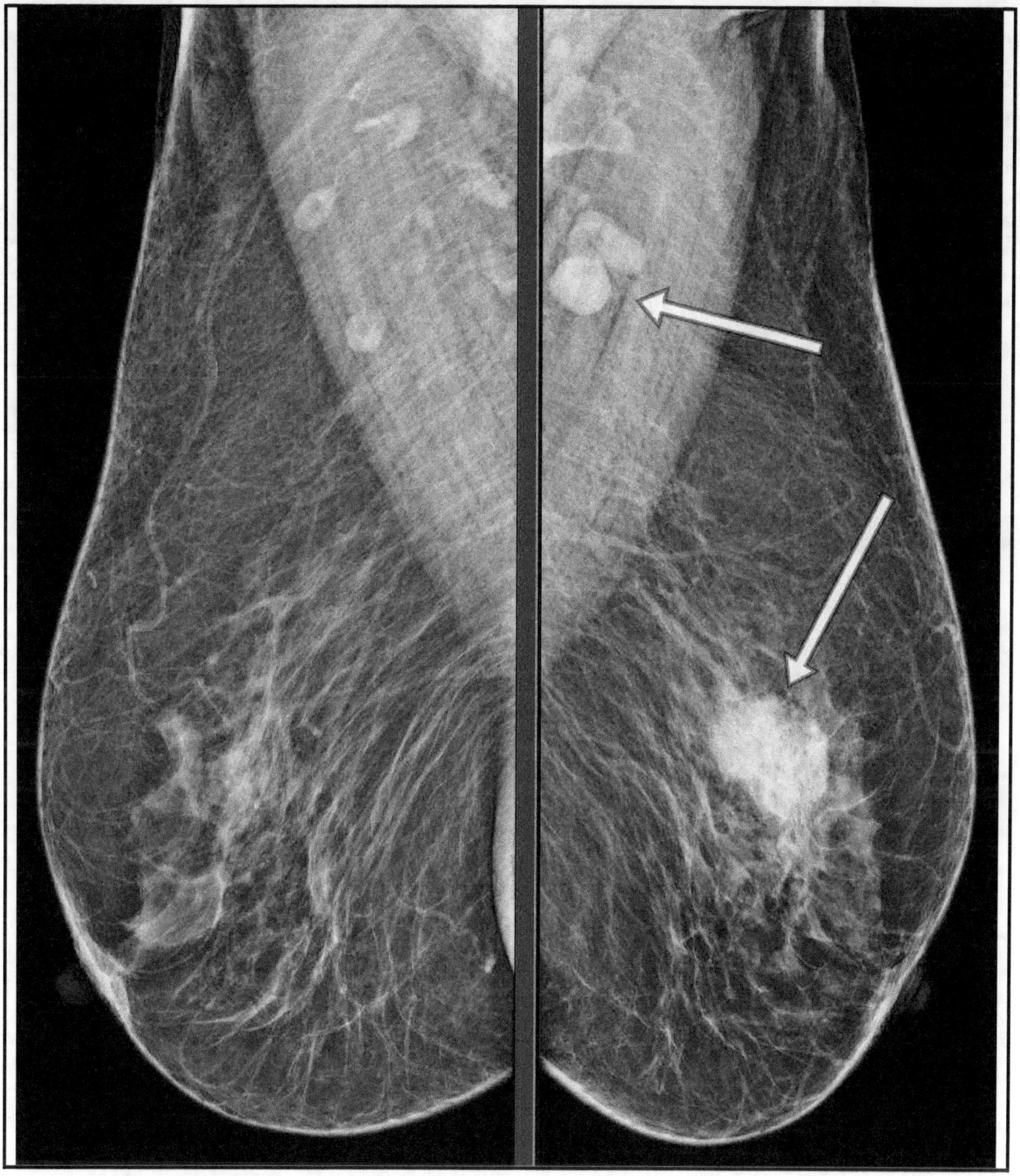

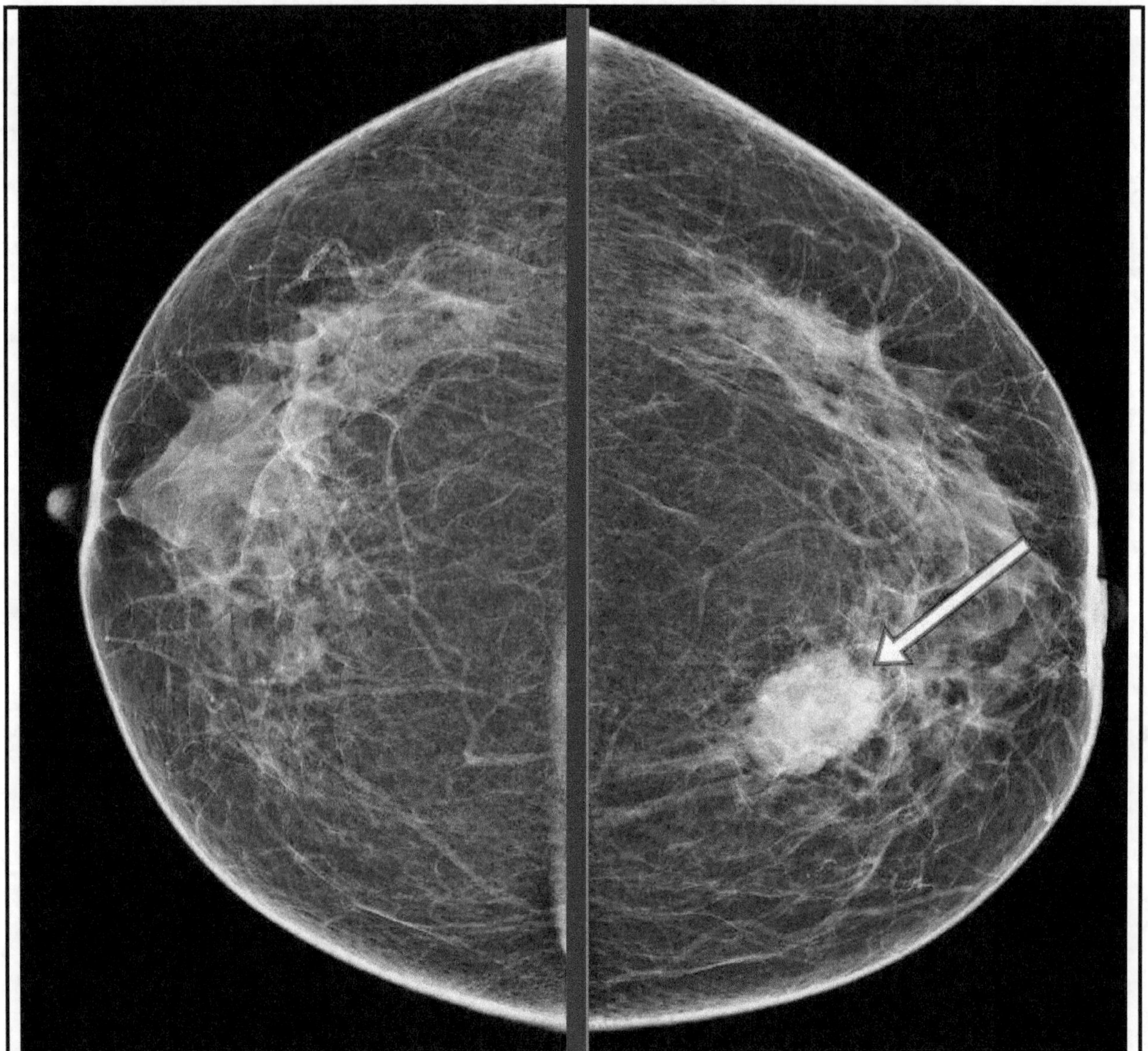

RIGHT BREAST	
Breast Parenchymal Density	***Scattered areas of fibroglandular density (ACR B)***
Focal Mass	None
Asymmetric Density	None
Parenchymal Distortion	None
Calcification	None
Skin Thickening	None
Axillary Nodes	None

LEFT BREAST	
Breast Parenchymal Density	***Scattered areas of fibroglandular density (ACR B)***
Focal Mass	***UIQ oval indistinct Mass Lesion***
Asymmetric Density	None
Parenchymal Distortion	None
Calcification	None
Skin Thickening	None
Axillary Nodes	***lymphadenopathy***

IMPRESSION:

RIGHT BREAST: (BI-RADS 1)
LEFT BREAST: (BI-RADS 4C)

RECOMMENDATION: Histopathological Correlation

CASE 27: 57-year-old female/ Diagnostic	
Right MLO	Left MLO

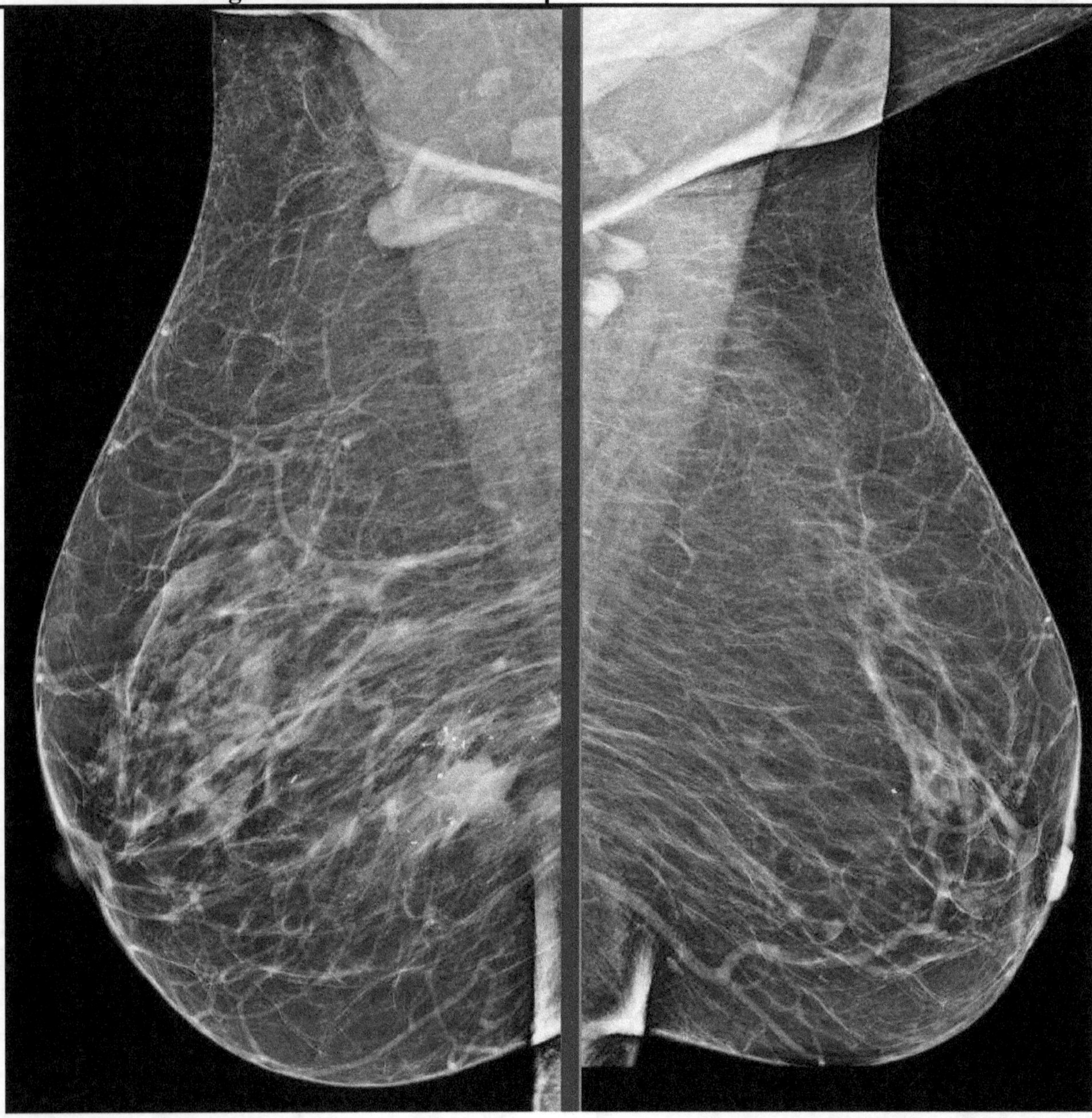

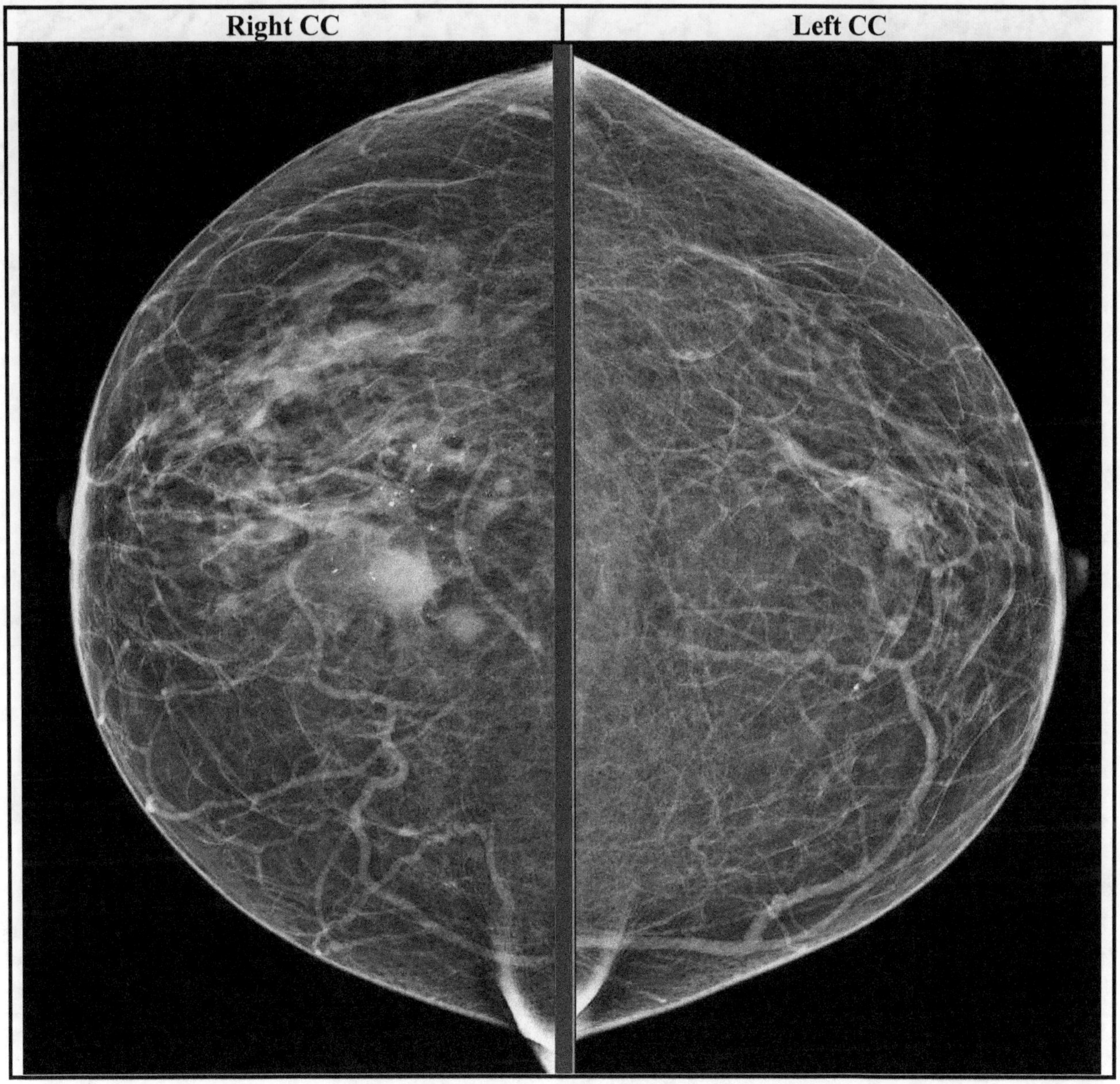
Right CC
Left CC

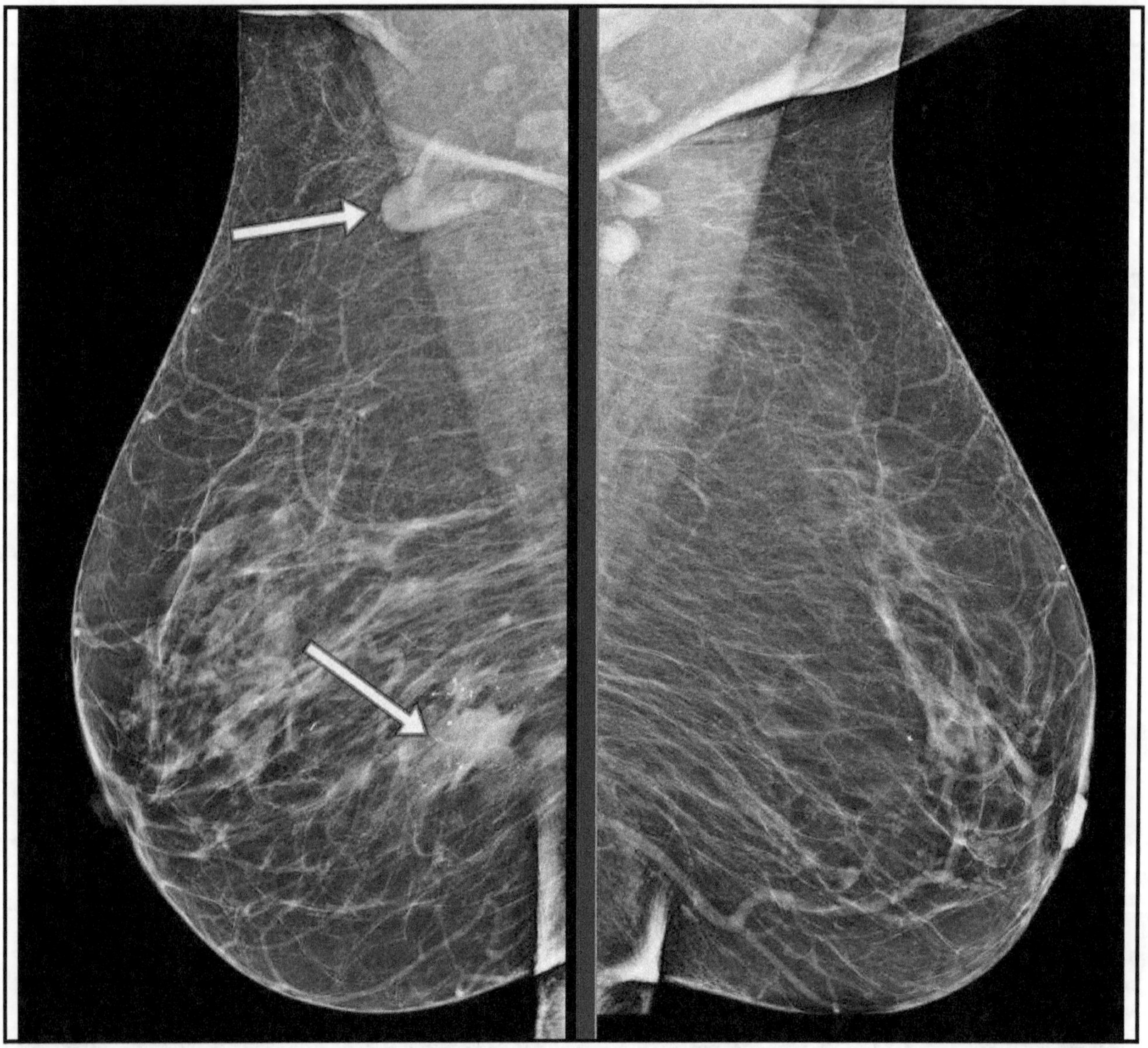

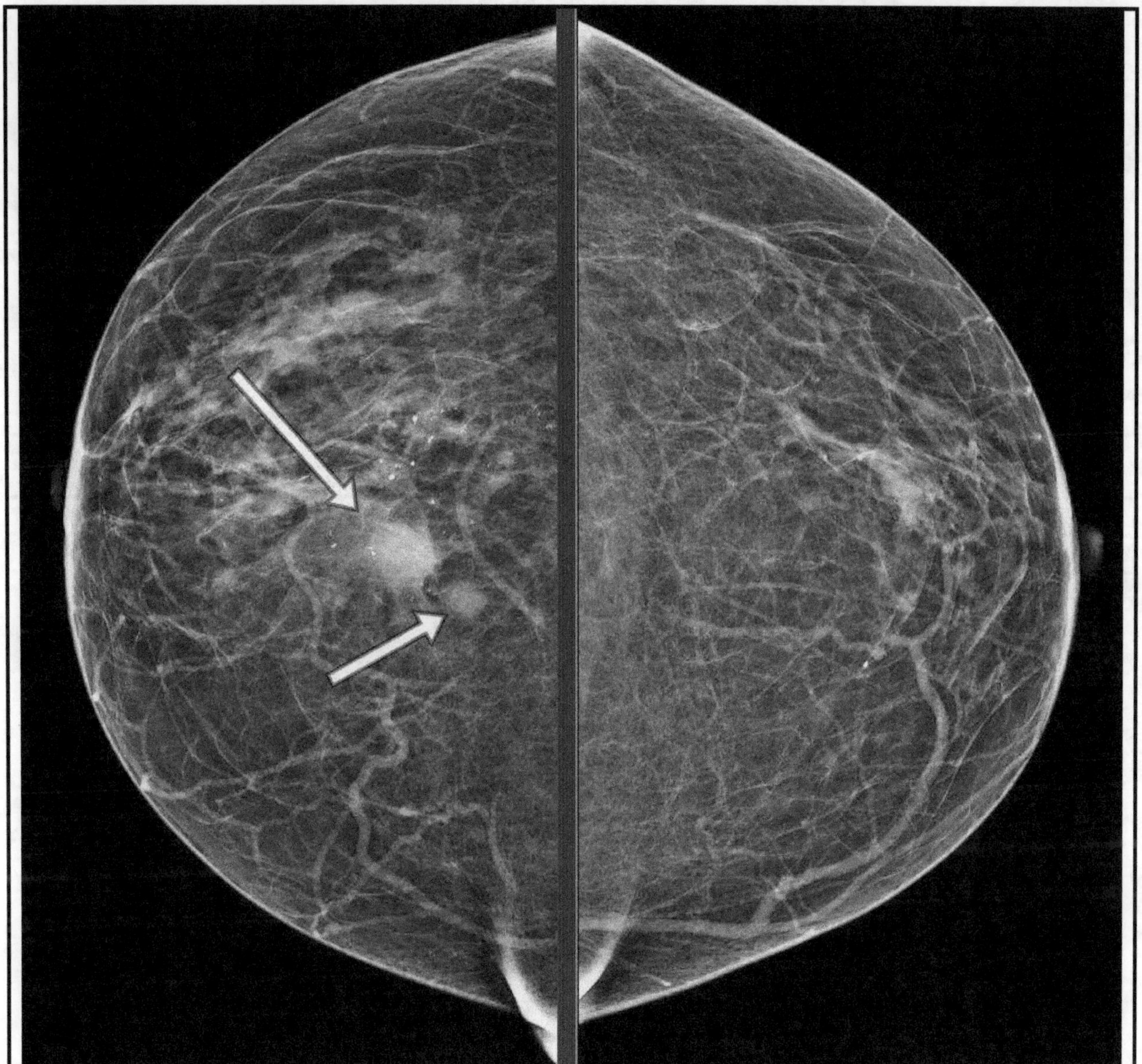

RIGHT BREAST	
Breast Parenchymal Density	***Scattered areas of fibroglandular density (ACR B)***
Focal Mass	***lower central (6 o'clock) multifocal mass lesion with micro-calcification***
Asymmetric Density	None
Parenchymal Distortion	None
Calcification	None
Skin Thickening	None
Axillary Nodes	***lymphadenopathy***

LEFT BREAST	
Breast Parenchymal Density	***Scattered areas of fibroglandular density (ACR B)***
Focal Mass	None
Asymmetric Density	None
Parenchymal Distortion	None
Calcification	None
Skin Thickening	None
Axillary Nodes	None

IMPRESSION:

RIGHT BREAST: (BI-RADS 4C)
LEFT BREAST: (BI-RADS 1)

RECOMMENDATION: Histopathological Correlation

CASE 28: 71-year-old female/ Diagnostic

Right MLO	**Left MLO**

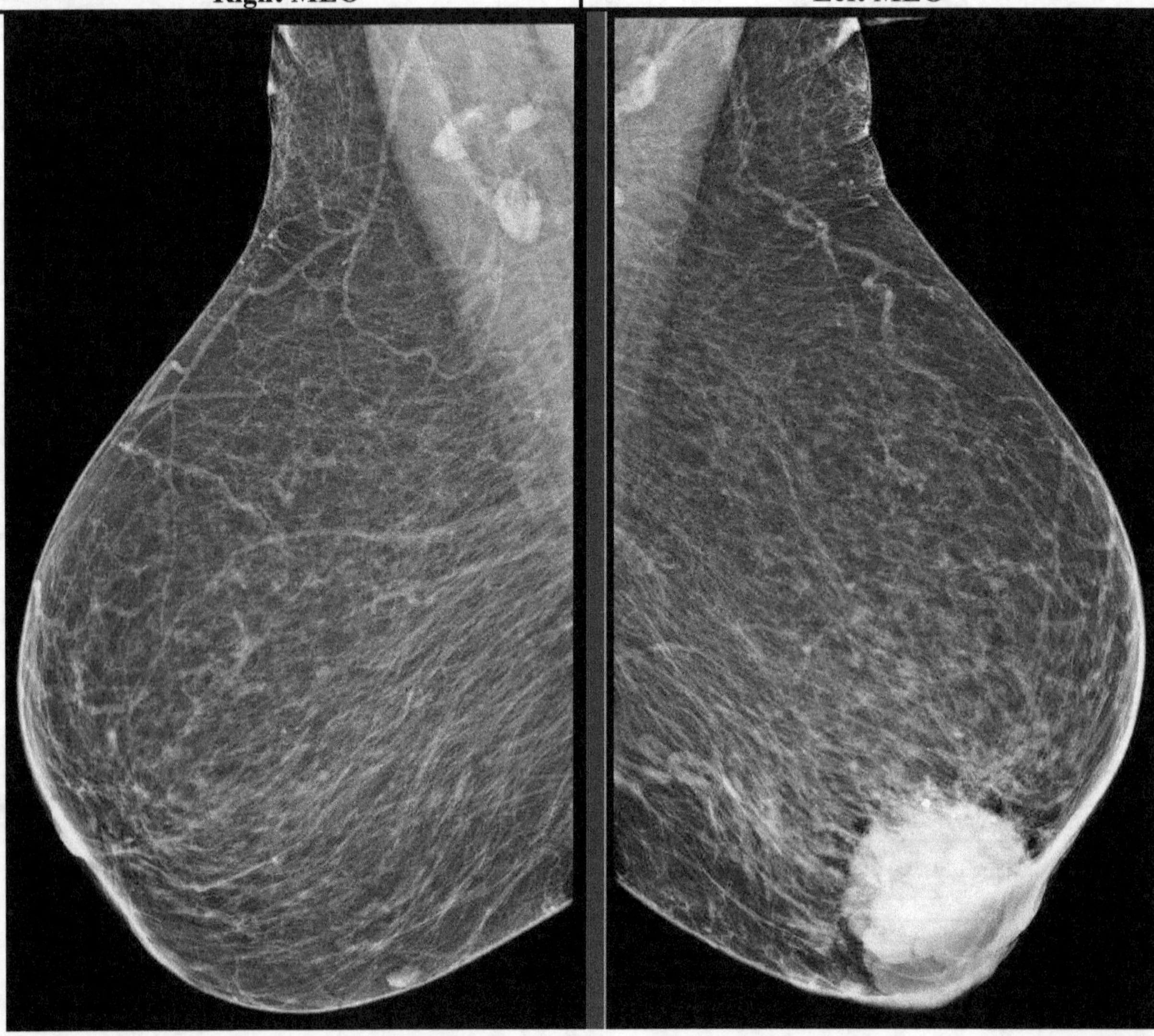

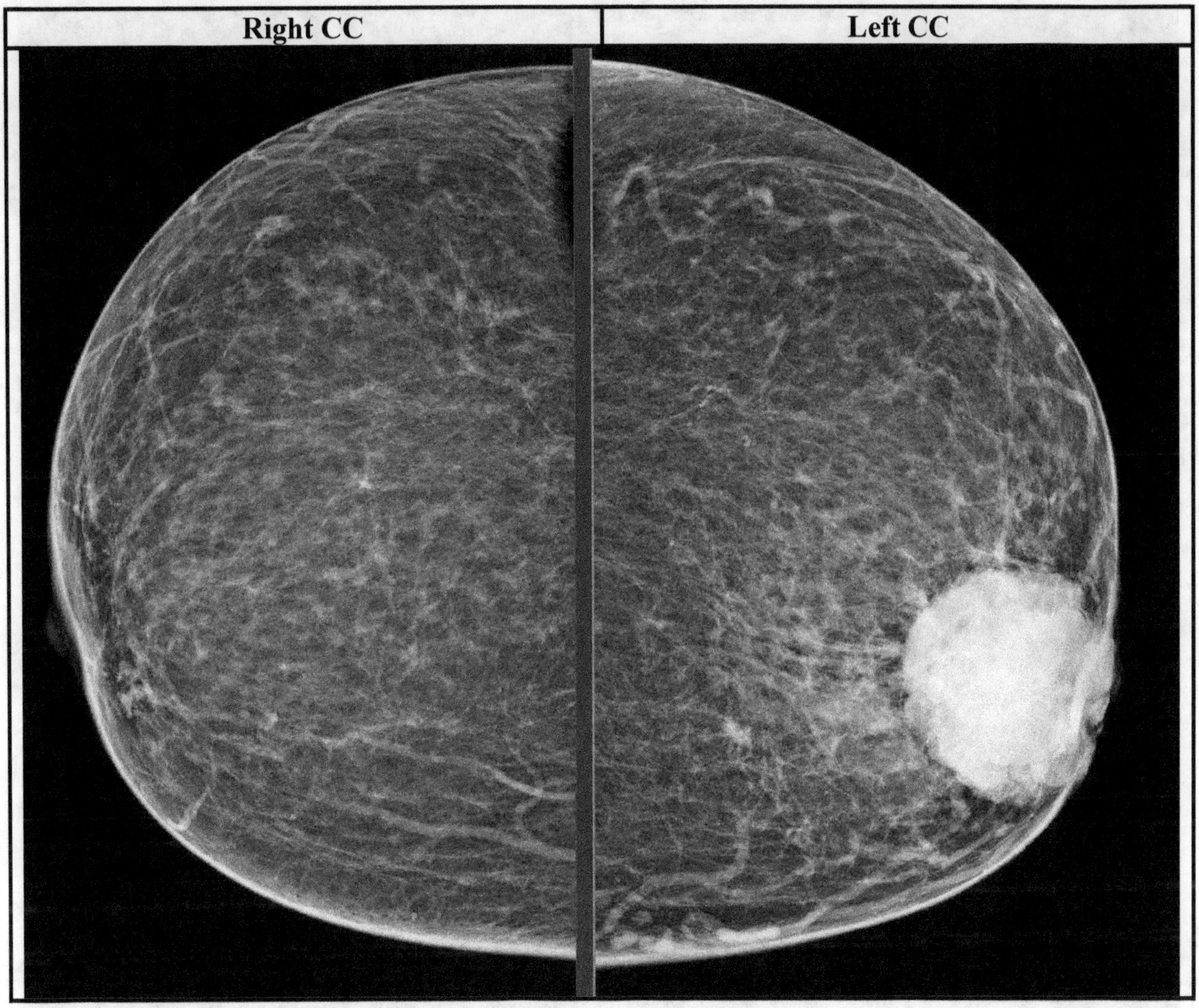
Right CC
Left CC

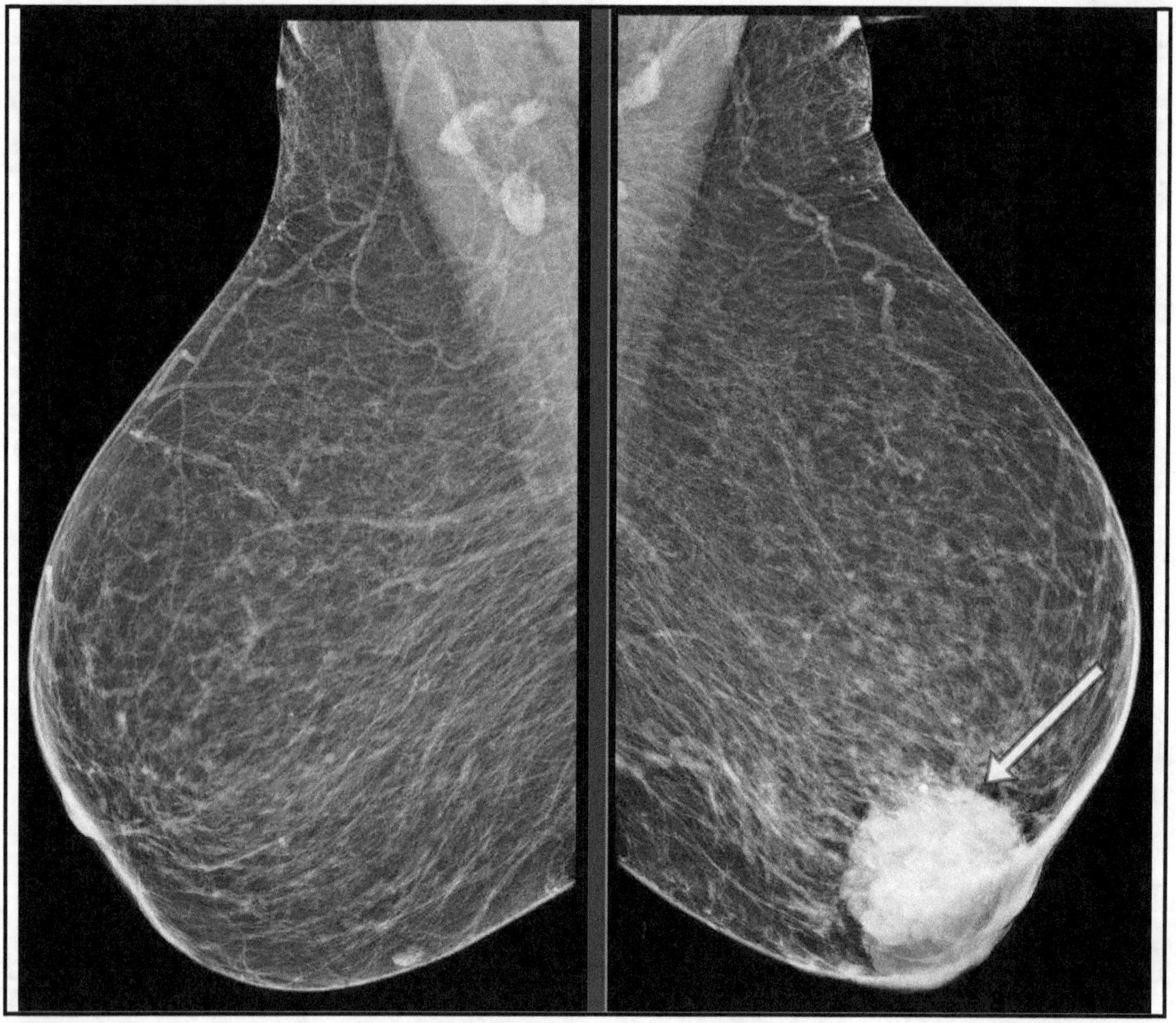

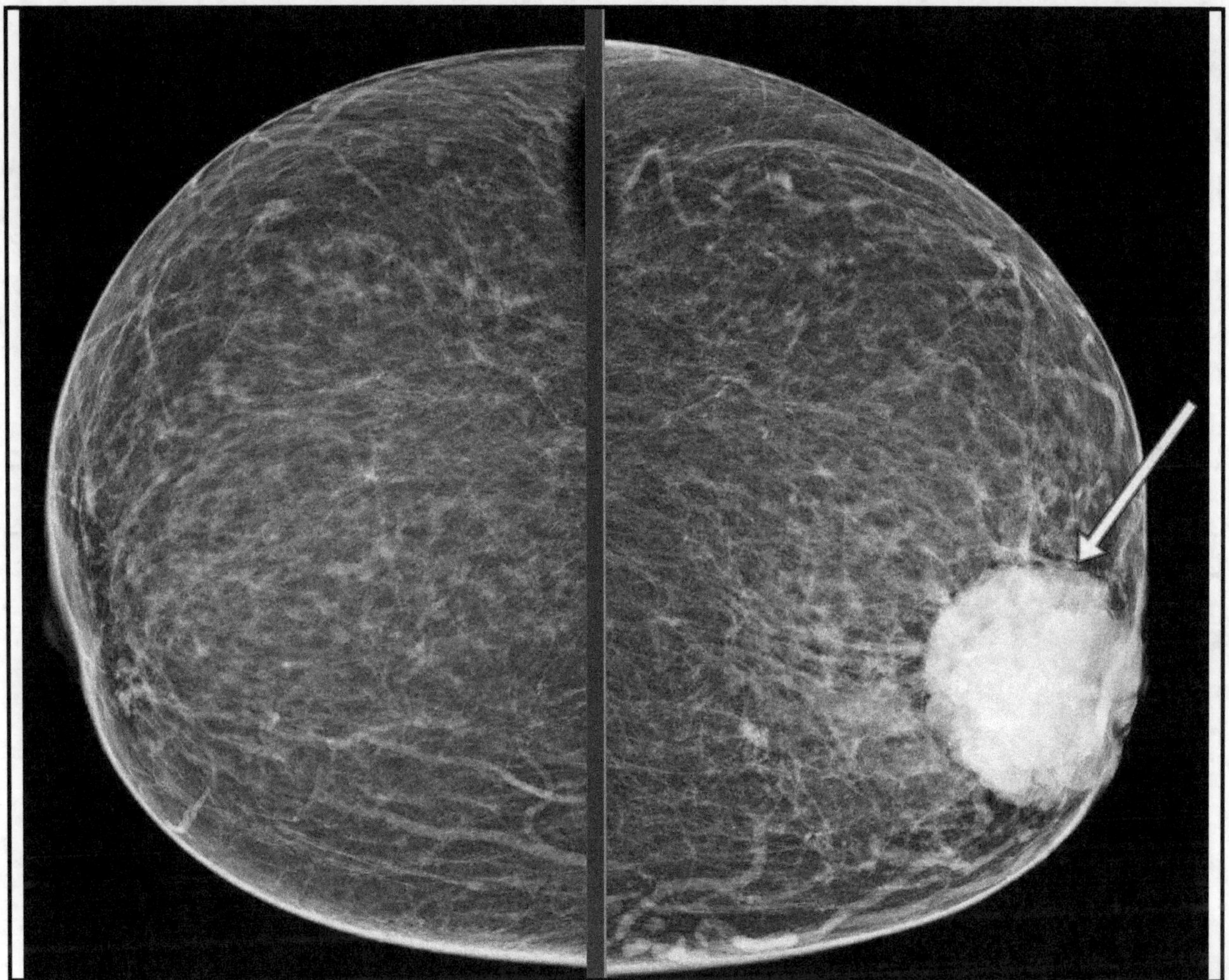

RIGHT BREAST	
Breast Parenchymal Density	***Scattered areas of fibroglandular density (ACR B)***
Focal Mass	None
Asymmetric Density	None
Parenchymal Distortion	None
Calcification	None
Skin Thickening	None
Axillary Nodes	None

LEFT BREAST	
Breast Parenchymal Density	***Scattered areas of fibroglandular density (ACR B)***
Focal Mass	***Nipple areola round complex lobulated mass lesion***
Asymmetric Density	None
Parenchymal Distortion	None
Calcification	None
Skin Thickening	None
Axillary Nodes	***Lymphadenopathy***

IMPRESSION:

RIGHT BREAST: (BI-RADS 1)
LEFT BREAST: (BI-RADS 5)

RECOMMENDATION: Histopathological Correlation

CASE 29: 44-year-old female/ Diagnostic

Right MLO	Left MLO

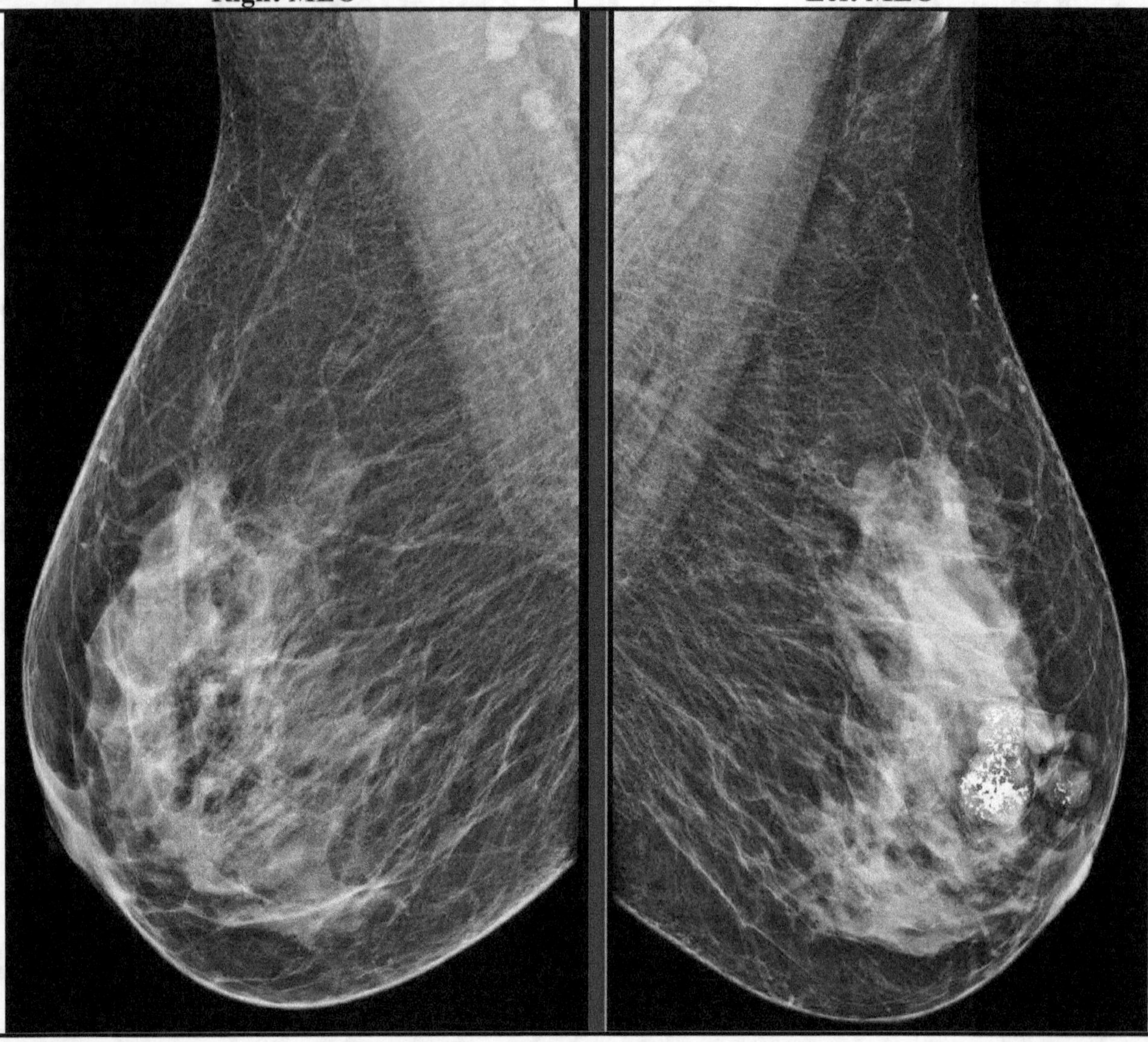

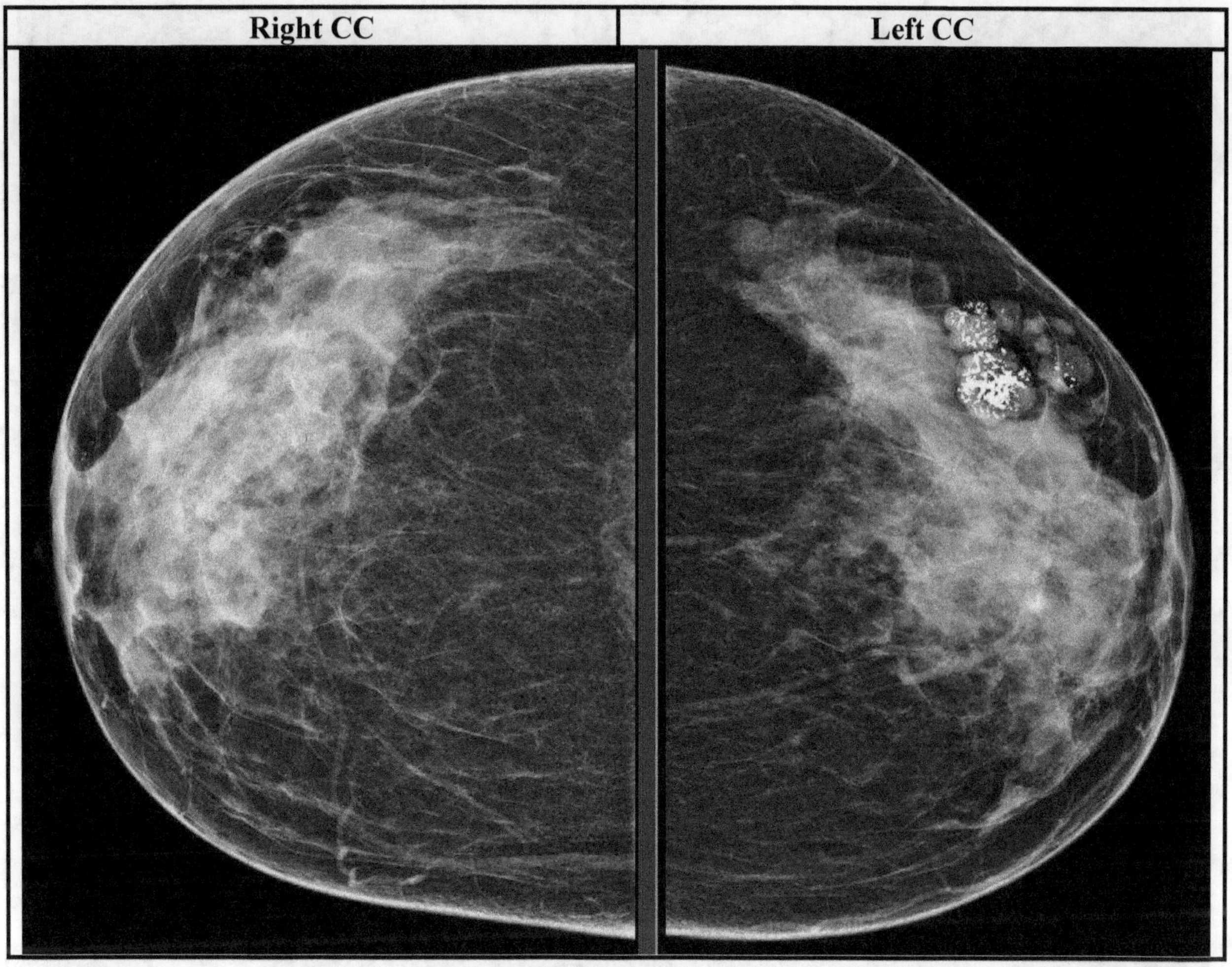
Right CC
Left CC

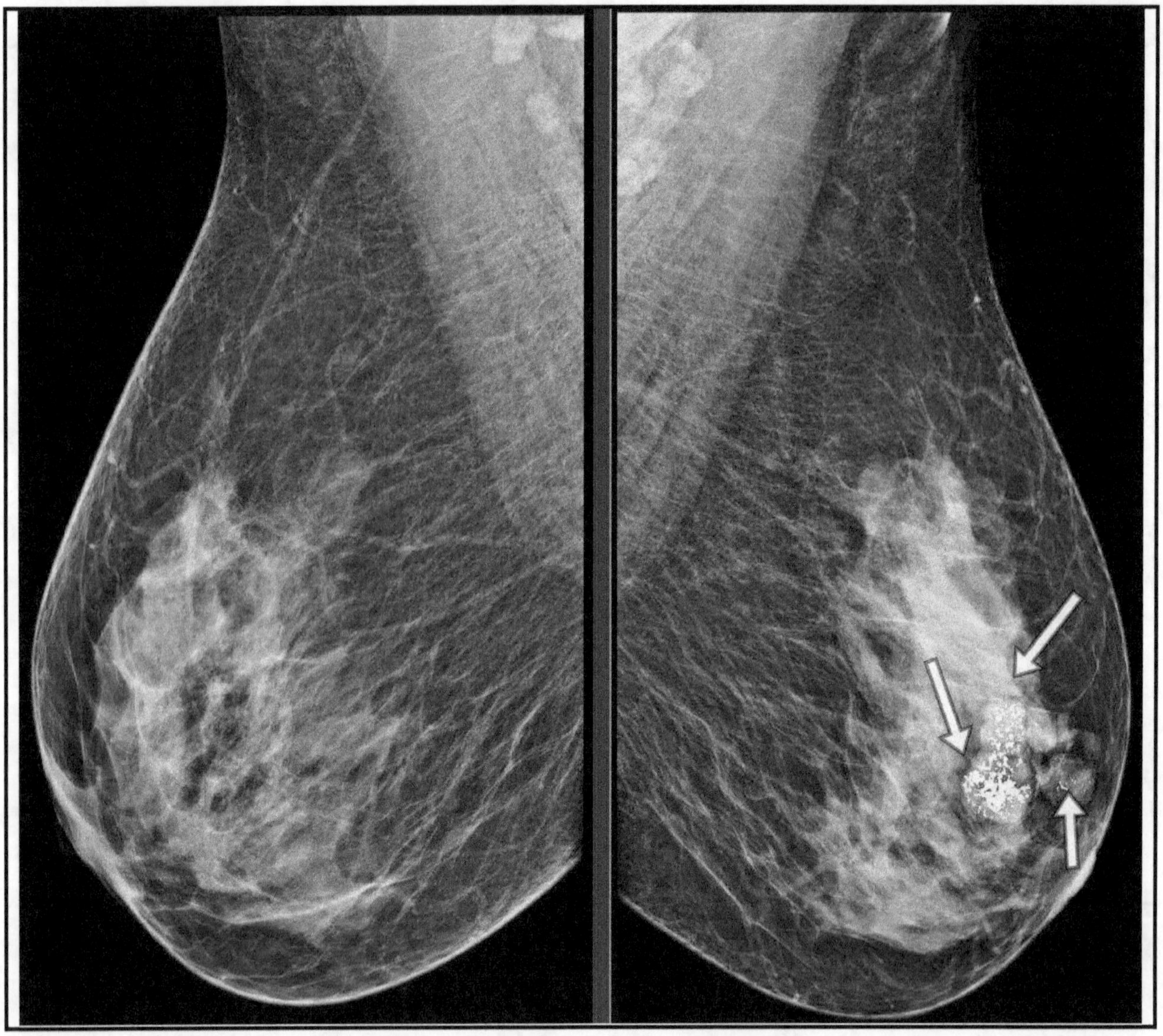

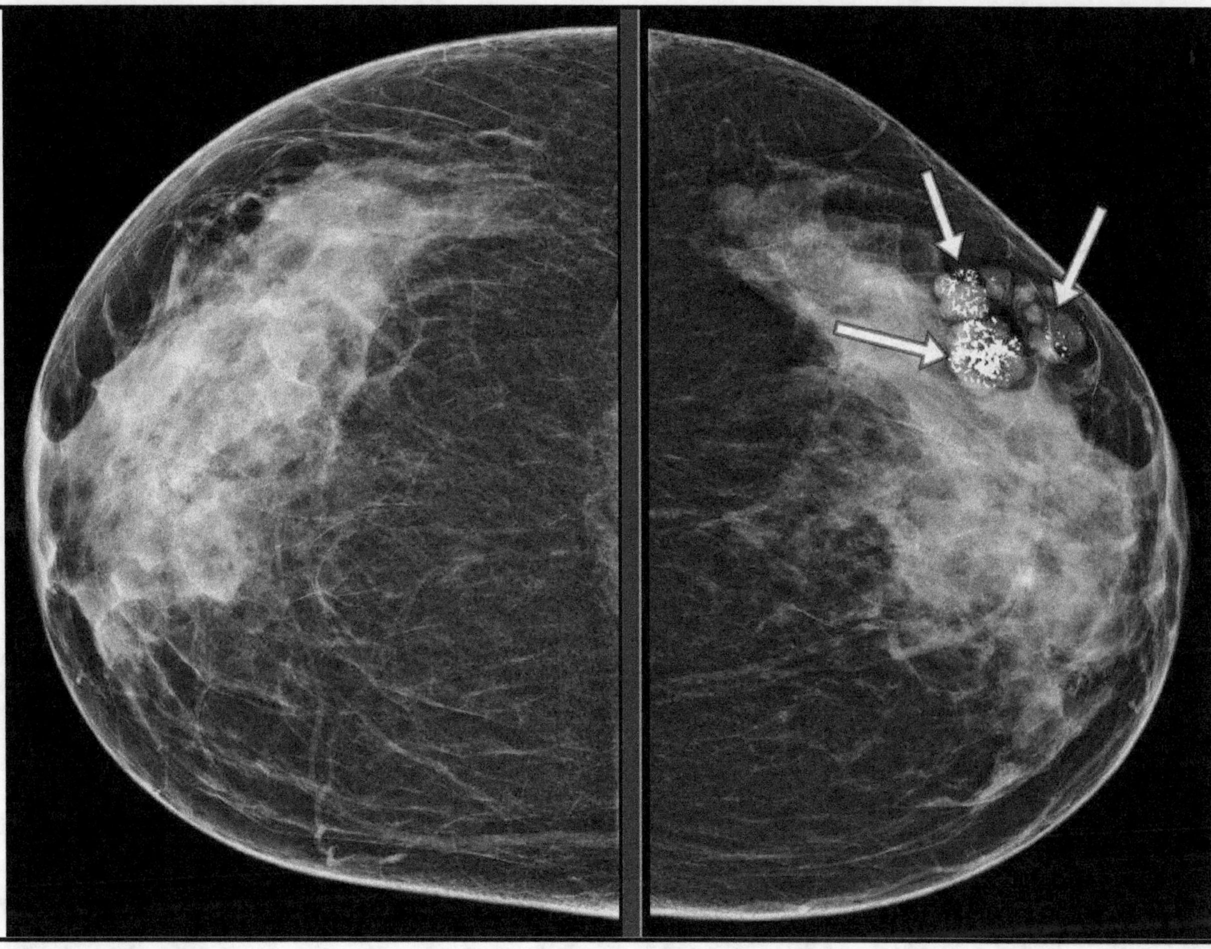

RIGHT BREAST	
Breast Parenchymal Density	***Heterogeneously dense, may obscure small masses (ACR C)***
Focal Mass	None
Asymmetric Density	None
Parenchymal Distortion	None
Calcification	None
Skin Thickening	None
Axillary Nodes	None

LEFT BREAST	
Breast Parenchymal Density	***Heterogeneously dense, may obscure small masses (ACR C)***
Focal Mass	***UOQ multiple involuted fibroadenomas (Coarse calcifications)***
Asymmetric Density	None
Parenchymal Distortion	None
Calcification	***UOQ Coarse calcifications***
Skin Thickening	None
Axillary Nodes	None

IMPRESSION:

RIGHT BREAST: (BI-RADS 1) LEFT BREAST: (BI-RADS 2) **RECOMMENDATION:** Routine Annual screening

CASE 30: 58-year-old female/ Diagnostic	
Right MLO	**Left MLO**

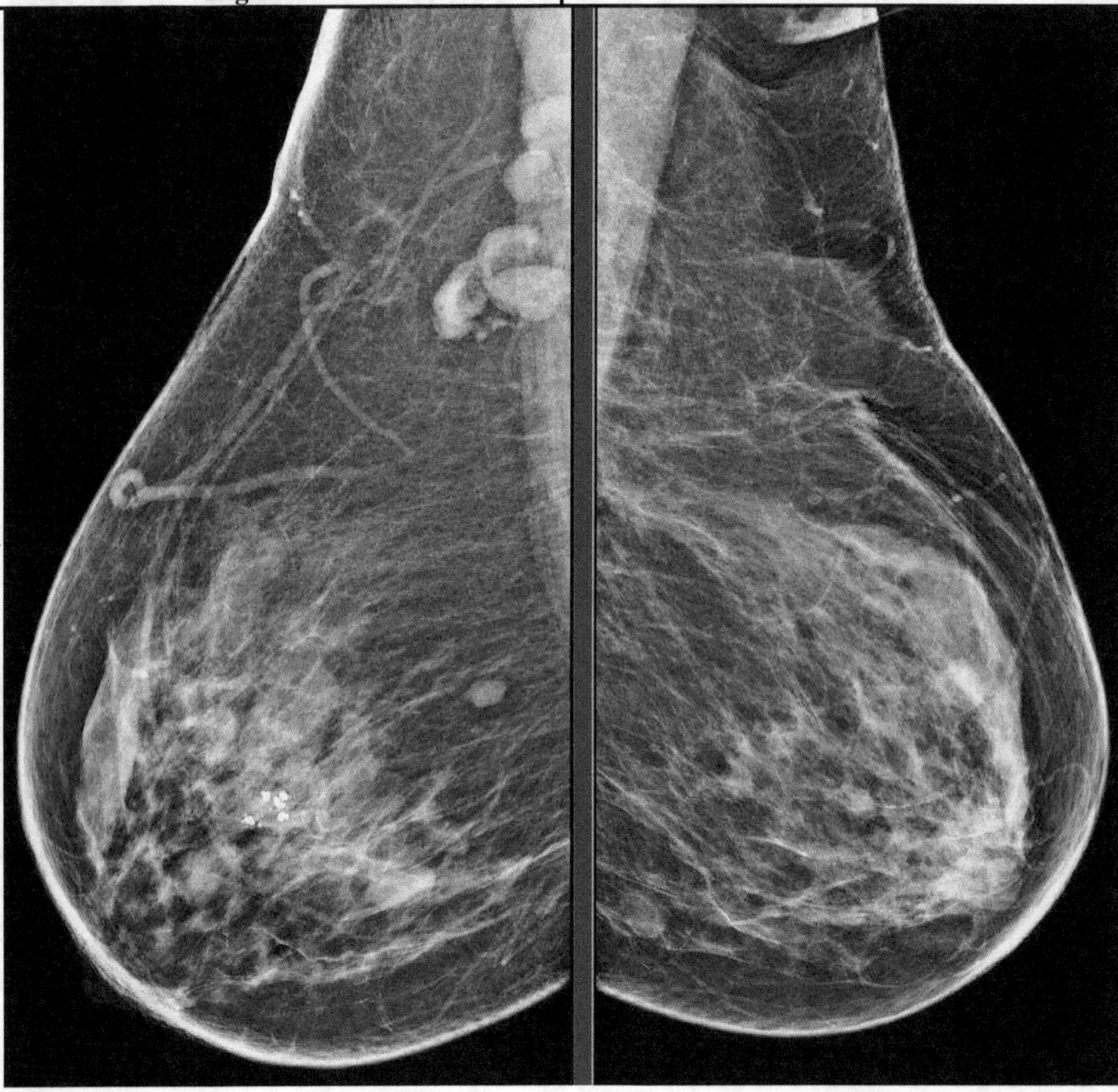

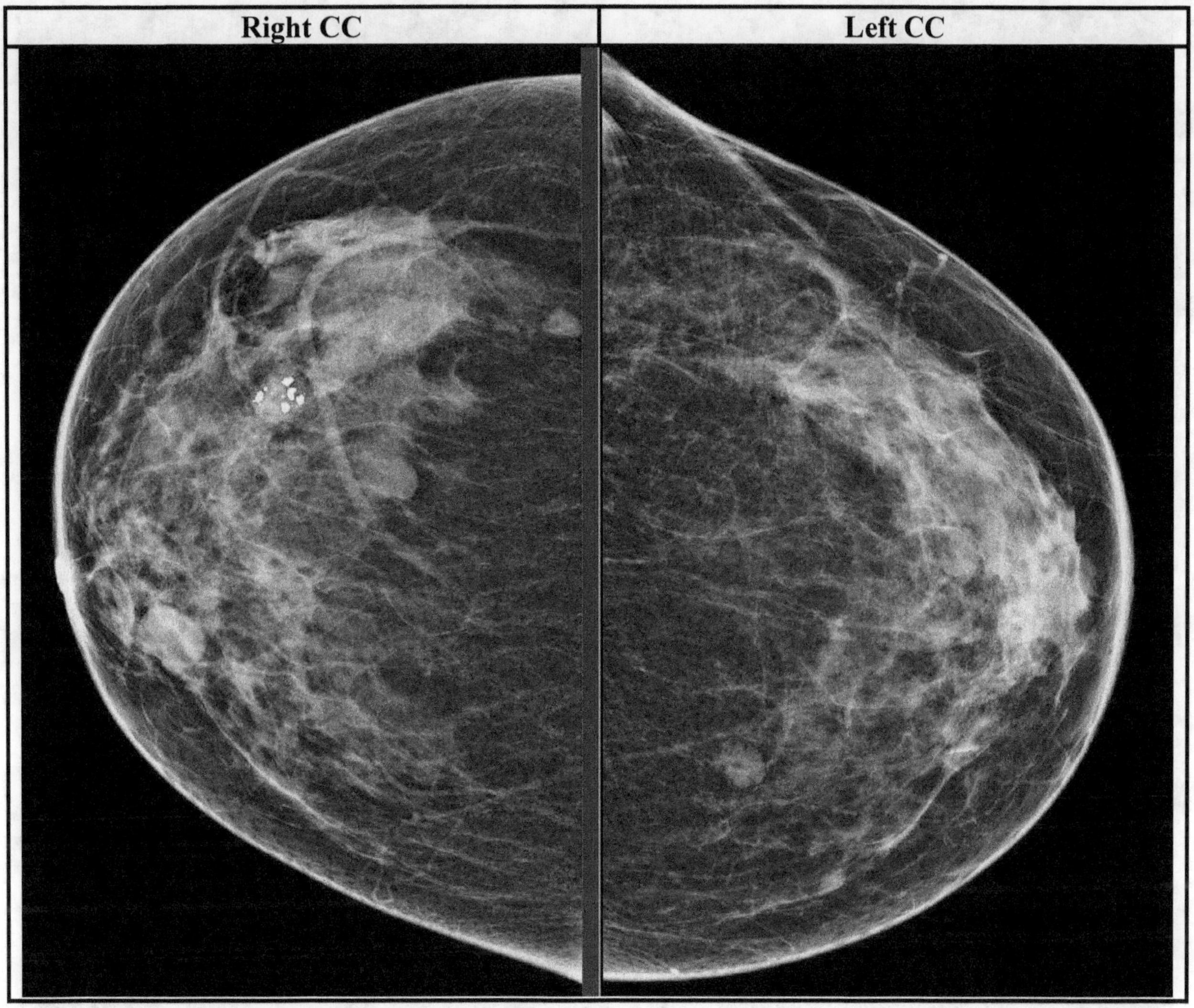
Right CC
Left CC

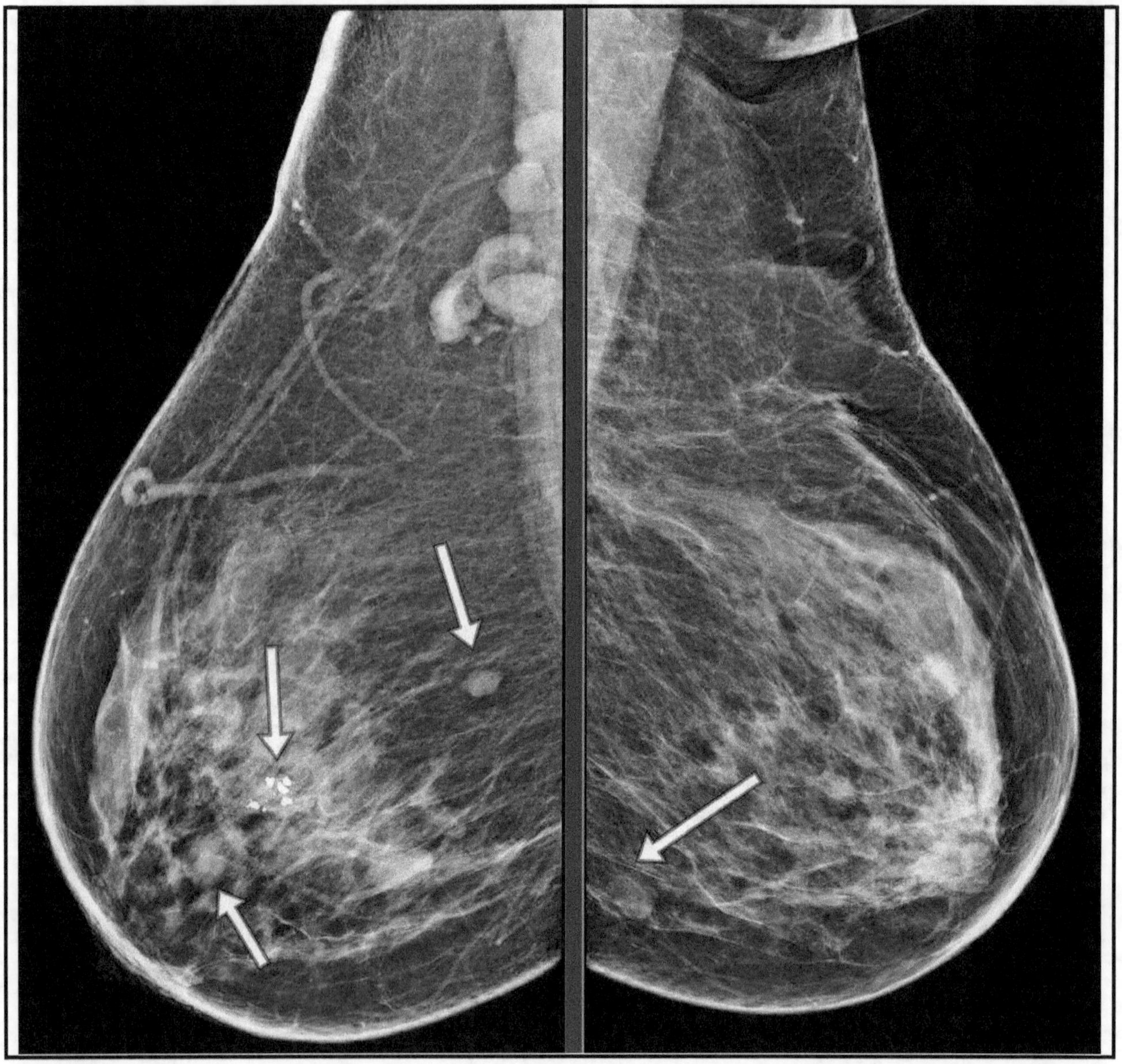

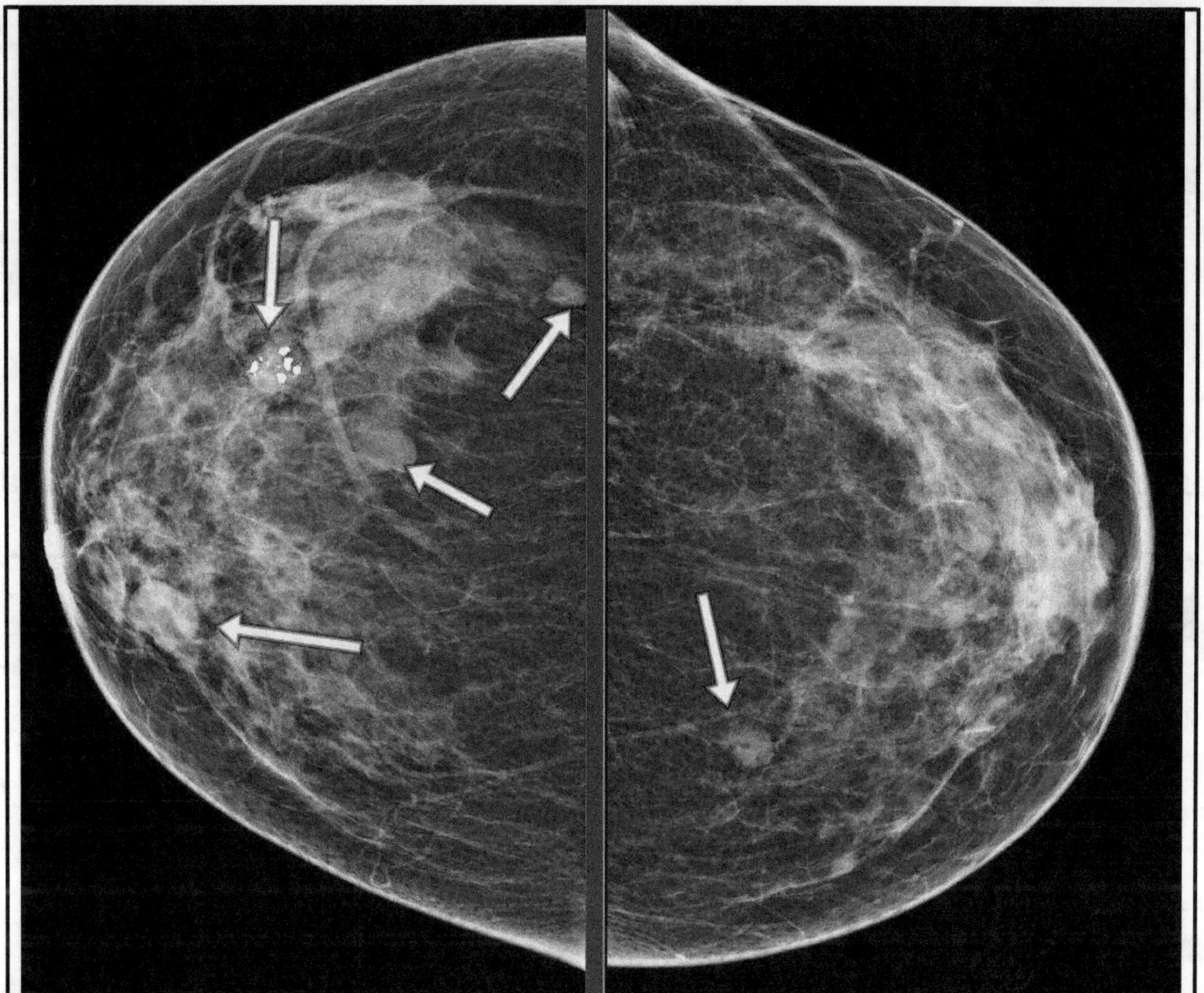

RIGHT BREAST	
Breast Parenchymal Density	***Heterogeneously dense, may obscure small masses (ACR C)***
Focal Mass	***Multiple oval circumscribed mass lesions***
Asymmetric Density	None
Parenchymal Distortion	None
Calcification	***UOQ Coarse calcification (involuted fibroadenomas)***
Skin Thickening	None
Axillary Nodes	None

LEFT BREAST	
Breast Parenchymal Density	***Heterogeneously dense, may obscure small masses (ACR C)***
Focal Mass	***LIQ Oval circumscribed mass lesions***
Asymmetric Density	None
Parenchymal Distortion	None
Calcification	None
Skin Thickening	None
Axillary Nodes	None

IMPRESSION:
RIGHT BREAST: (BI-RADS 0)
LEFT BREAST: (BI-RADS 0)

RECOMMENDATION: US Correlation

US demonstrate bilateral multiple fibroadenomas for short term follow-up

CASE 31: 43-year-old female/ Diagnostic

Right MLO	Left MLO

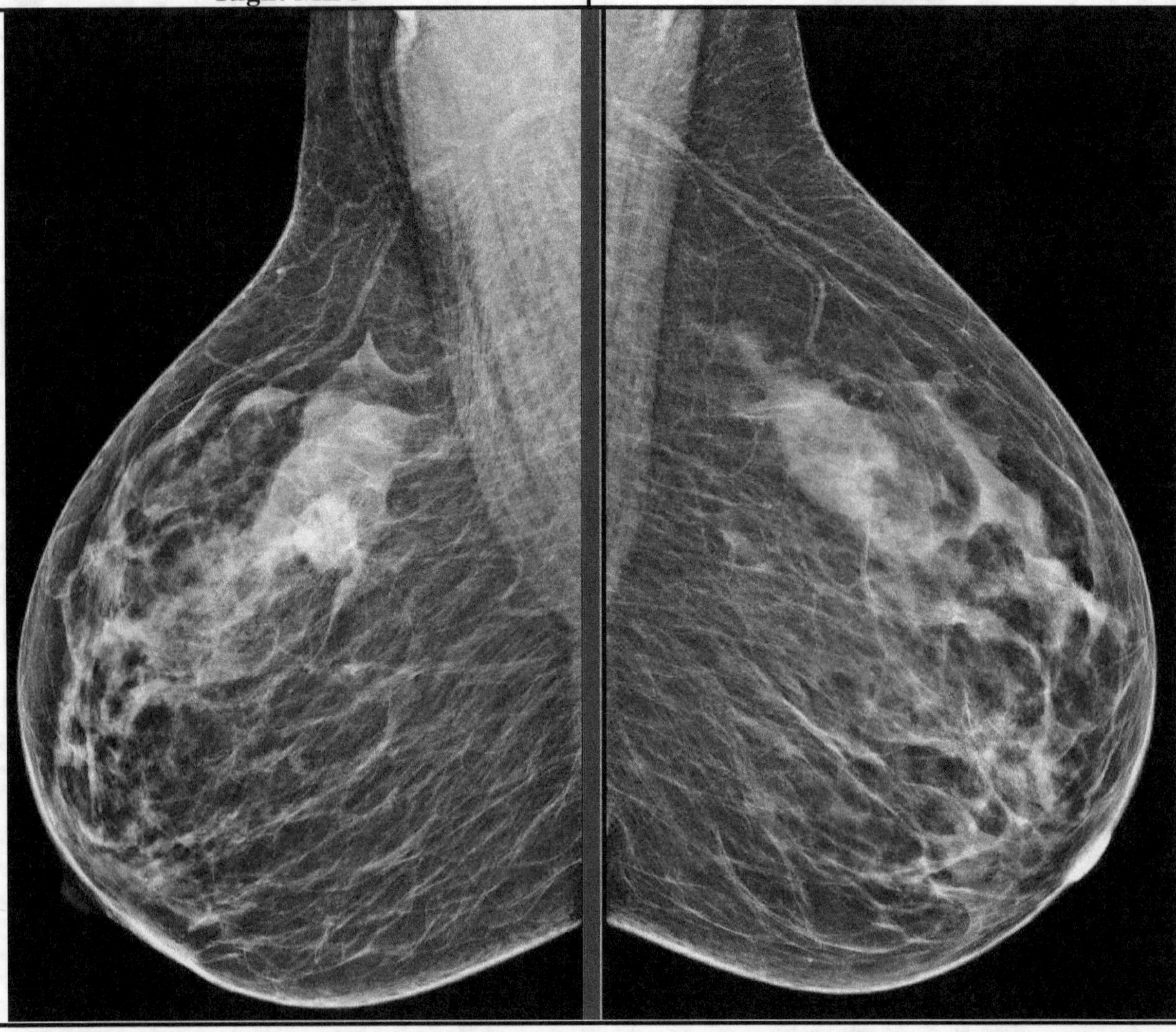

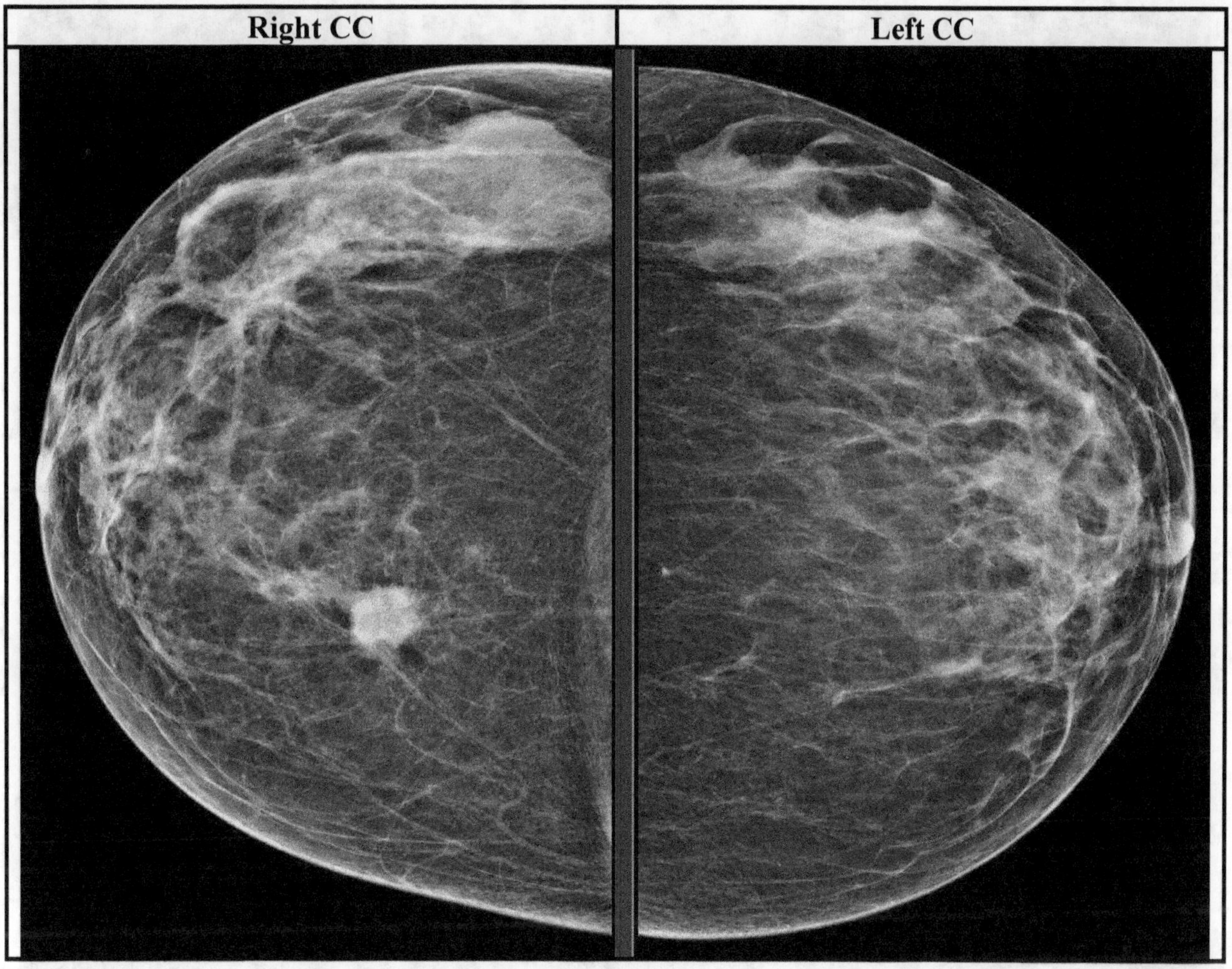
Right CC
Left CC

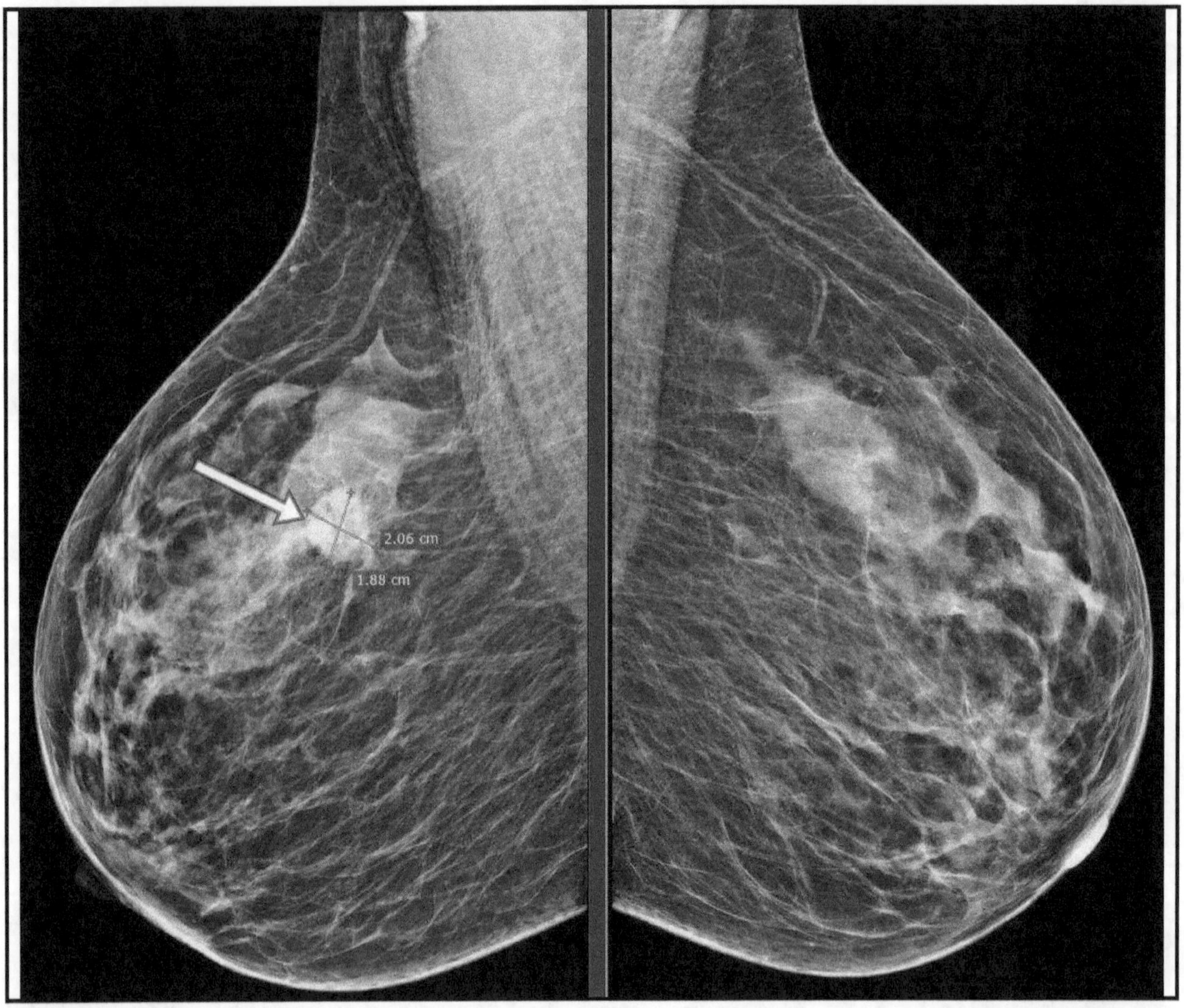
2.06 cm
1.88 cm

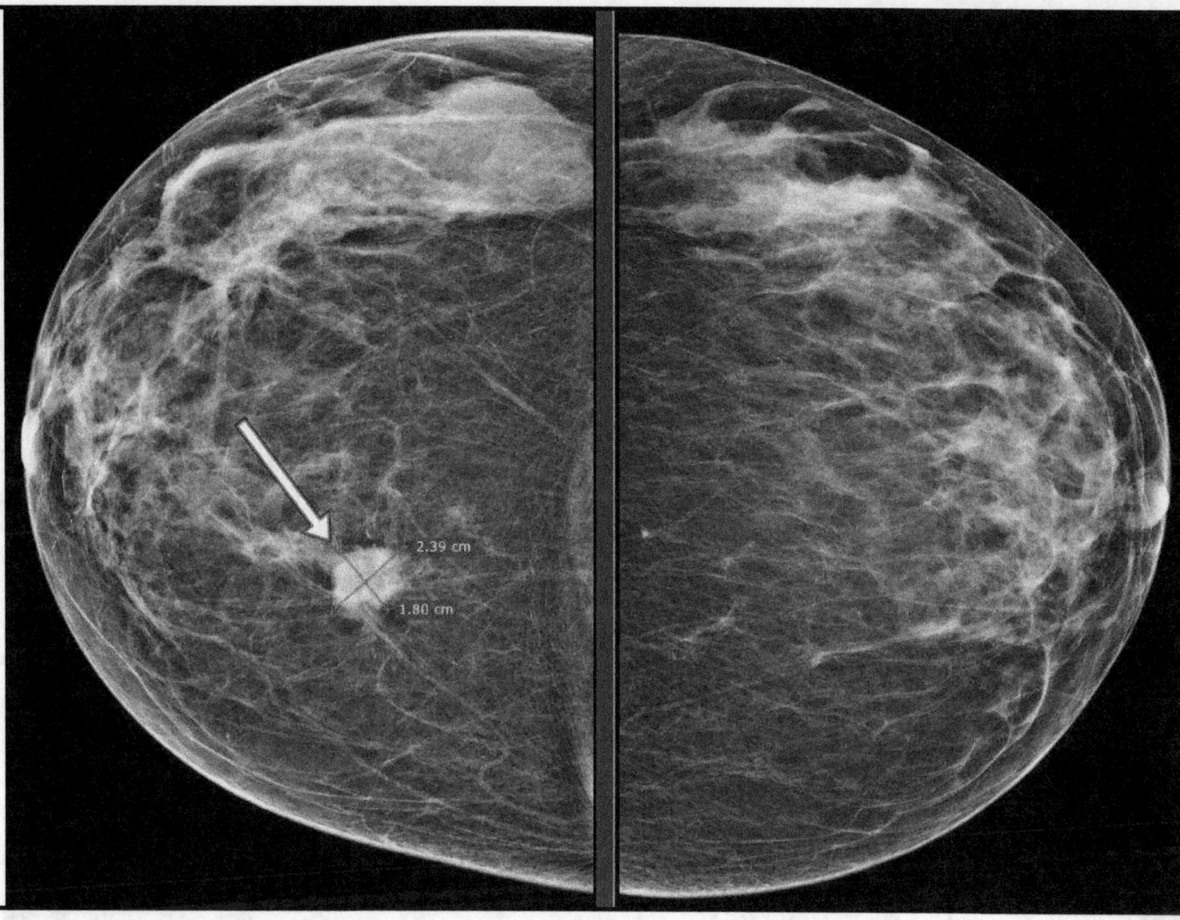

RIGHT BREAST	
Breast Parenchymal Density	***Heterogeneously dense, may obscure small masses (ACR C)***
Focal Mass	***UIQ irregular lobulated mass lesion measure(x)***
Asymmetric Density	None
Parenchymal Distortion	None
Calcification	None
Skin Thickening	None
Axillary Nodes	None

LEFT BREAST	
Breast Parenchymal Density	***Heterogeneously dense, may obscure small masses (ACR C)***
Focal Mass	None
Asymmetric Density	None
Parenchymal Distortion	None
Calcification	None
Skin Thickening	None
Axillary Nodes	None

IMPRESSION:

RIGHT BREAST: (BI-RADS 4B)

LEFT BREAST: (BI-RADS 1)
RECOMMENDATION: Histopathological Correlation

CASE 32: 59-year-old female/ Diagnostic

Right MLO	Left MLO

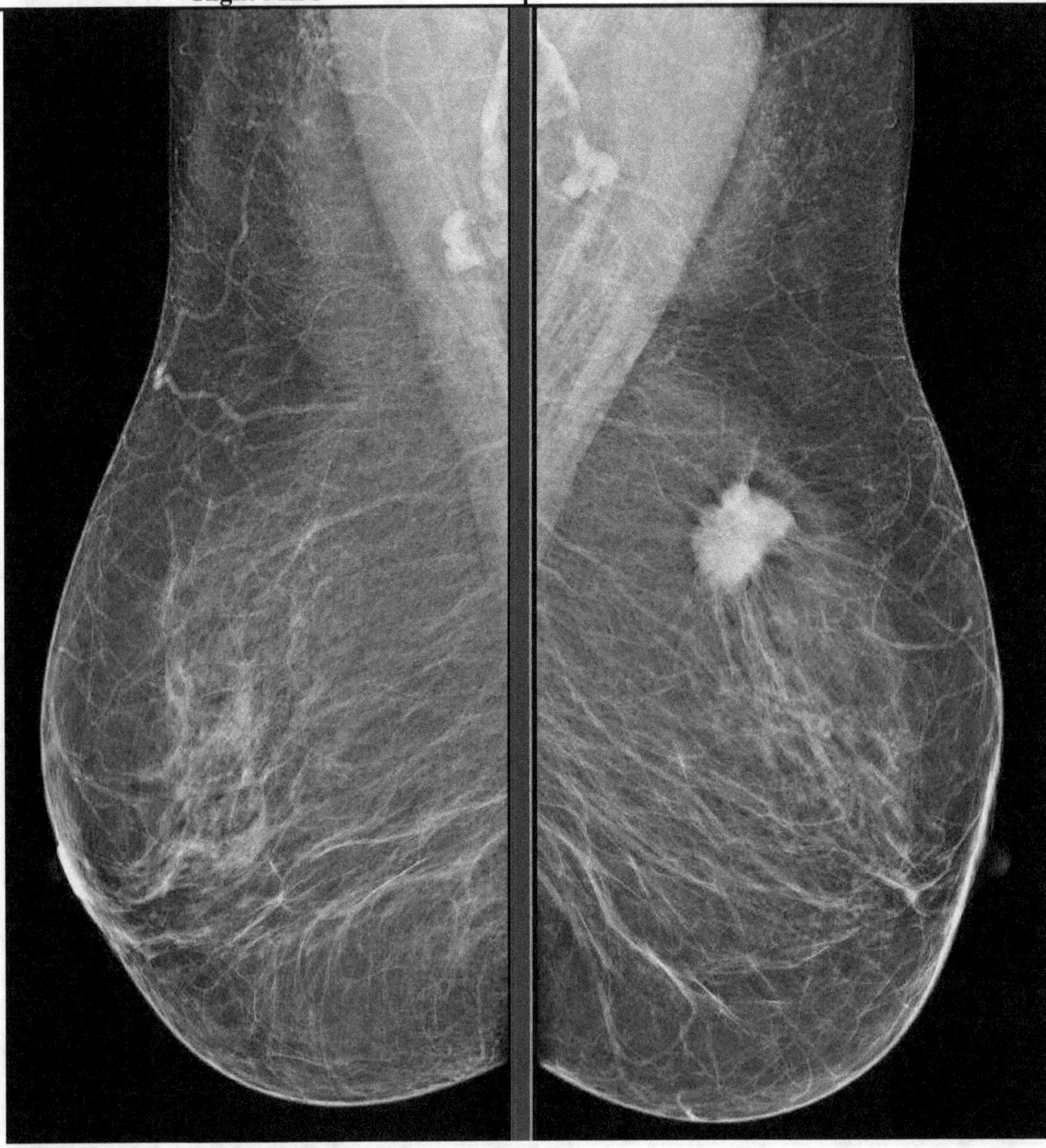

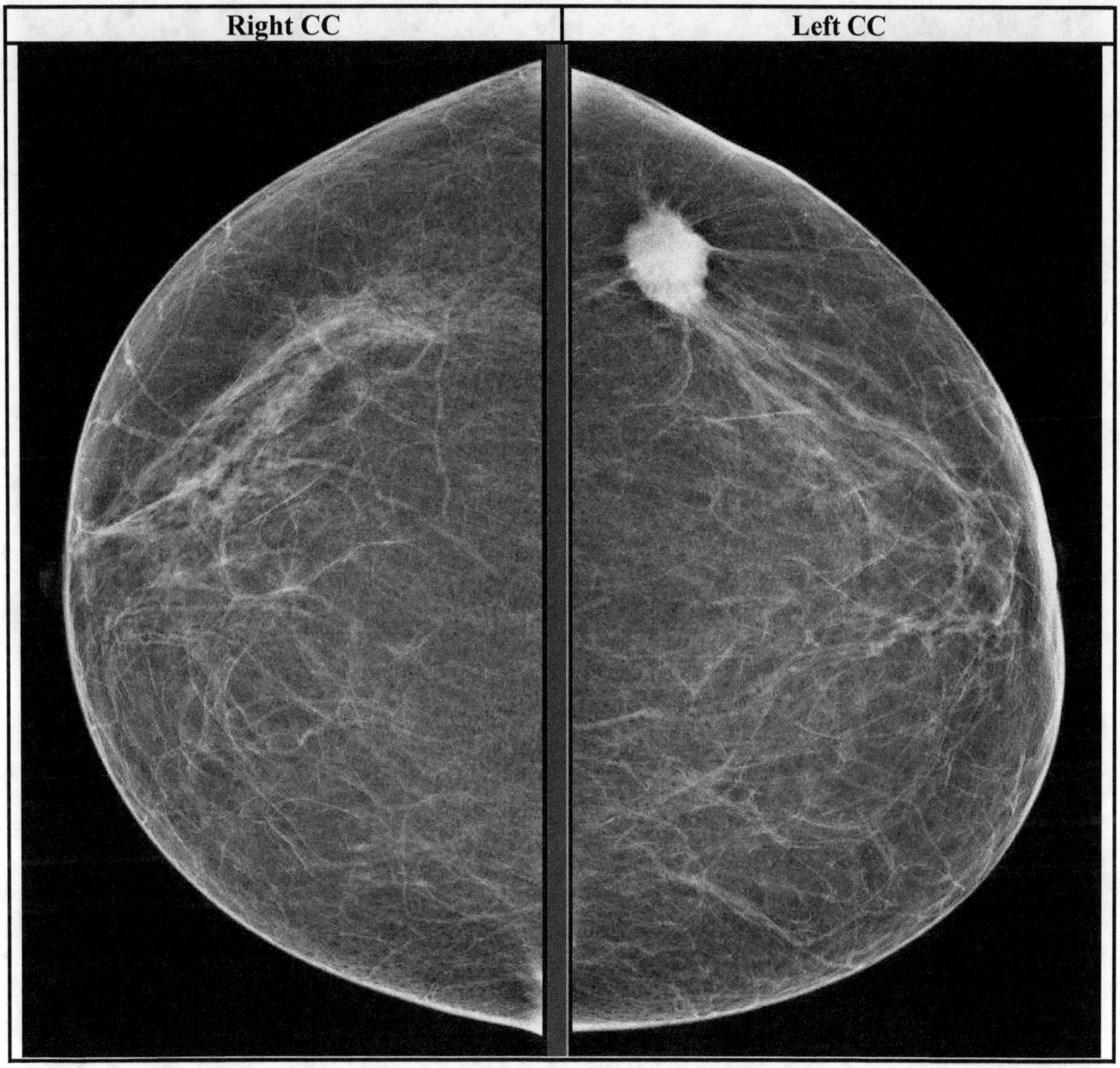
Right CC
Left CC

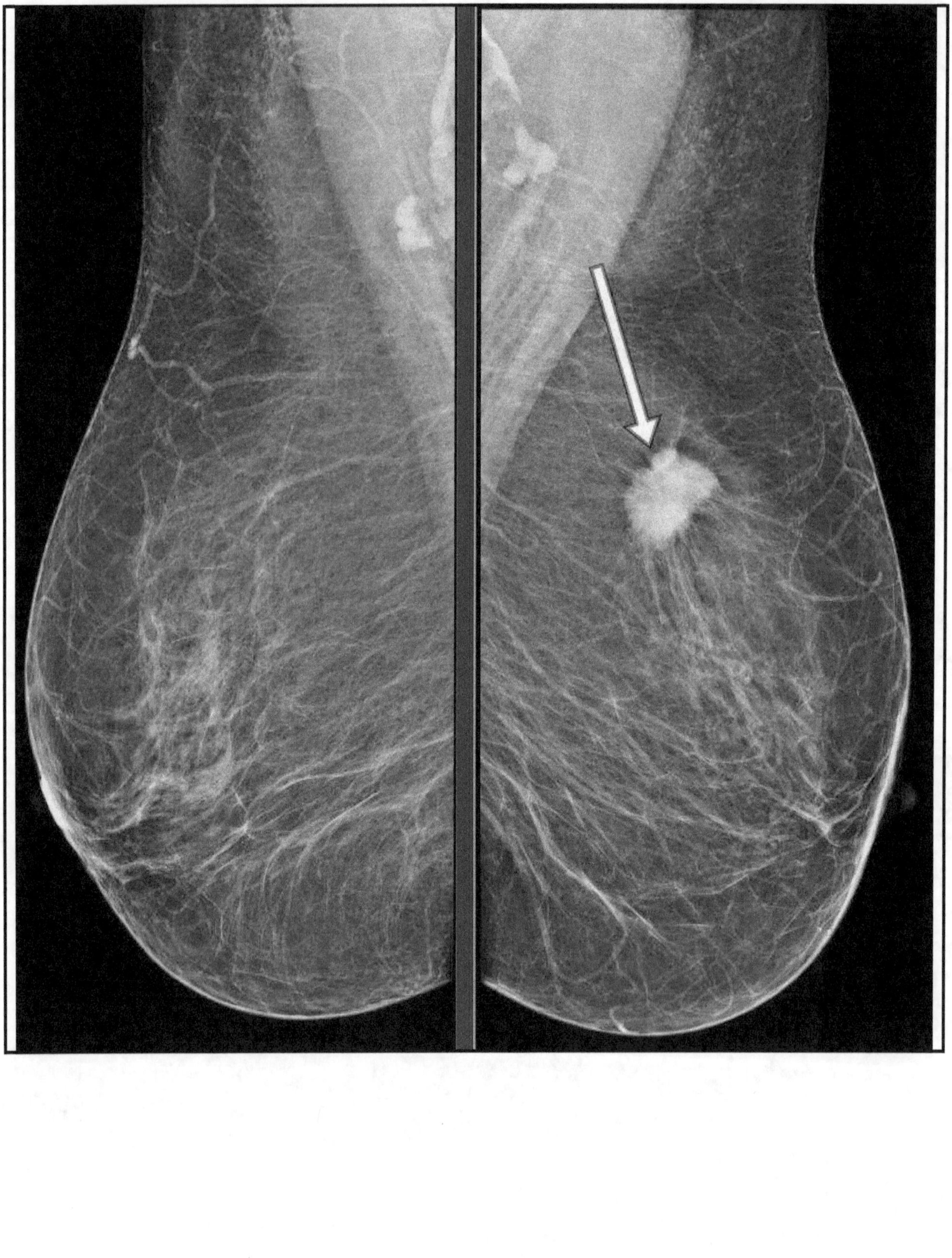

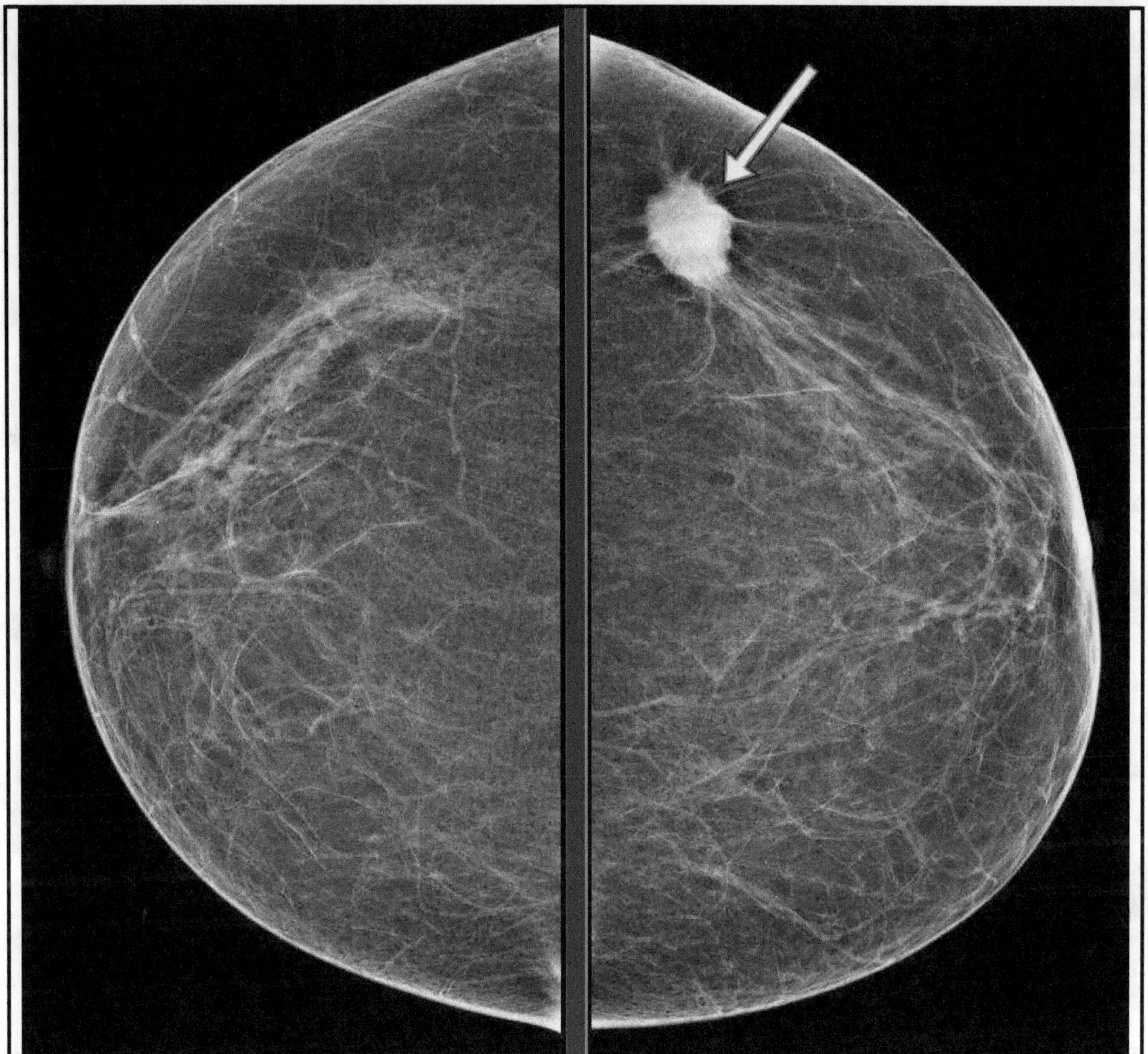

RIGHT BREAST	
Breast Parenchymal Density	***Scattered areas of fibroglandular density (ACR B)***
Focal Mass	None
Asymmetric Density	None
Parenchymal Distortion	None
Calcification	None
Skin Thickening	None
Axillary Nodes	None

LEFT BREAST	
Breast Parenchymal Density	***Scattered areas of fibroglandular density (ACR B)***
Focal Mass	***UOQ Oval Spiculated Mass Lesion***
Asymmetric Density	None
Parenchymal Distortion	None
Calcification	None
Skin Thickening	None
Axillary Nodes	None

IMPRESSION:

RIGHT BREAST: (BI-RADS 1)
LEFT BREAST: (BI-RADS 5)

RECOMMENDATION: Histopathological Correlation

CASE 33: 69-year-old female/screening	
Right MLO	Left MLO

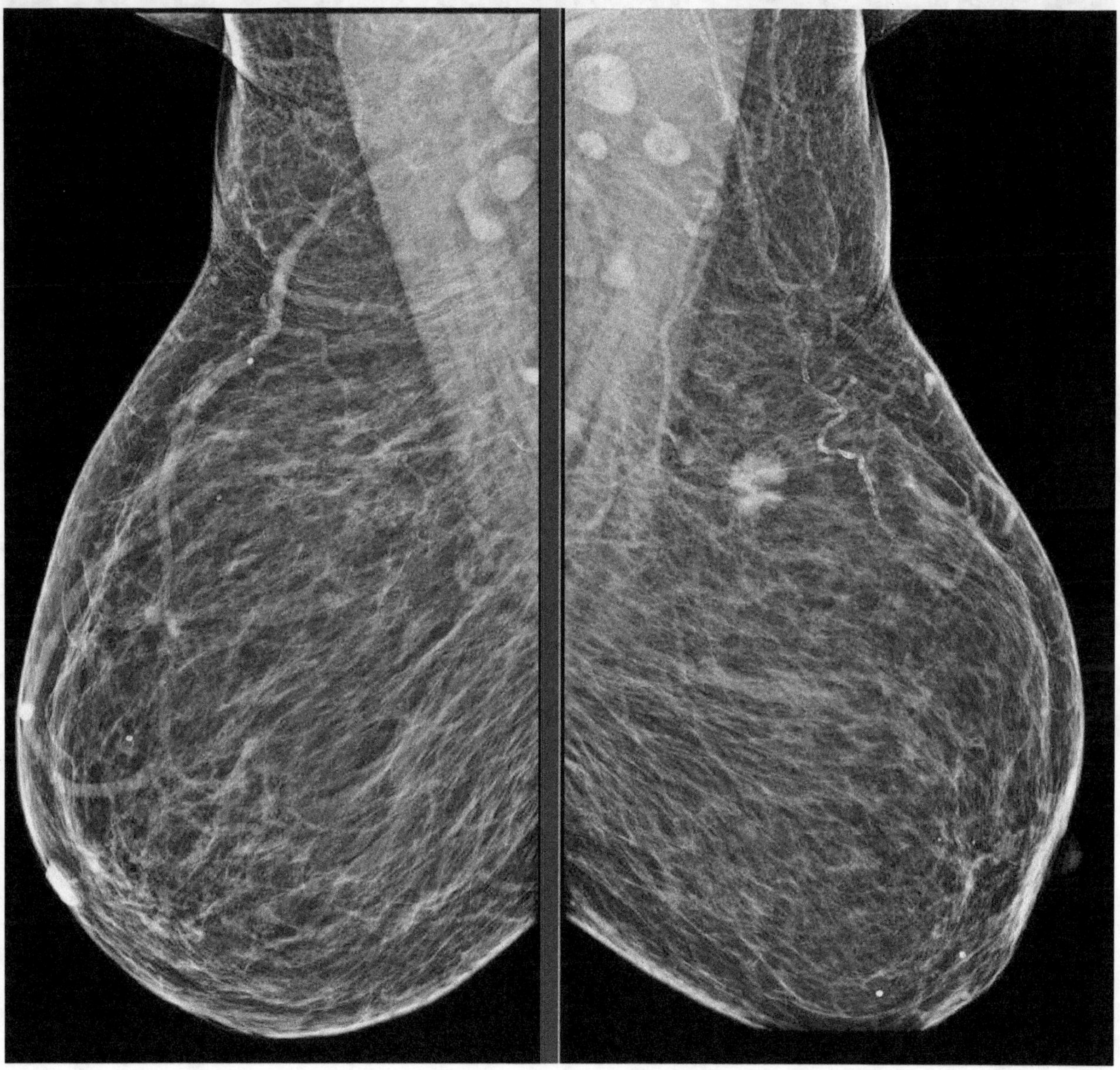

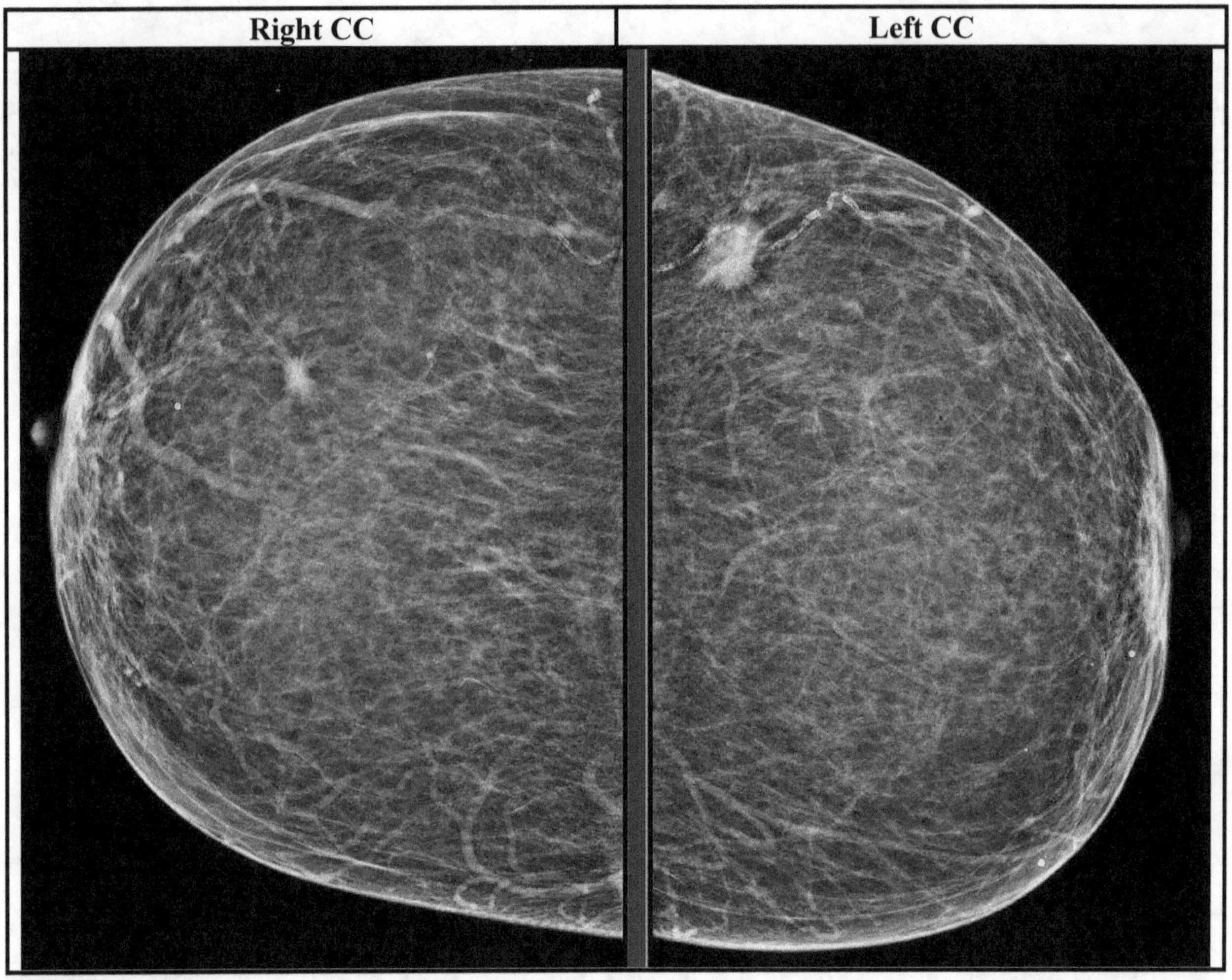
Right CC
Left CC

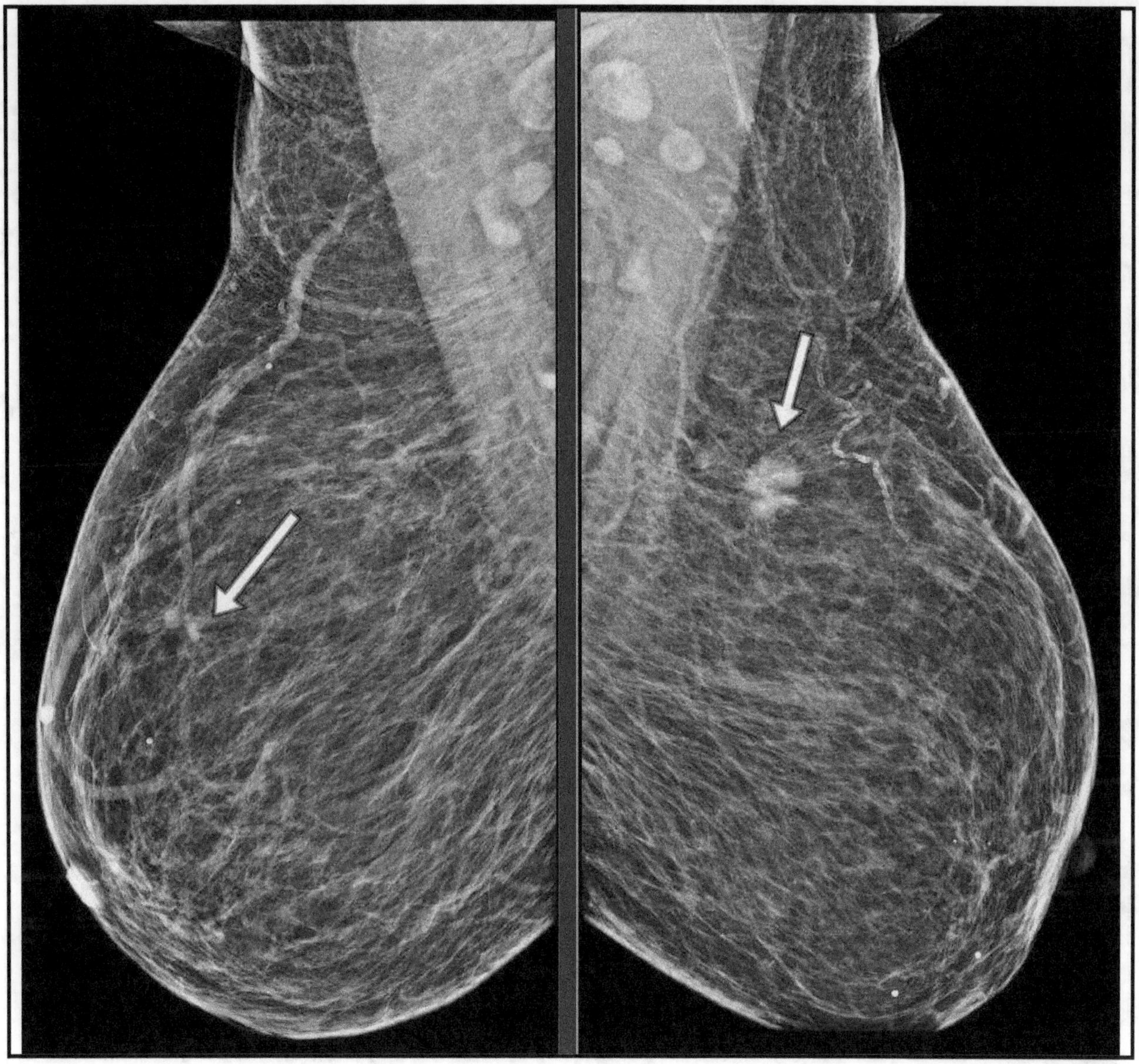

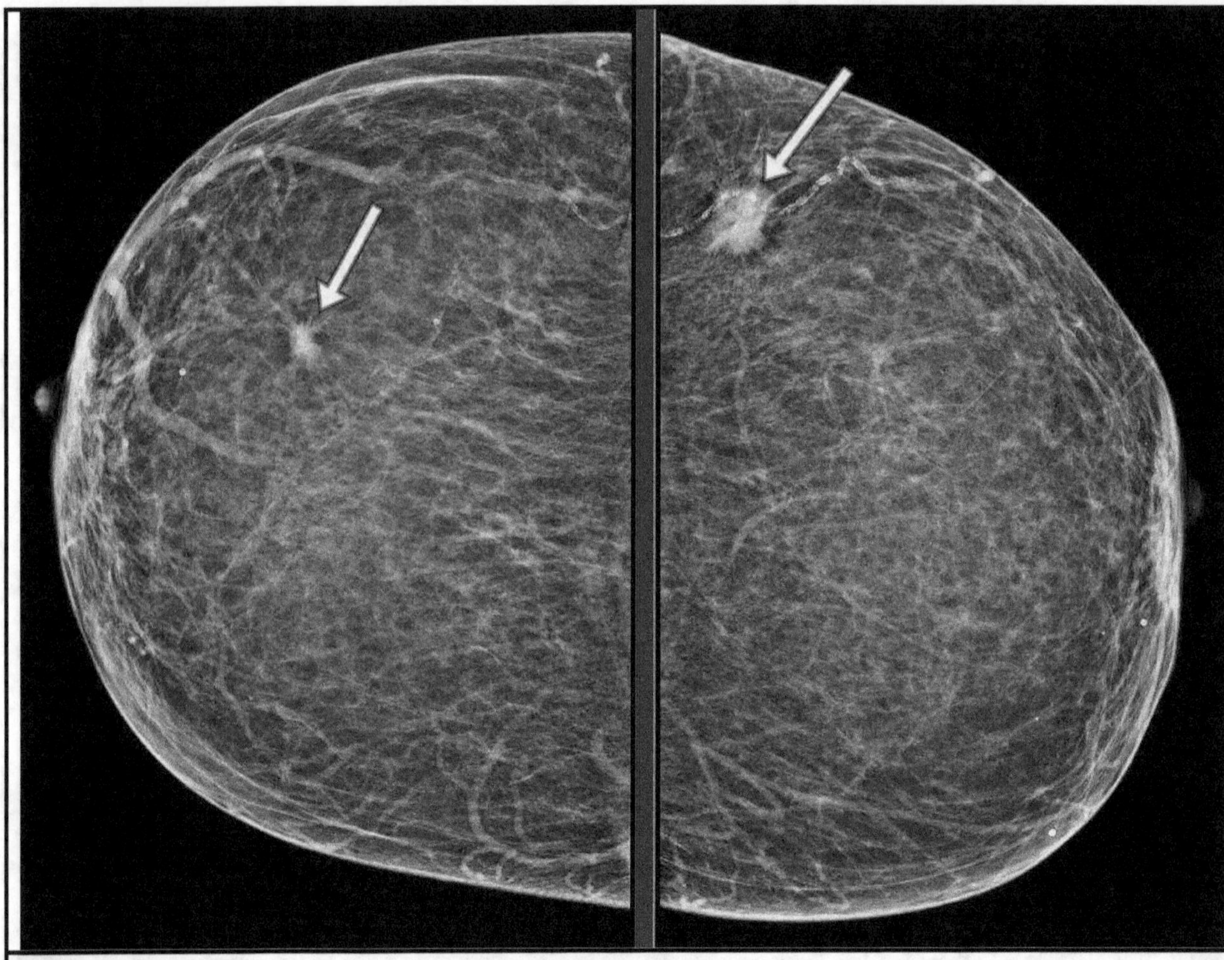

RIGHT BREAST	
Breast Parenchymal Density	***Scattered areas of fibroglandular density (ACR B)***
Focal Mass	***UOQ irregular Spiculated Mass Lesion***
Asymmetric Density	None
Parenchymal Distortion	None
Calcification	***vascular calcification***
Skin Thickening	None
Axillary Nodes	None

LEFT BREAST	
Breast Parenchymal Density	***Scattered areas of fibroglandular density (ACR B)***
Focal Mass	***UOQ irregular Spiculated Mass Lesion***
Asymmetric Density	None
Parenchymal Distortion	None
Calcification	***vascular calcification***
Skin Thickening	None
Axillary Nodes	None

IMPRESSION:

RIGHT BREAST: (BI-RADS 5)
LEFT BREAST: (BI-RADS 5)

RECOMMENDATION: Histopathological Correlation

CASE 34: 47-year-old female/ Diagnostic

Right MLO	Left MLO

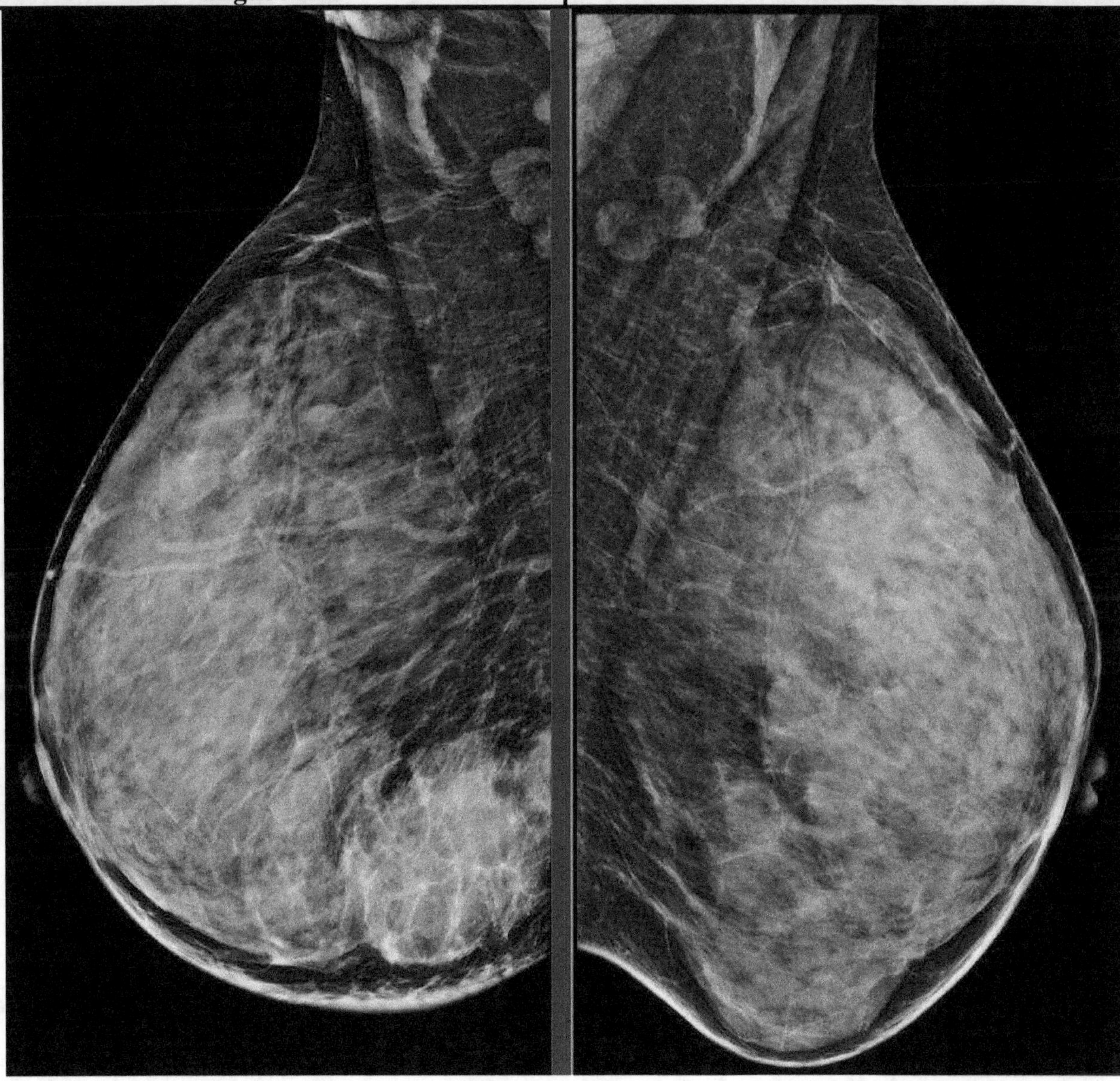

Right CC	Left CC
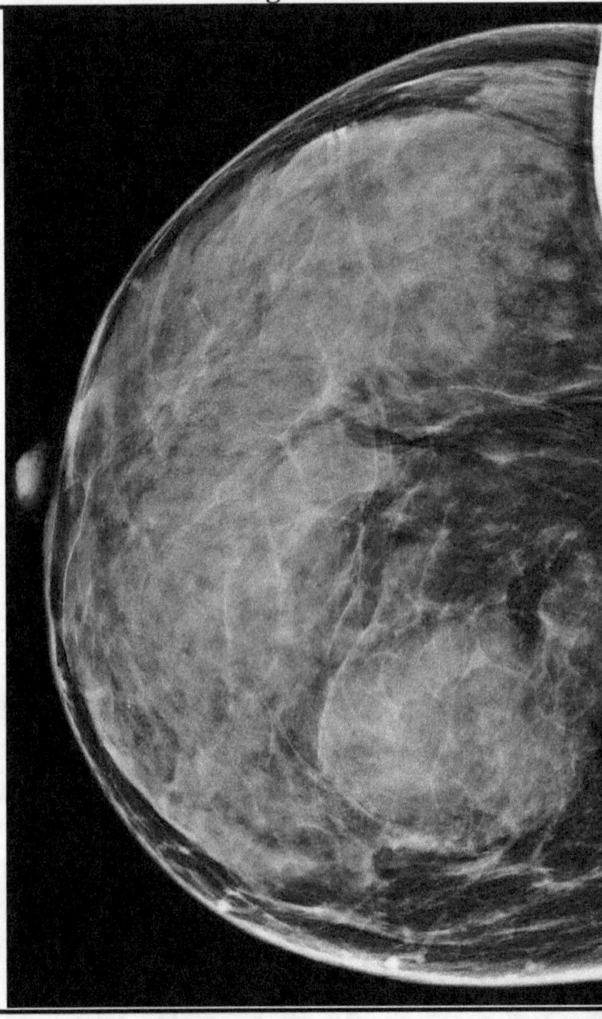	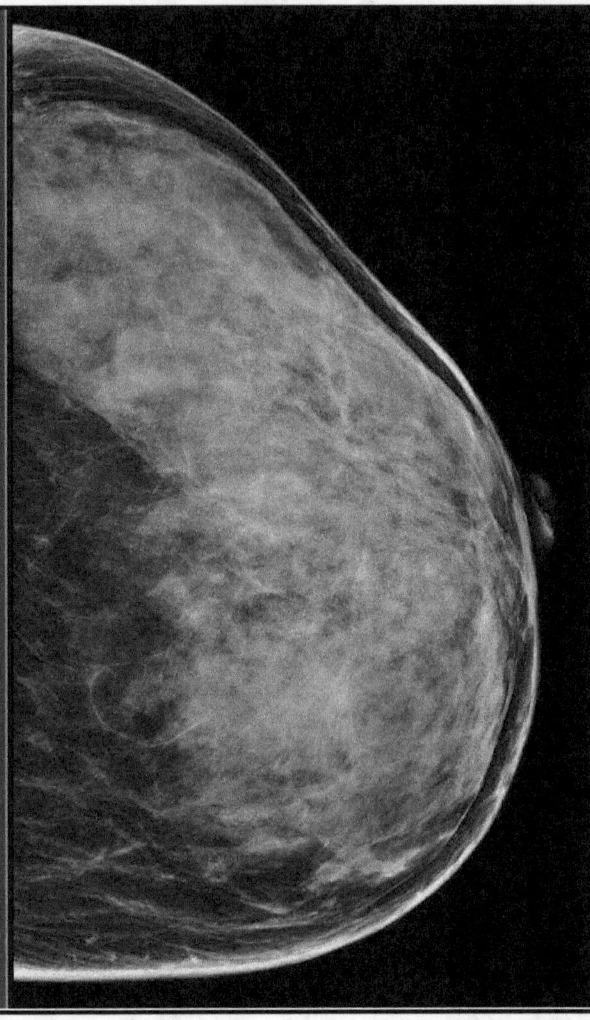

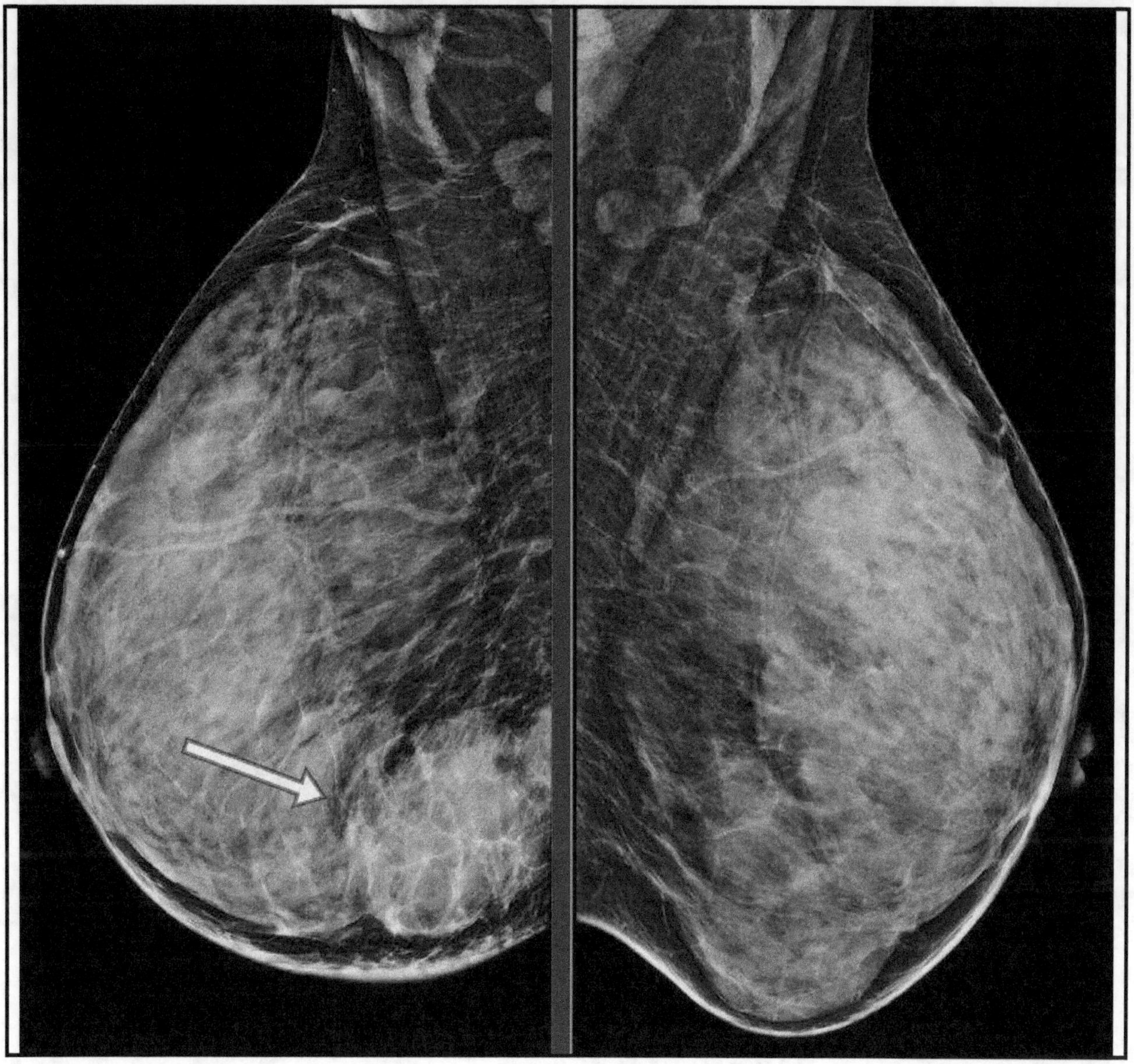

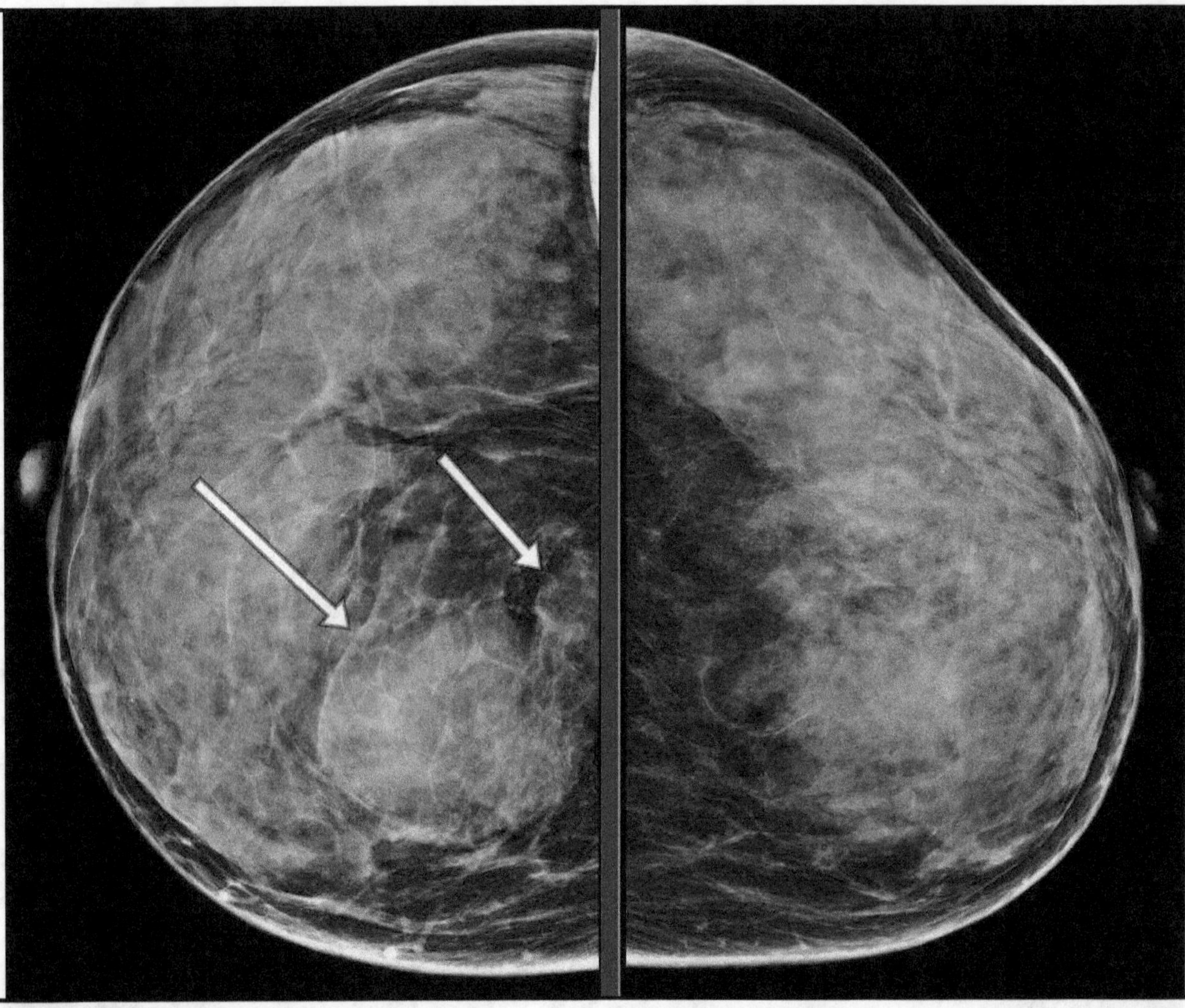

RIGHT BREAST	
Breast Parenchymal Density	***Extremely dense, which lowers the sensitivity of mammography (ACR D)***
Focal Mass	***LIQ Oval obscured mass lesion***
Asymmetric Density	None
Parenchymal Distortion	None
Calcification	None
Skin Thickening	None
Axillary Nodes	None

LEFT BREAST	
Breast Parenchymal Density	***Extremely dense, which lowers the sensitivity of mammography (ACR D)***
Focal Mass	None
Asymmetric Density	None
Parenchymal Distortion	None
Calcification	None
Skin Thickening	None
Axillary Nodes	None

IMPRESSION:

RIGHT BREAST: (BI-RADS 0)
LEFT BREAST: (BI-RADS 0)

RECOMMENDATION: US Correlation

CASE 35: 70-year-old female/ Diagnostic	
Right MLO	Left MLO

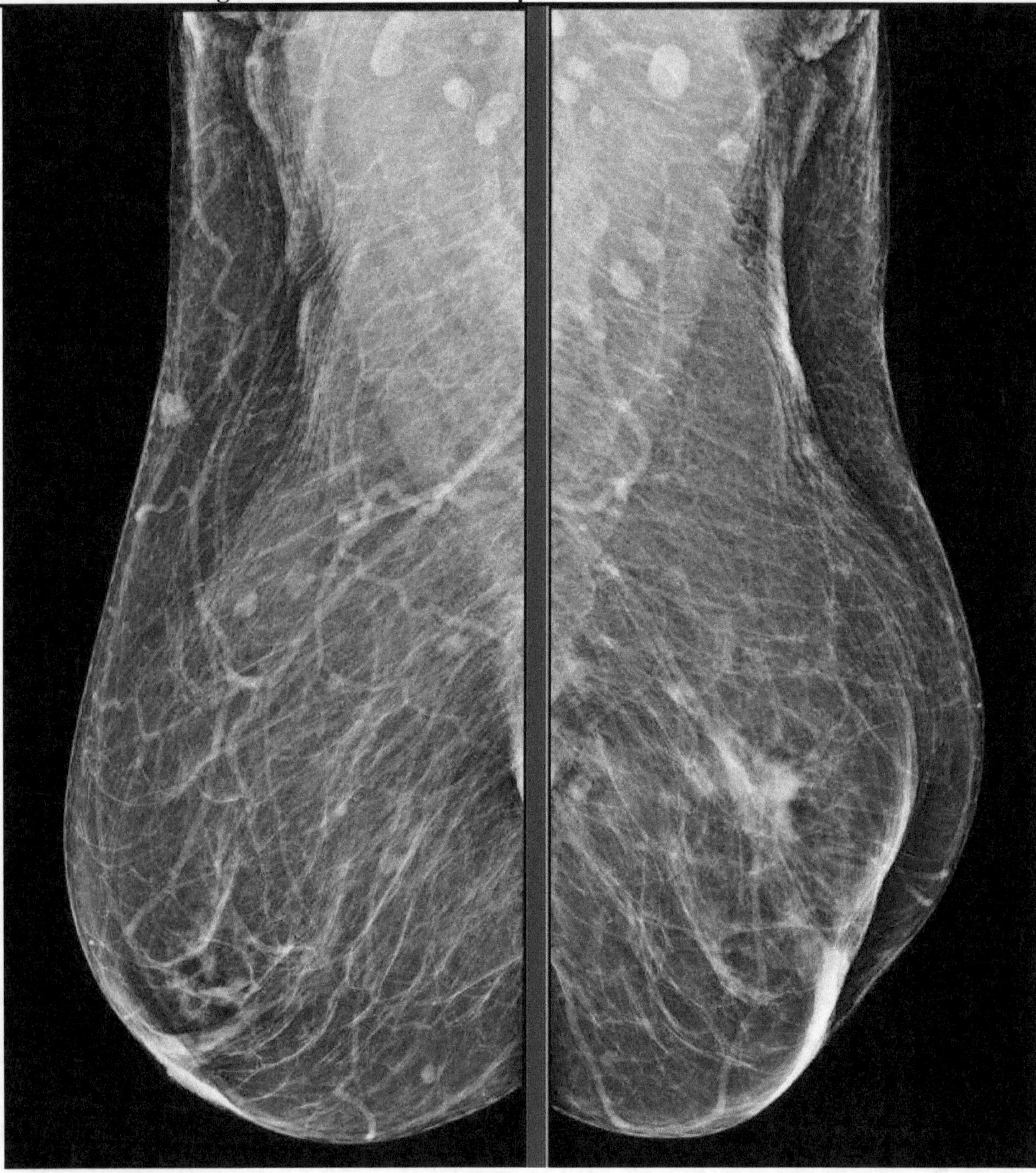

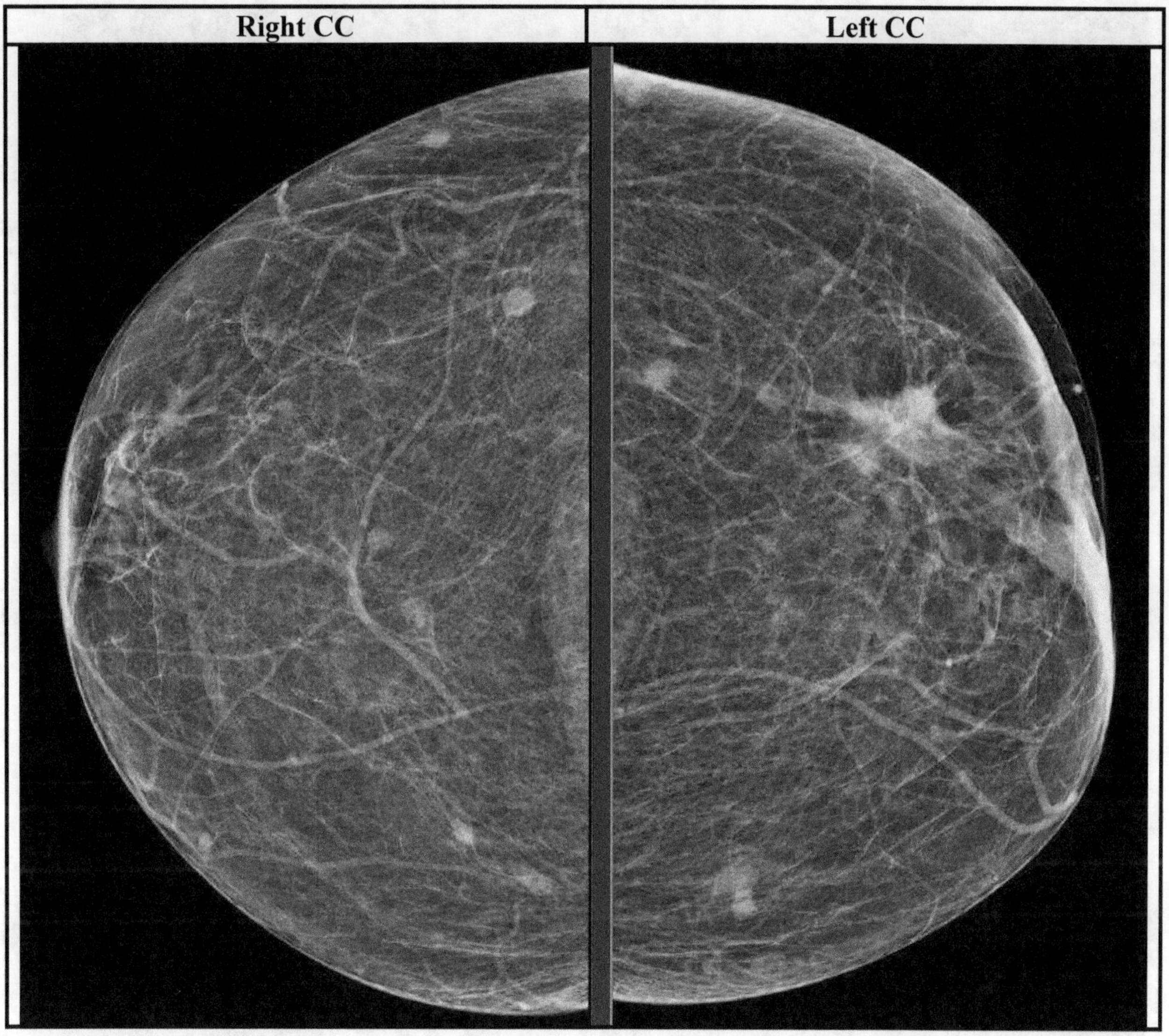
Right CC
Left CC

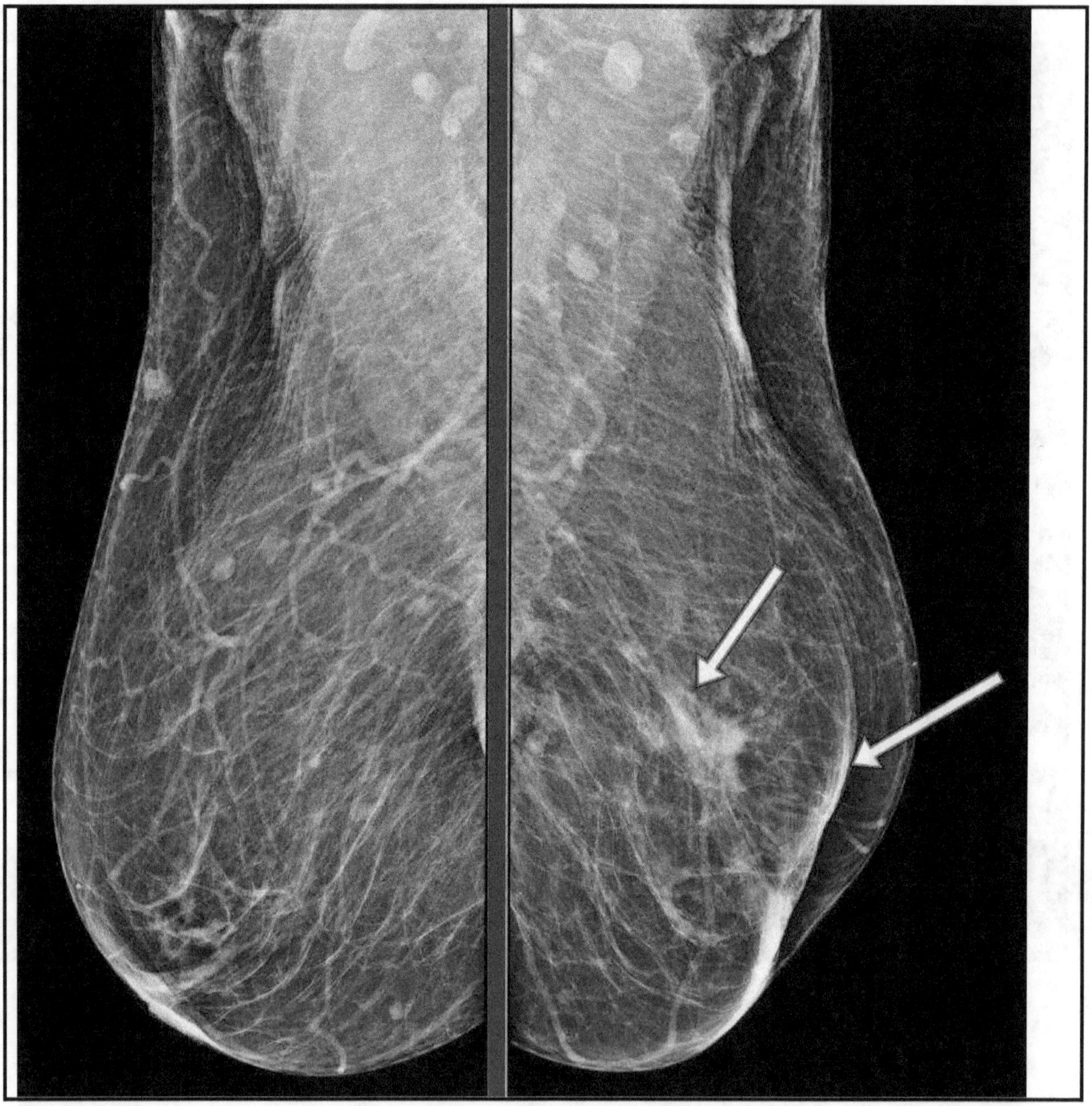

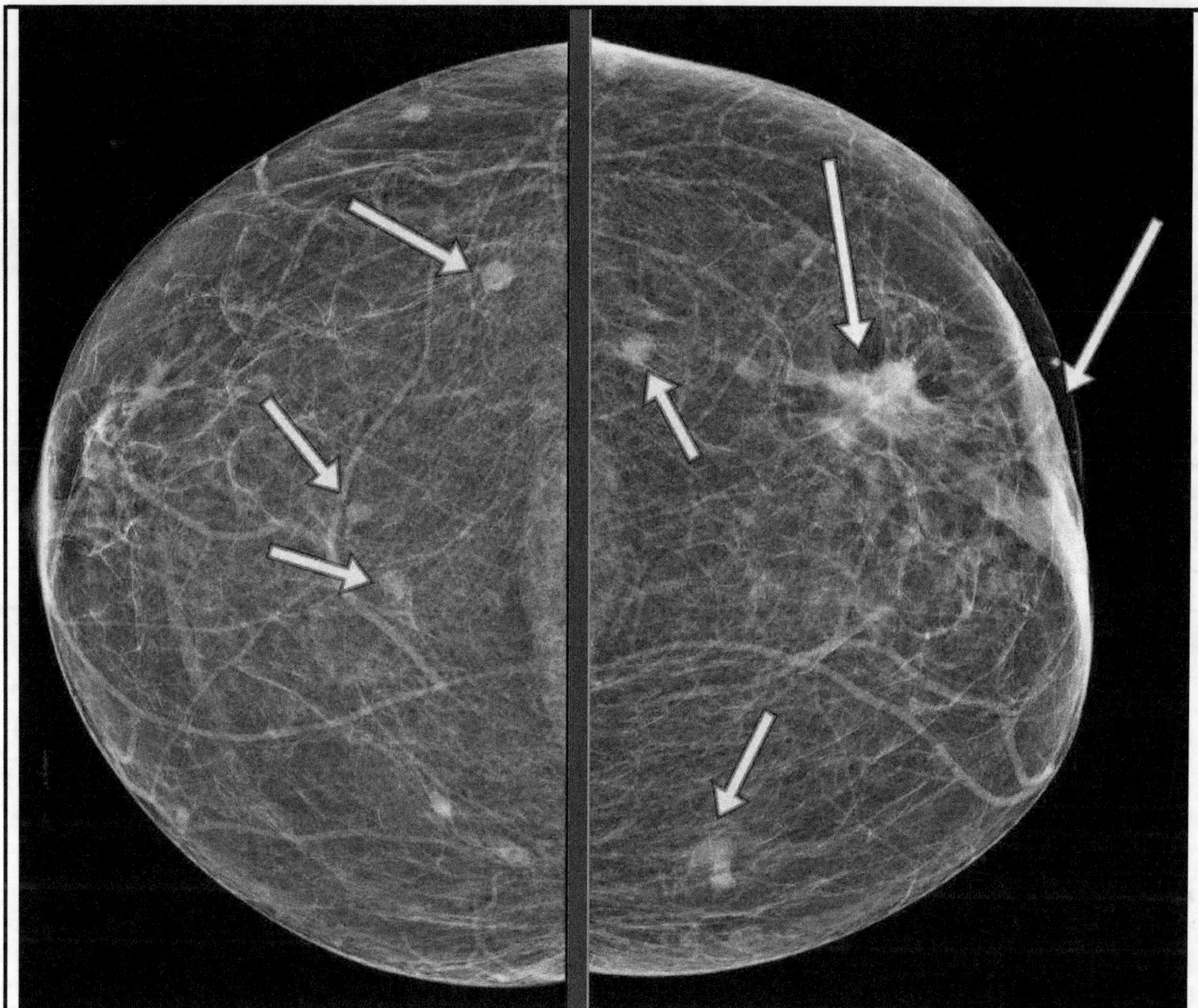

RIGHT BREAST	
Breast Parenchymal Density	***Scattered areas of fibroglandular density (ACR B)***
Focal Mass	***UOQ irregular indistinct mass lesion associated with corresponding nipple and skin retraction***
Asymmetric Density	None
Parenchymal Distortion	None
Calcification	None
Skin Thickening	None
Axillary Nodes	None / ***Multiple IMLN (green arrows)***

LEFT BREAST	
Breast Parenchymal Density	***Scattered areas of fibroglandular density (ACR B)***
Focal Mass	None
Asymmetric Density	None
Parenchymal Distortion	None
Calcification	None
Skin Thickening	None
Axillary Nodes	None / ***Multiple IMLN (green arrows)***

IMPRESSION:

RIGHT BREAST: (BI-RADS 5)
LEFT BREAST: (BI-RADS 1)

RECOMMENDATION: Histopathological Correlation

CASE 36: 62-year-old female/ Diagnostic	
Right MLO	**Left MLO**

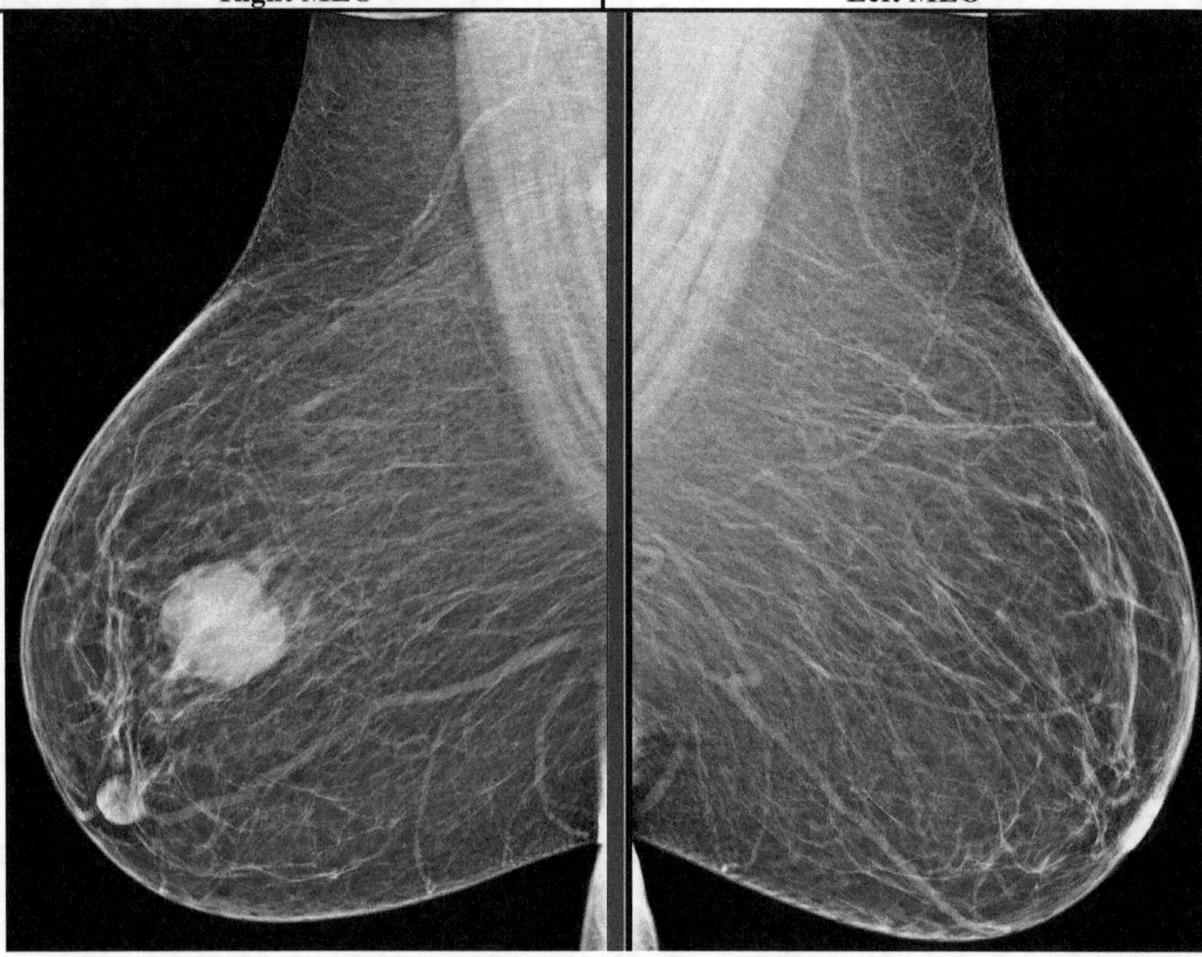

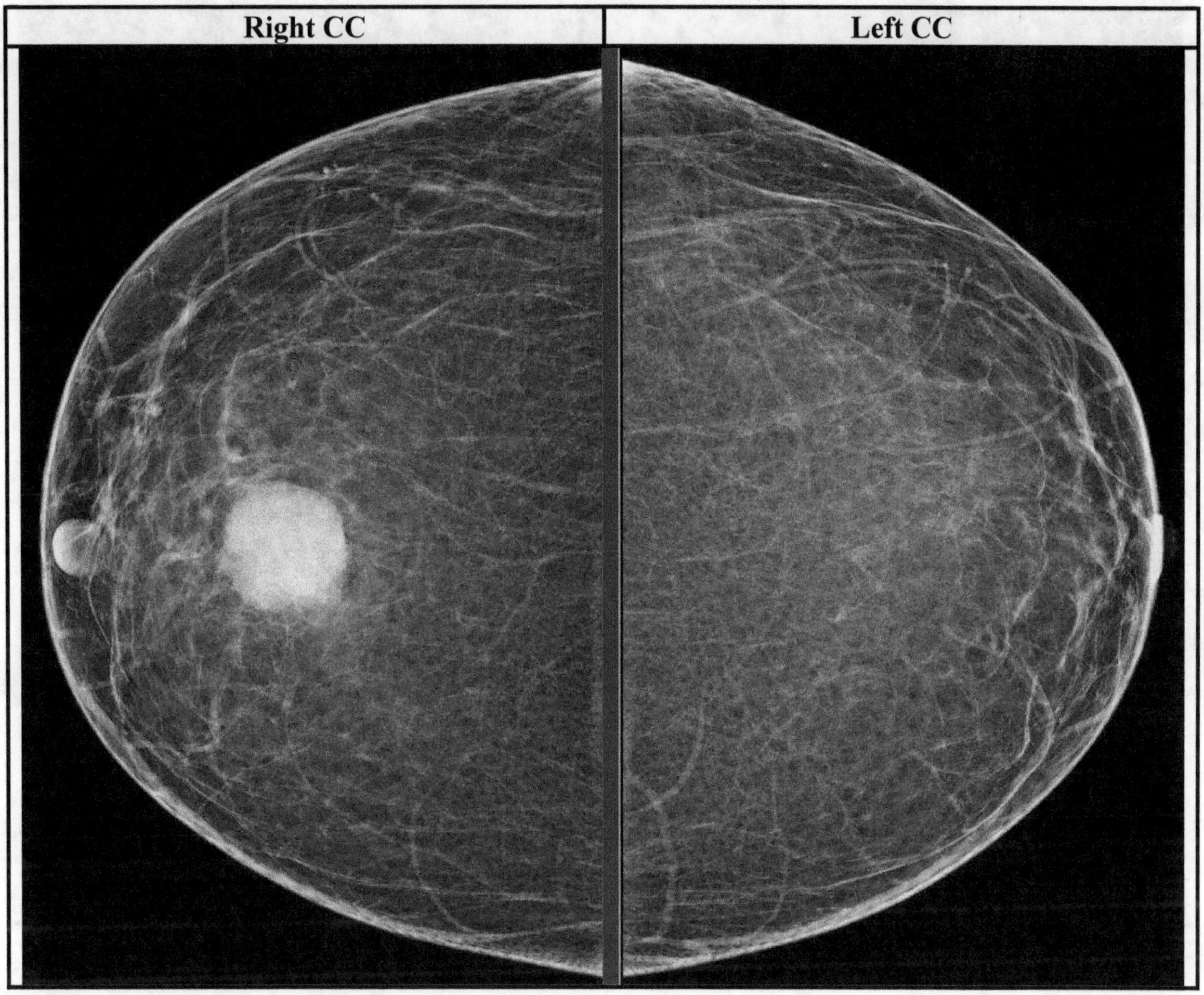
Right CC
Left CC

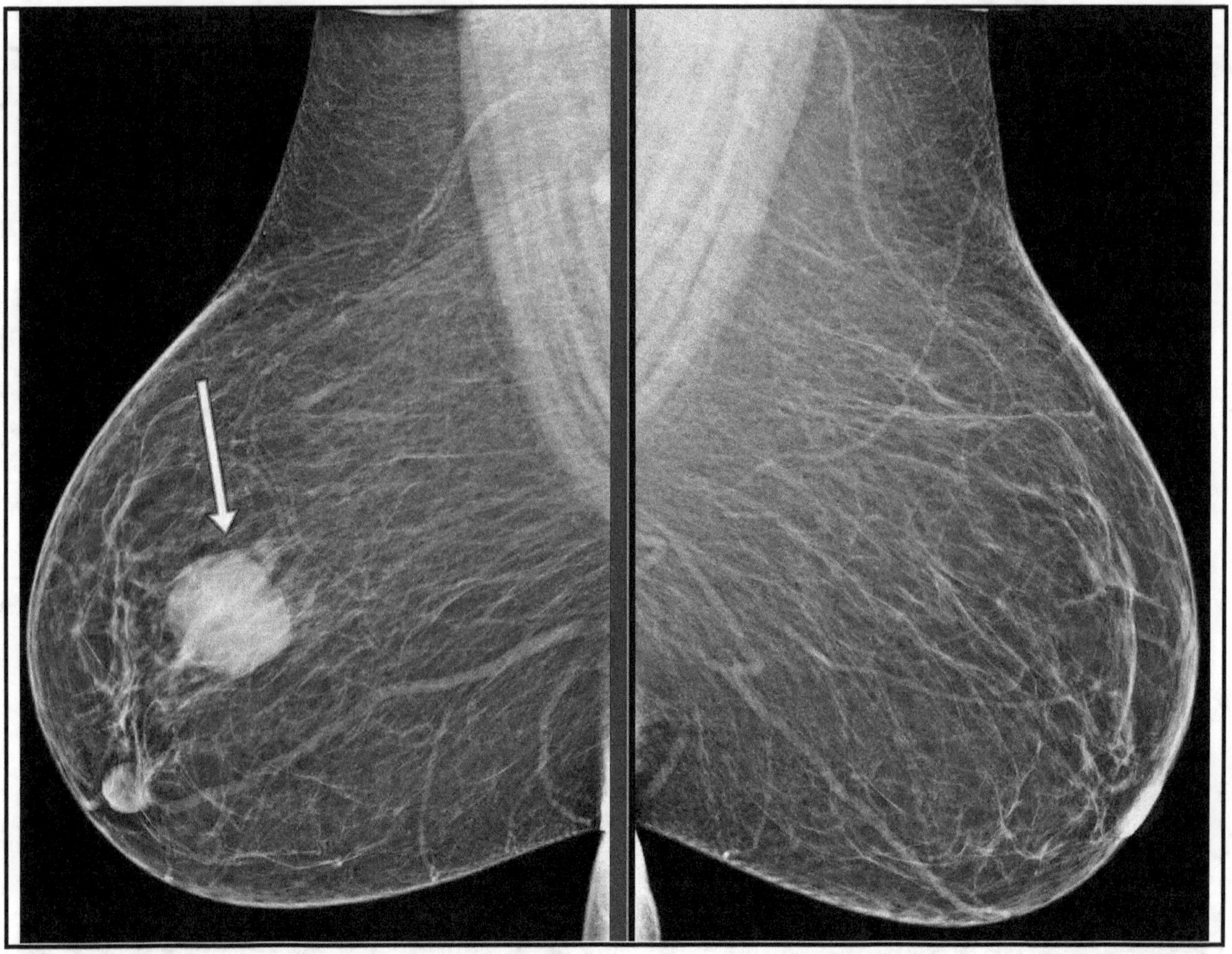

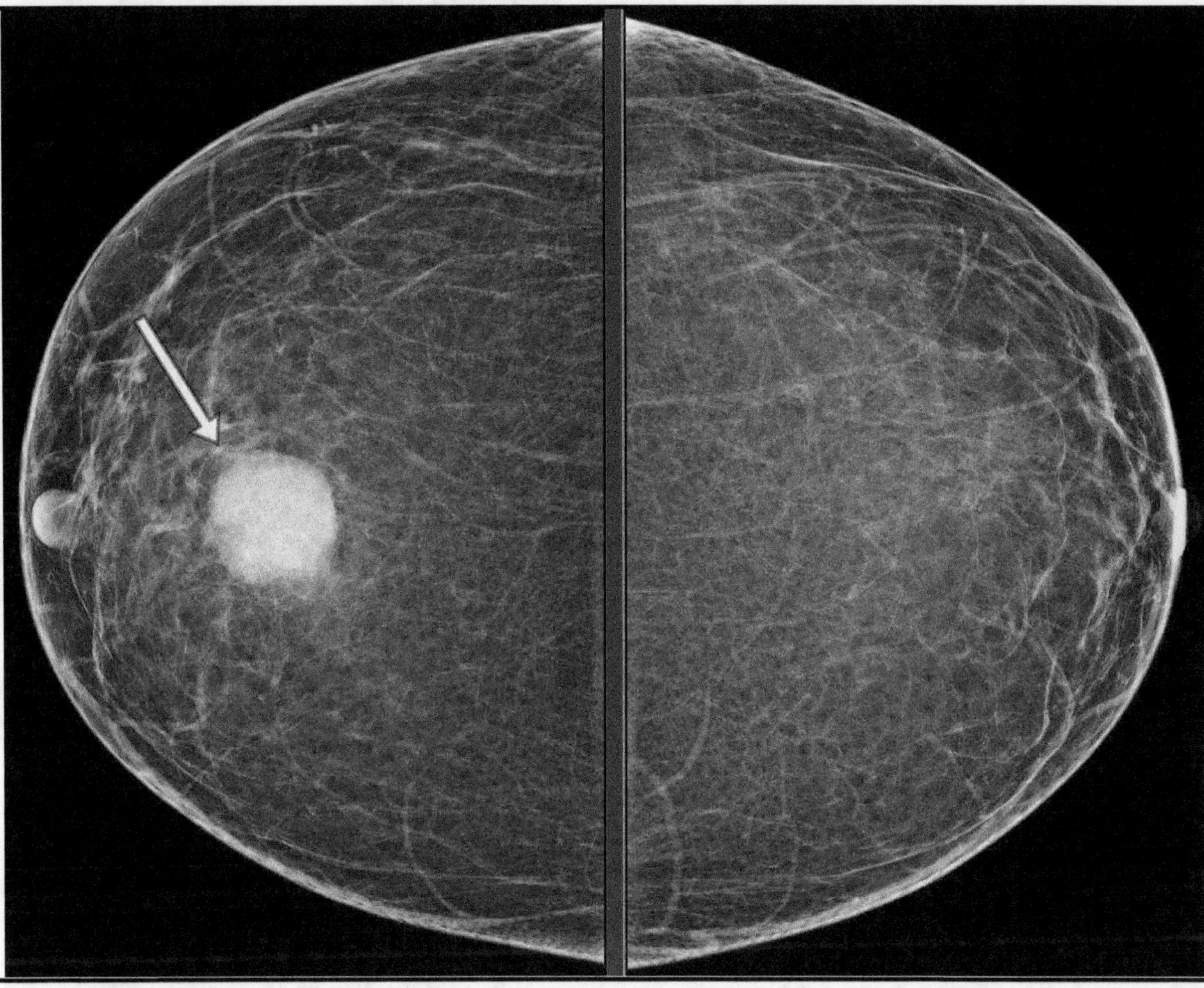

RIGHT BREAST	
Breast Parenchymal Density	***Almost entirely fatty (ACR A)***
Focal Mass	***Upper central (12 o'clock) round lobulated mass lesion***
Asymmetric Density	None
Parenchymal Distortion	None
Calcification	None
Skin Thickening	None
Axillary Nodes	None

LEFT BREAST	
Breast Parenchymal Density	***Almost entirely fatty (ACR A)***
Focal Mass	None
Asymmetric Density	None
Parenchymal Distortion	None
Calcification	None
Skin Thickening	None
Axillary Nodes	None

IMPRESSION:
RIGHT BREAST: (BI-RADS 4B)
LEFT BREAST: (BI-RADS 1)

RECOMMENDATION: Histopathological Correlation

CASE 37: 45 -year-old female/ Diagnostic

Right MLO	Left MLO

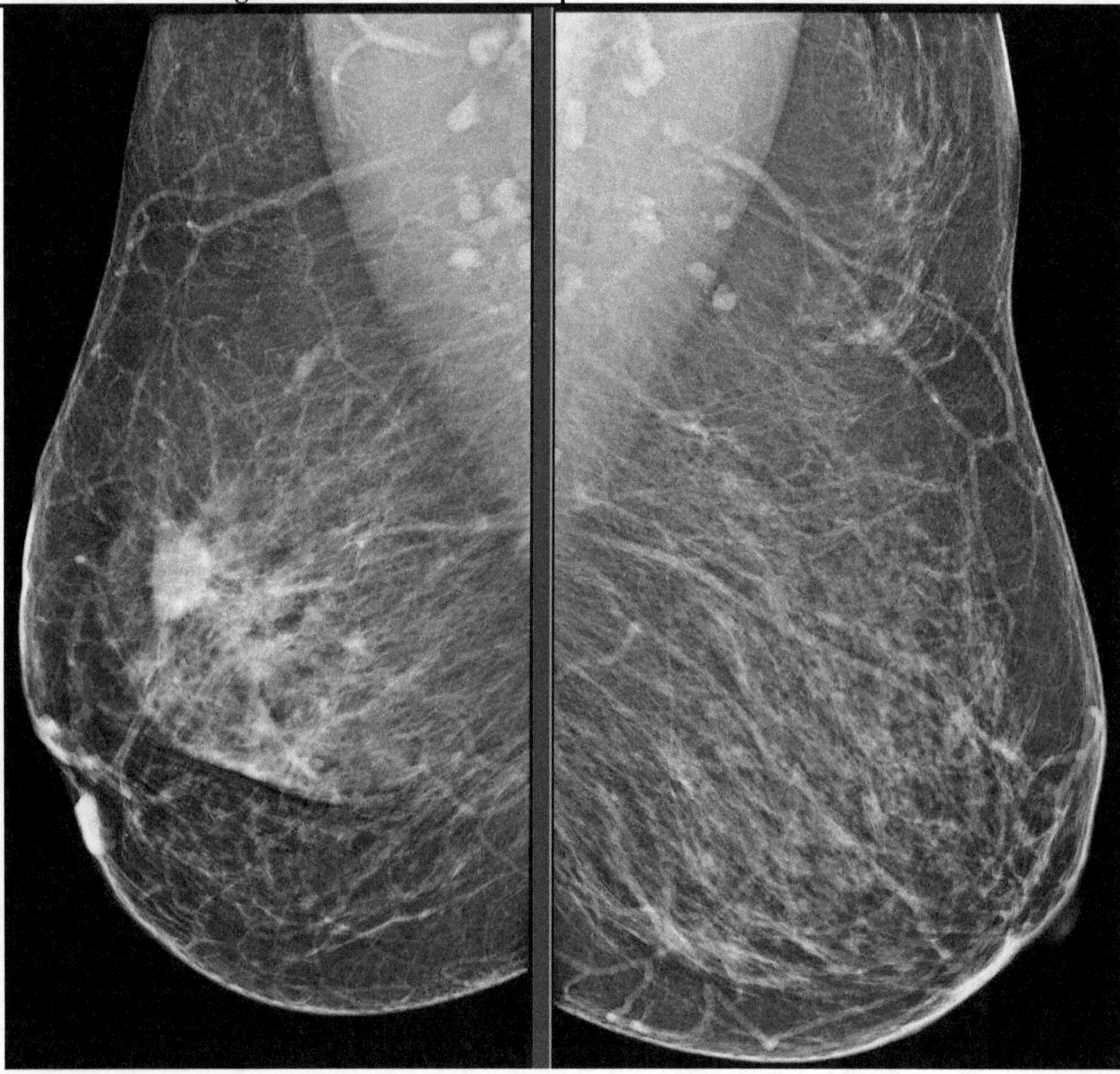

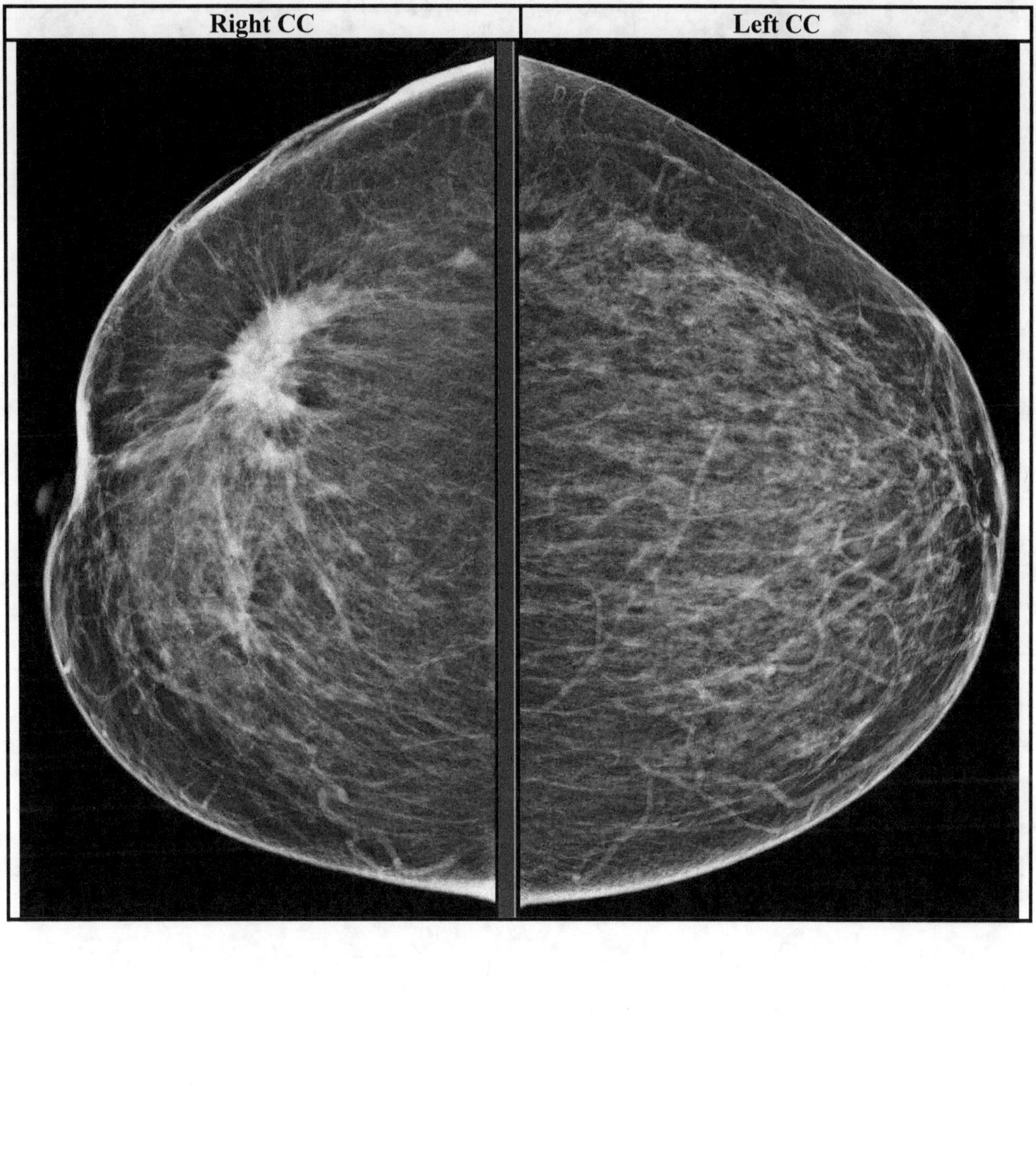
Right CC
Left CC

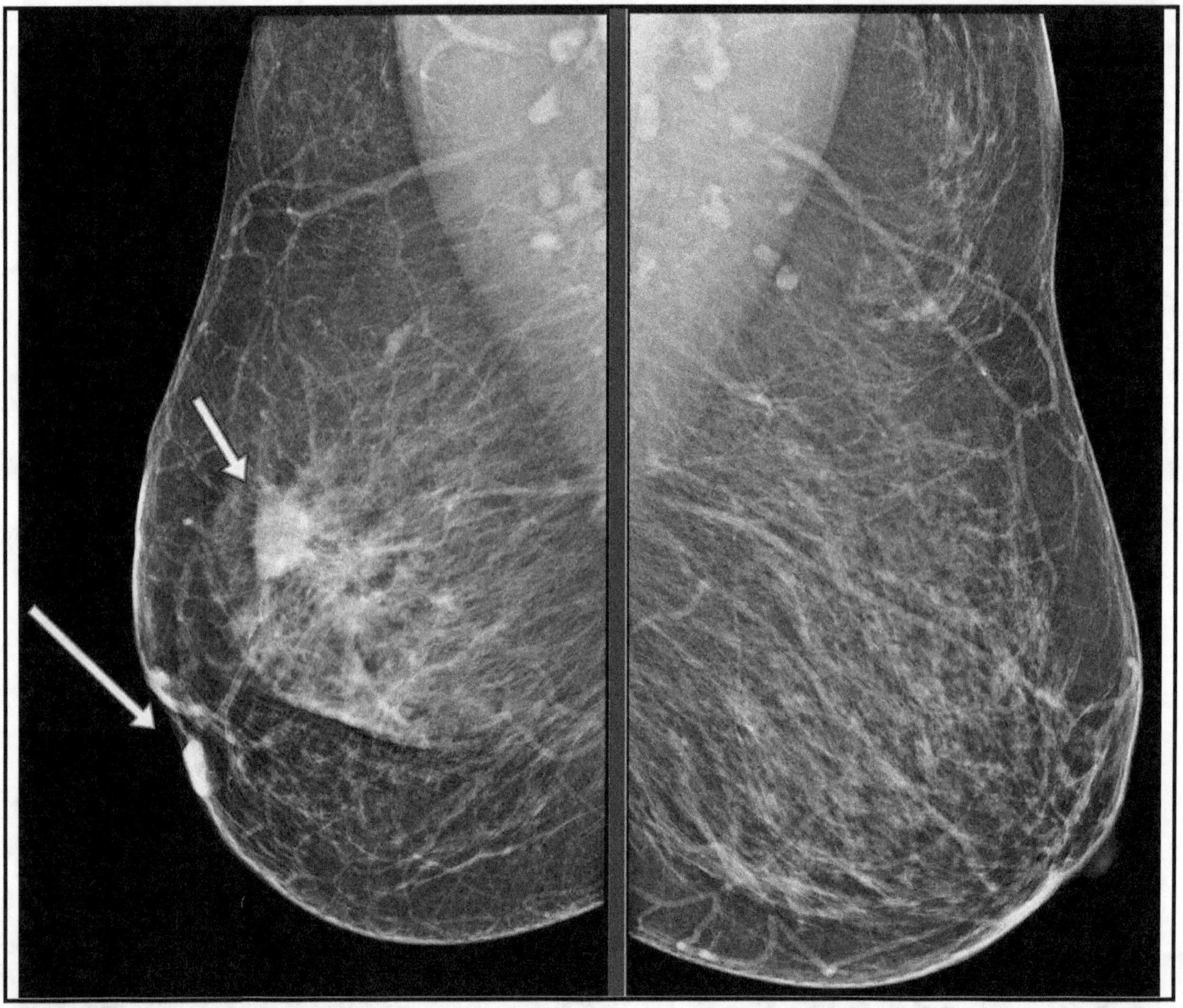

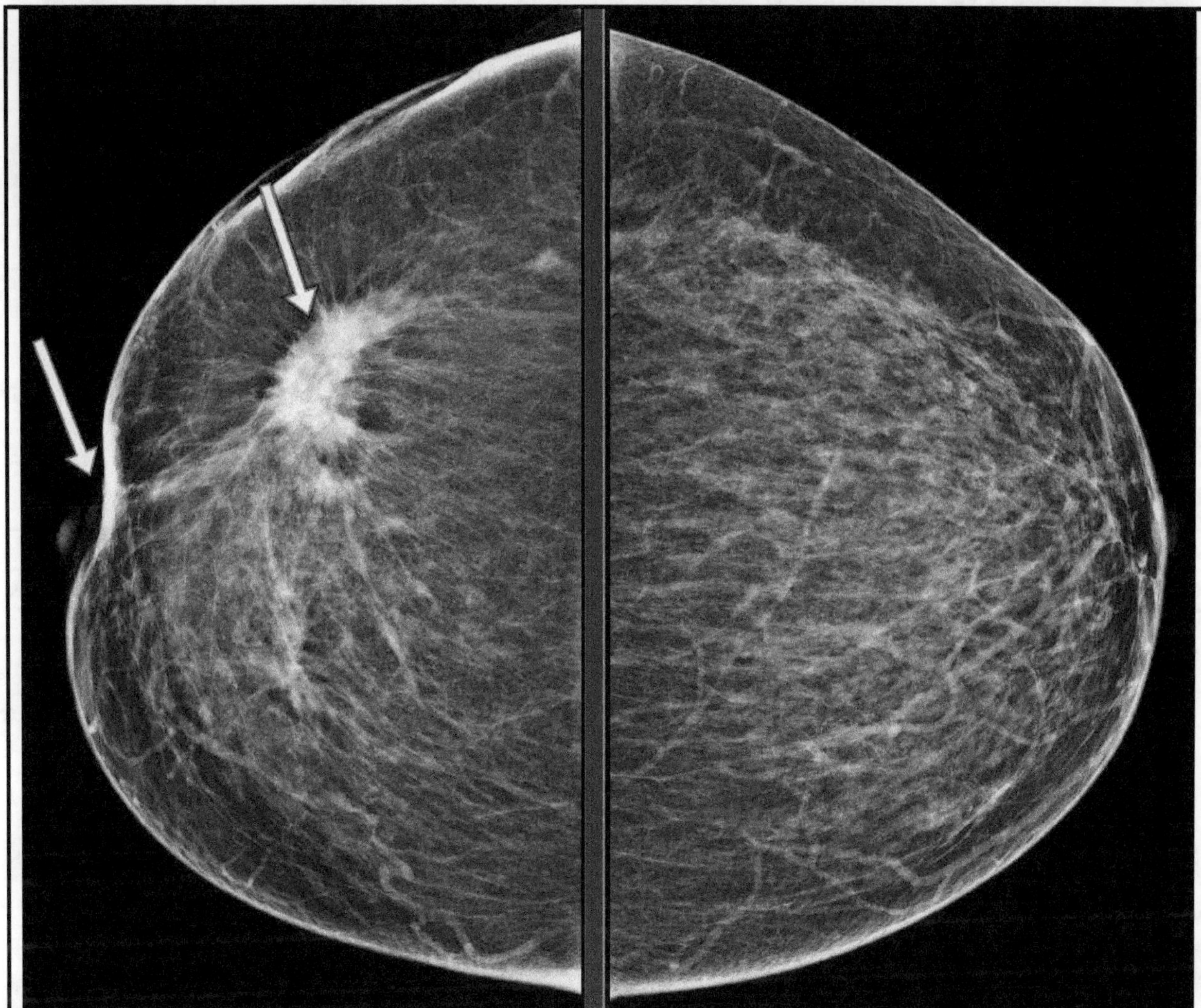

RIGHT BREAST	
Breast Parenchymal Density	***Scattered areas of fibroglandular density (ACR B)***
Focal Mass	***UOQ irregular spiculated mass lesion associate with nipple and skin retraction***
Asymmetric Density	None
Parenchymal Distortion	None
Calcification	None
Skin Thickening	None
Axillary Nodes	None

LEFT BREAST	
Breast Parenchymal Density	***Scattered areas of fibroglandular density (ACR B)***
Focal Mass	None
Asymmetric Density	None
Parenchymal Distortion	None
Calcification	None
Skin Thickening	None
Axillary Nodes	None

IMPRESSION:

RIGHT BREAST: (BI-RADS 5)
LEFT BREAST: (BI-RADS 1)

RECOMMENDATION: Histopathological Correlation

CASE 38: 75-year-old female/ Diagnostic

Right MLO	**Left MLO**
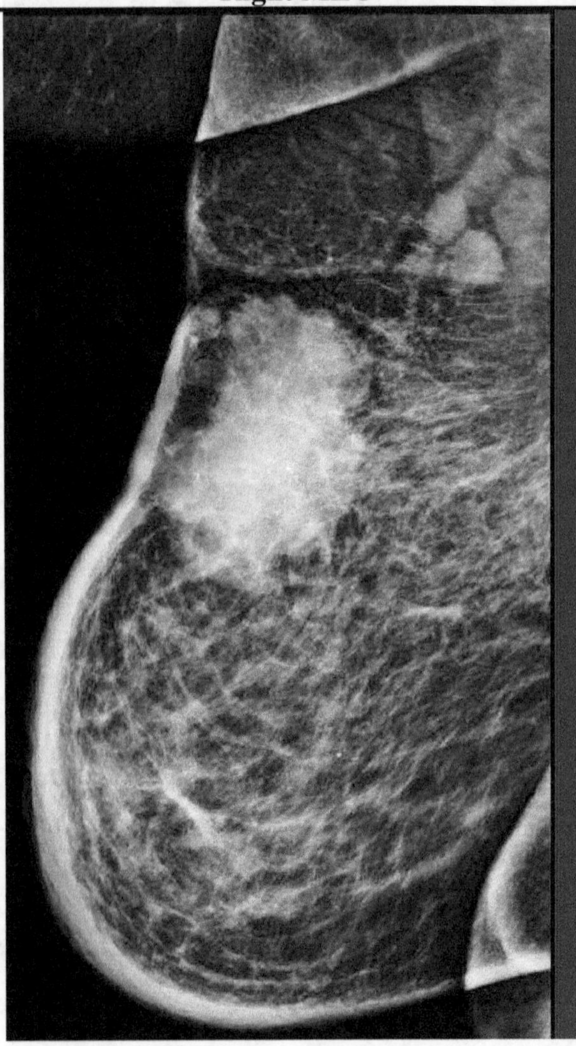	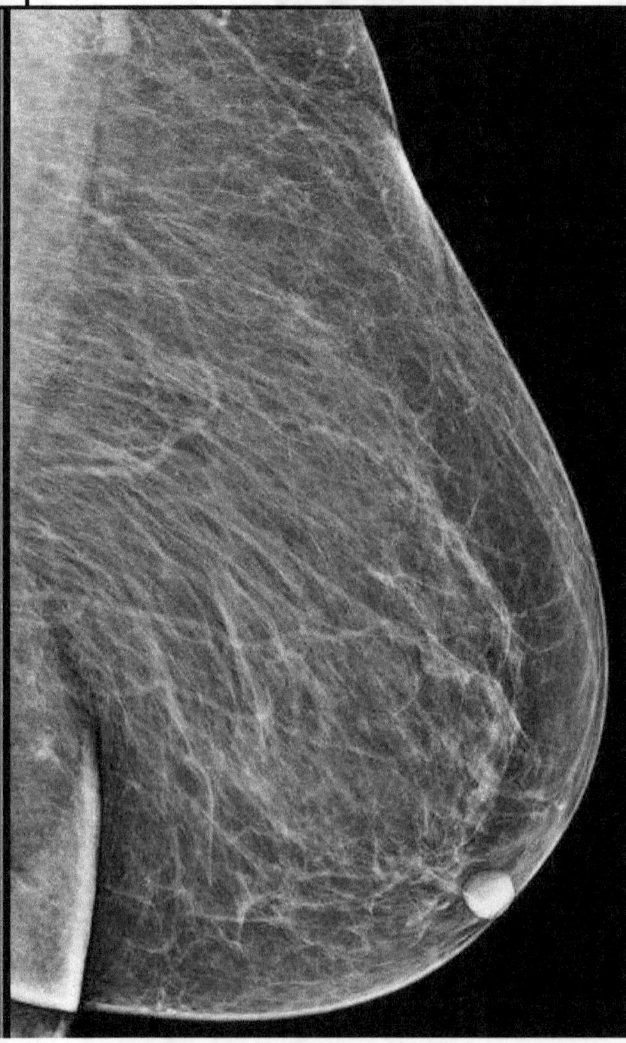

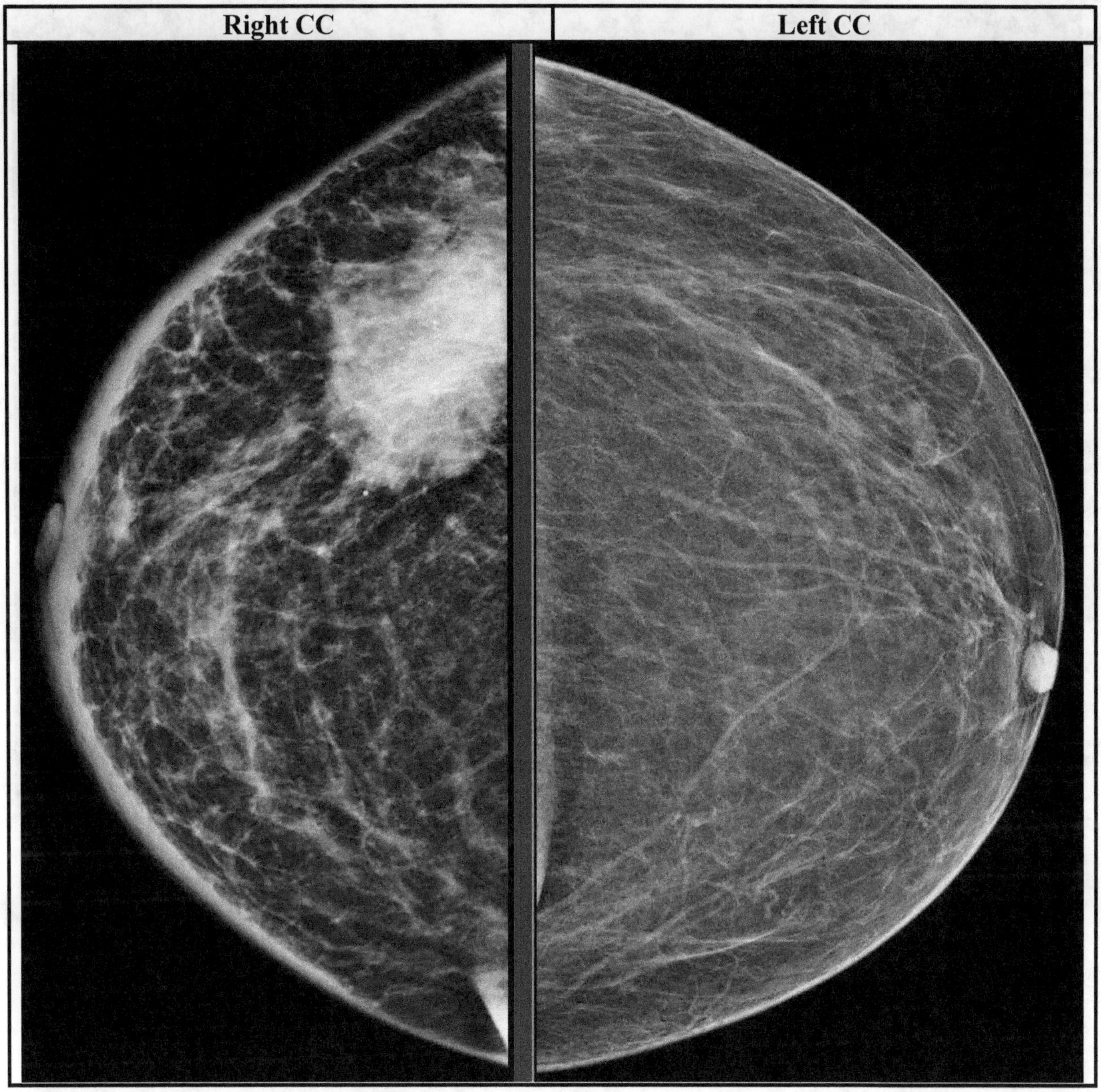
Right CC
Left CC

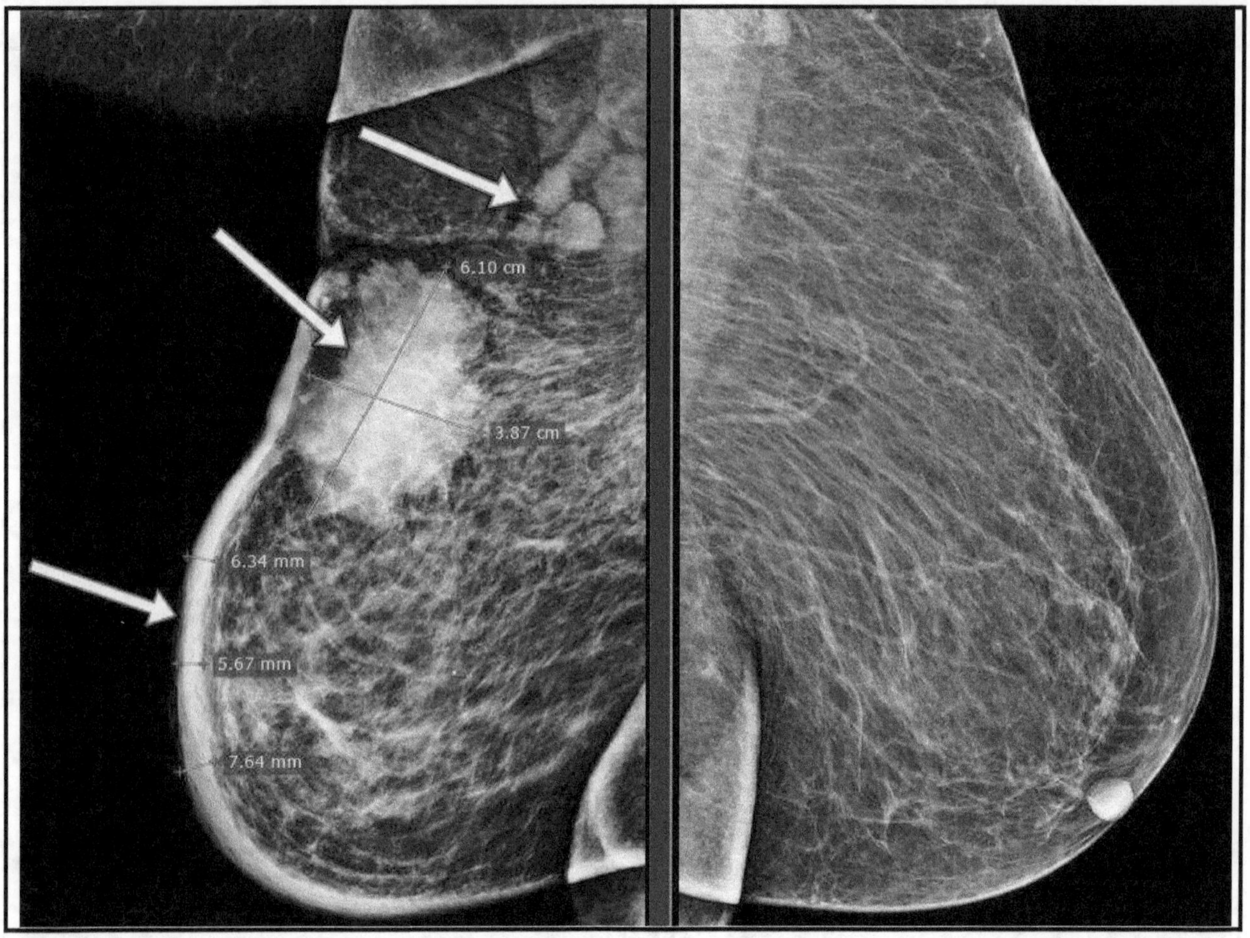
6.10 cm
3.87 cm
6.34 mm
5.67 mm
7.64 mm

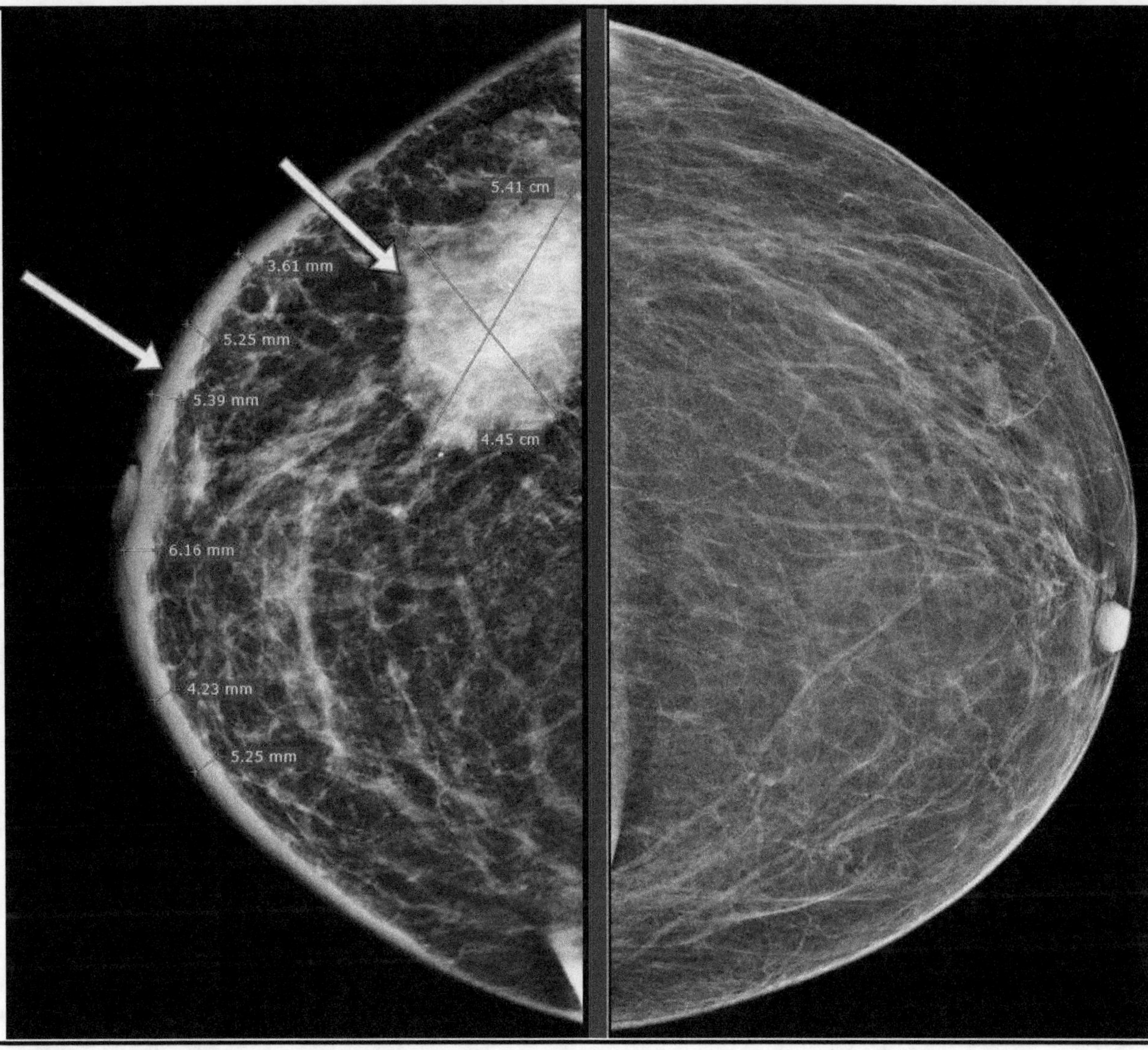

RIGHT BREAST	
Breast Parenchymal Density	***Almost entirely fatty (ACR A)***
Focal Mass	***UOQ irregular indistinct mass lesion associated with trabecular edema***
Asymmetric Density	None
Parenchymal Distortion	None
Calcification	None
Skin Thickening	***Positive (normal equal or less than 2 mm)***
Axillary Nodes	***Lymphadenopathy***

LEFT BREAST	
Breast Parenchymal Density	***Almost entirely fatty (ACR A)***
Focal Mass	None
Asymmetric Density	None
Parenchymal Distortion	None
Calcification	None
Skin Thickening	None
Axillary Nodes	None

IMPRESSION:

RIGHT BREAST: (BI-RADS 5)
LEFT BREAST: (BI-RADS 1)

RECOMMENDATION: Histopathological Correlation

CASE 39: 64-year-old female/ Diagnostic	
Right MLO	**Left MLO**
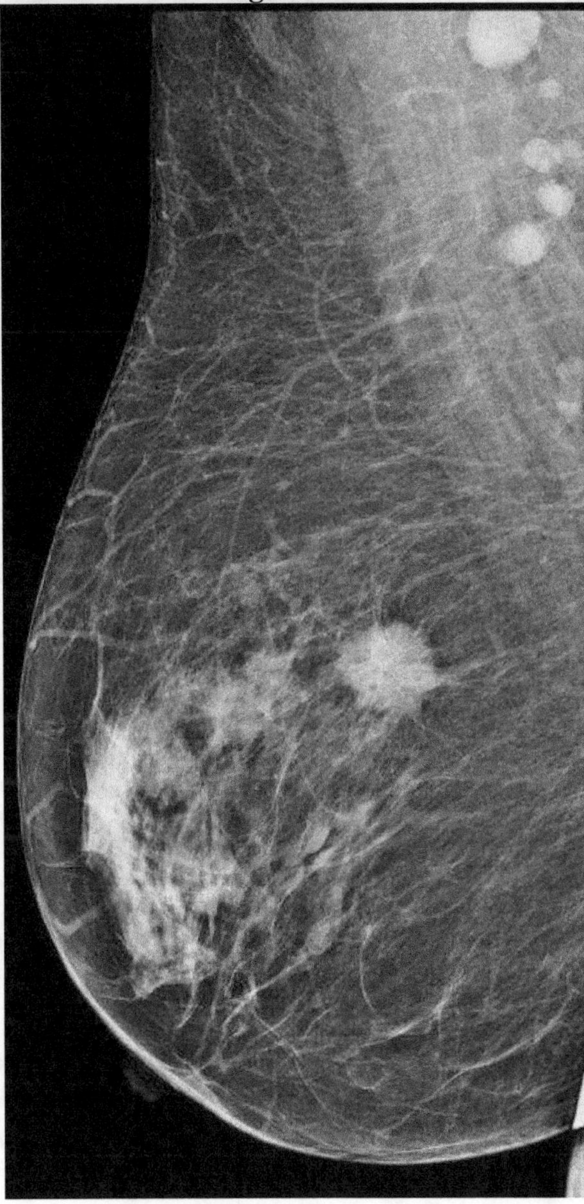	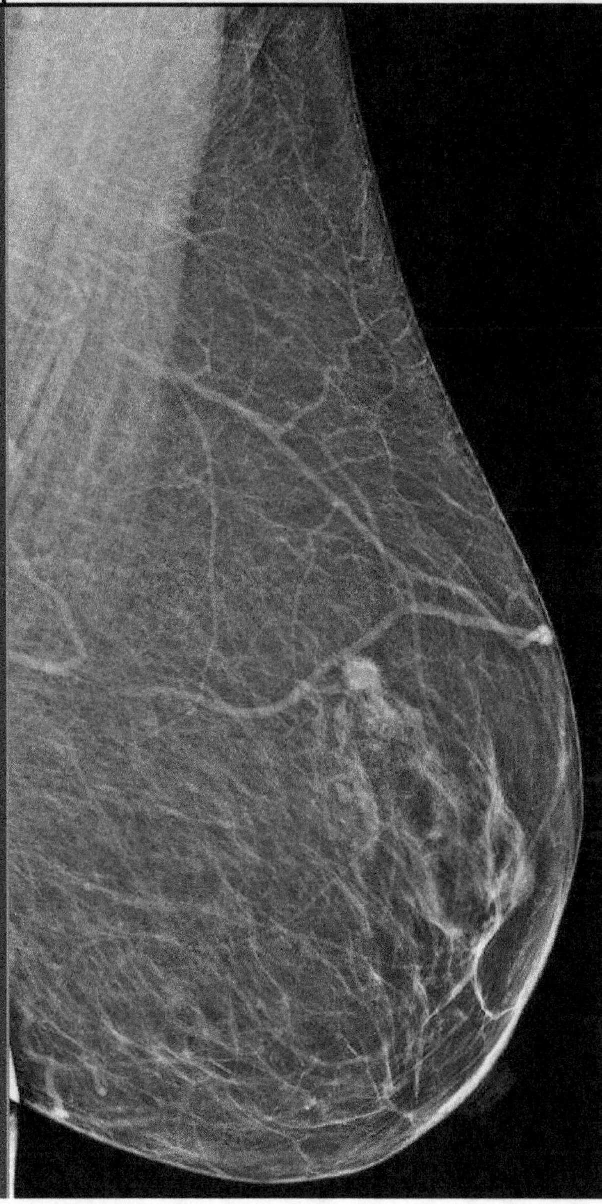

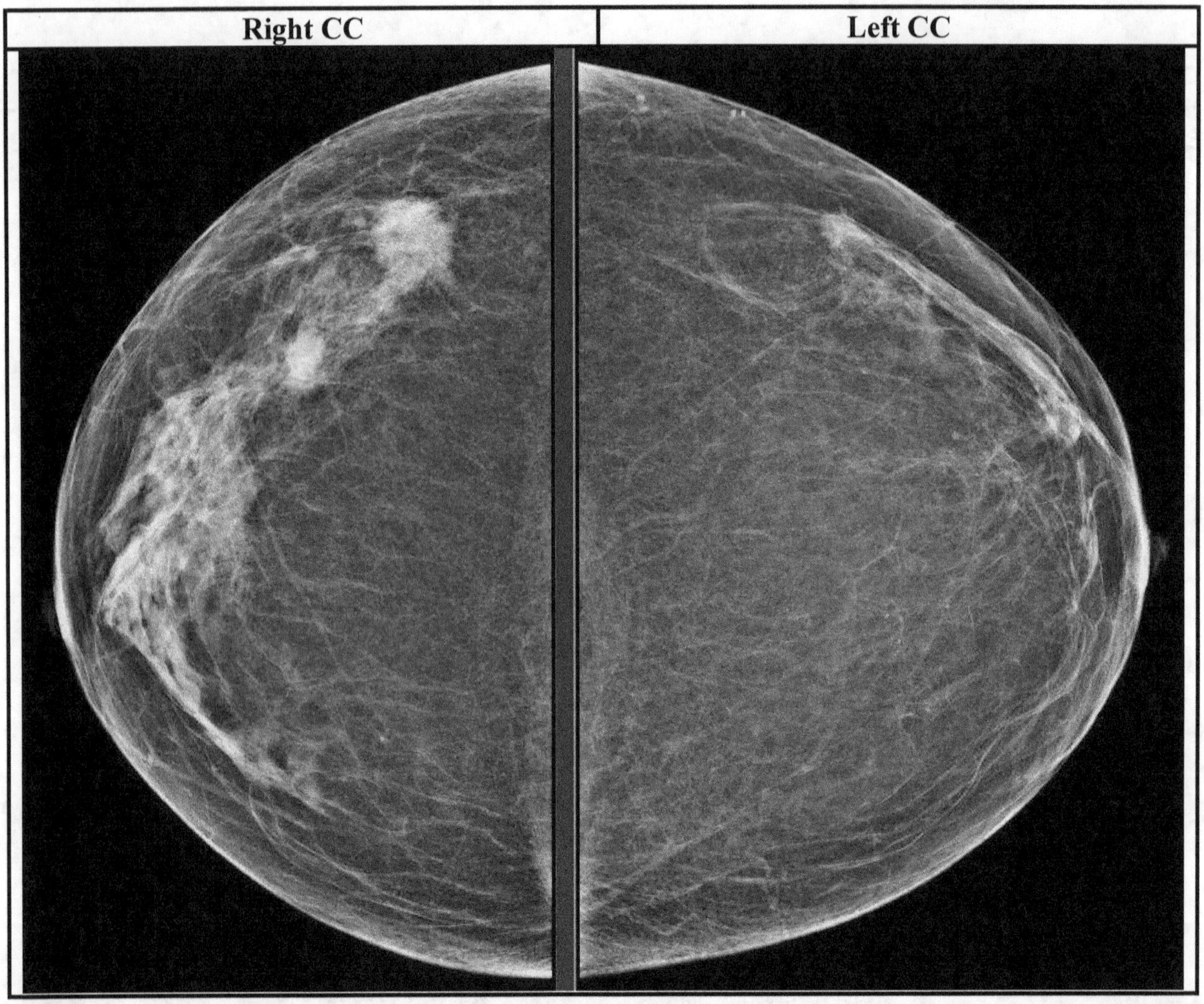
Right CC
Left CC

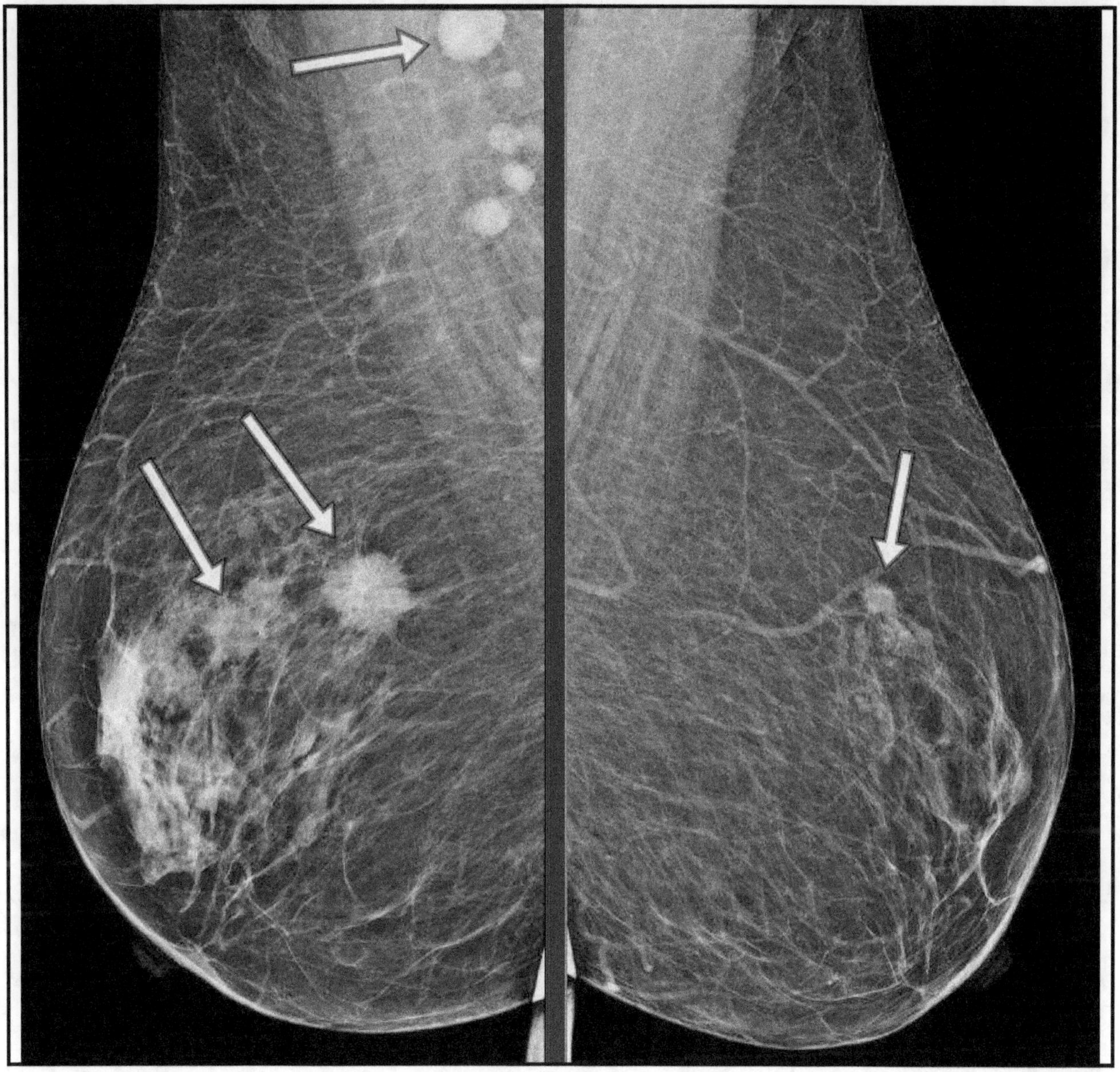

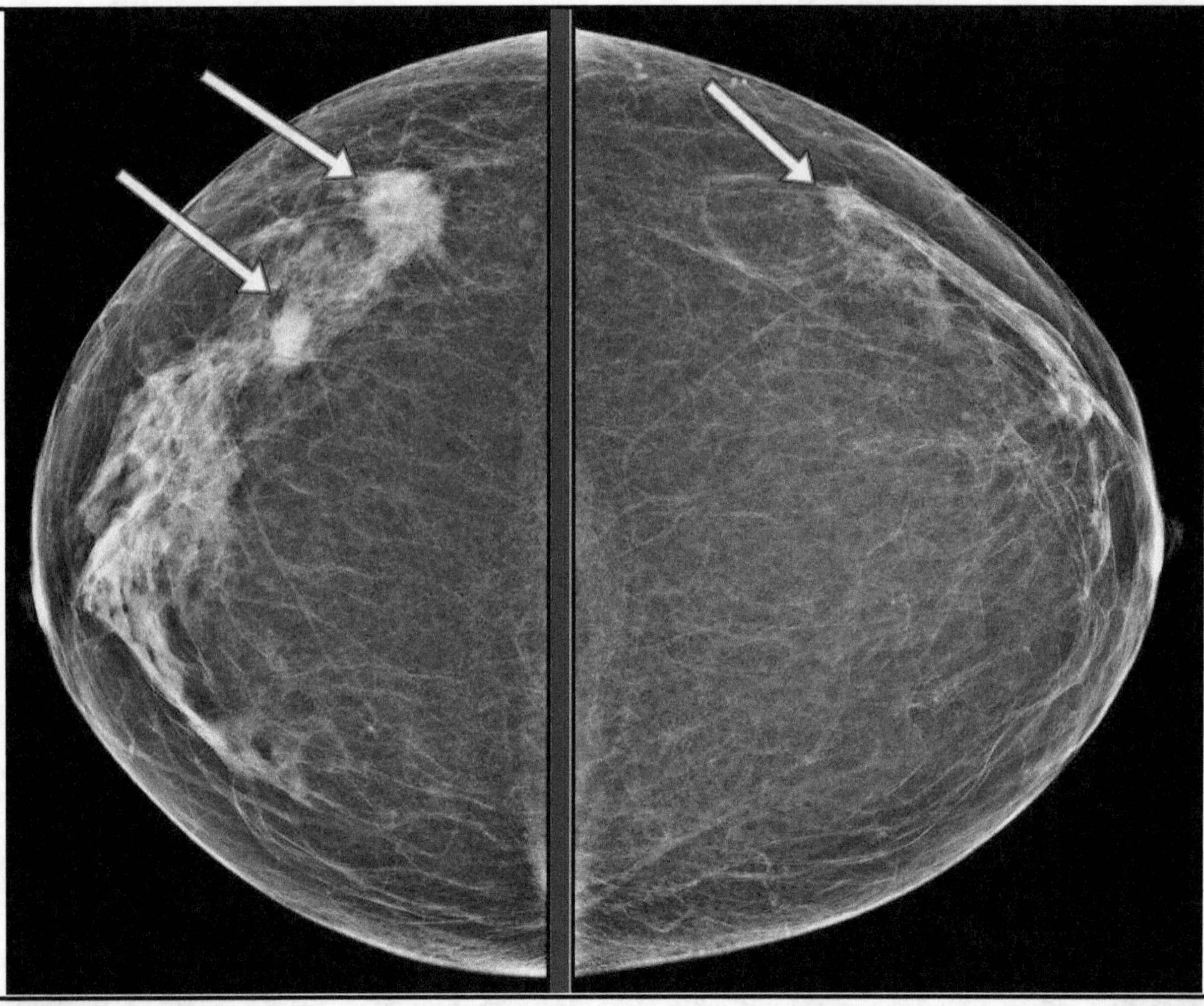

RIGHT BREAST	
Breast Parenchymal Density	***Scattered areas of fibroglandular density (ACR B)***
Focal Mass	***UOQ multifocal round spiculated mass lesions***
Asymmetric Density	None
Parenchymal Distortion	None
Calcification	None
Skin Thickening	None
Axillary Nodes	***Lymphadenopathy***

LEFT BREAST	
Breast Parenchymal Density	***Scattered areas of fibroglandular density (ACR B)***
Focal Mass	***UOQ round spiculated mass lesion***
Asymmetric Density	None
Parenchymal Distortion	None
Calcification	None
Skin Thickening	None
Axillary Nodes	None

IMPRESSION:

RIGHT BREAST: (BI-RADS 5)
LEFT BREAST: (BI-RADS 5)

RECOMMENDATION: Histopathological Correlation

CASE 40: 45-year-old female/ Diagnostic	
Right MLO	Left MLO

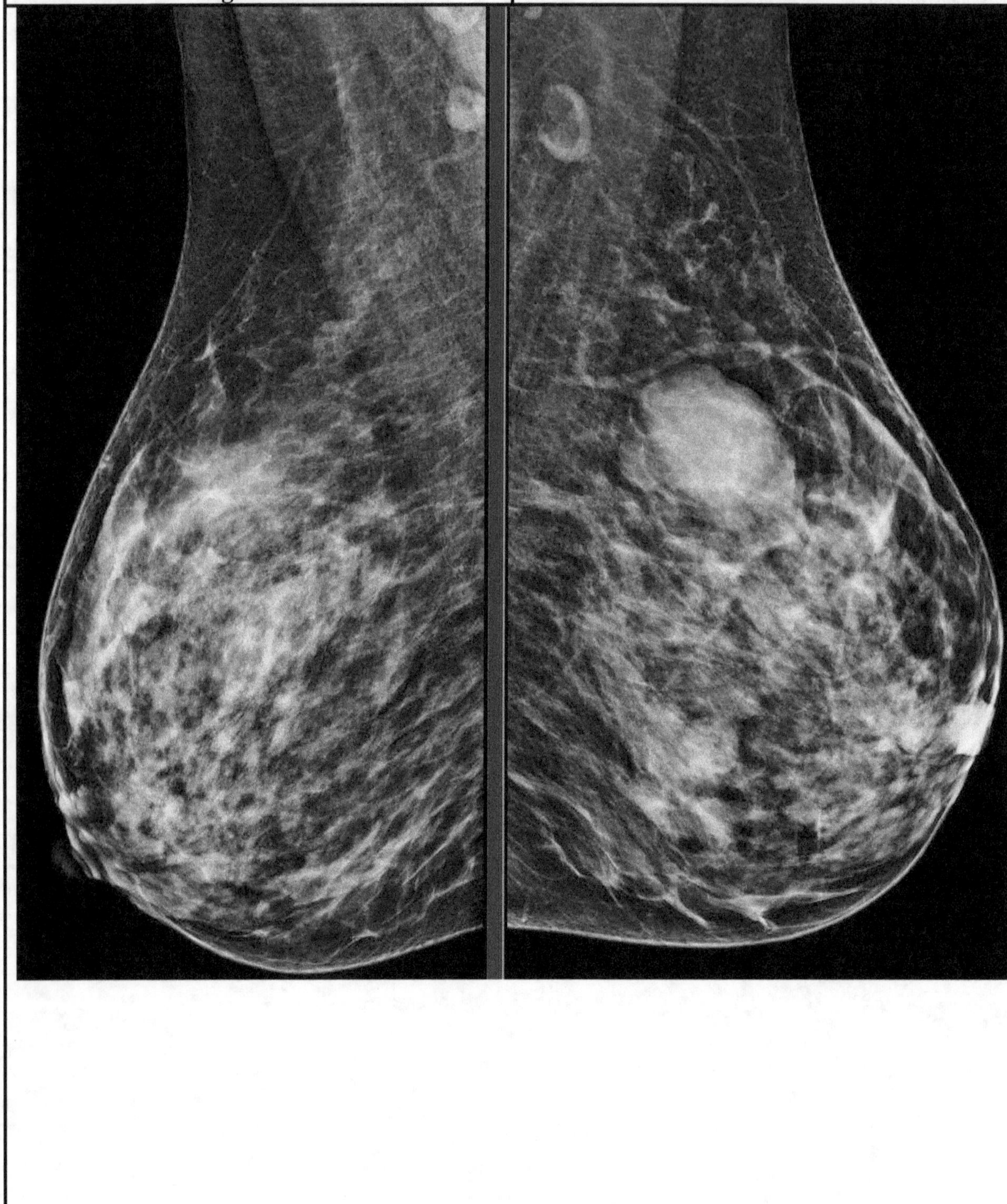

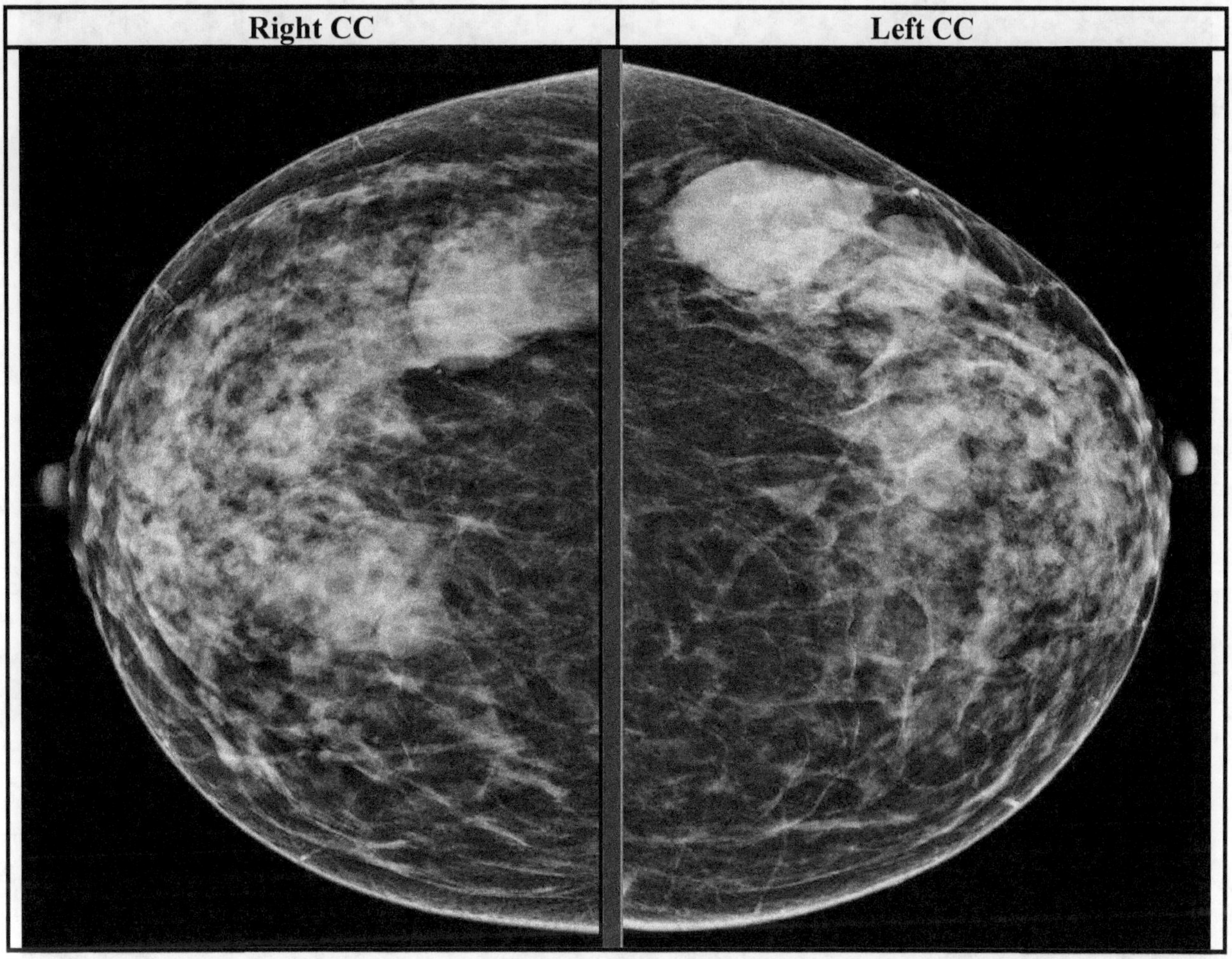
Right CC
Left CC

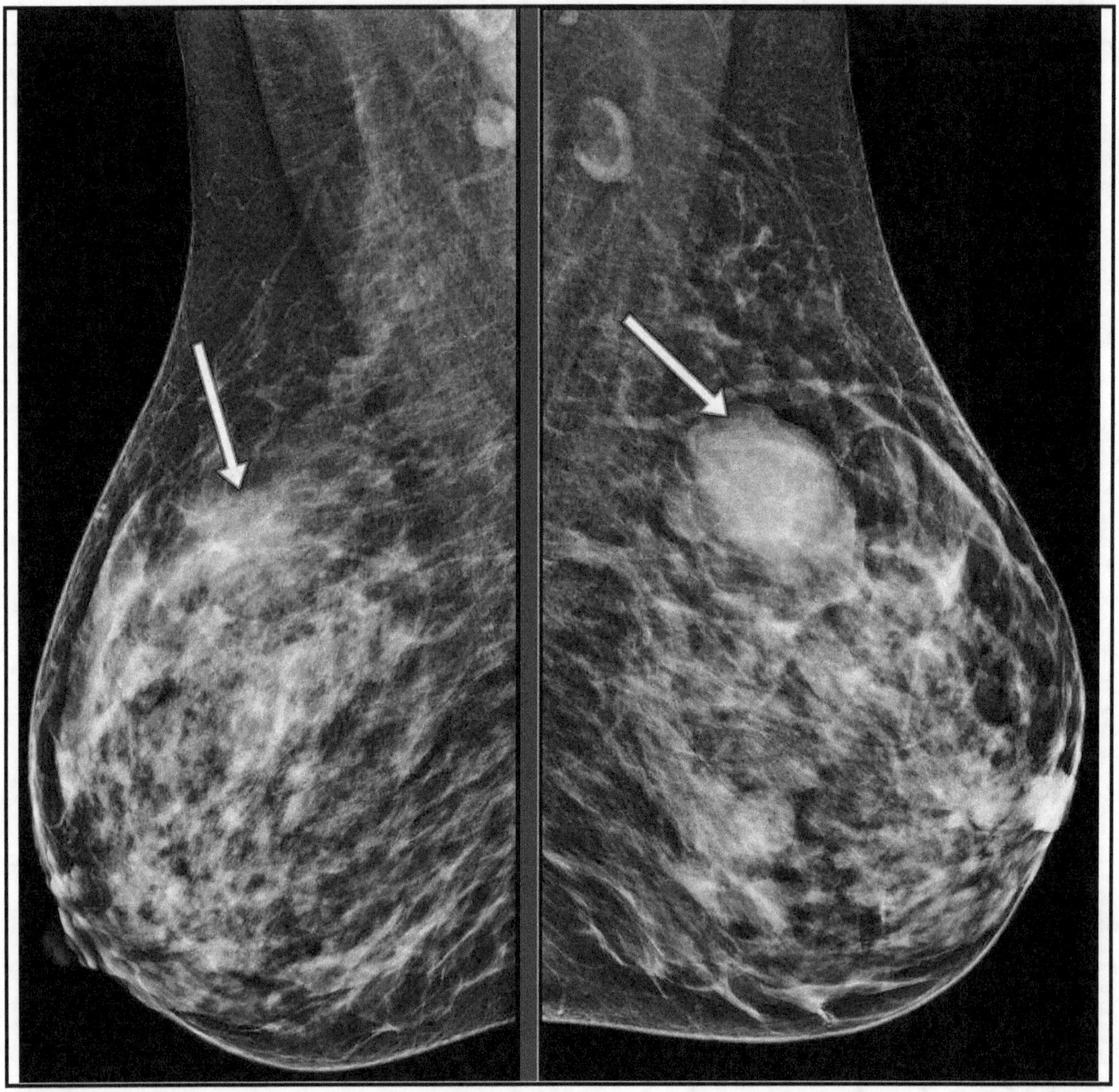

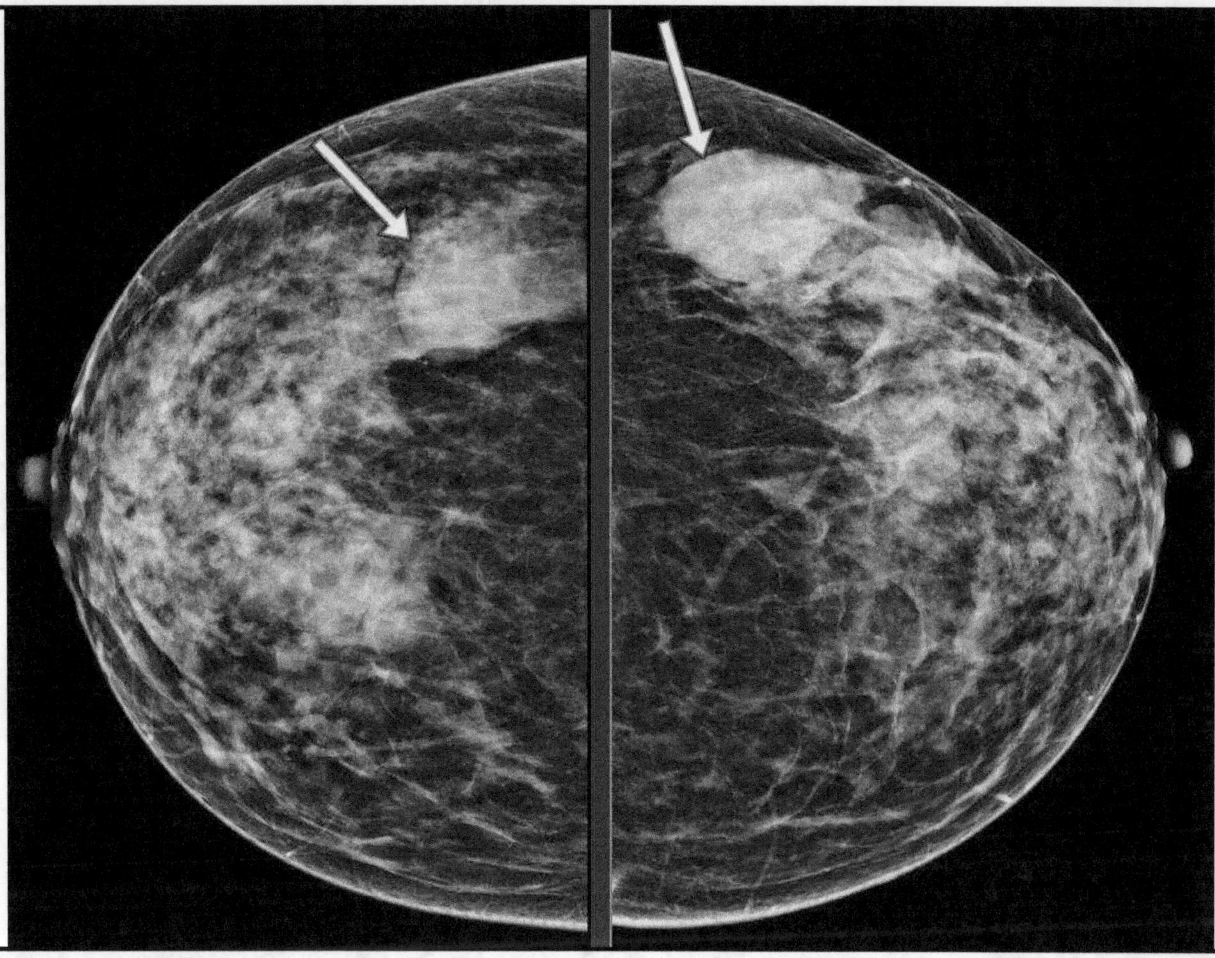

RIGHT BREAST	
Breast Parenchymal Density	***Heterogeneously dense, may obscure small masses (ACR C)***
Focal Mass	***Multiple oval circumscribed mass lesions***
Asymmetric Density	None
Parenchymal Distortion	None
Calcification	None
Skin Thickening	None
Axillary Nodes	None

LEFT BREAST	
Breast Parenchymal Density	***Heterogeneously dense, may obscure small masses (ACR C)***
Focal Mass	***Multiple oval circumscribed mass lesions***
Asymmetric Density	None
Parenchymal Distortion	None
Calcification	None
Skin Thickening	None
Axillary Nodes	None

IMPRESSION:

RIGHT BREAST: (BI-RADS 0)
LEFT BREAST: (BI-RADS 0)

RECOMMENDATION: US Correlation

US demonstrated bilateral multiple simple cysts =fibrocystic c hanges = BI-RADS 3

CASE 41: 59-year-old female/ Diagnostic	
Right MLO	**Left MLO**

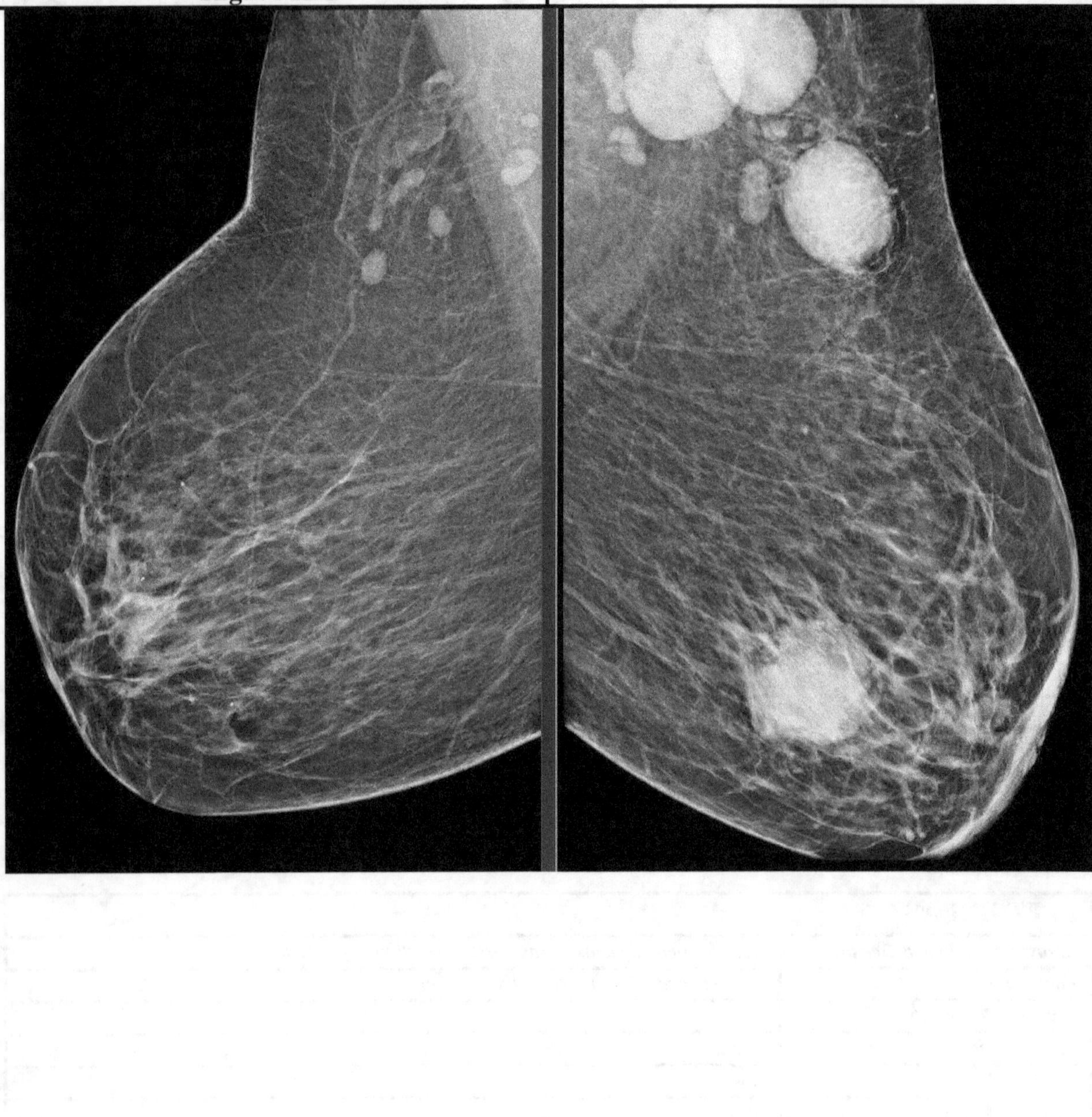

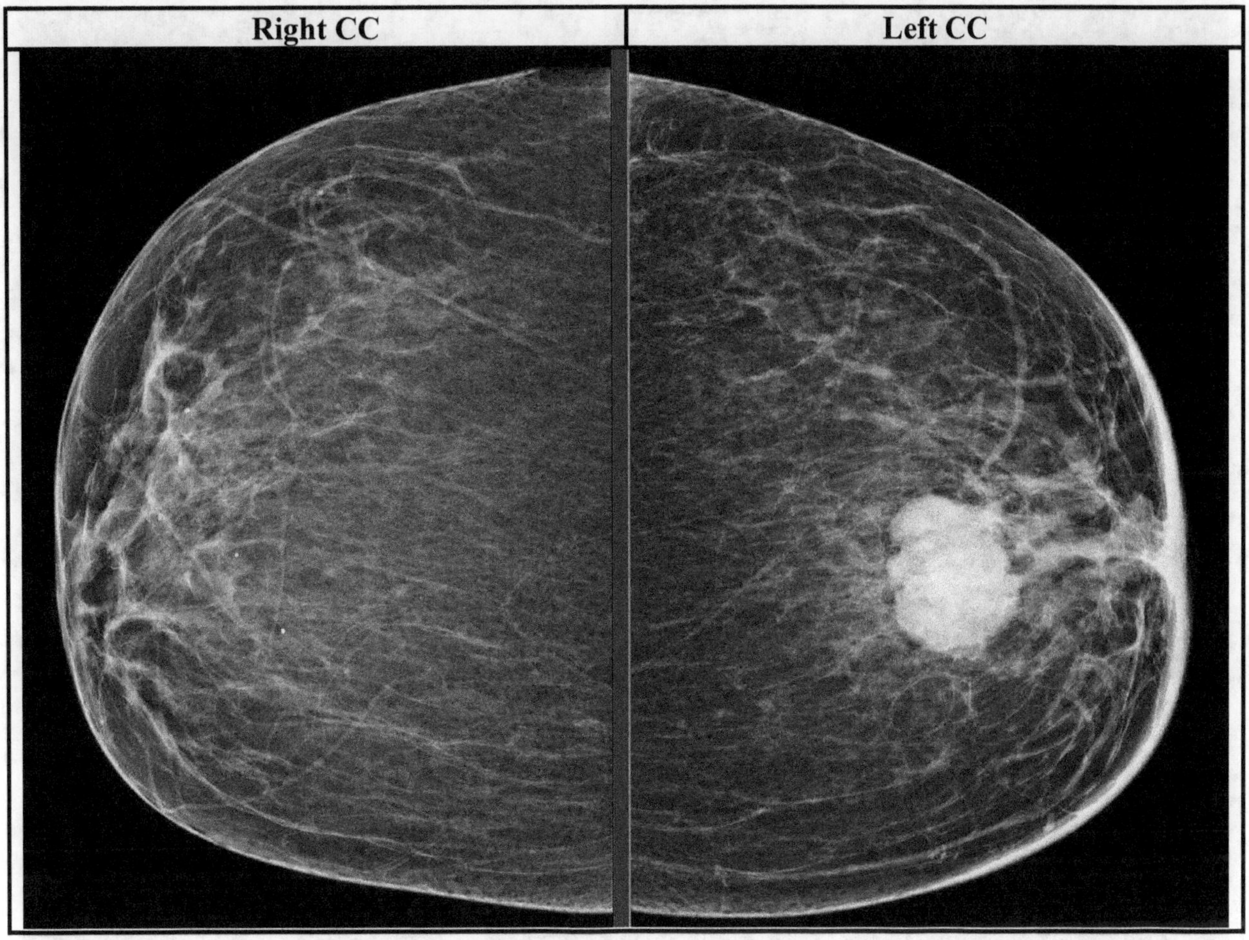
Right CC
Left CC

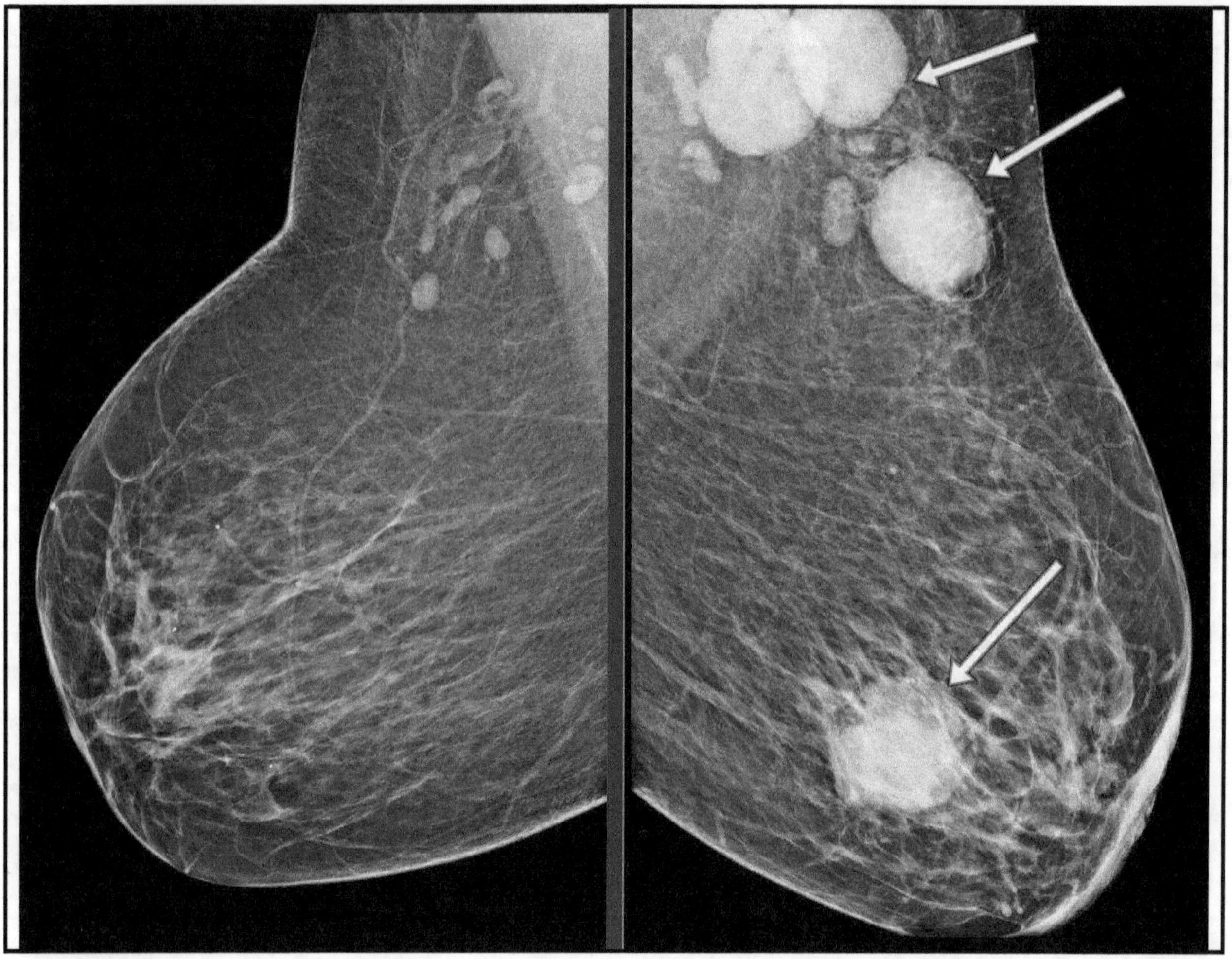

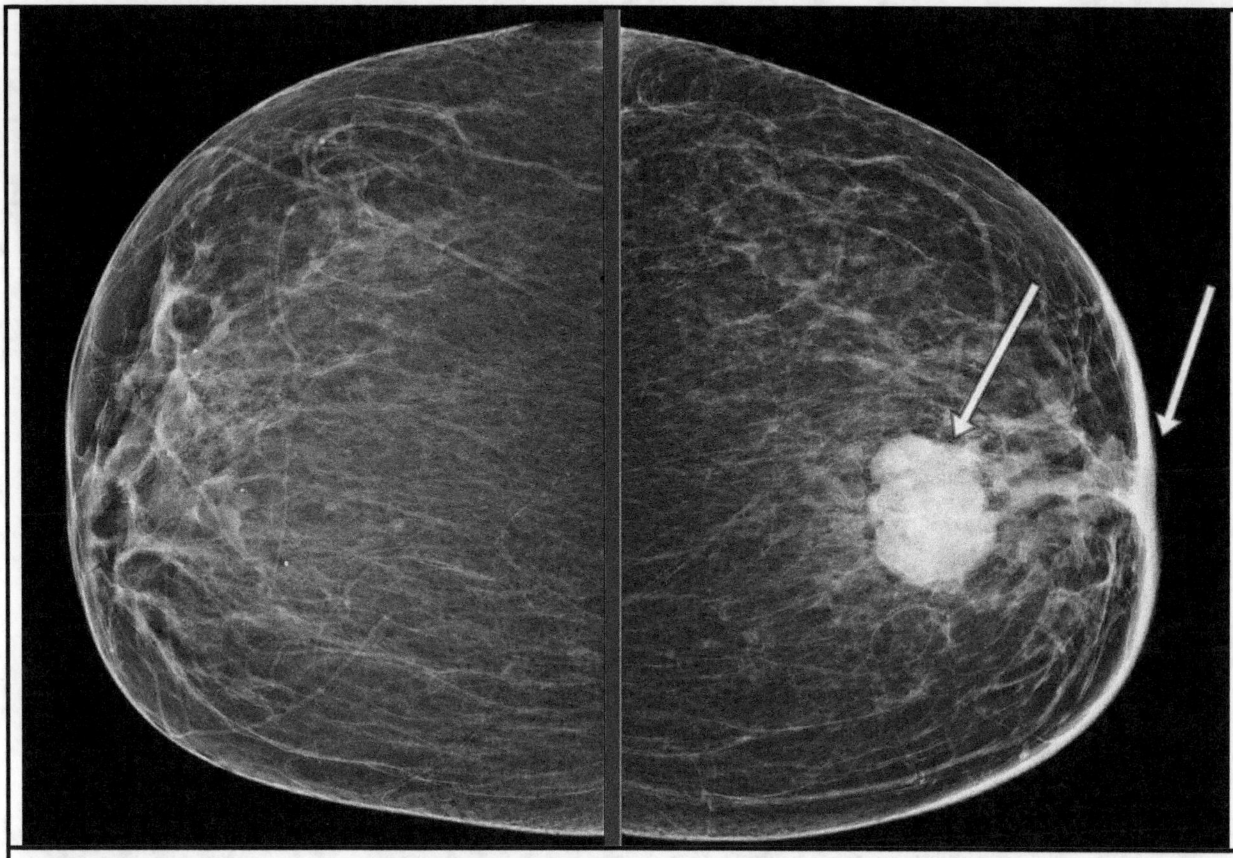

RIGHT BREAST	
Breast Parenchymal Density	***Scattered areas of fibroglandular density (ACR B)***
Focal Mass	None
Asymmetric Density	None
Parenchymal Distortion	None
Calcification	***Skin calcifications***
Skin Thickening	None
Axillary Nodes	None

LEFT BREAST	
Breast Parenchymal Density	***Scattered areas of fibroglandular density (ACR B)***
Focal Mass	***Lower central (6 o'clock) rounded micro-lobulated /obscured mass lesion***
Asymmetric Density	None
Parenchymal Distortion	None
Calcification	None
Skin Thickening	***Positive***
Axillary Nodes	***Multiple enlarged LNs***

IMPRESSION:

RIGHT BREAST: (BI-RADS 2)
LEFT BREAST: (BI-RADS 5)

RECOMMENDATION: Histopathological Correlation

CASE 42: 38-year-old female/ Diagnostic	
Right MLO	**Left MLO**

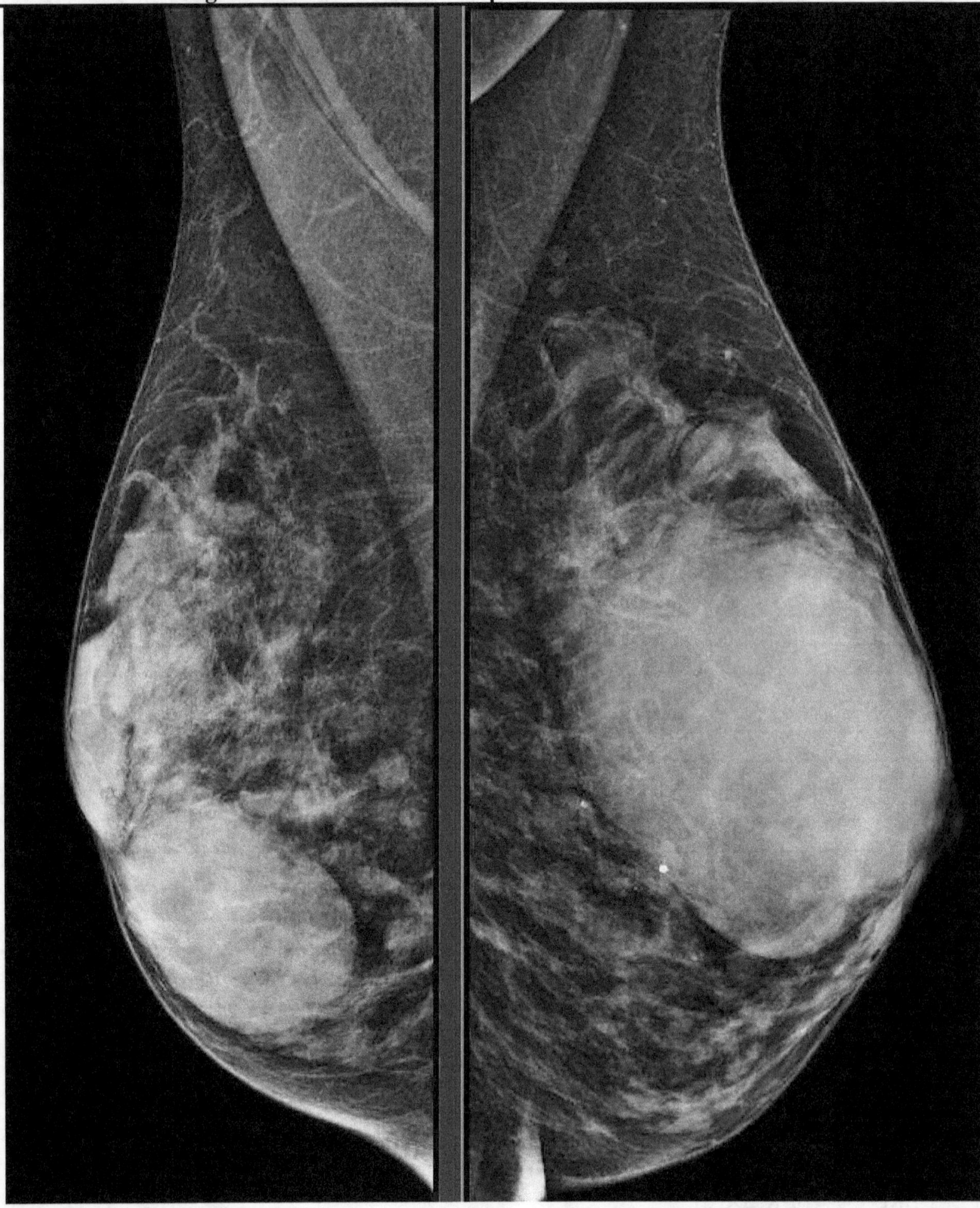

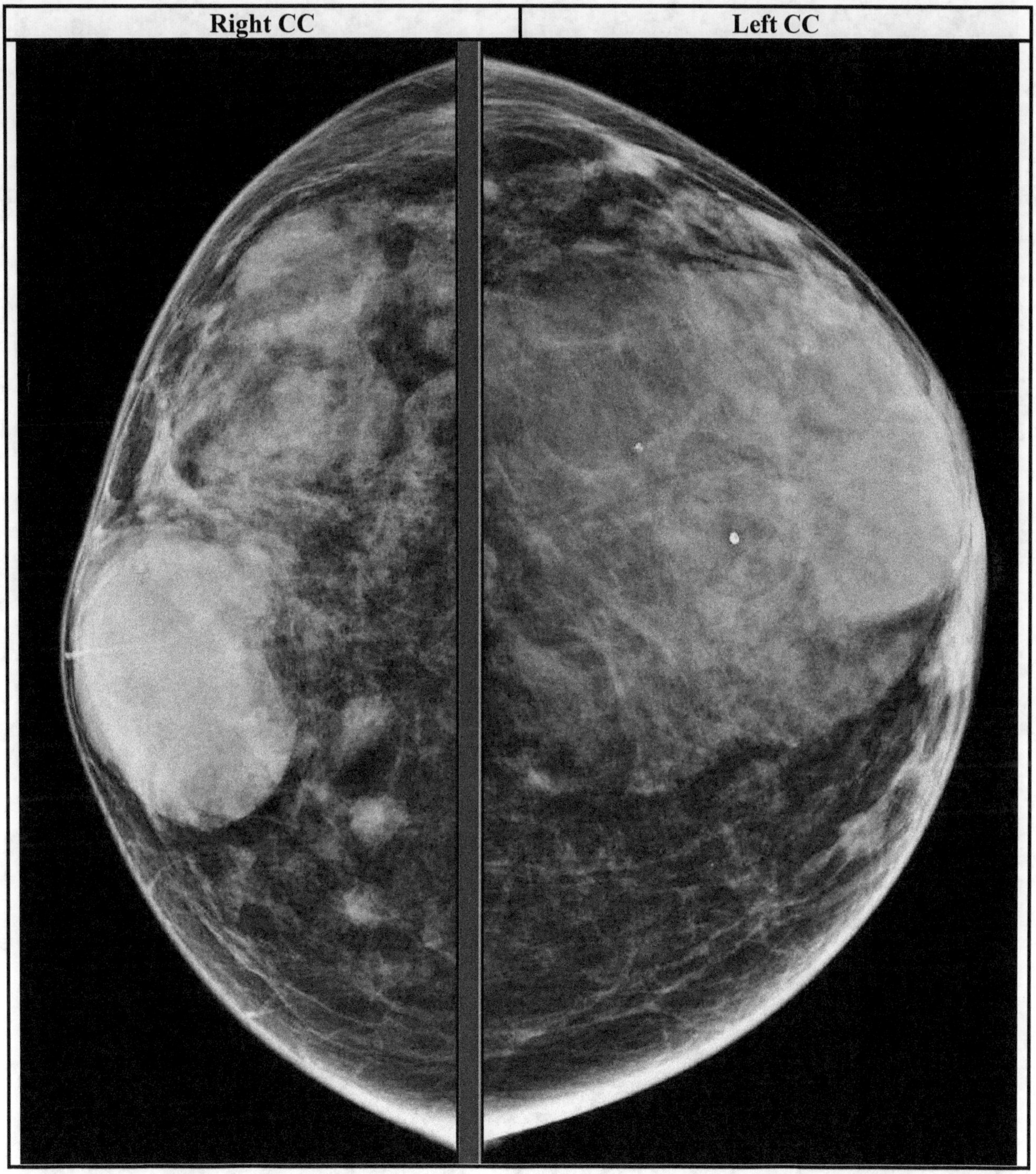
Right CC
Left CC

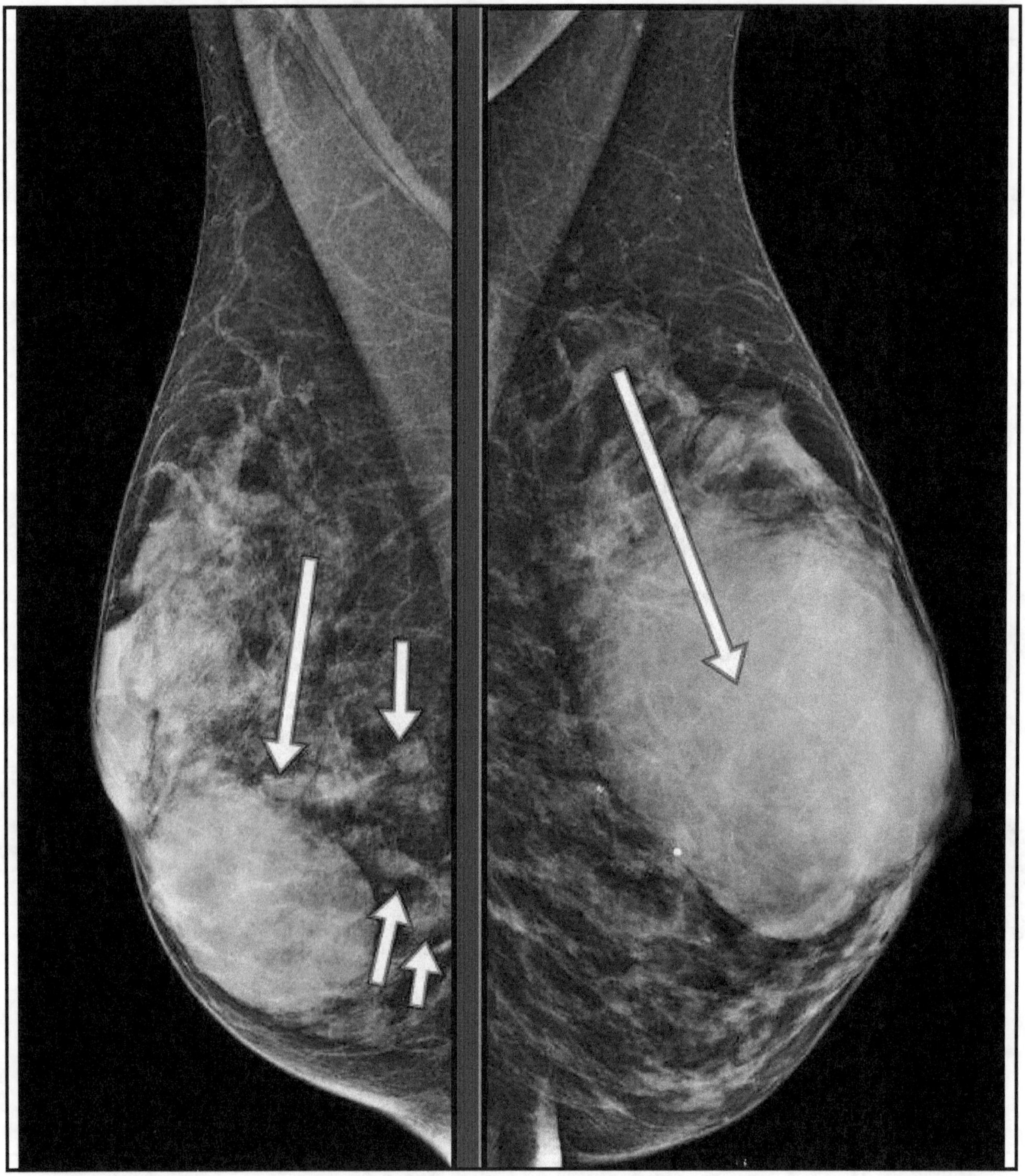

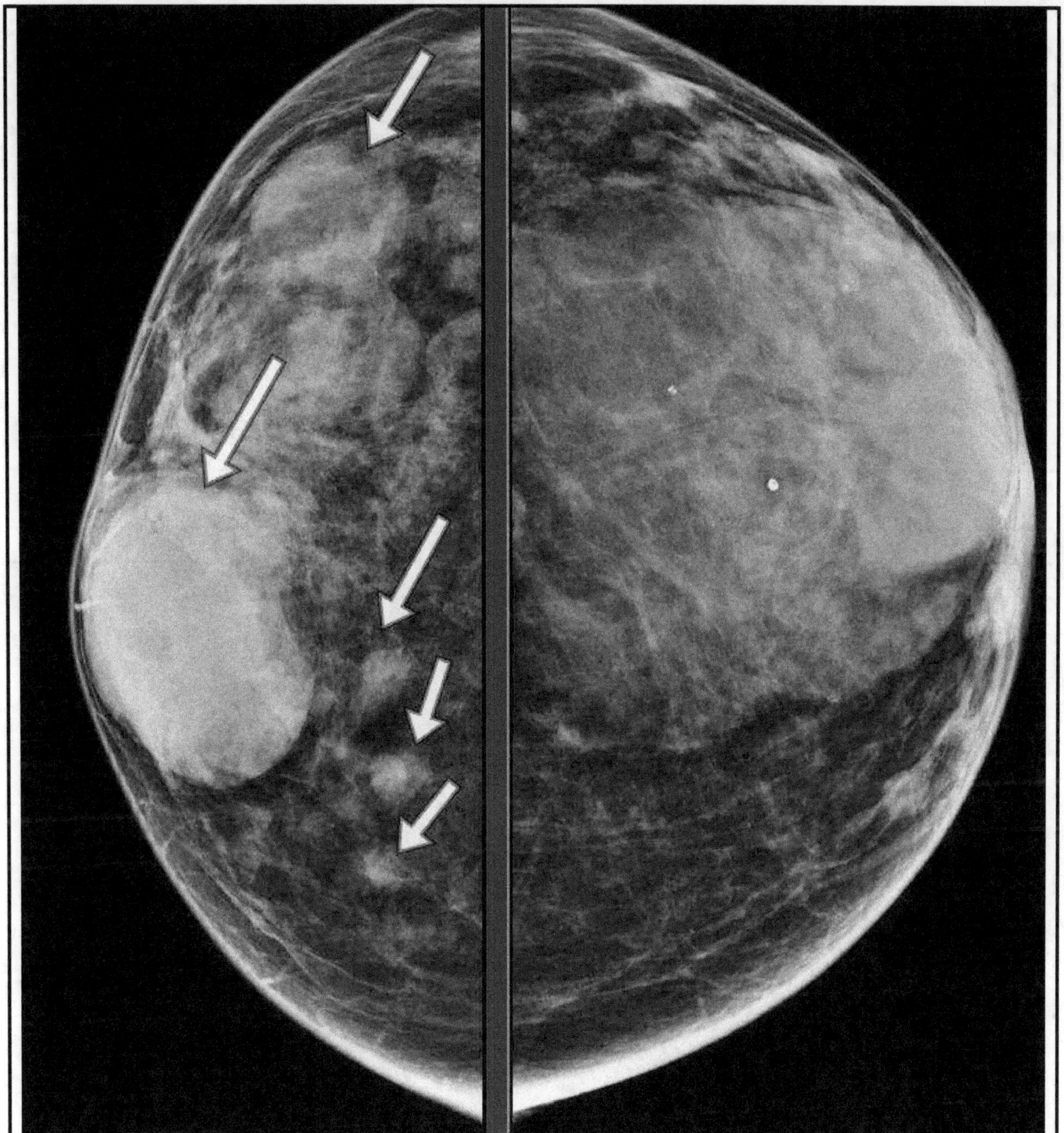

RIGHT BREAST	
Breast Parenchymal Density	***Extremely dense, which lowers the sensitivity of mammography (ACR D)***
Focal Mass	***Bilateral multiple masses oval /rounded circumscribed/ indistinct mass lesions***
Asymmetric Density	None
Parenchymal Distortion	None
Calcification	None
Skin Thickening	None
Axillary Nodes	None

LEFT BREAST	
Breast Parenchymal Density	***Extremely dense, which lowers the sensitivity of mammography (ACR D)***
Focal Mass	***Large oval circumscribed mass lesion***
Asymmetric Density	*None*
Parenchymal Distortion	*None*
Calcification	***Skin calcification***
Skin Thickening	*None*
Axillary Nodes	*None*

IMPRESSION:
RIGHT BREAST: (BI-RADS 0)
LEFT BREAST: (BI-RADS 0)

RECOMMENDATION: US Correlation

CASE 43: 63-year-old female/ Diagnostic	
Right MLO	**Left MLO**

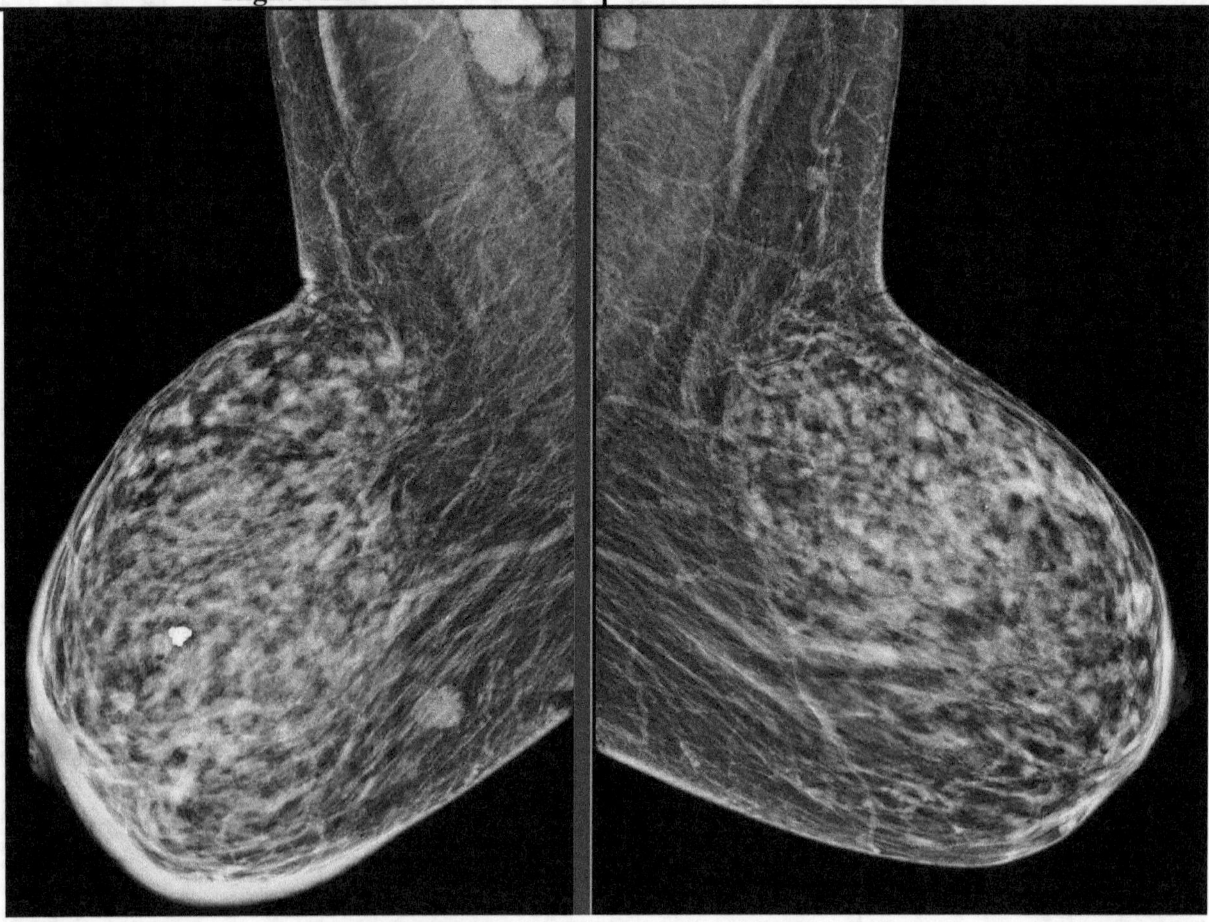

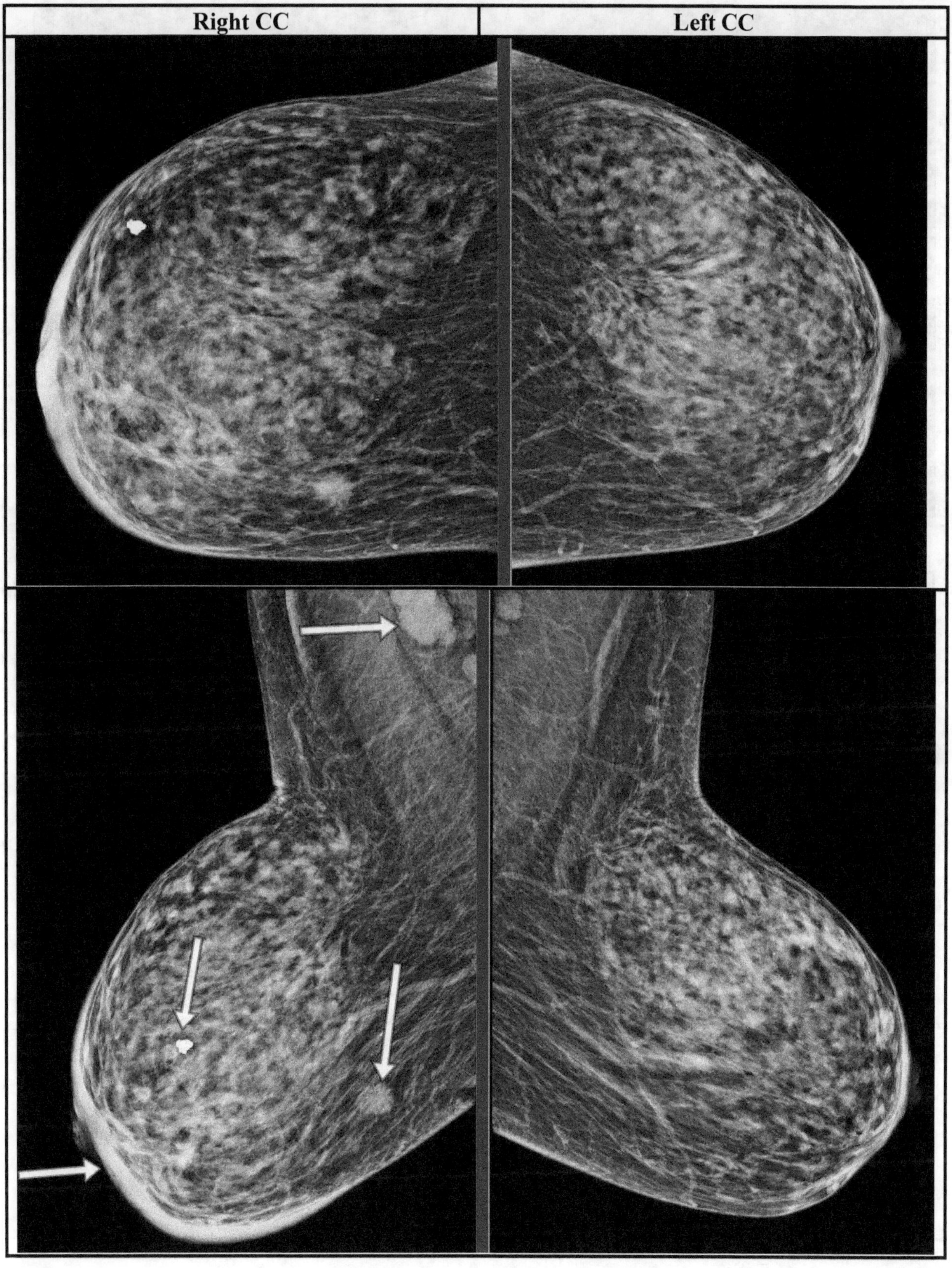
Right CC
Left CC

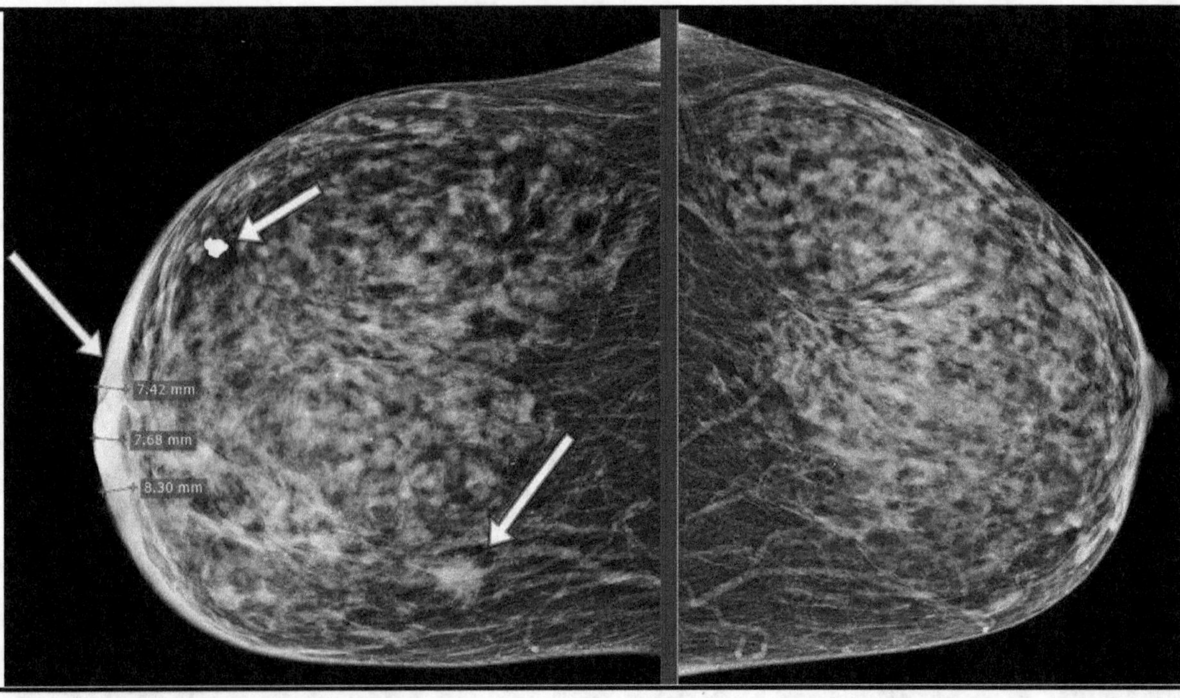

RIGHT BREAST	
Breast Parenchymal Density	***Heterogeneously dense, may obscure small masses (ACR C)***
Focal Mass	***LIQ irregular spiculated mass lesion / UOQ involuted fibroadenoma with coarse (=popcorn calcification)***
Asymmetric Density	None
Parenchymal Distortion	None
Calcification	***UOQ course (=popcorn calcification)***
Skin Thickening	***Positive***
Axillary Nodes	***Lymphadenopathy***

LEFT BREAST	
Breast Parenchymal Density	***Heterogeneously dense, may obscure small masses (ACR C)***
Focal Mass	None
Asymmetric Density	None
Parenchymal Distortion	None
Calcification	None
Skin Thickening	None
Axillary Nodes	None

IMPRESSION:
RIGHT BREAST: (BI-RADS 5)
LEFT BREAST: (BI-RADS 1)

RECOMMENDATION: Histopathological Correlation

CASE 44: 59-year-old female/ Diagnostic

Right MLO

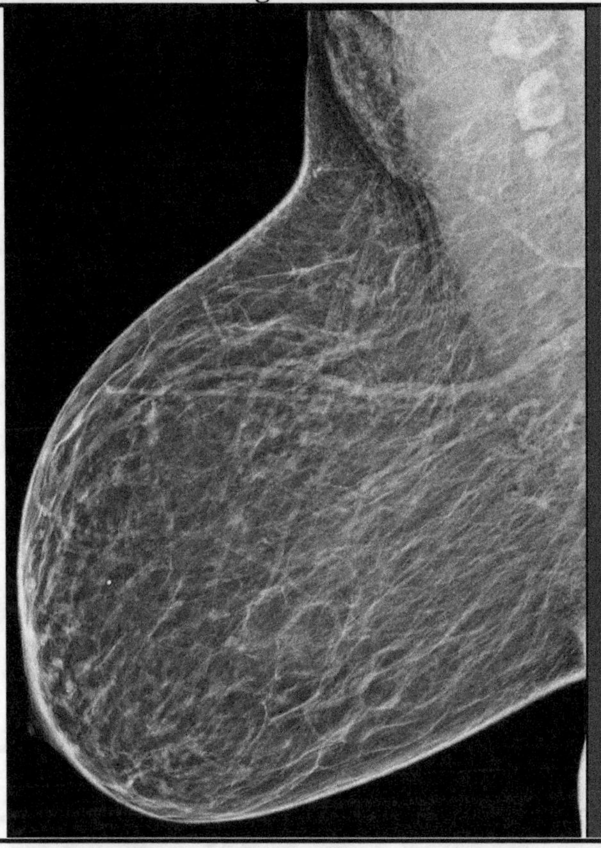

Left MLO

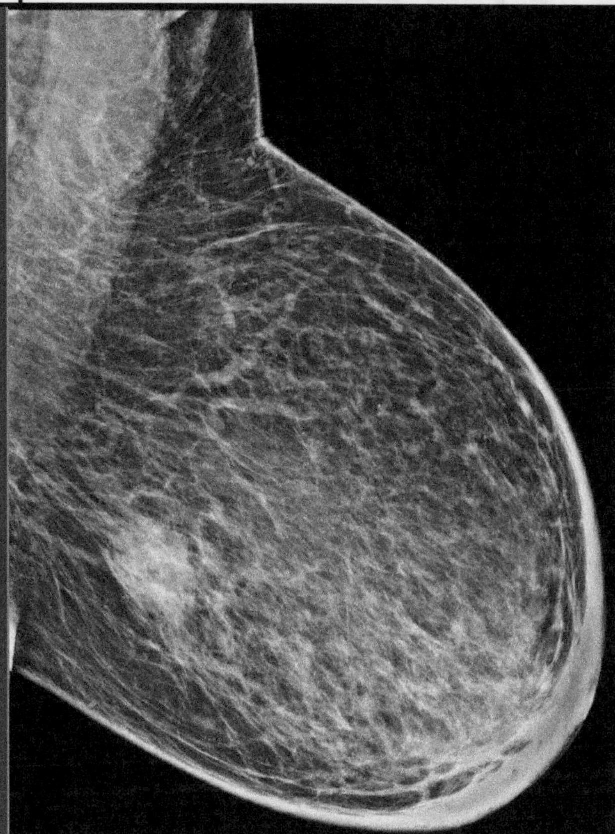

Right CC

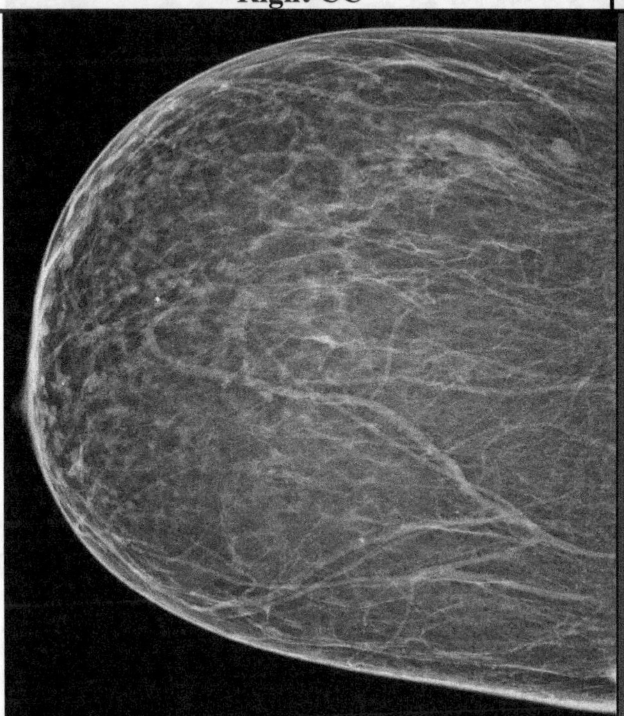

Left CC

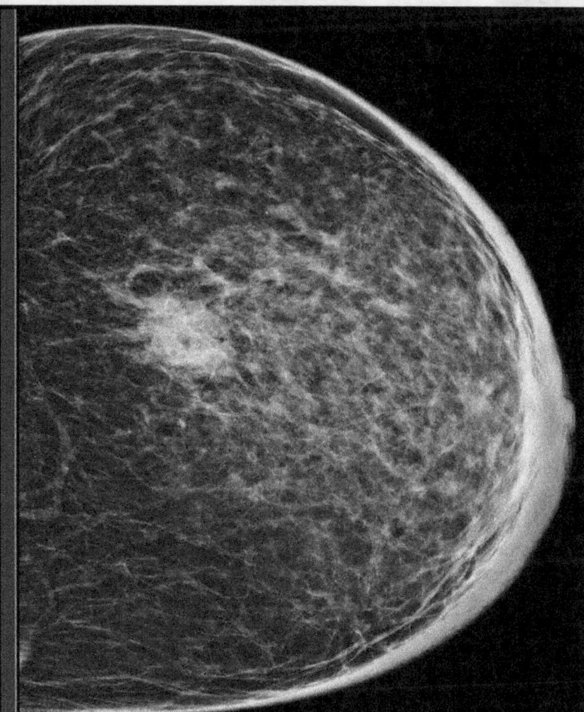

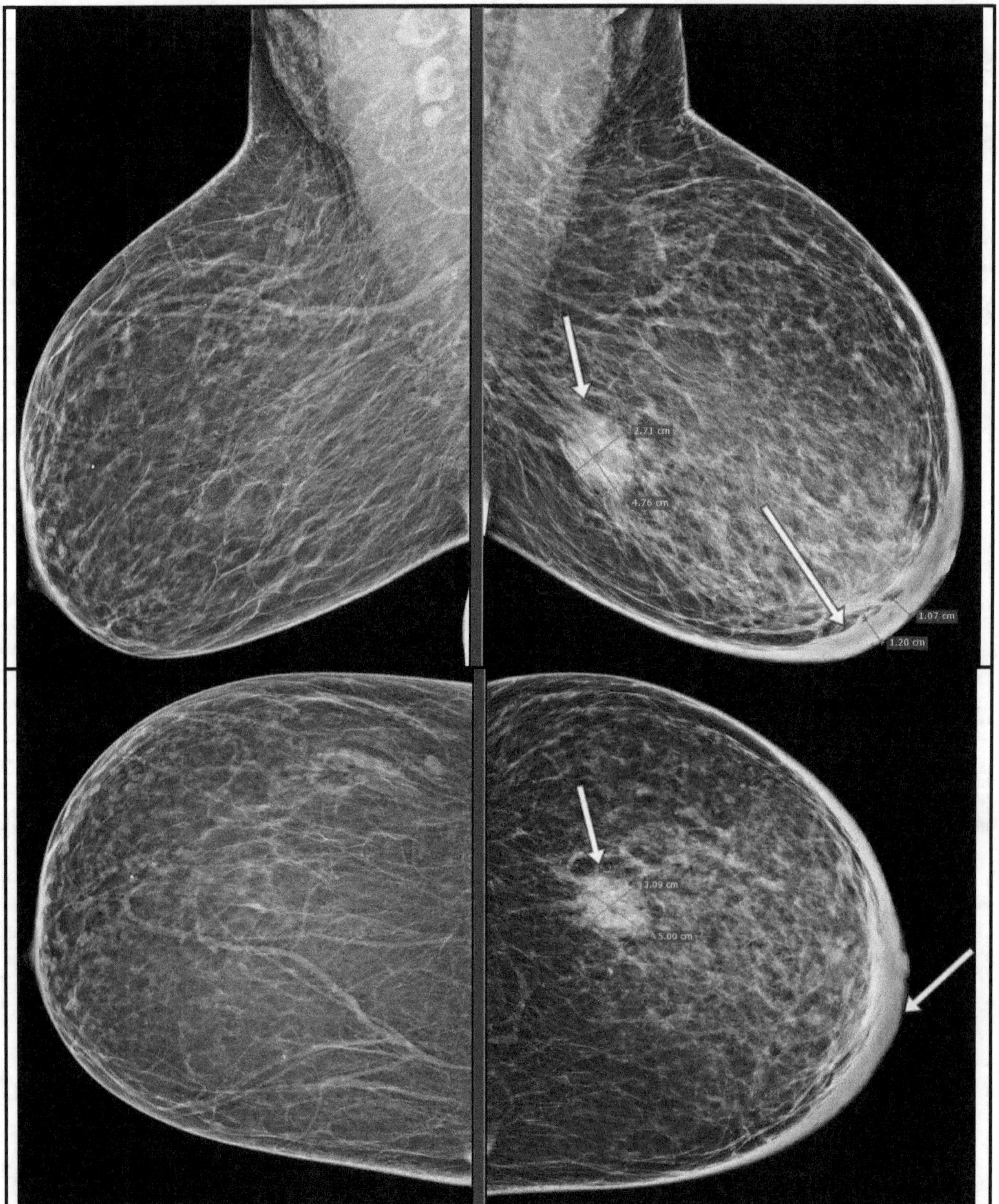

RIGHT BREAST	
Breast Parenchymal Density	***Scattered areas of fibroglandular density (ACR B)***
Focal Mass	None
Asymmetric Density	None

Parenchymal Distortion	None
Calcification	None
Skin Thickening	None
Axillary Nodes	None

LEFT BREAST	
Breast Parenchymal Density	***Scattered areas of fibroglandular density (ACR B)/ Trabecular Edema***
Focal Mass	***LOQ irregular indistinct focal mass lesion measures (x)***
Asymmetric Density	None
Parenchymal Distortion	None
Calcification	None
Skin Thickening	***Positive***
Axillary Nodes	None

IMPRESSION:
RIGHT BREAST: (BI-RADS 1)
LEFT BREAST: (BI-RADS 5)

RECOMMENDATION: Histopathological Correlation

CASE 45: 29-year-old female/ Diagnostic	
Right MLO	Left MLO

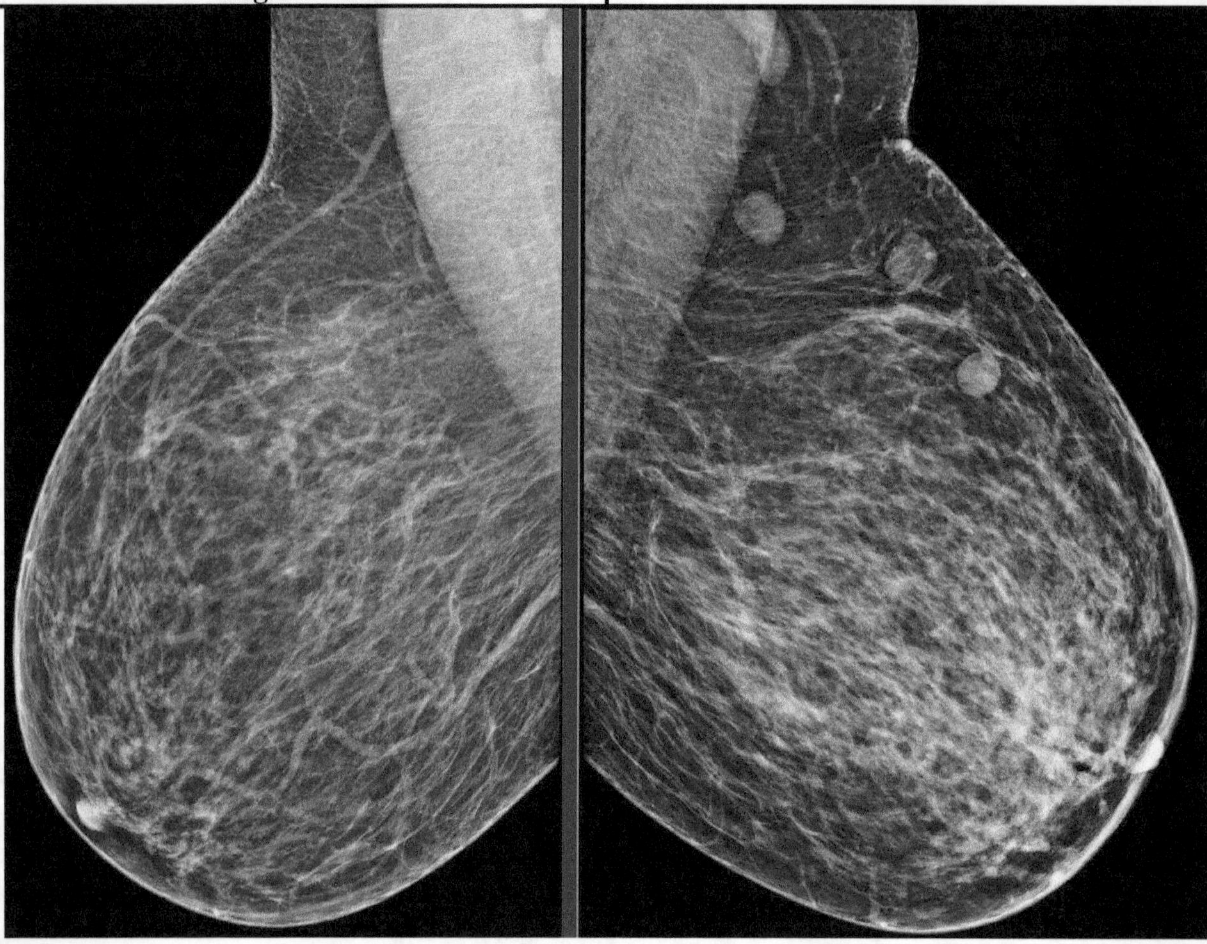

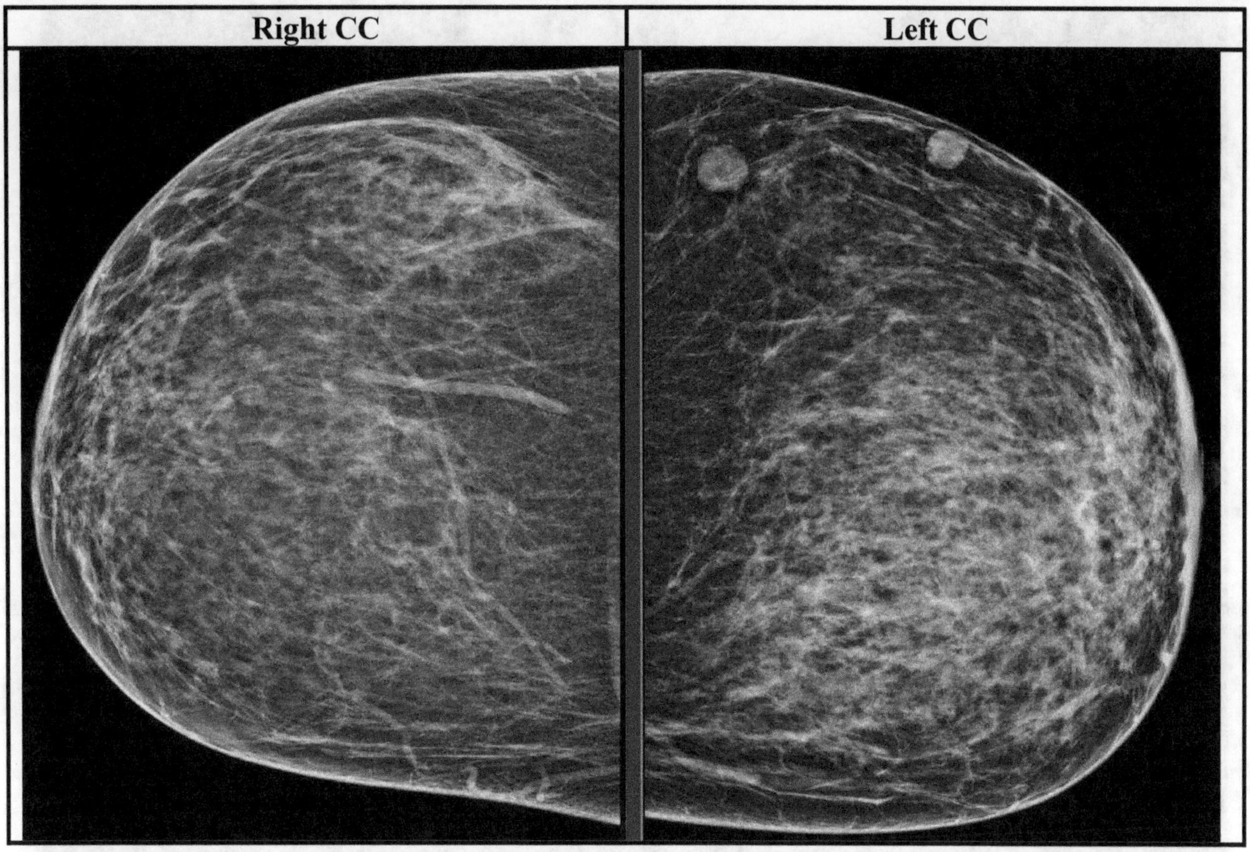
Right CC
Left CC

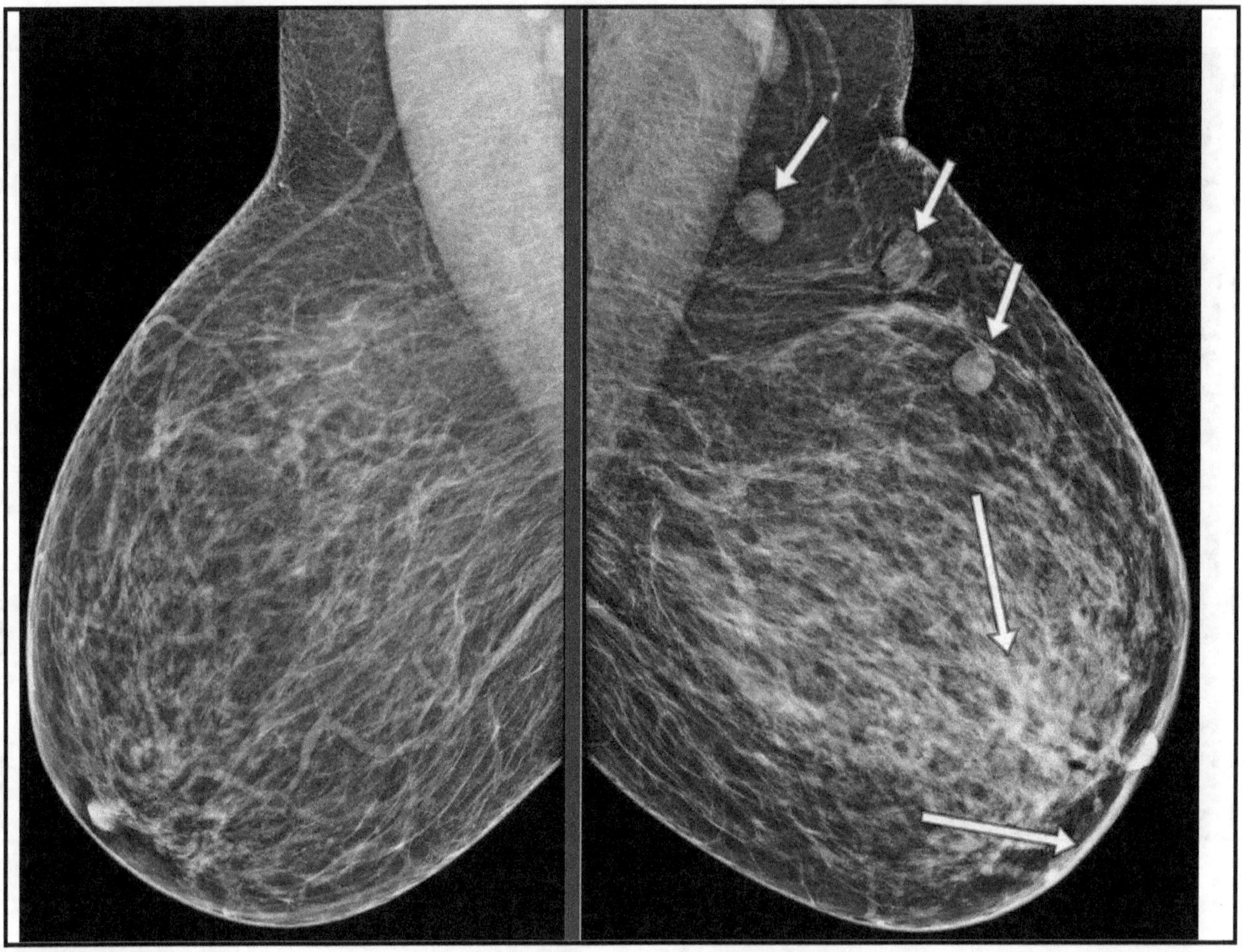

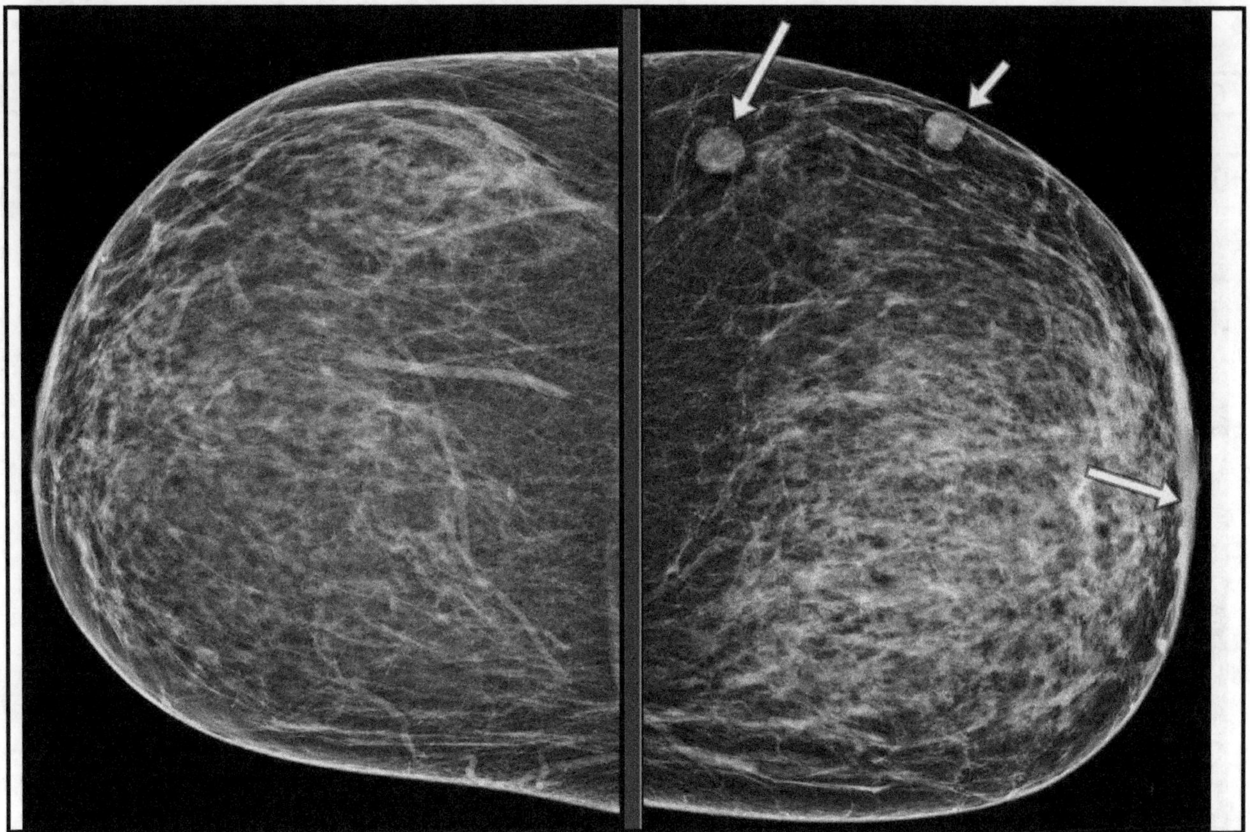

RIGHT BREAST	
Breast Parenchymal Density	***Scattered areas of fibroglandular density (ACR B)***
Focal Mass	None
Asymmetric Density	None
Parenchymal Distortion	None
Calcification	None
Skin Thickening	None
Axillary Nodes	None

LEFT BREAST	
Breast Parenchymal Density	***Scattered areas of fibroglandular density (ACR B) /Trabecular Edema***
Focal Mass	None
Asymmetric Density	None
Parenchymal Distortion	None
Calcification	None
Skin Thickening	***Positive***
Axillary Nodes	***Multiple Enlarged IMLNs=Reactive***

IMPRESSION:
RIGHT BREAST: (BI-RADS 1)
LEFT BREAST: (BI-RADS 3) = **Mastitis**

RECOMMENDATION: Short Term Follow-Up by US

CASE 46: 64-year-old female/ Left Breast Conservative Surgery	
Right MLO	Left MLO

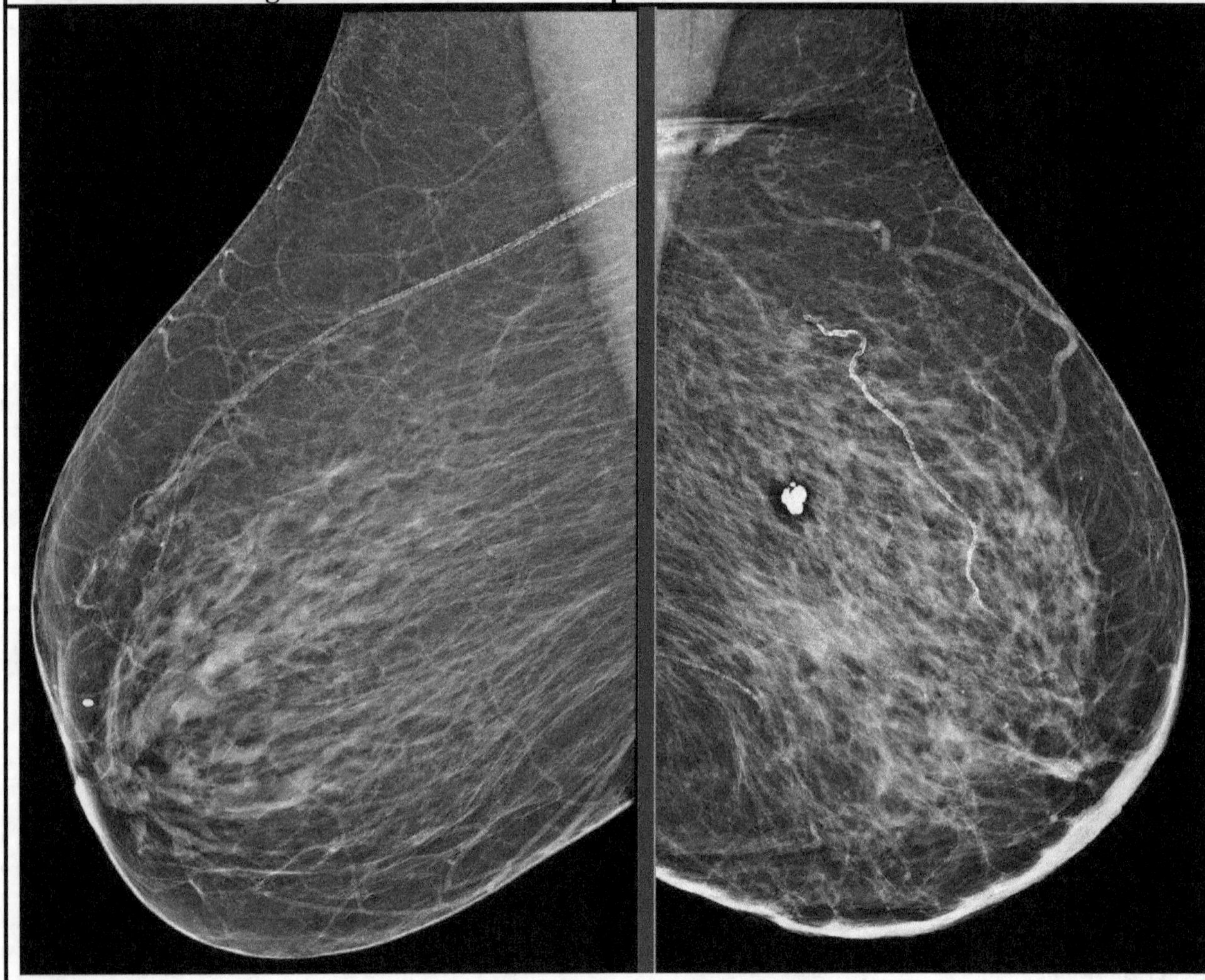

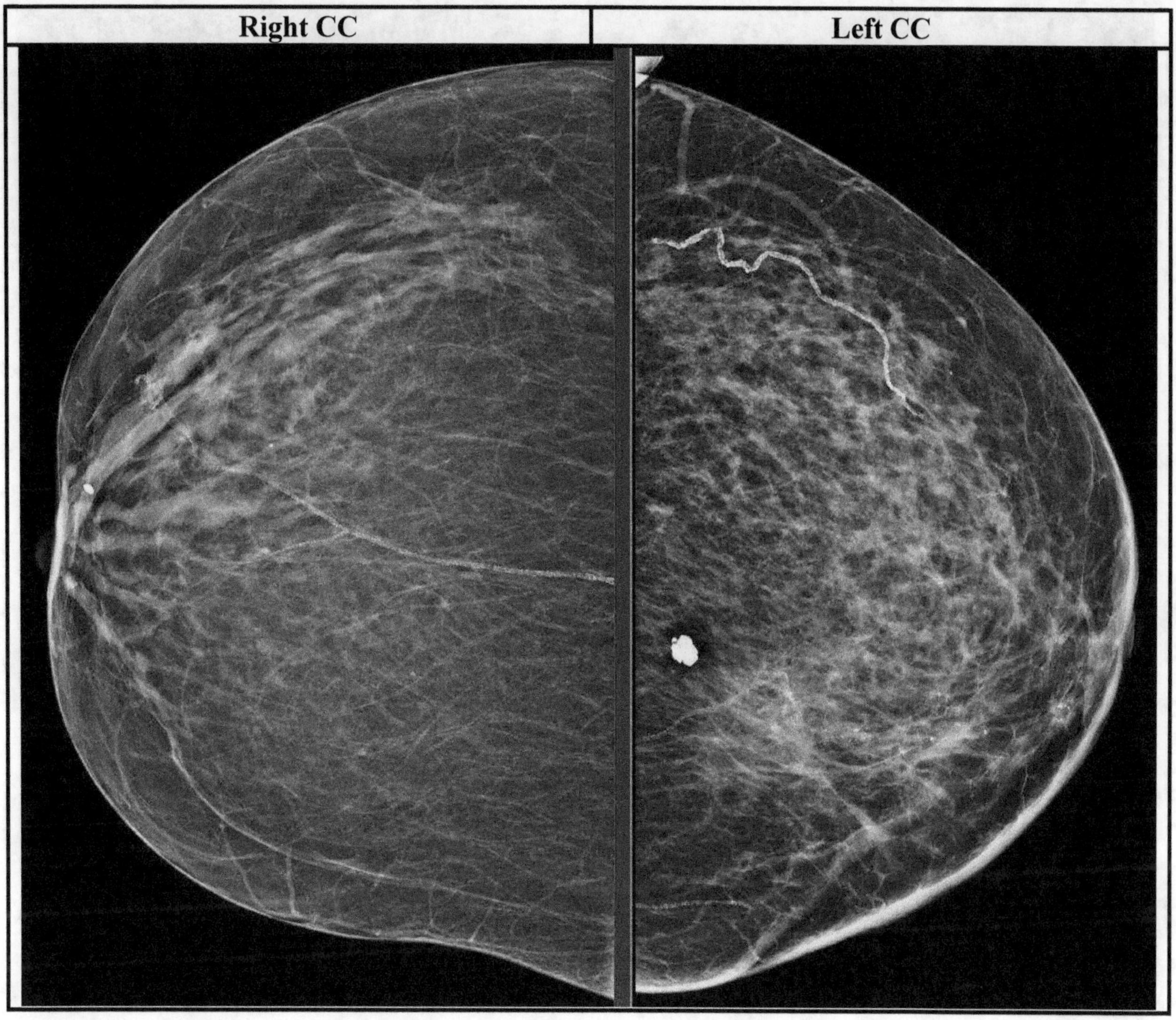
Right CC
Left CC

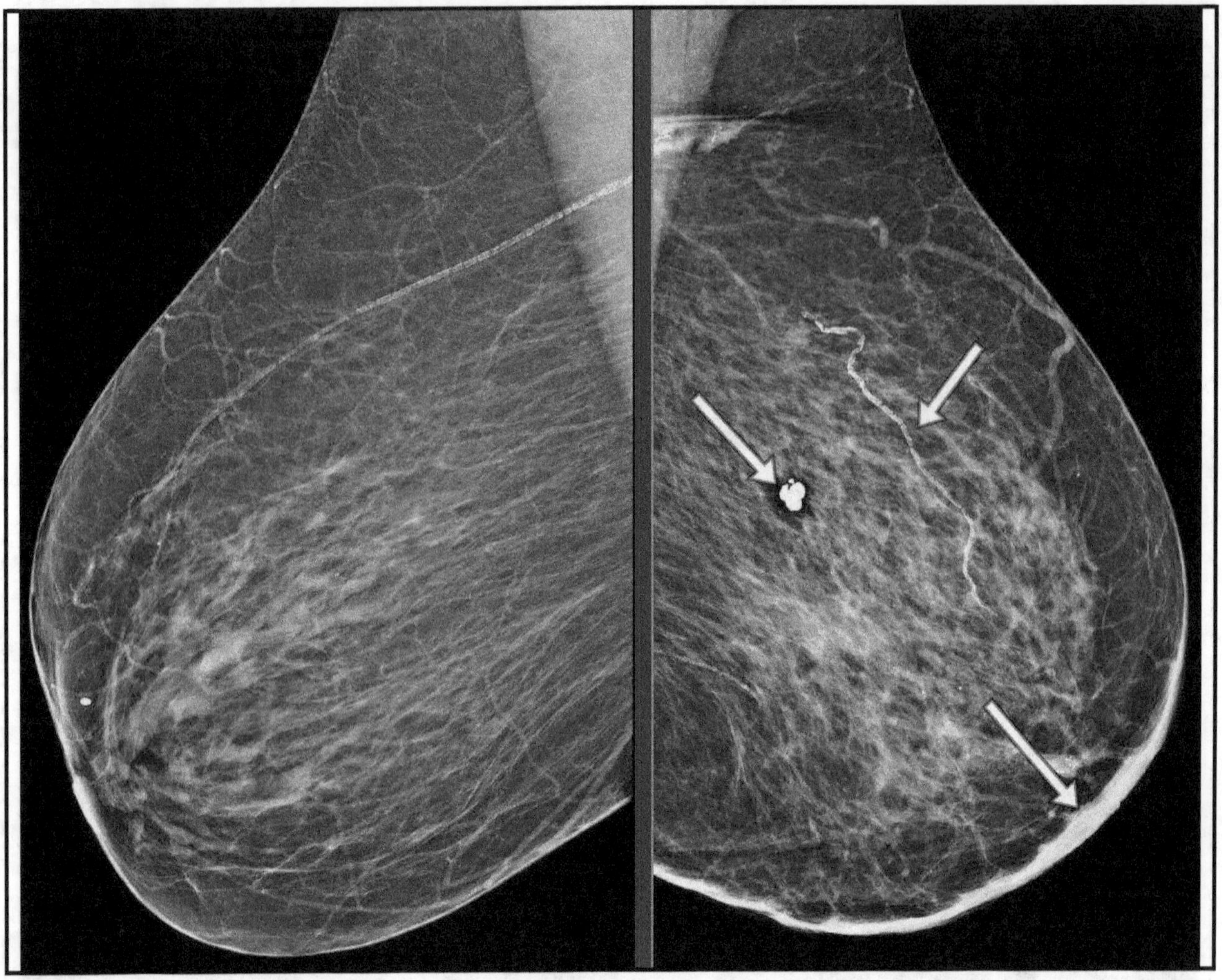

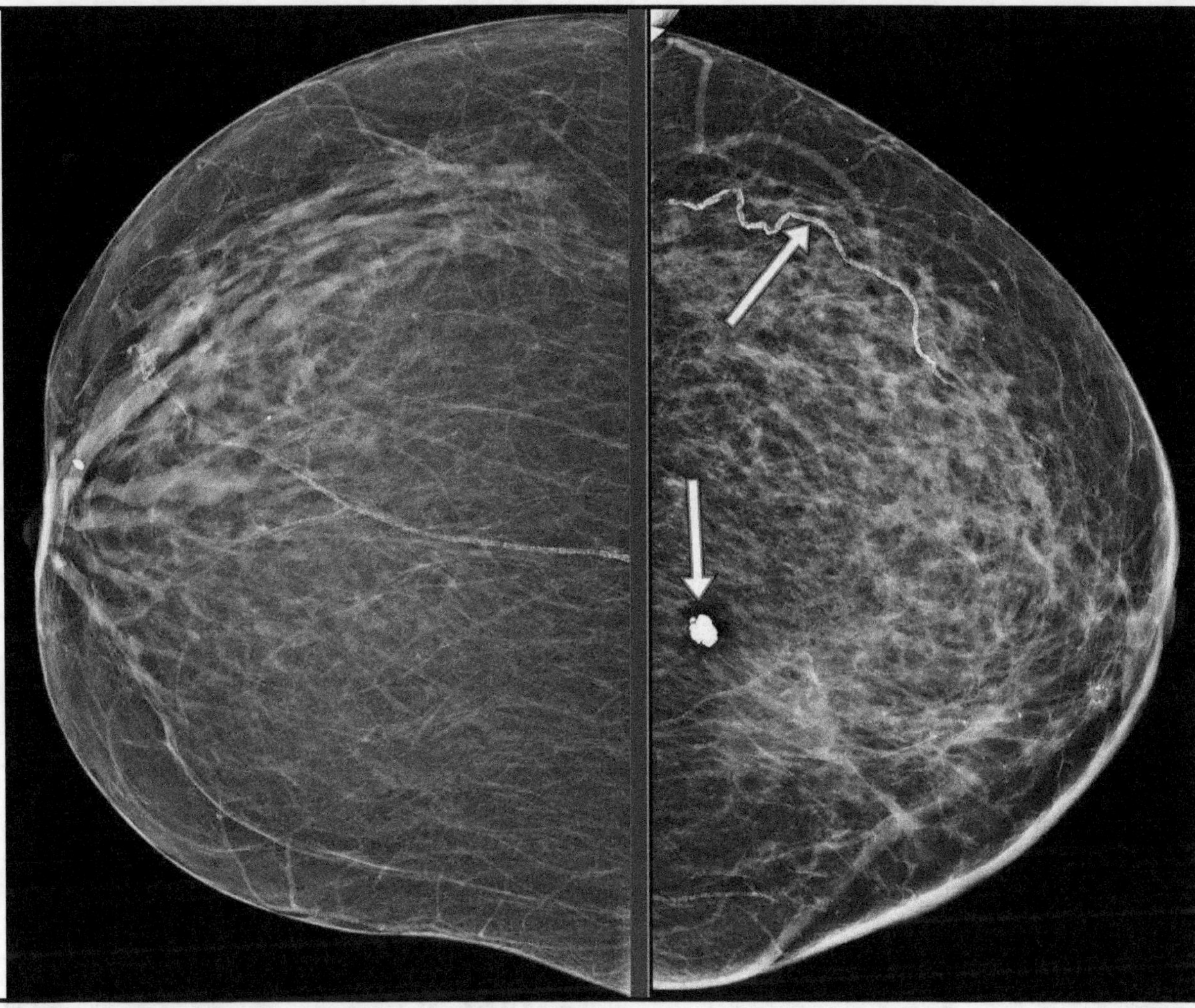

RIGHT BREAST	
Breast Parenchymal Density	***Scattered areas of fibroglandular density (ACR B)***
Focal Mass	None
Asymmetric Density	None
Parenchymal Distortion	None
Calcification	**Skin /Vascular Calcifications**
Skin Thickening	None
Axillary Nodes	None

LEFT BREAST	
Breast Parenchymal Density	***Scattered areas of fibroglandular density (ACR B)/Trabecular edema***
Focal Mass	***UIQ involuted fibroadenoma***
Asymmetric Density	None
Parenchymal Distortion	None
Calcification	***Skin /Vascular /Coarse Calcifications***
Skin Thickening	***Positive***
Axillary Nodes	None

IMPRESSION:

RIGHT BREAST: (BI-RADS 2)

LEFT BREAST: (BI-RADS 2) =***Post Interventional /Radiation Changes***

RECOMMENDATION: Annual Follow-Up

CASE 47: 43-year-old female/screening	
Right MLO	Left MLO

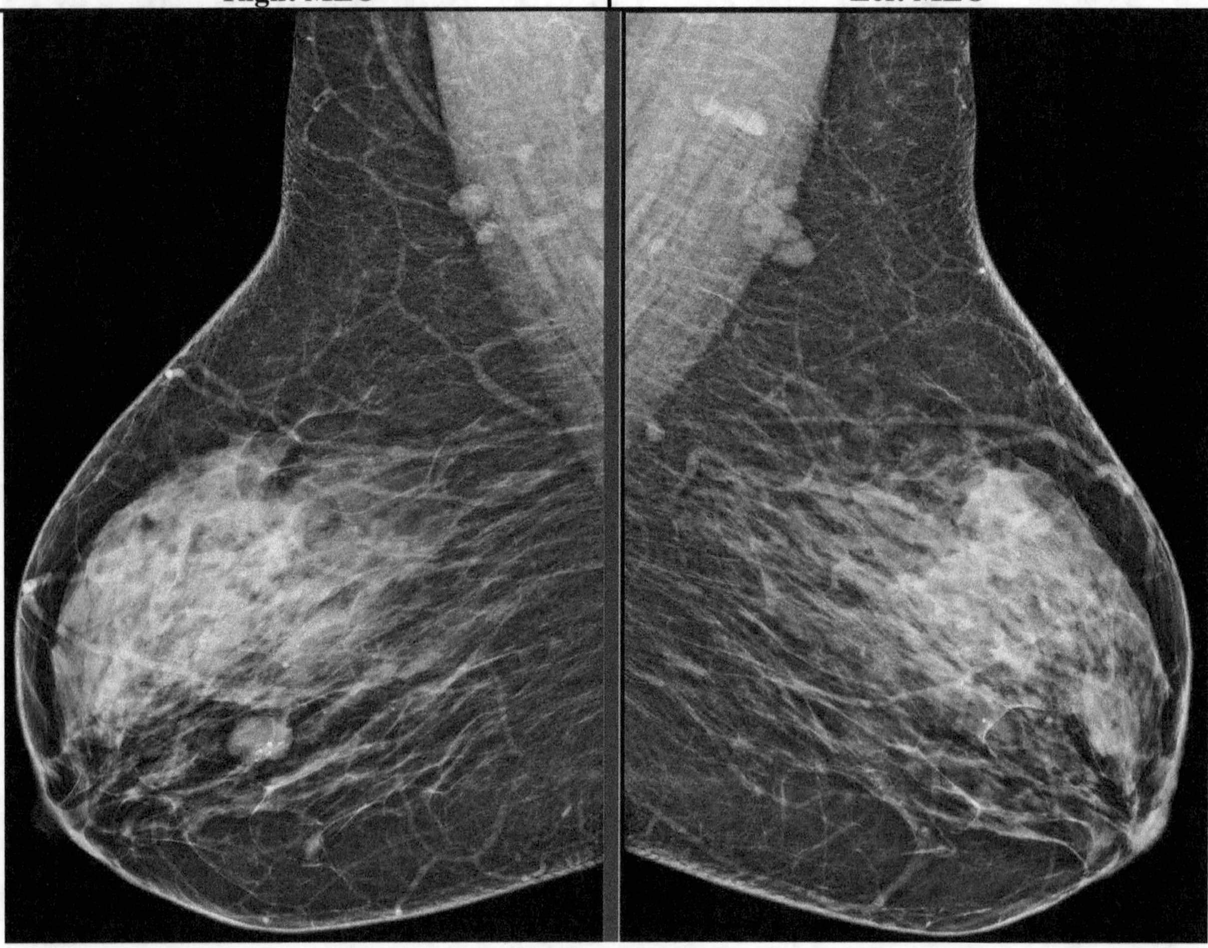

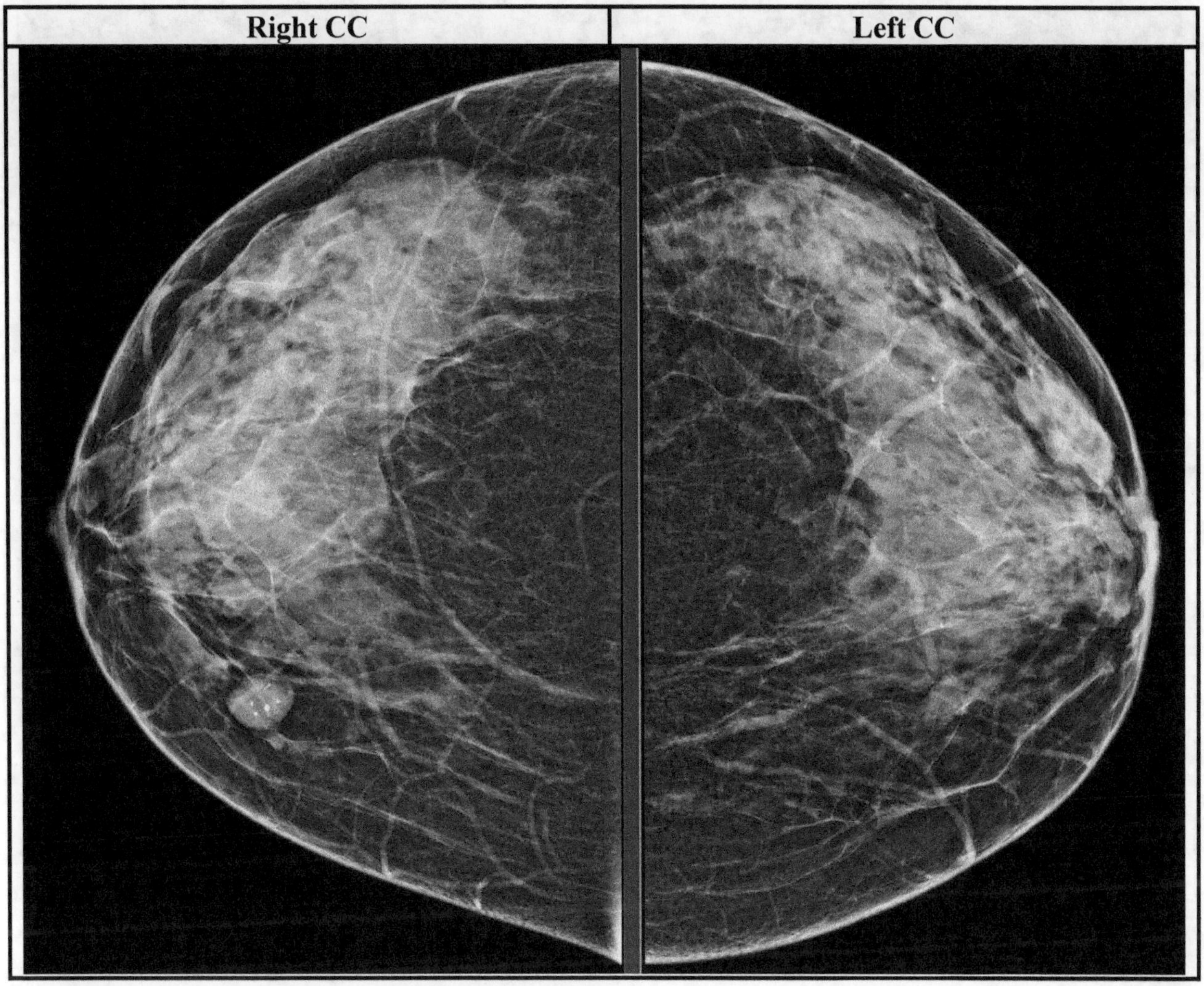
Right CC
Left CC

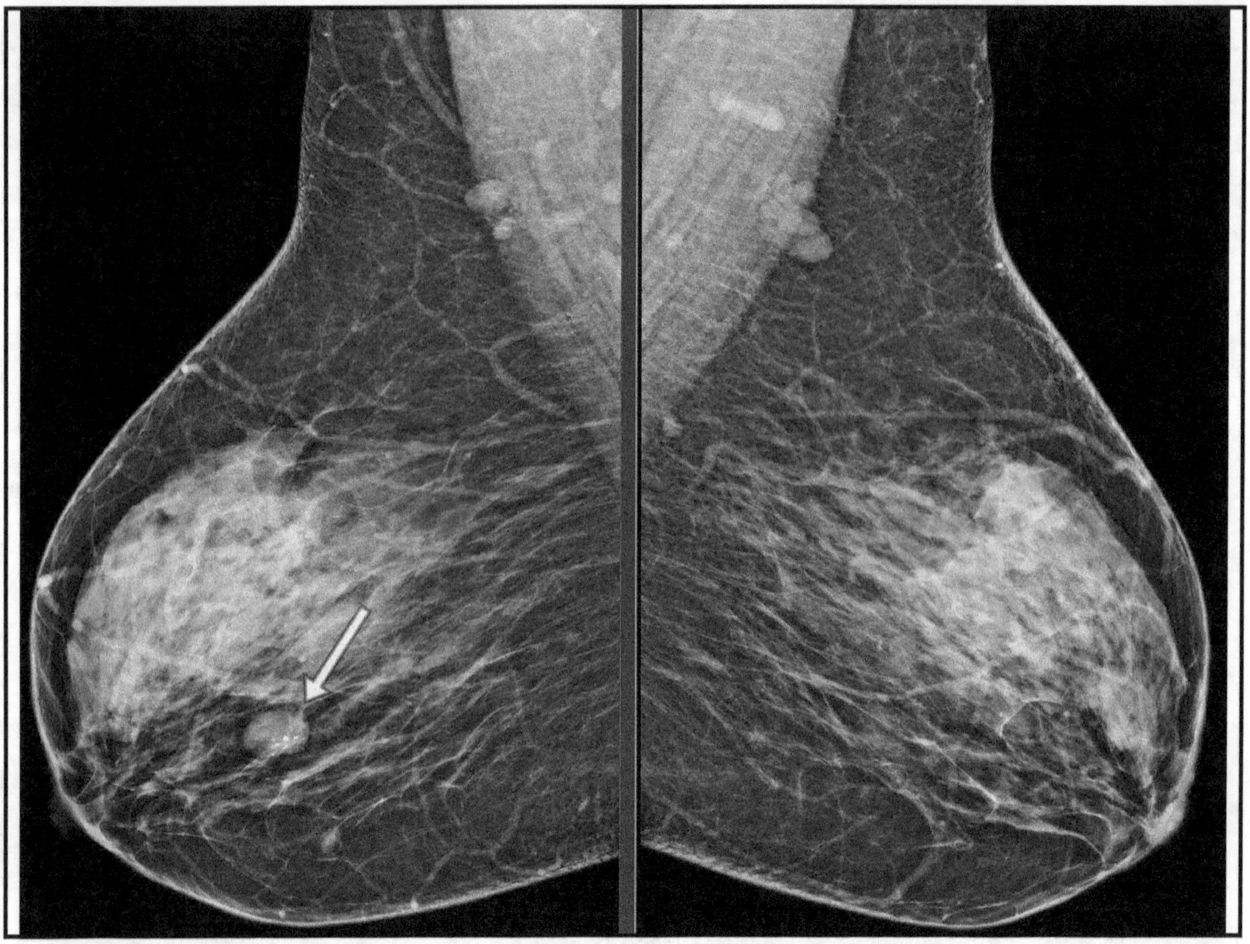

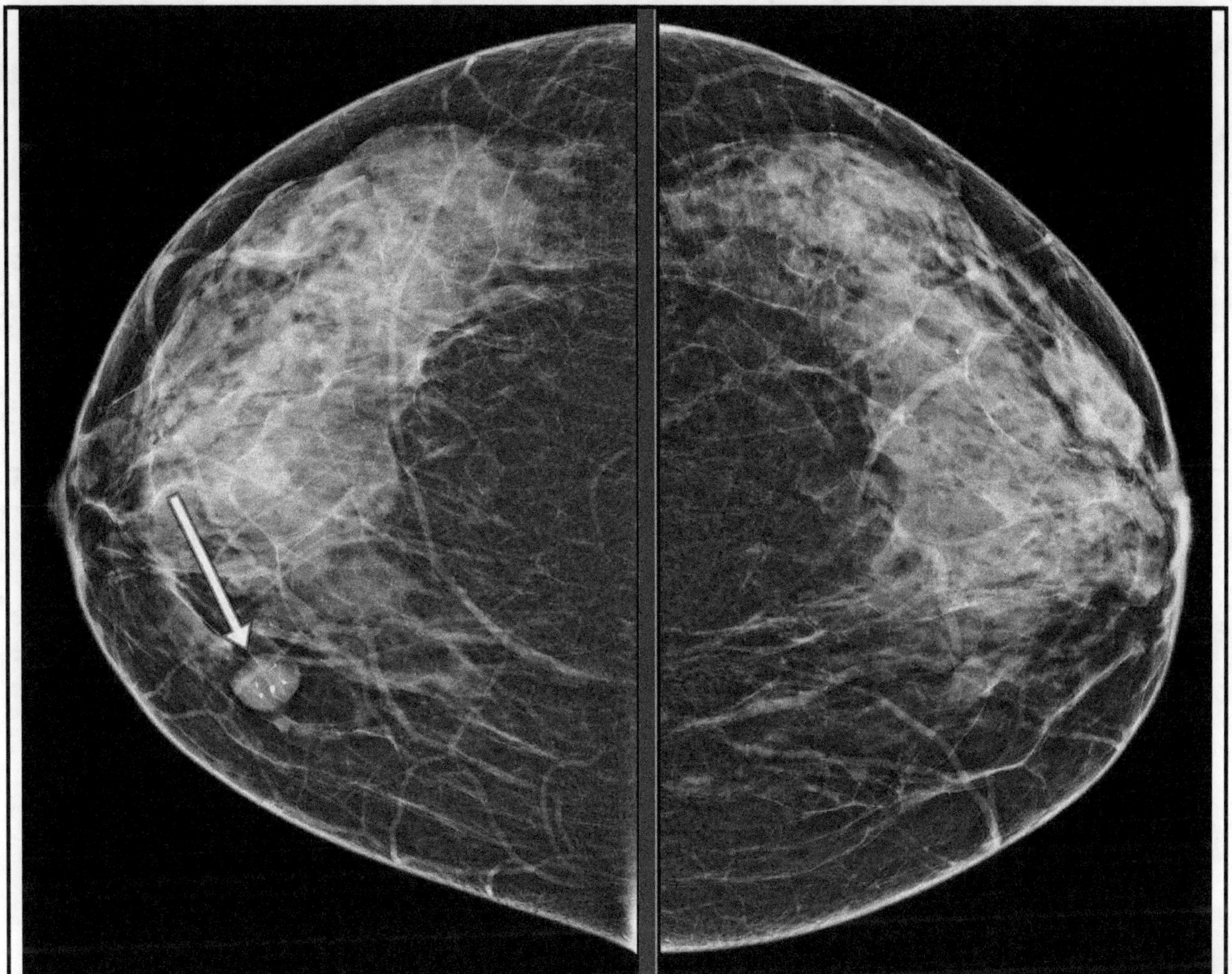

RIGHT BREAST	
Breast Parenchymal Density	***Heterogeneously dense, may obscure small masses (ACR C)***
Focal Mass	***LIQ oval circumscribed with coarse calcification (involuted fibroadenoma)***
Asymmetric Density	None
Parenchymal Distortion	None
Calcification	***coarse calcification***
Skin Thickening	None
Axillary Nodes	None

LEFT BREAST	
Breast Parenchymal Density	***Heterogeneously dense, may obscure small masses (ACR C)***
Focal Mass	None
Asymmetric Density	None
Parenchymal Distortion	None
Calcification	None
Skin Thickening	None
Axillary Nodes	None

IMPRESSION:

RIGHT BREAST: (BI-RADS 2)
LEFT BREAST: (BI-RADS 1)

RECOMMENDATION: Routine Annual screening

CASE 48: 44-year-old female/ Diagnostic	
Right MLO	**Left MLO**

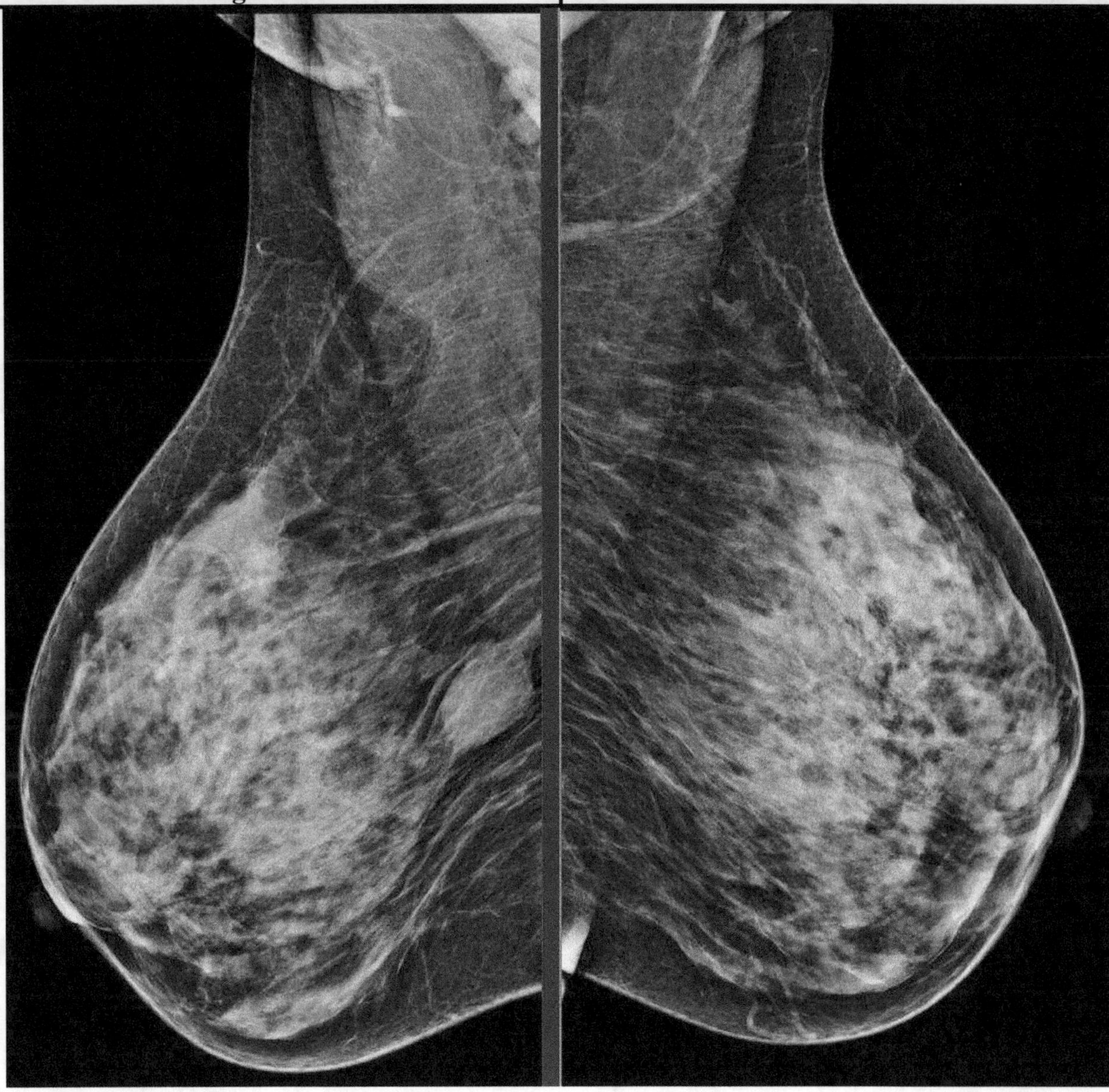

Right CC	Left CC

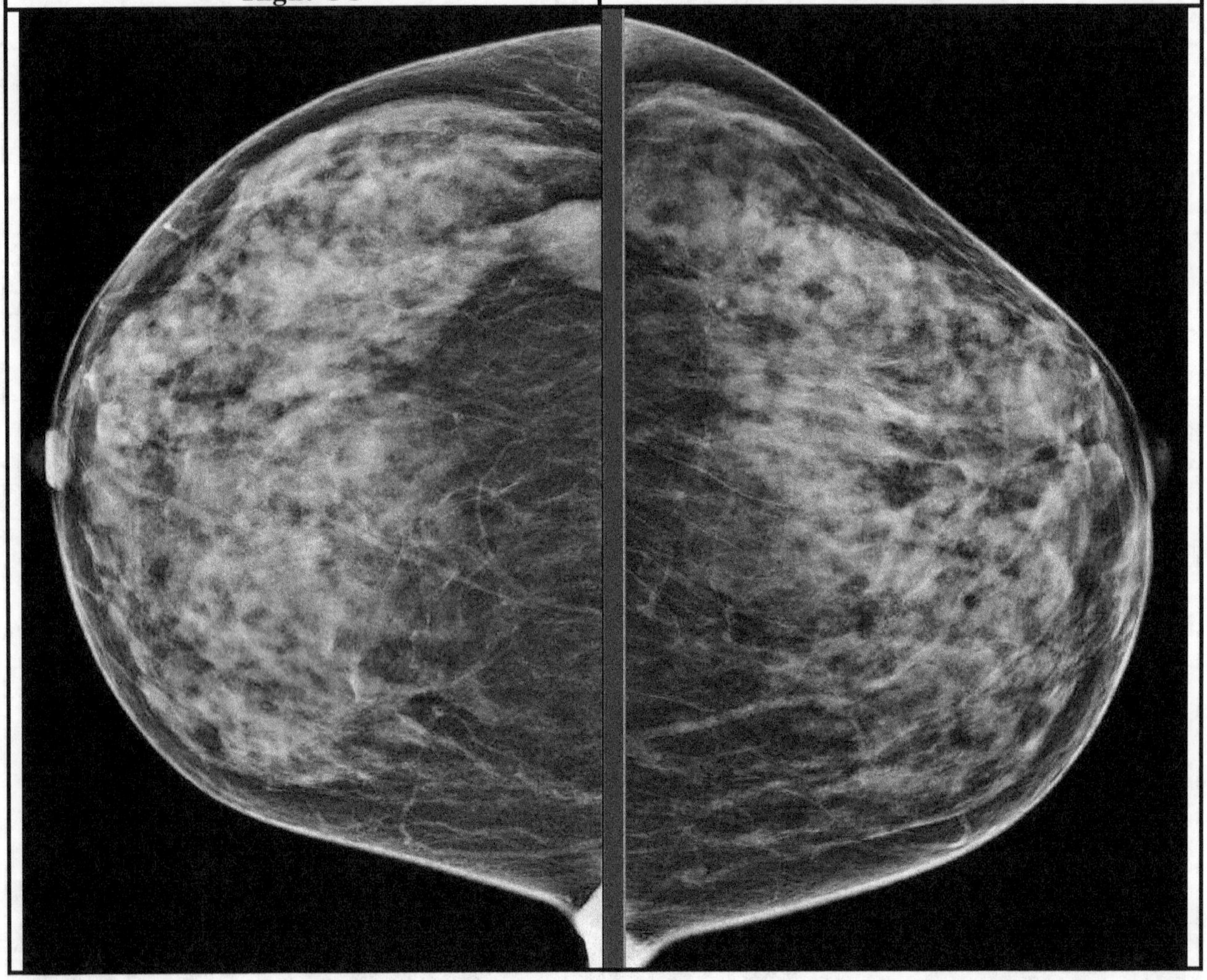

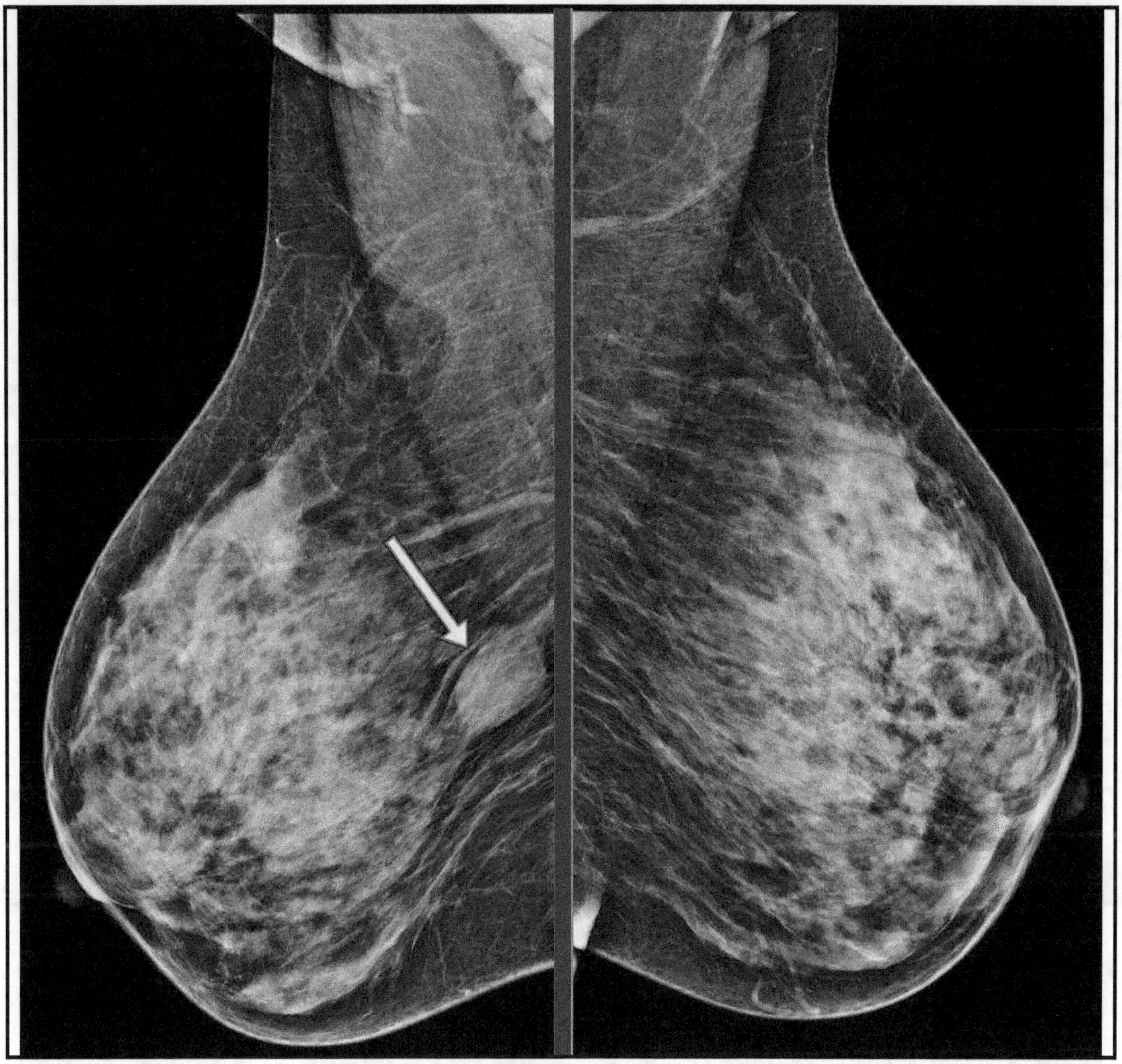

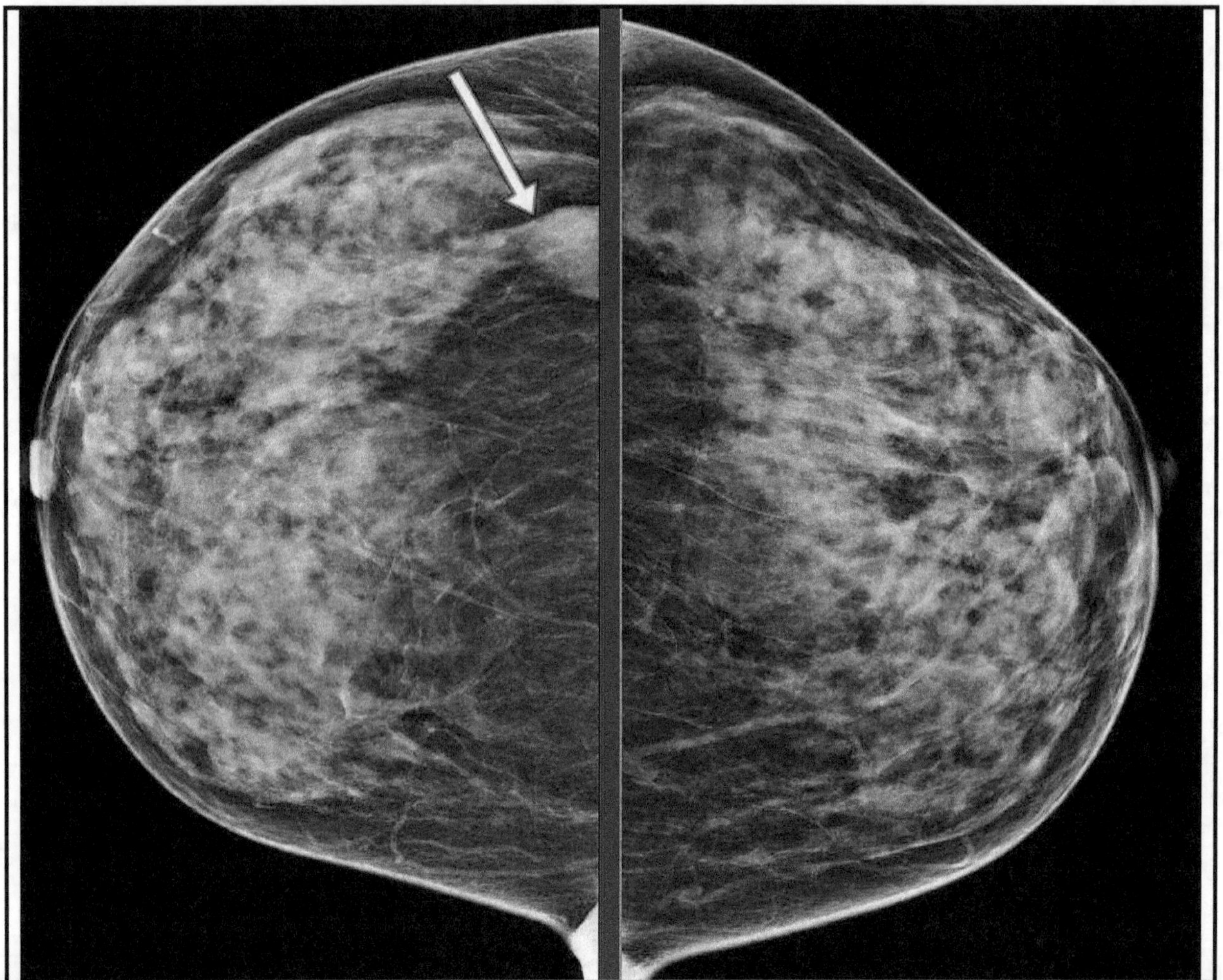

RIGHT BREAST	
Breast Parenchymal Density	***Extremely dense, which lowers the sensitivity of mammography (ACR D)***
Focal Mass	***UOQ oval obscured mass lesion***
Asymmetric Density	None
Parenchymal Distortion	None
Calcification	None
Skin Thickening	None
Axillary Nodes	None

LEFT BREAST	
Breast Parenchymal Density	***Extremely dense, which lowers the sensitivity of mammography (ACR D)***
Focal Mass	None
Asymmetric Density	None
Parenchymal Distortion	None
Calcification	None
Skin Thickening	None
Axillary Nodes	None

IMPRESSION:

RIGHT BREAST: (BI-RADS 0)
LEFT BREAST: (BI-RADS 0)

RECOMMENDATION: US Correlation

CASE 49: 33-year-old female/Diagnostic

Right MLO	Left MLO

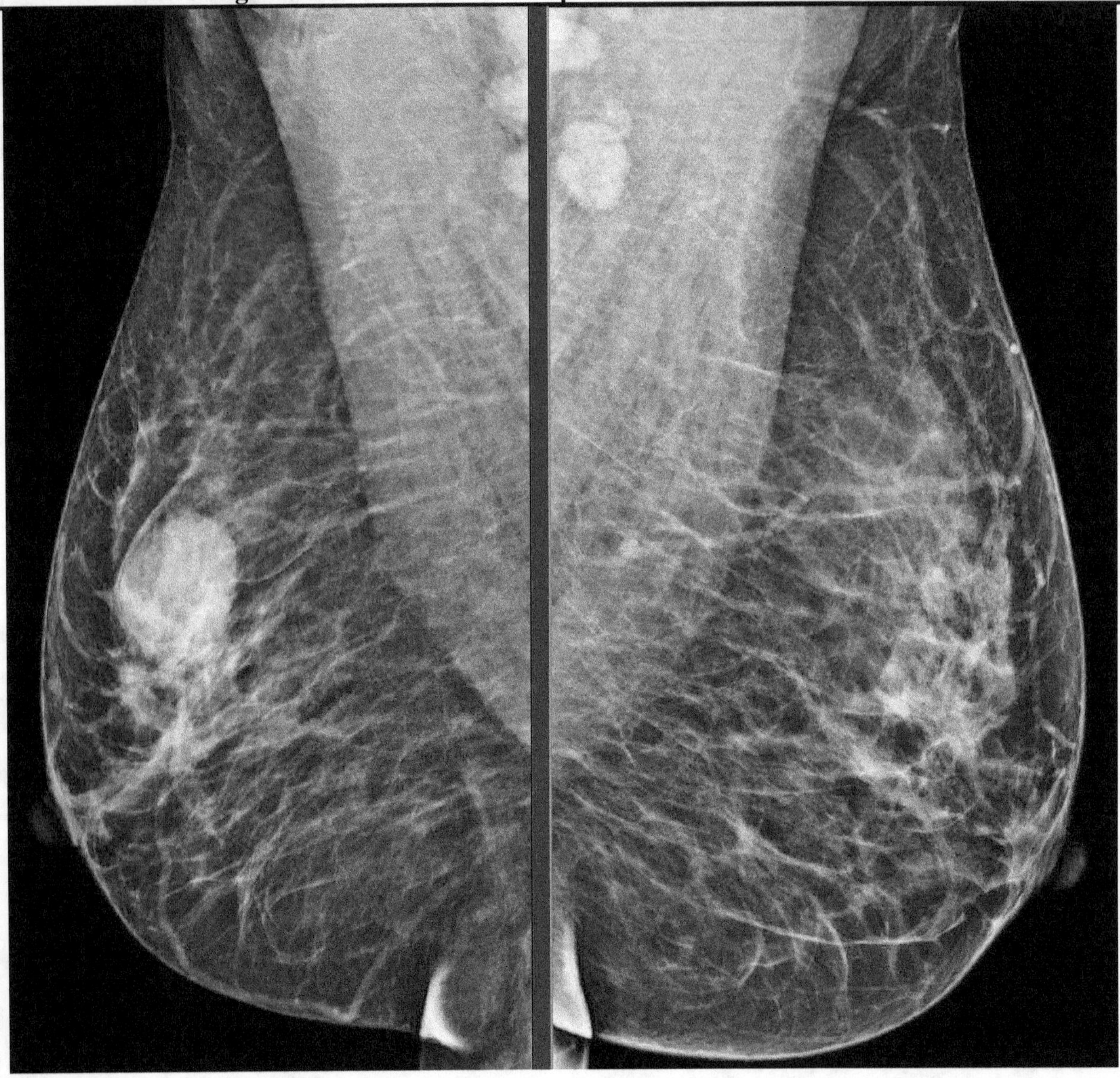

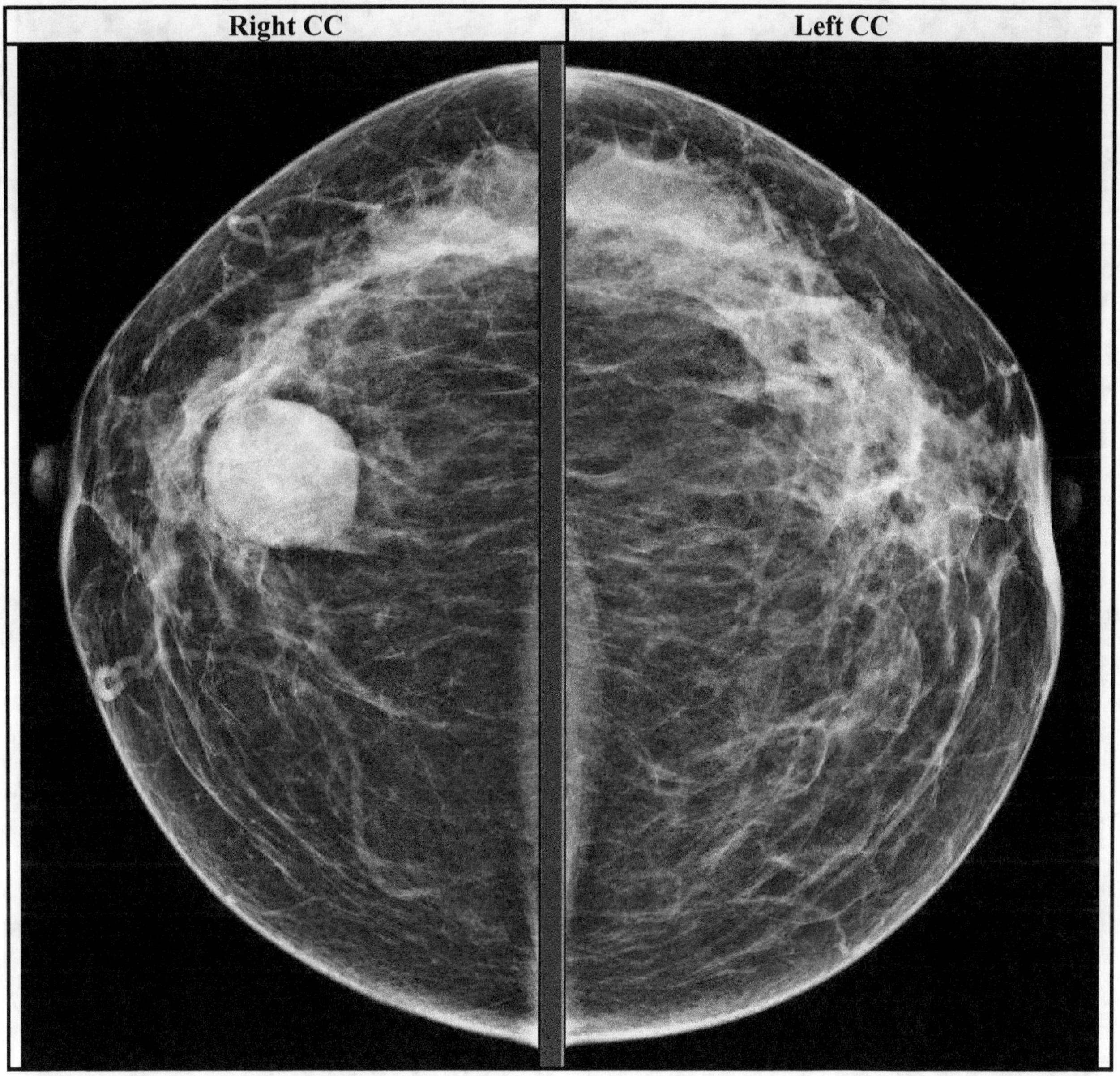
Right CC
Left CC

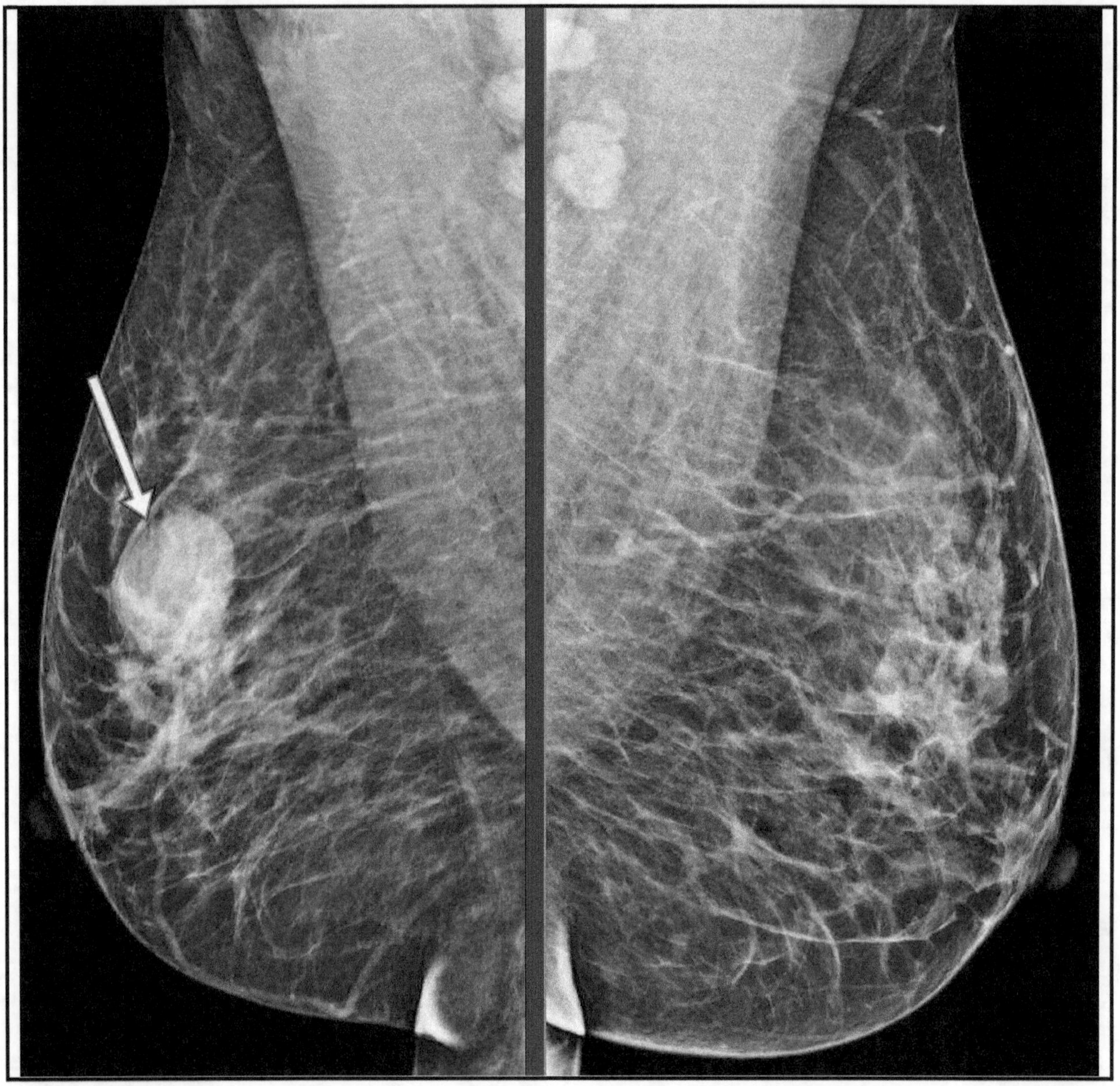

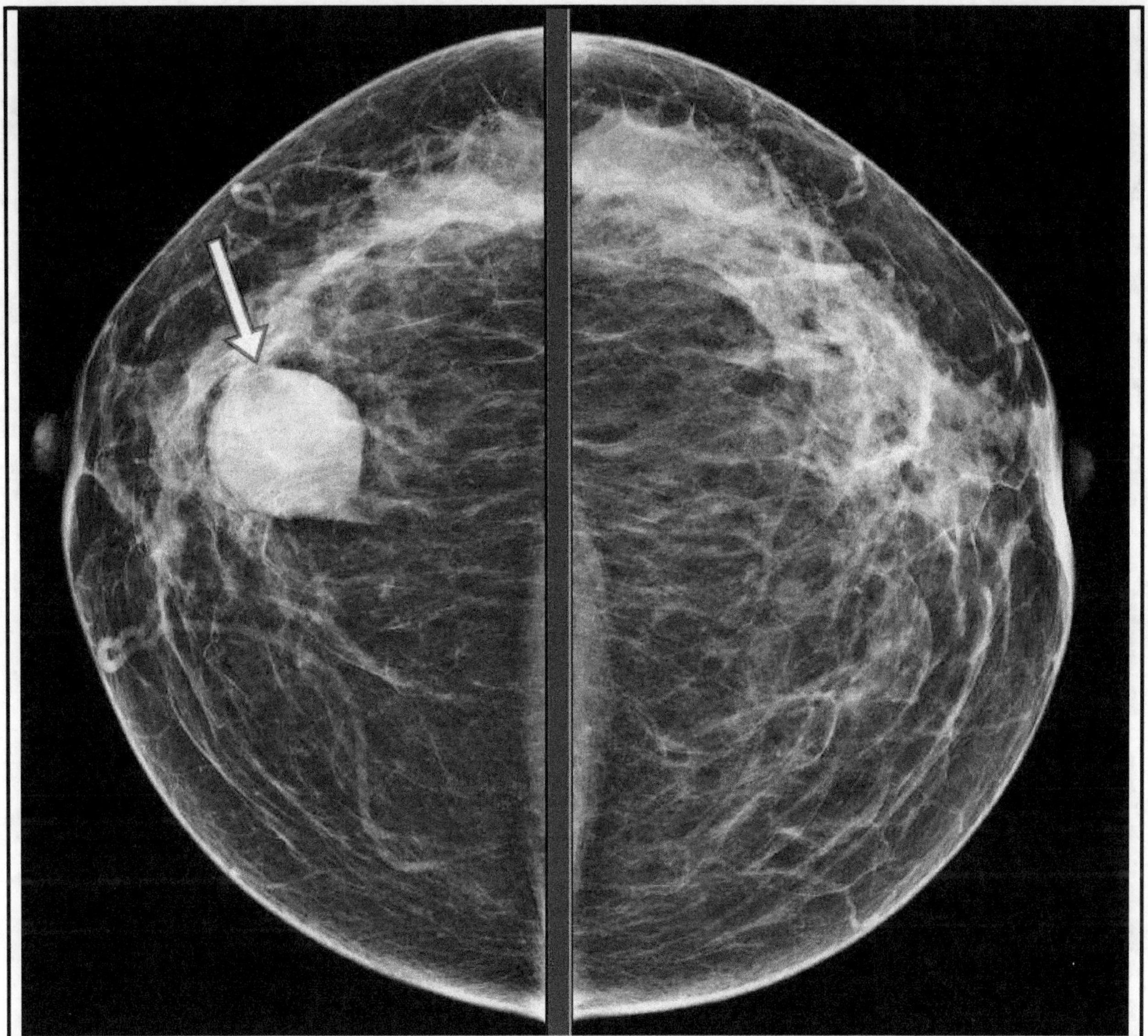

RIGHT BREAST	
Breast Parenchymal Density	***Scattered areas of fibroglandular density (ACR B)***
Focal Mass	***Upper central round obscured mass lesion***
Asymmetric Density	None
Parenchymal Distortion	None
Calcification	None
Skin Thickening	None
Axillary Nodes	None

LEFT BREAST	
Breast Parenchymal Density	***Scattered areas of fibroglandular density (ACR B)***
Focal Mass	None
Asymmetric Density	None
Parenchymal Distortion	None
Calcification	None
Skin Thickening	None
Axillary Nodes	None

IMPRESSION:

RIGHT BREAST: (BI-RADS 0)
LEFT BREAST: (BI-RADS 1)

RECOMMENDATION: US Correlation

US demonstrated simple cyst

CASE 50: 48-year-old female/ Diagnostic	
Right MLO	**Left MLO**

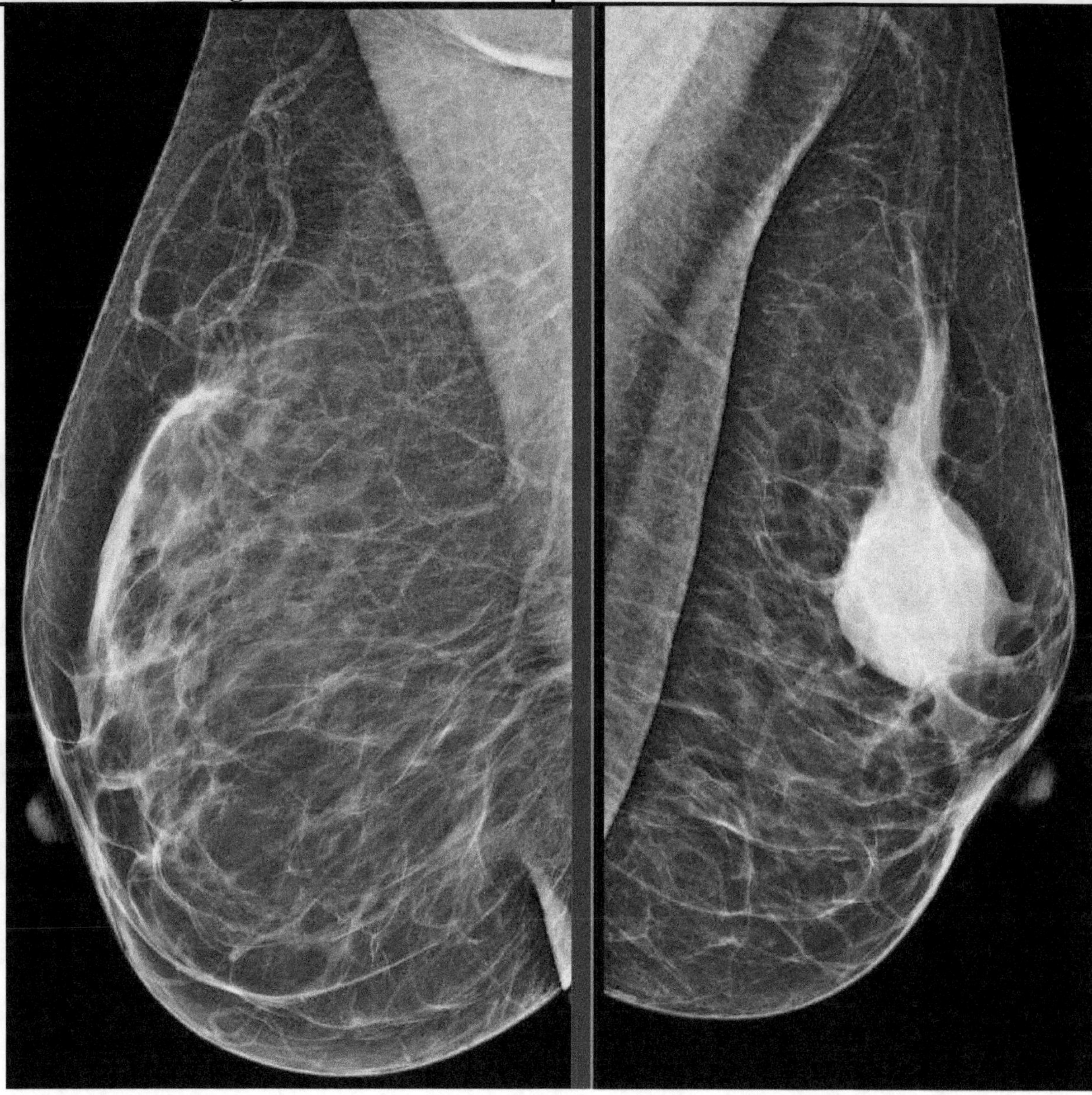

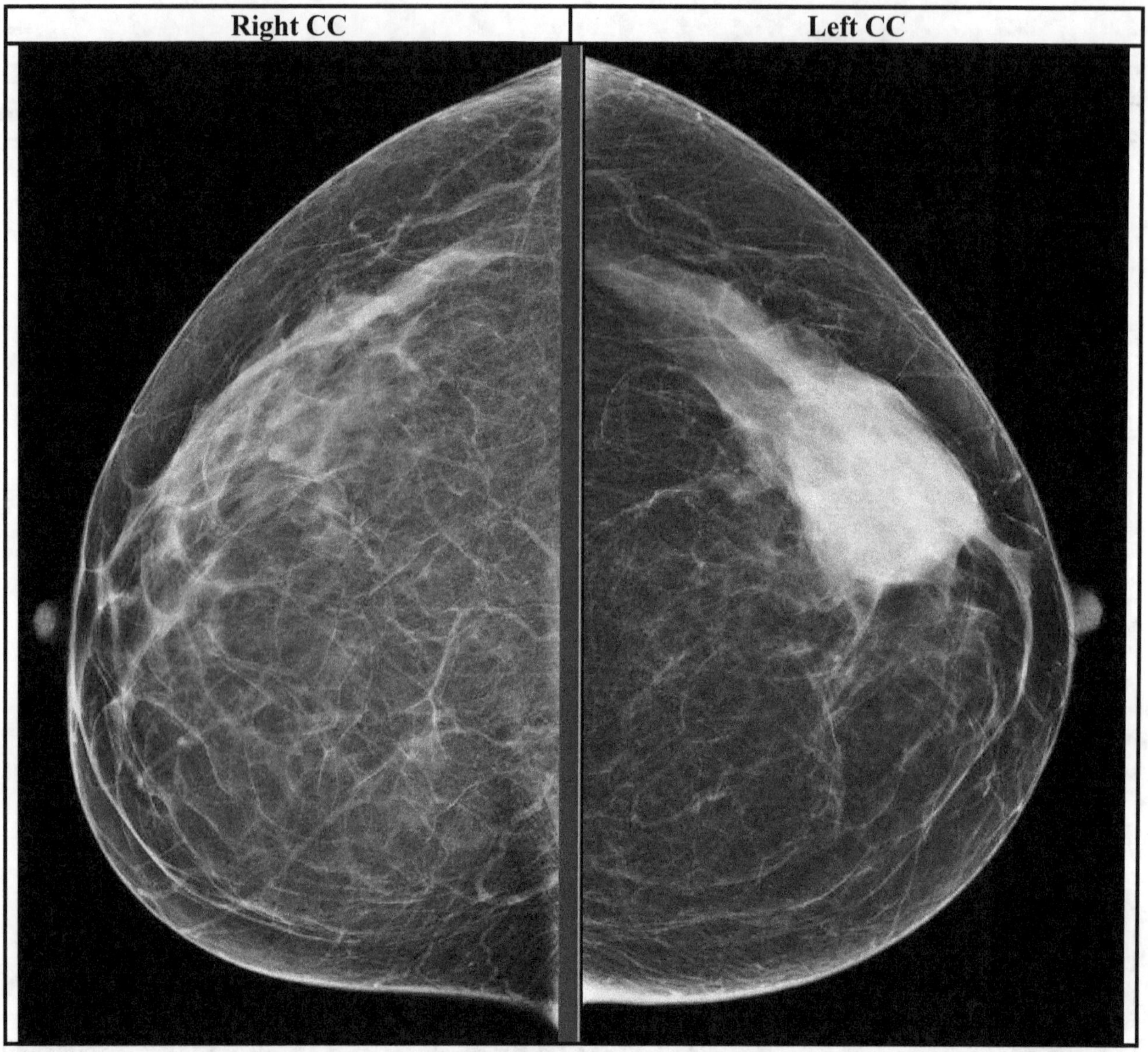
Right CC
Left CC

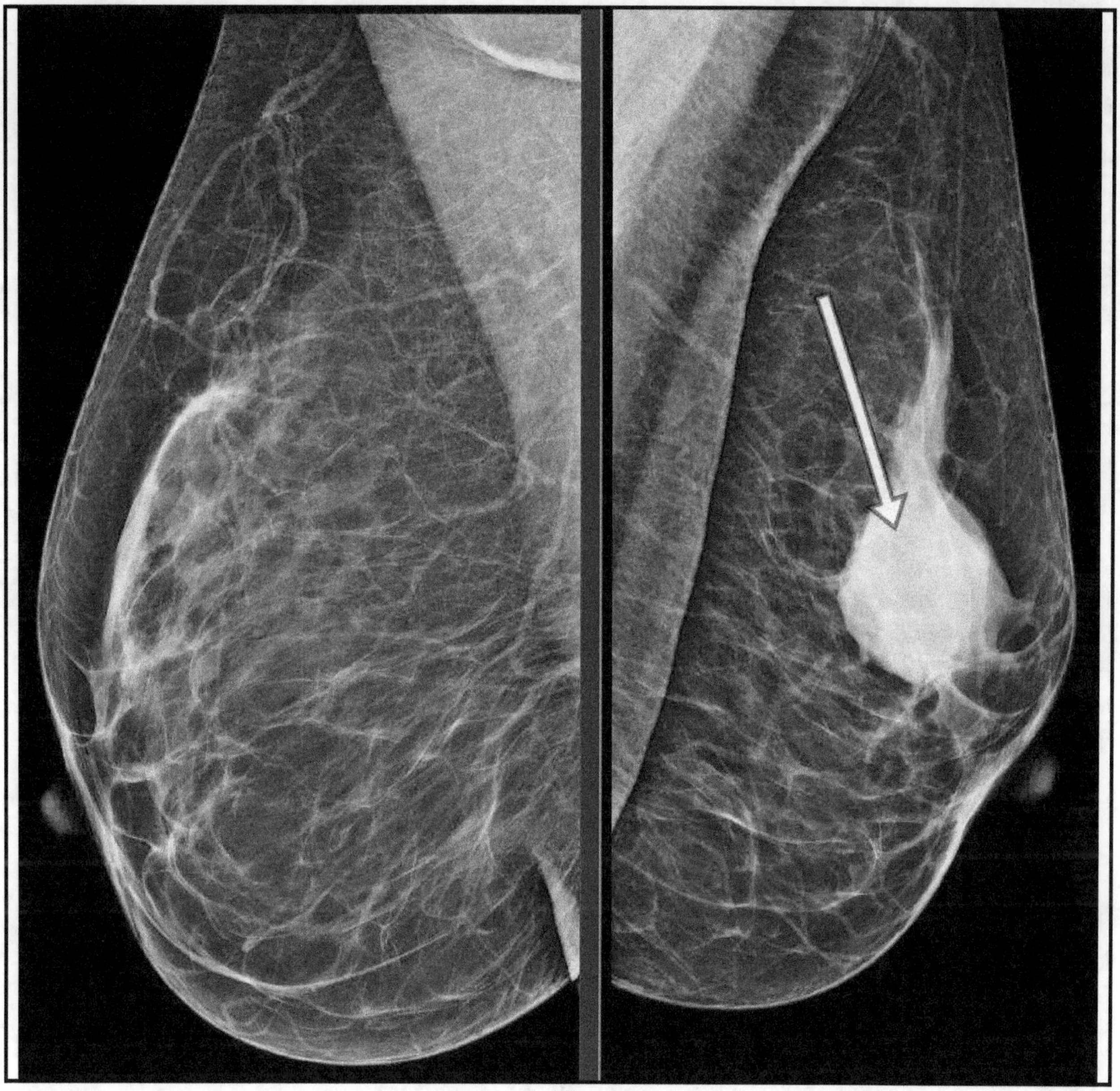

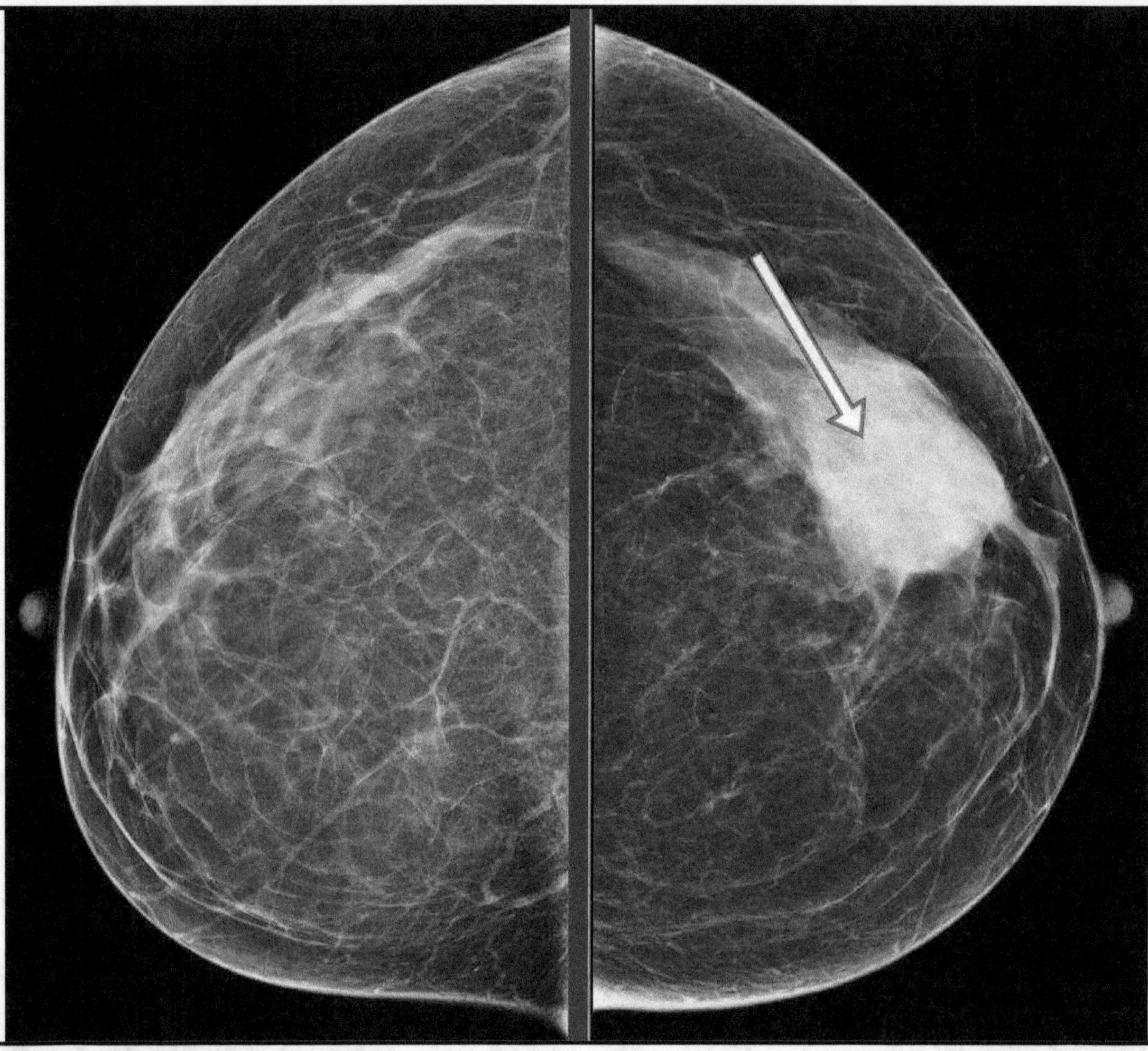

RIGHT BREAST	
Breast Parenchymal Density	***Scattered areas of fibroglandular density (ACR B)***
Focal Mass	None
Asymmetric Density	None
Parenchymal Distortion	None
Calcification	None
Skin Thickening	None
Axillary Nodes	None

LEFT BREAST	
Breast Parenchymal Density	***Scattered areas of fibroglandular density (ACR B)***
Focal Mass	***UOQ oval obscured mass lesion***
Asymmetric Density	None
Parenchymal Distortion	None
Calcification	None
Skin Thickening	None
Axillary Nodes	None

IMPRESSION:
RIGHT BREAST: (BI-RADS 1)
LEFT BREAST: (BI-RADS 0)

RECOMMENDATION: US Correlation

CASE 51: 55 -year-old female/screening	
Right MLO	Left MLO

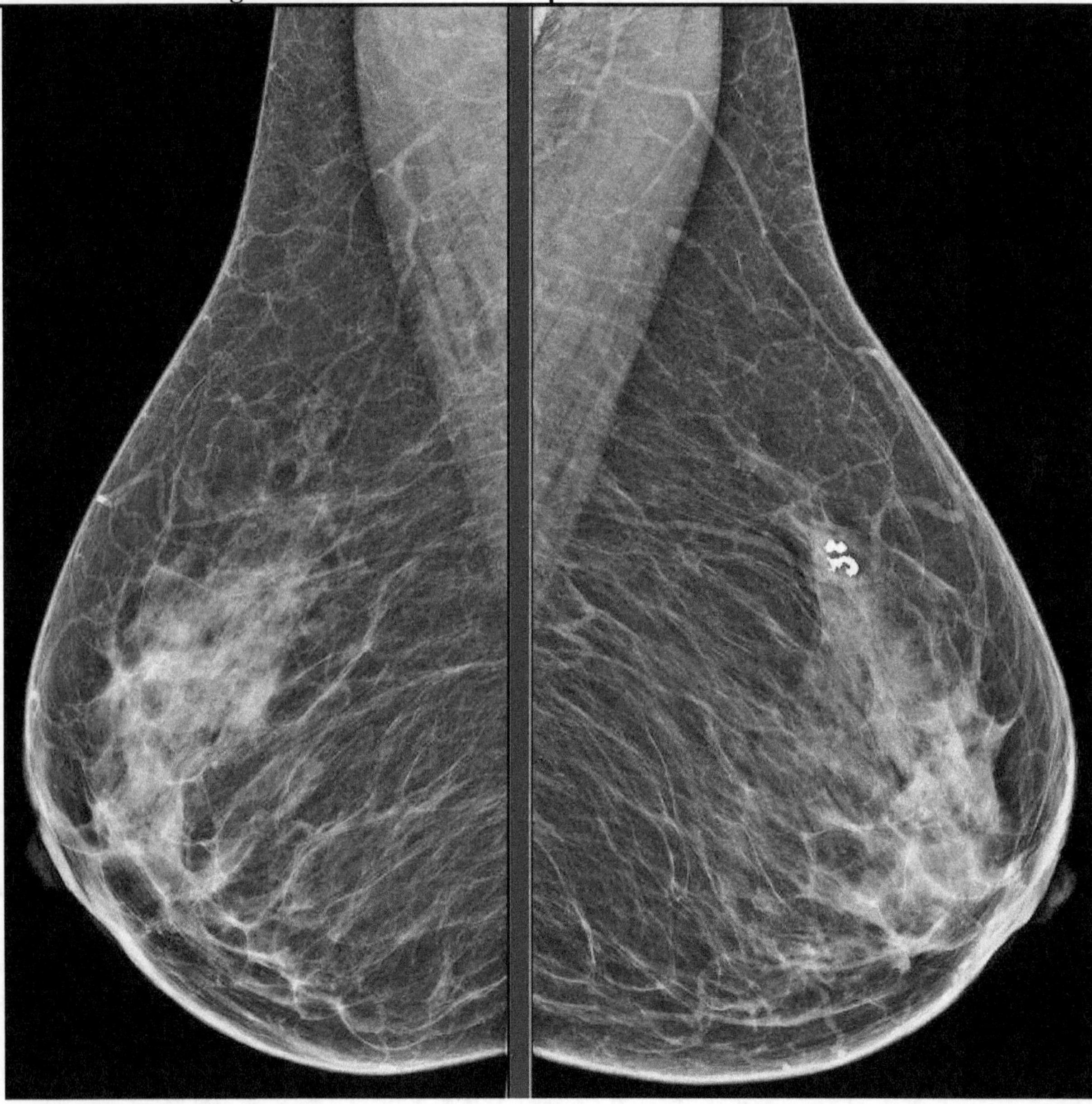

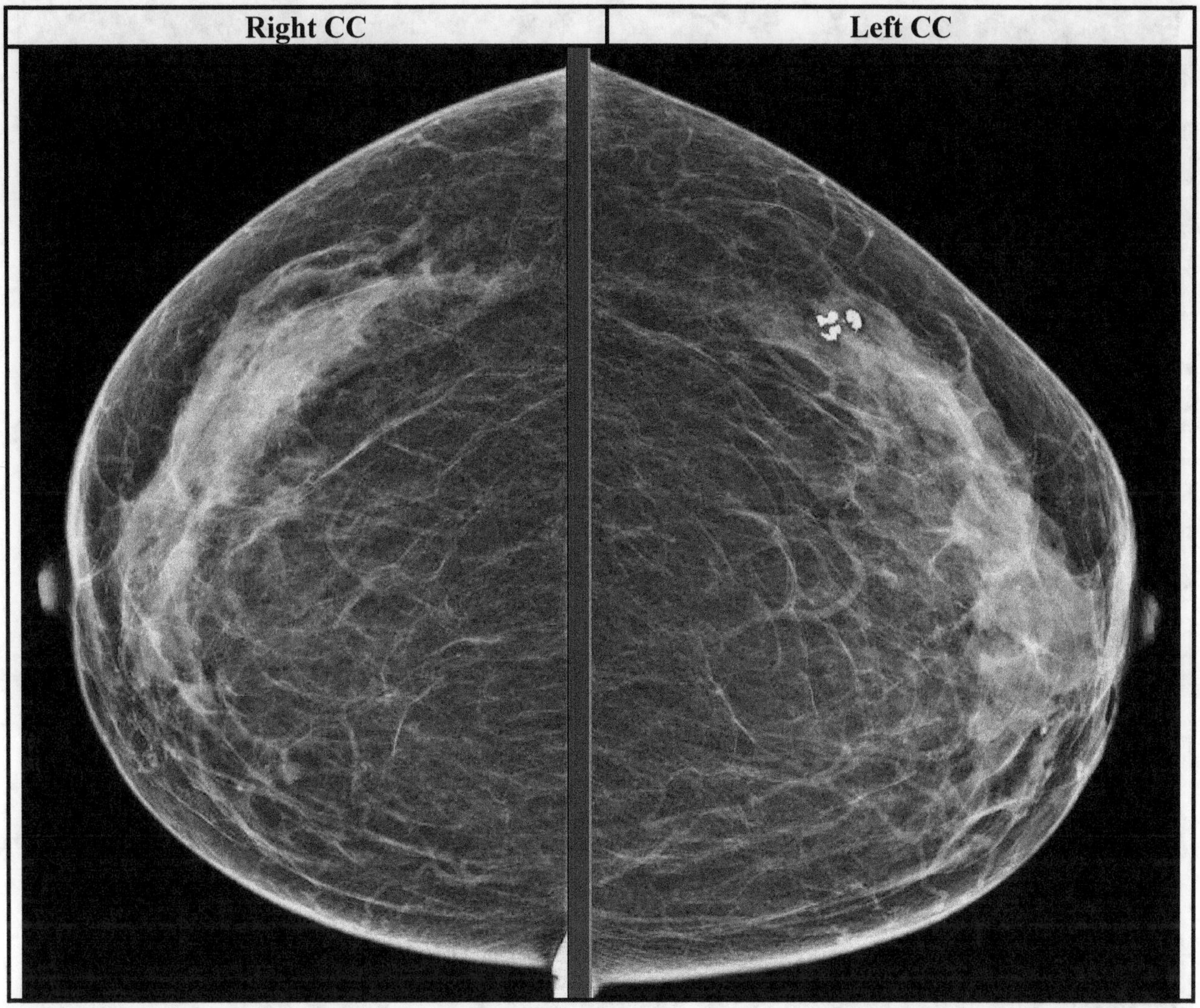
Right CC
Left CC

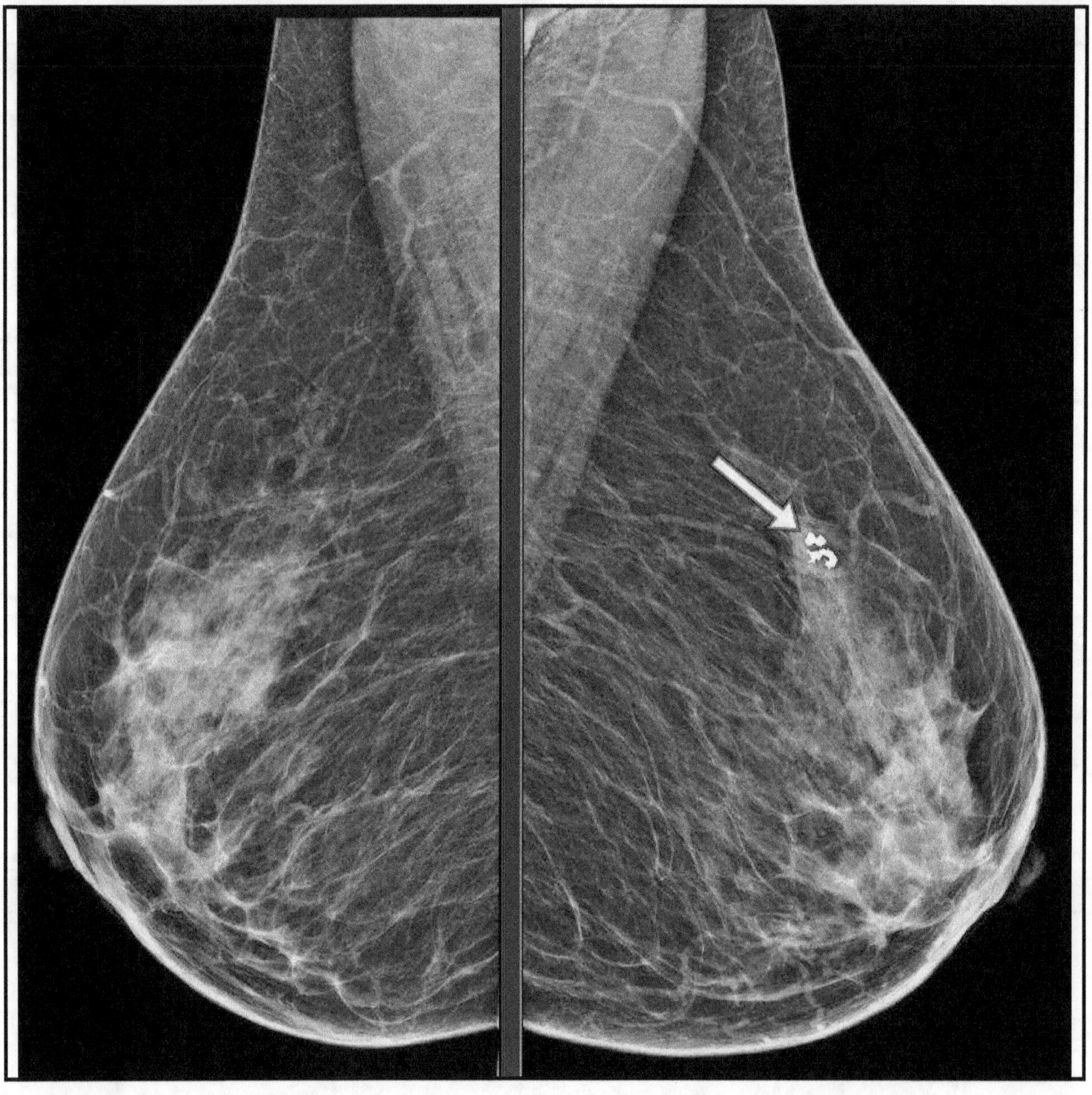

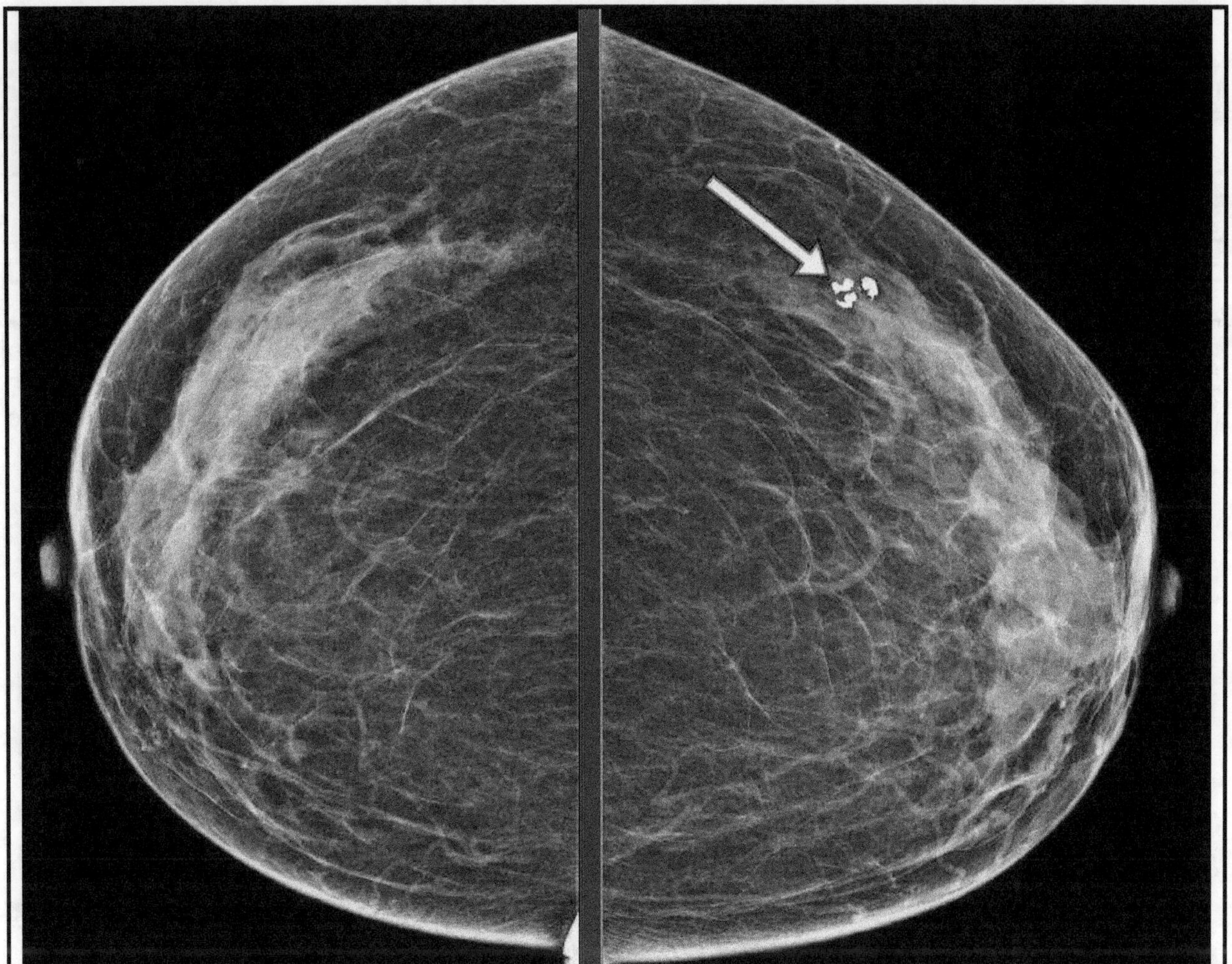

RIGHT BREAST	
Breast Parenchymal Density	***Heterogeneously dense, may obscure small masses (ACR C)***
Focal Mass	None
Asymmetric Density	None
Parenchymal Distortion	None
Calcification	None
Skin Thickening	None
Axillary Nodes	None

LEFT BREAST	
Breast Parenchymal Density	***Heterogeneously dense, may obscure small masses (ACR C)***
Focal Mass	***UOQ involuted fibroadenoma (with Coarse = popcorn calcification)***
Asymmetric Density	None
Parenchymal Distortion	None
Calcification	***UOQ Coarse = popcorn calcification***
Skin Thickening	None
Axillary Nodes	None

IMPRESSION:
RIGHT BREAST: (BI-RADS 1)
LEFT BREAST: (BI-RADS 2)

RECOMMENDATION: Routine Annual screening

CASE 52: 56 -year-old female/ Diagnostic

Right MLO	Left MLO
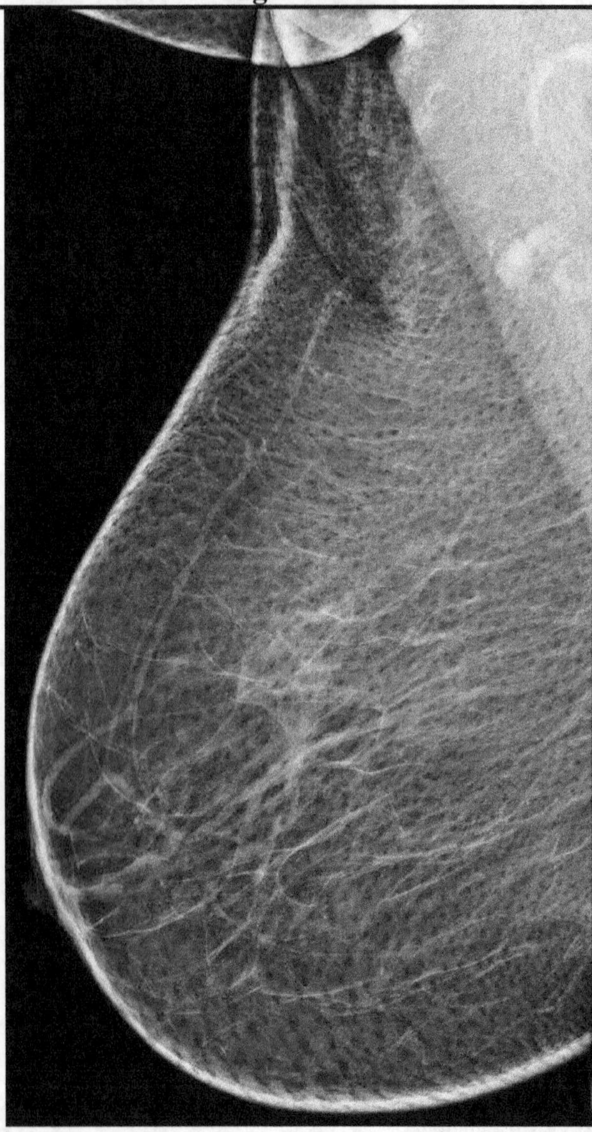	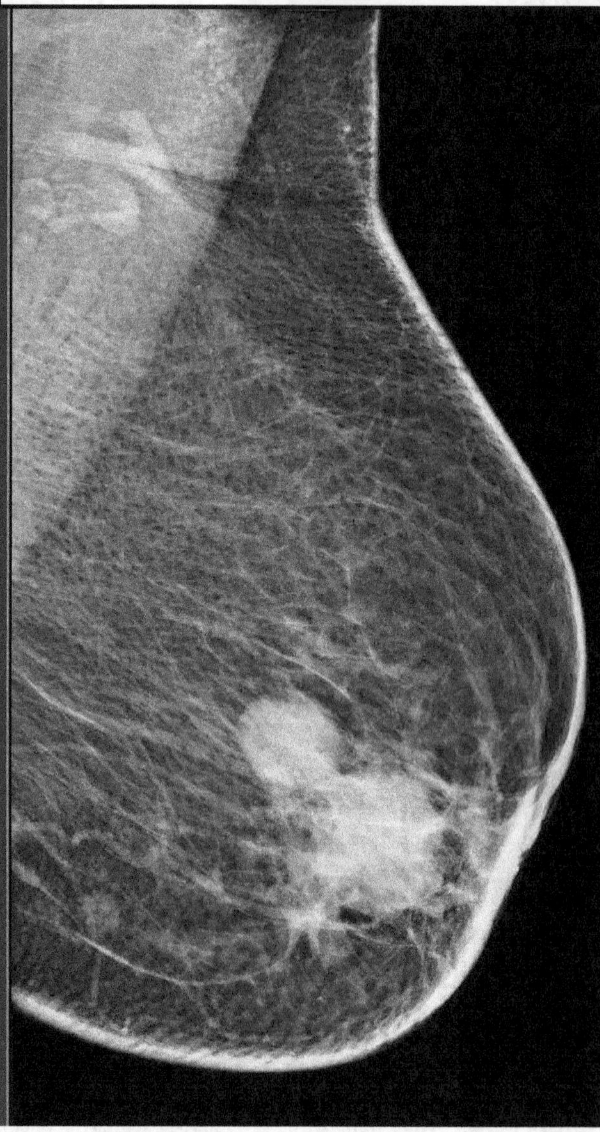

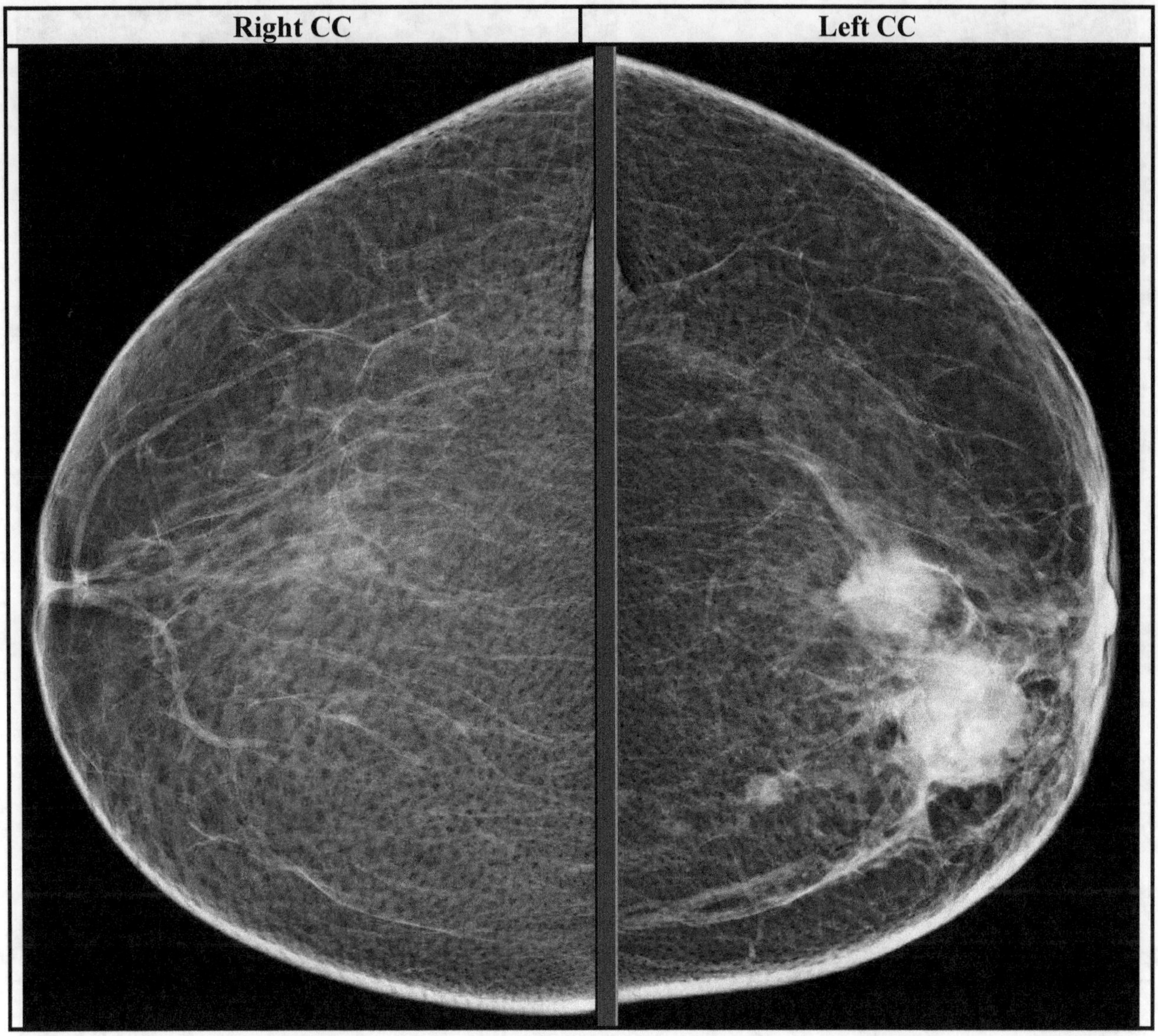
Right CC
Left CC

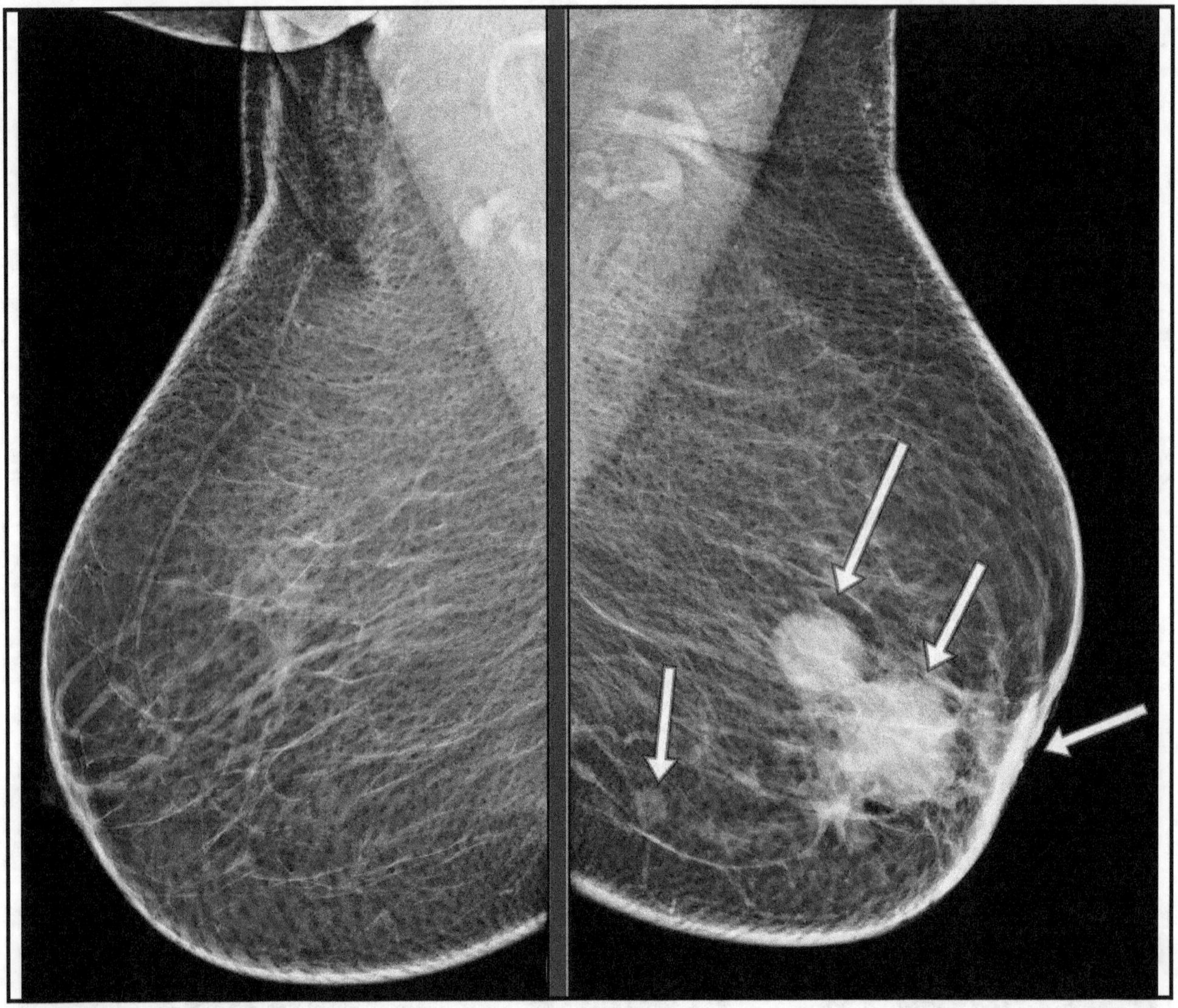

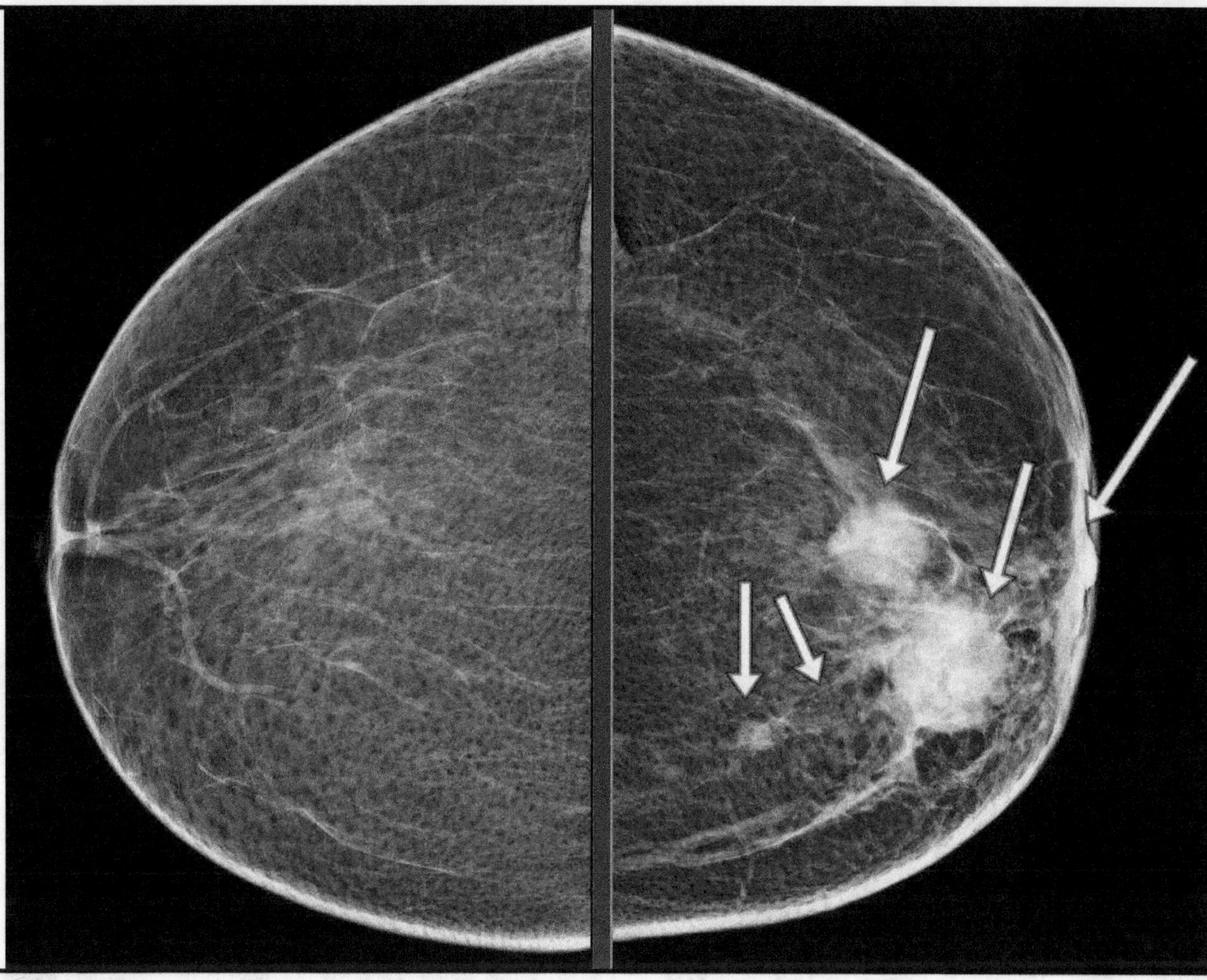

RIGHT BREAST	
Breast Parenchymal Density	***Almost entirely fatty (ACR A)***
Focal Mass	None
Asymmetric Density	None
Parenchymal Distortion	None
Calcification	None
Skin Thickening	None
Axillary Nodes	None

LEFT BREAST	
Breast Parenchymal Density	***Almost entirely fatty (ACR A)***
Focal Mass	***Retro-areolar/ LIQ multifocal round/oval obscured mass lesions***
Asymmetric Density	None
Parenchymal Distortion	None
Calcification	None
Skin Thickening	***Positive + nipple retraction***
Axillary Nodes	None

IMPRESSION:
RIGHT BREAST: (BI-RADS 1)
LEFT BREAST: (BI-RADS 5)

RECOMMENDATION: Histopathological Correlation

CASE 53: 47-year-old female/ Diagnostic

Right MLO	Left MLO

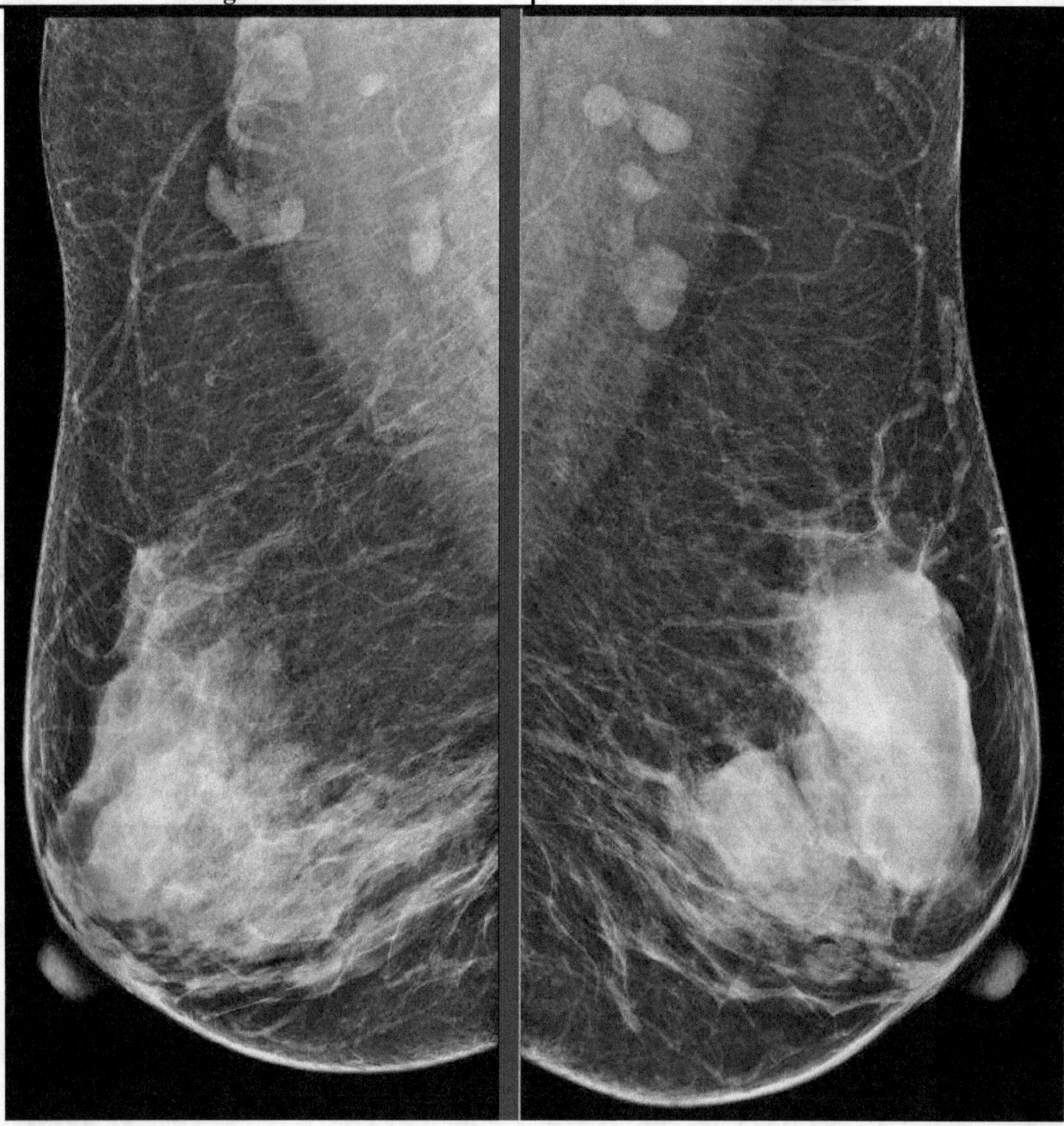

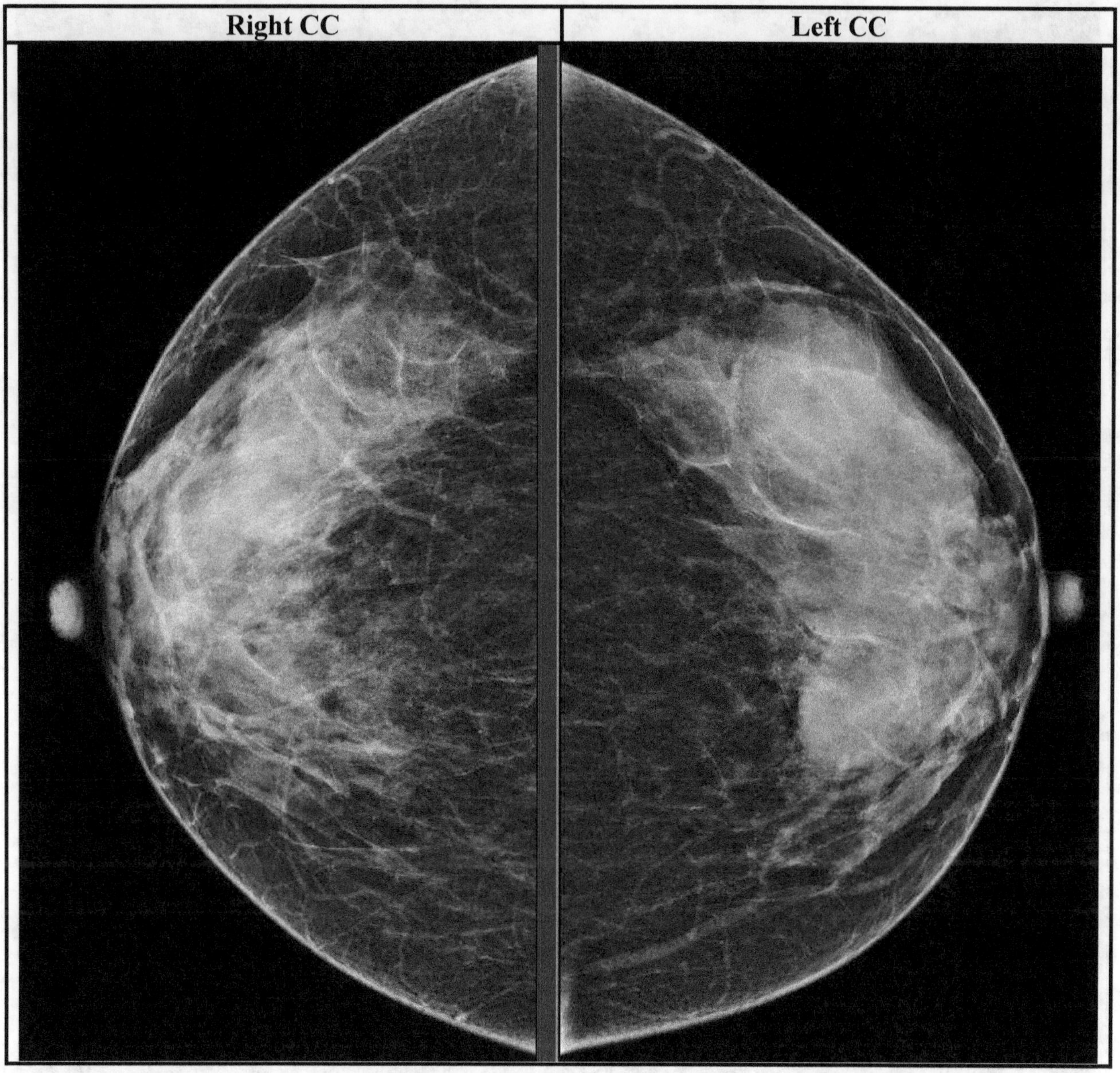
Right CC
Left CC

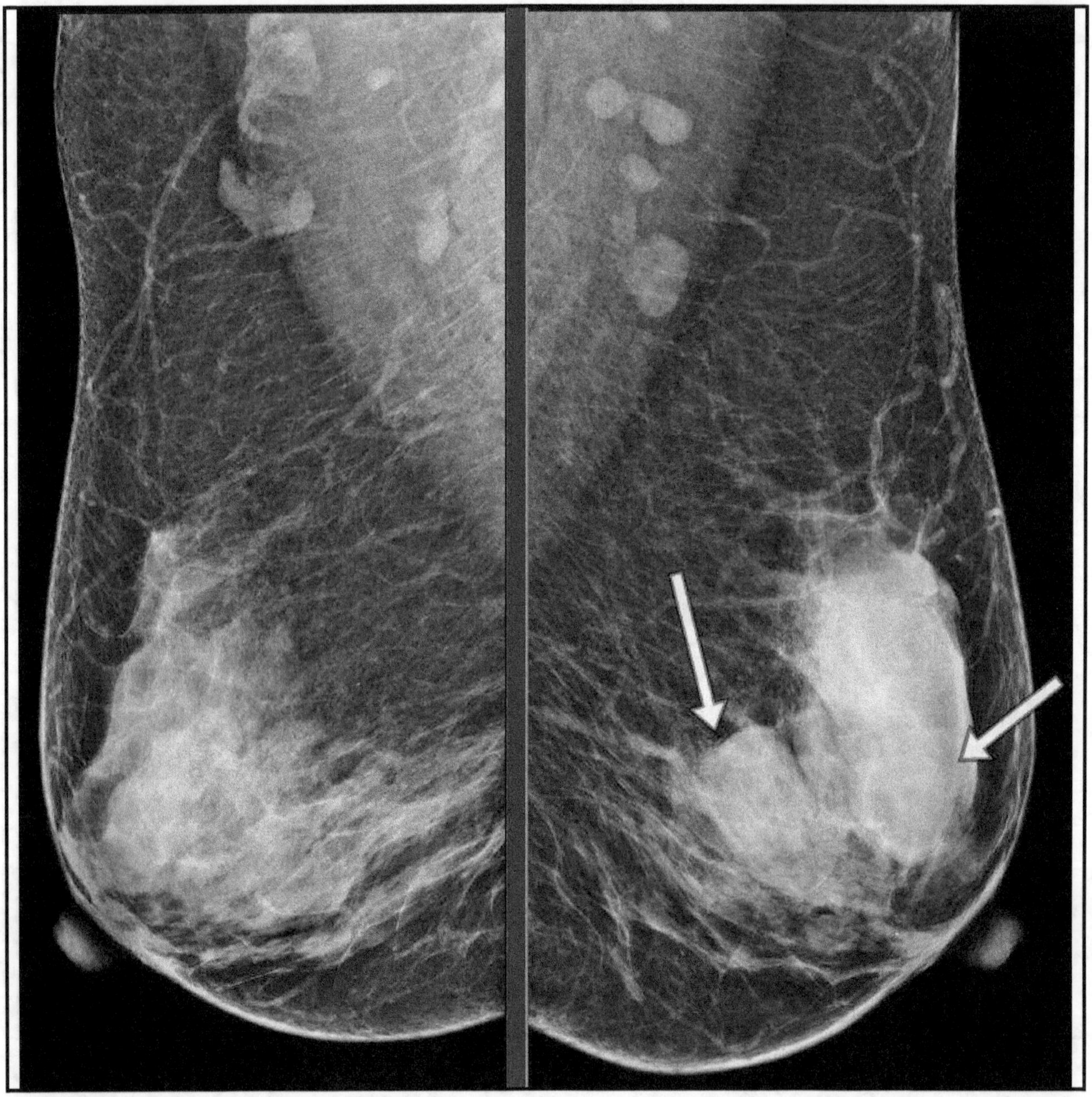

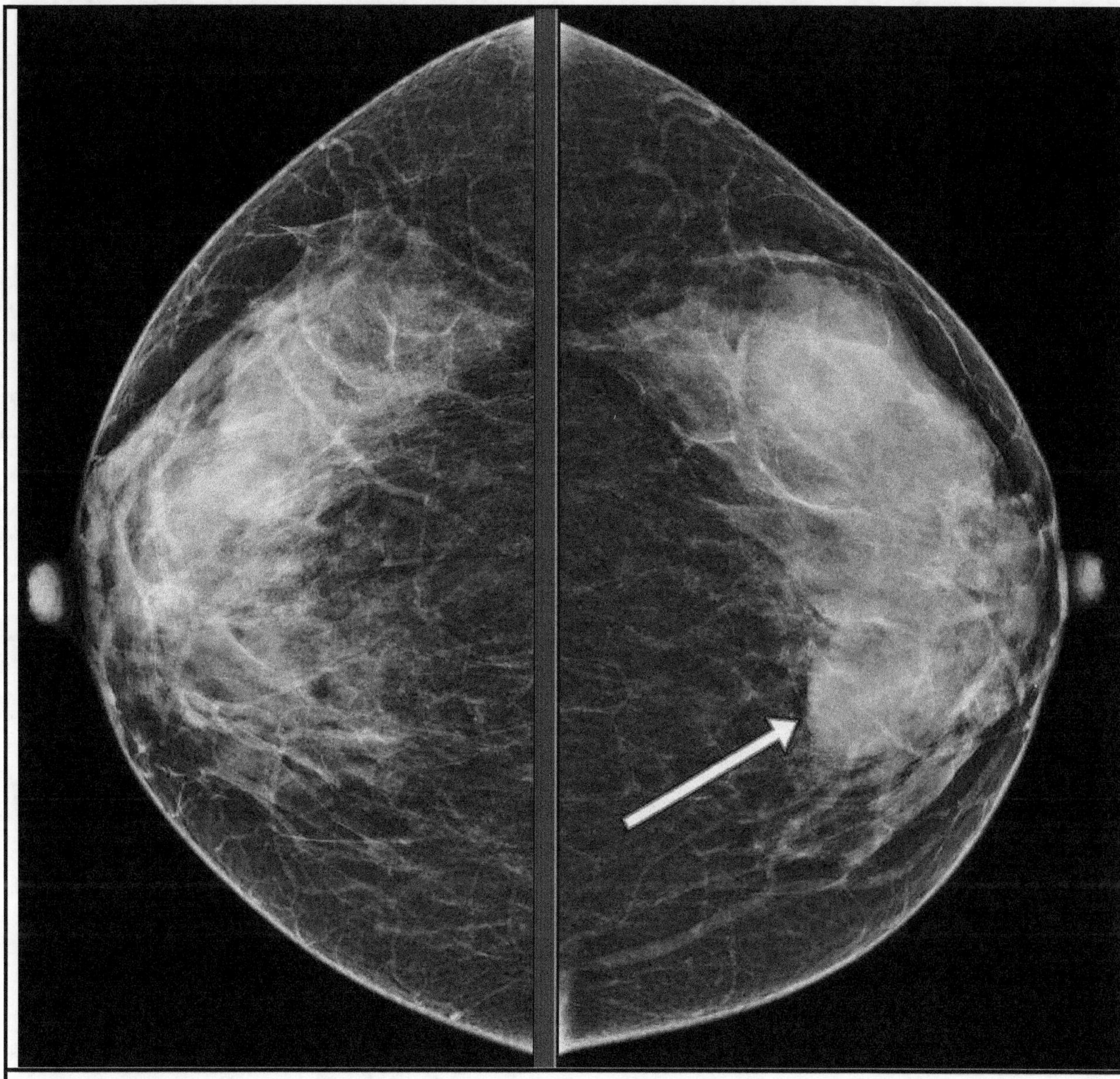

RIGHT BREAST	
Breast Parenchymal Density	***Heterogeneously dense, may obscure small masses (ACR C)***
Focal Mass	None
Asymmetric Density	None
Parenchymal Distortion	None
Calcification	None
Skin Thickening	None
Axillary Nodes	None

LEFT BREAST	
Breast Parenchymal Density	***Heterogeneously dense, may obscure small masses (ACR C)***
Focal Mass	***UOQ /LIQ oval obscured mass lesions***
Asymmetric Density	None
Parenchymal Distortion	None
Calcification	None
Skin Thickening	None
Axillary Nodes	None

IMPRESSION:

RIGHT BREAST: (BI-RADS 0)
LEFT BREAST: (BI-RADS 0)

RECOMMENDATION: US Correlation

CASE 54: 65-year-old female/ Diagnostic

Right MLO

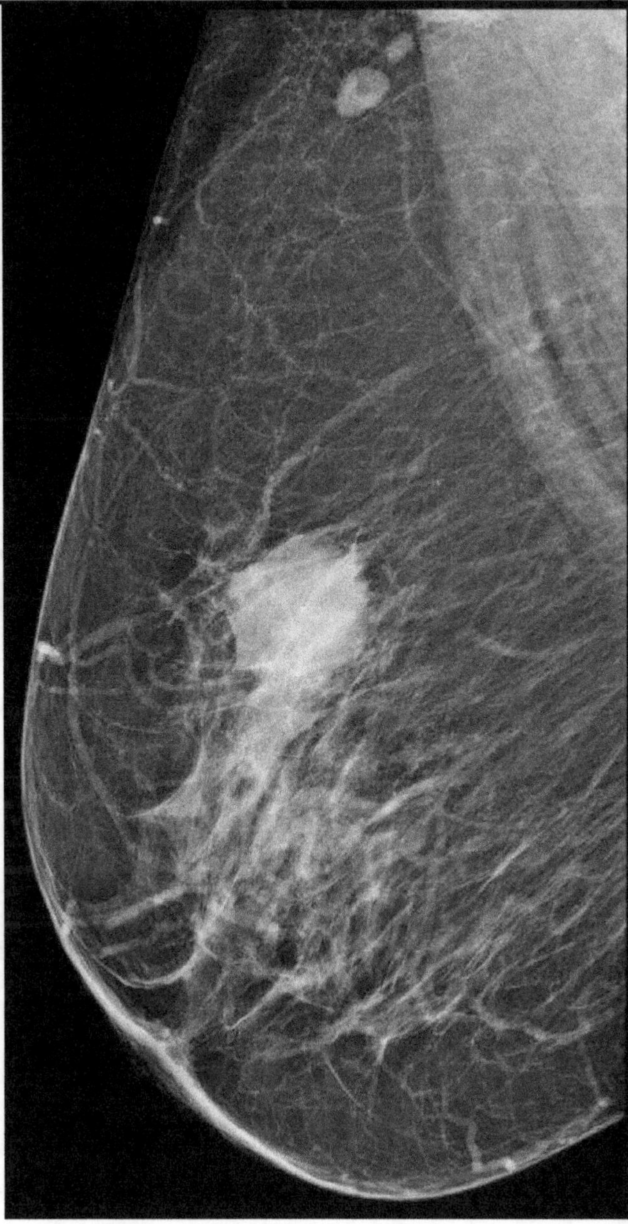

Left MLO

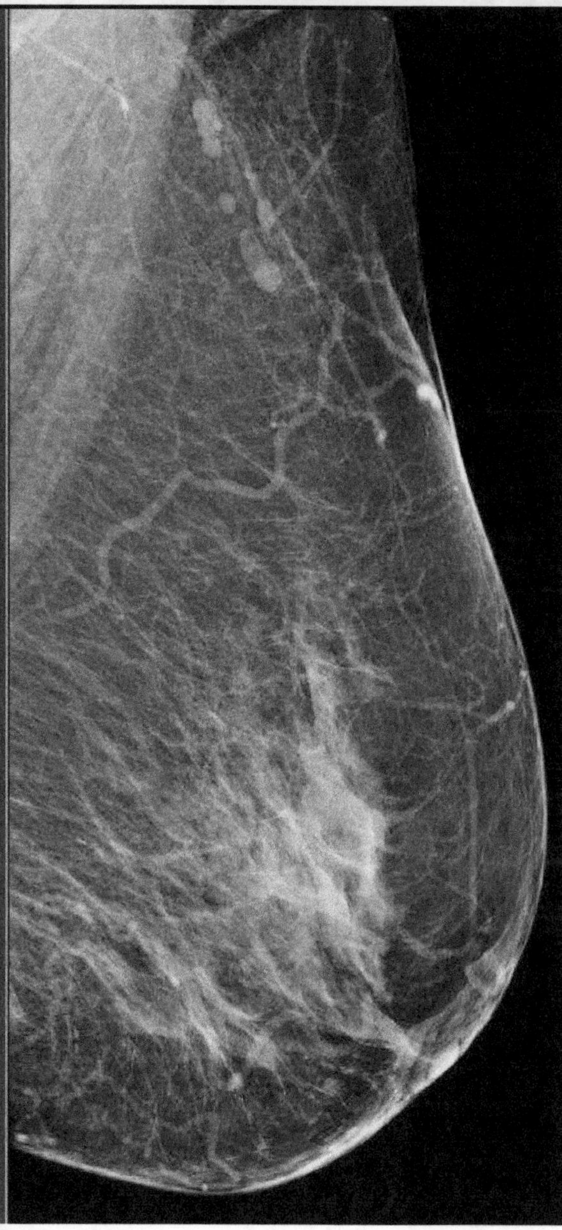

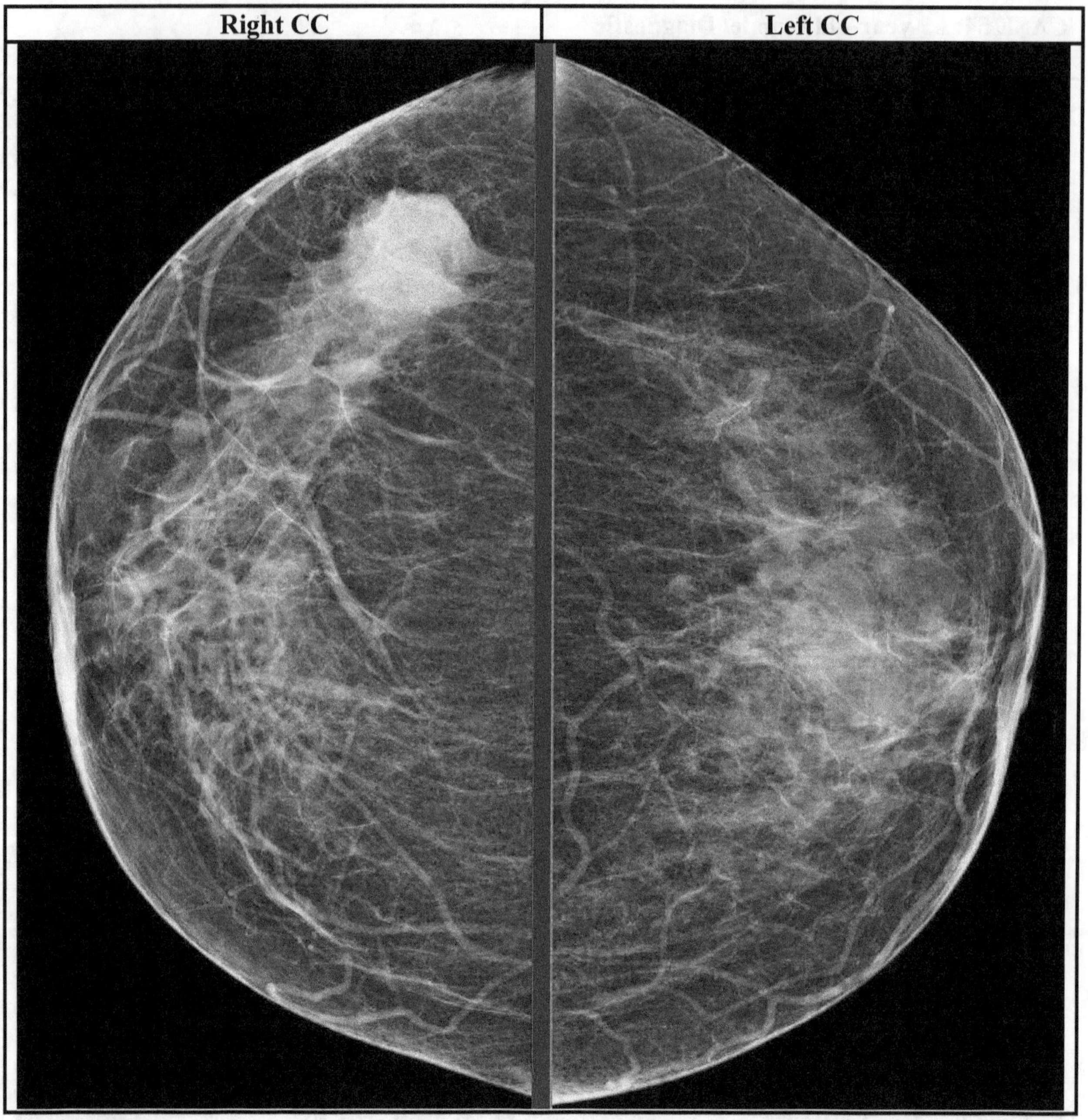
Right CC
Left CC

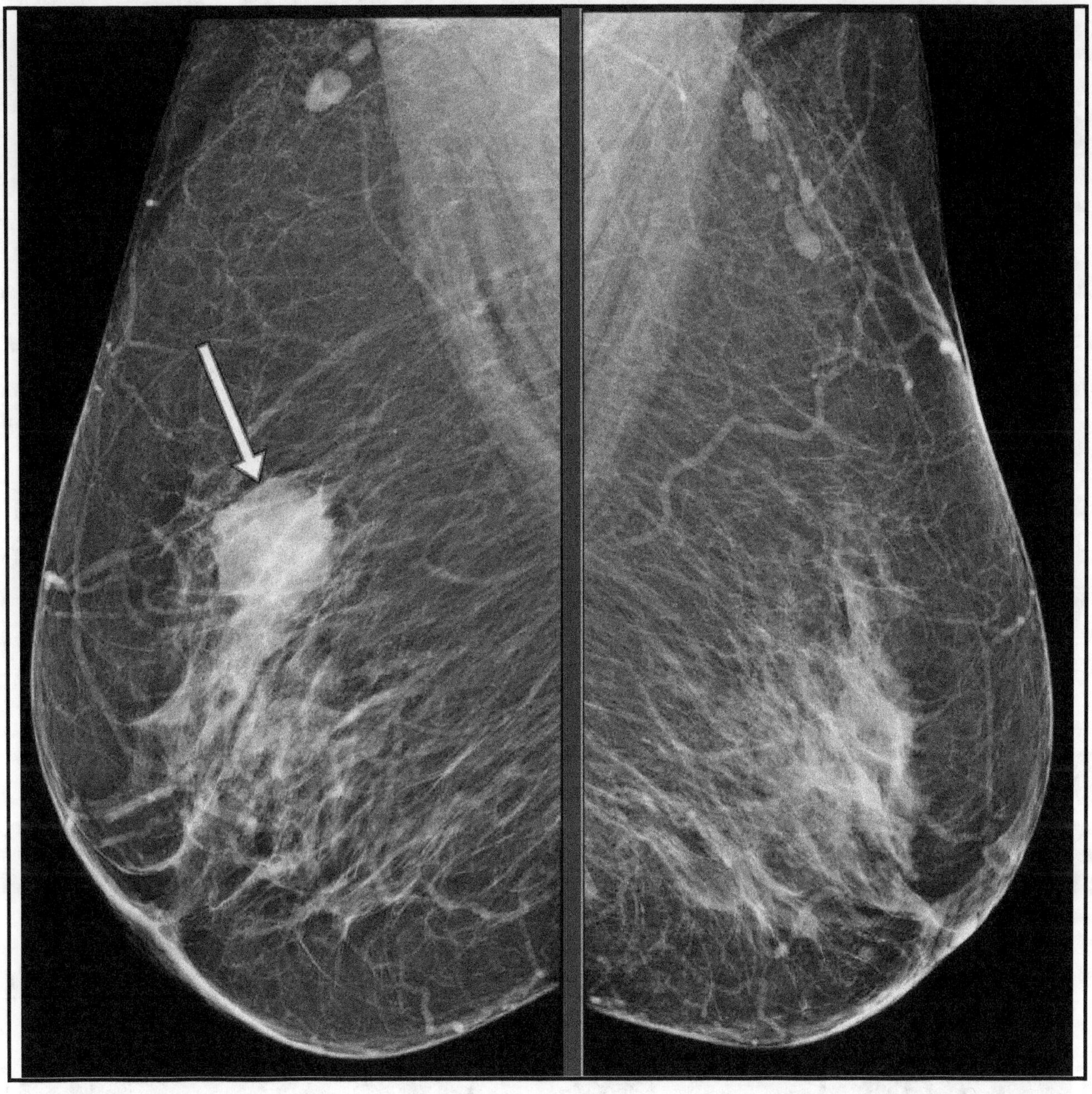

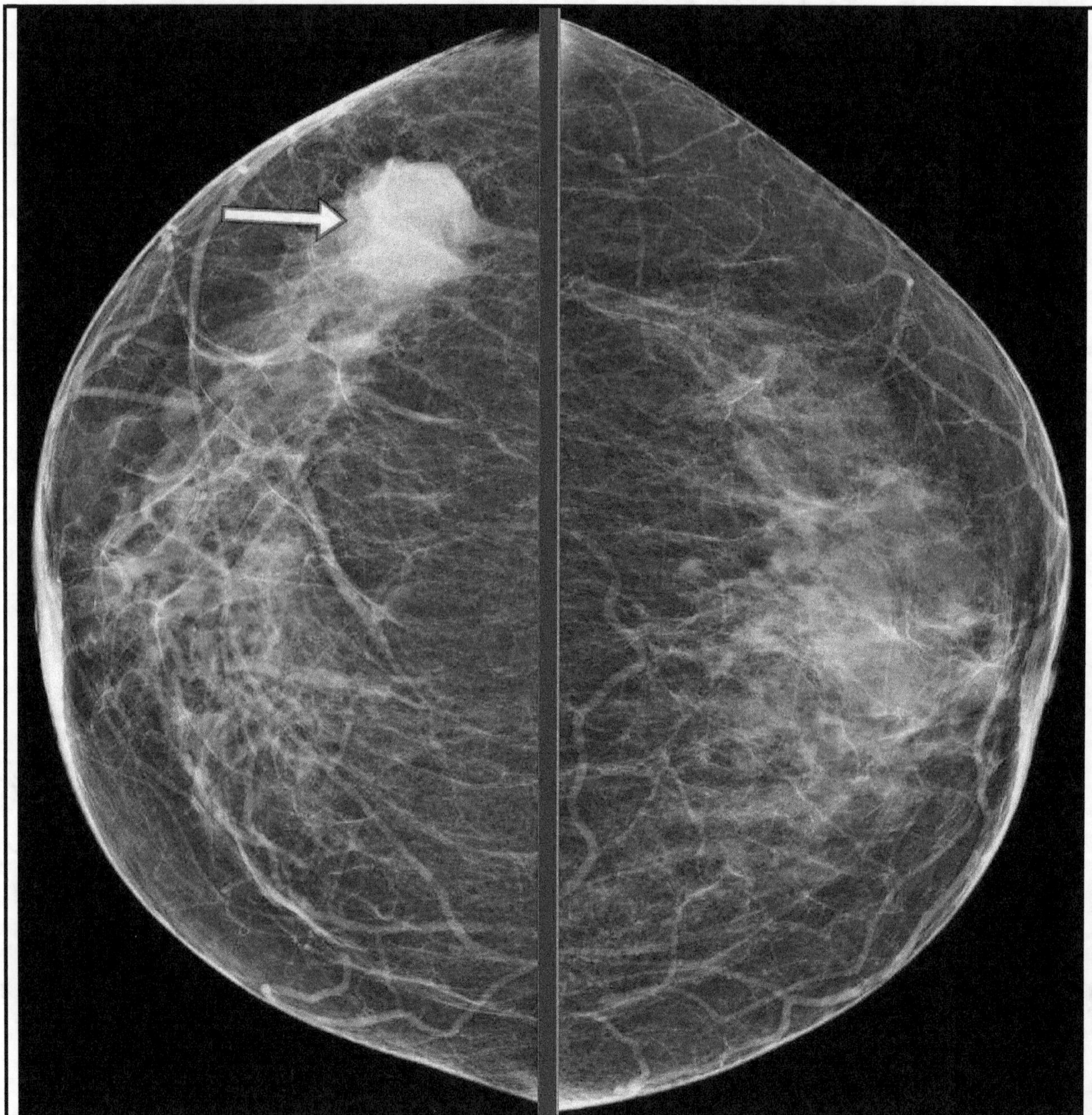

RIGHT BREAST	
Breast Parenchymal Density	***Scattered areas of fibroglandular density (ACR B)***
Focal Mass	***UOQ oval indistinct mass lesion***
Asymmetric Density	None
Parenchymal Distortion	None
Calcification	None
Skin Thickening	None
Axillary Nodes	None

LEFT BREAST	
Breast Parenchymal Density	***Scattered areas of fibroglandular density (ACR B)***
Focal Mass	None
Asymmetric Density	None
Parenchymal Distortion	None
Calcification	None
Skin Thickening	None
Axillary Nodes	None

IMPRESSION:

RIGHT BREAST: (BI-RADS 0)
LEFT BREAST: (BI-RADS 1)

RECOMMENDATION: US Correlation

CASE 55: 40-year-old female/ Diagnostic	
Right MLO	Left MLO

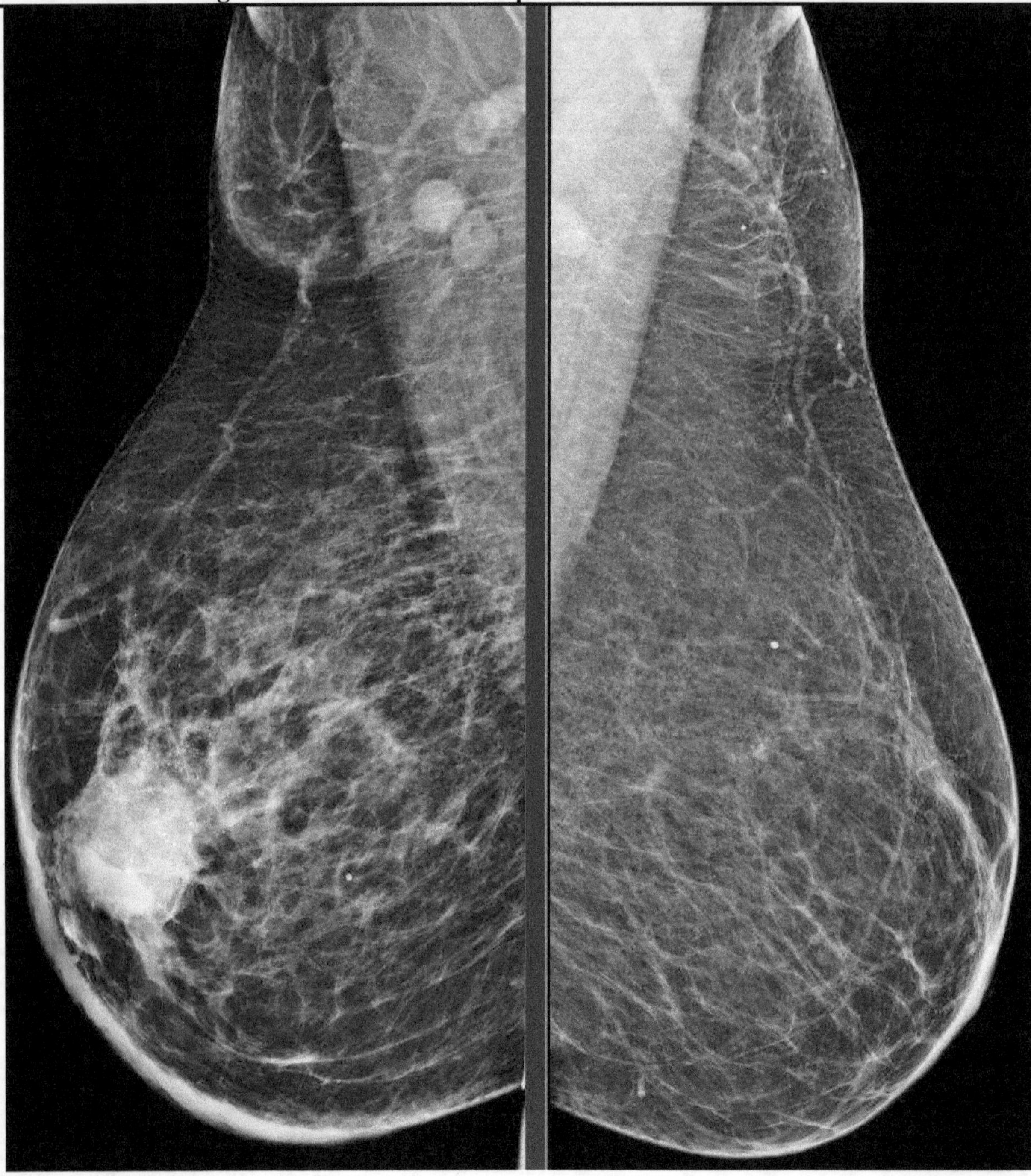

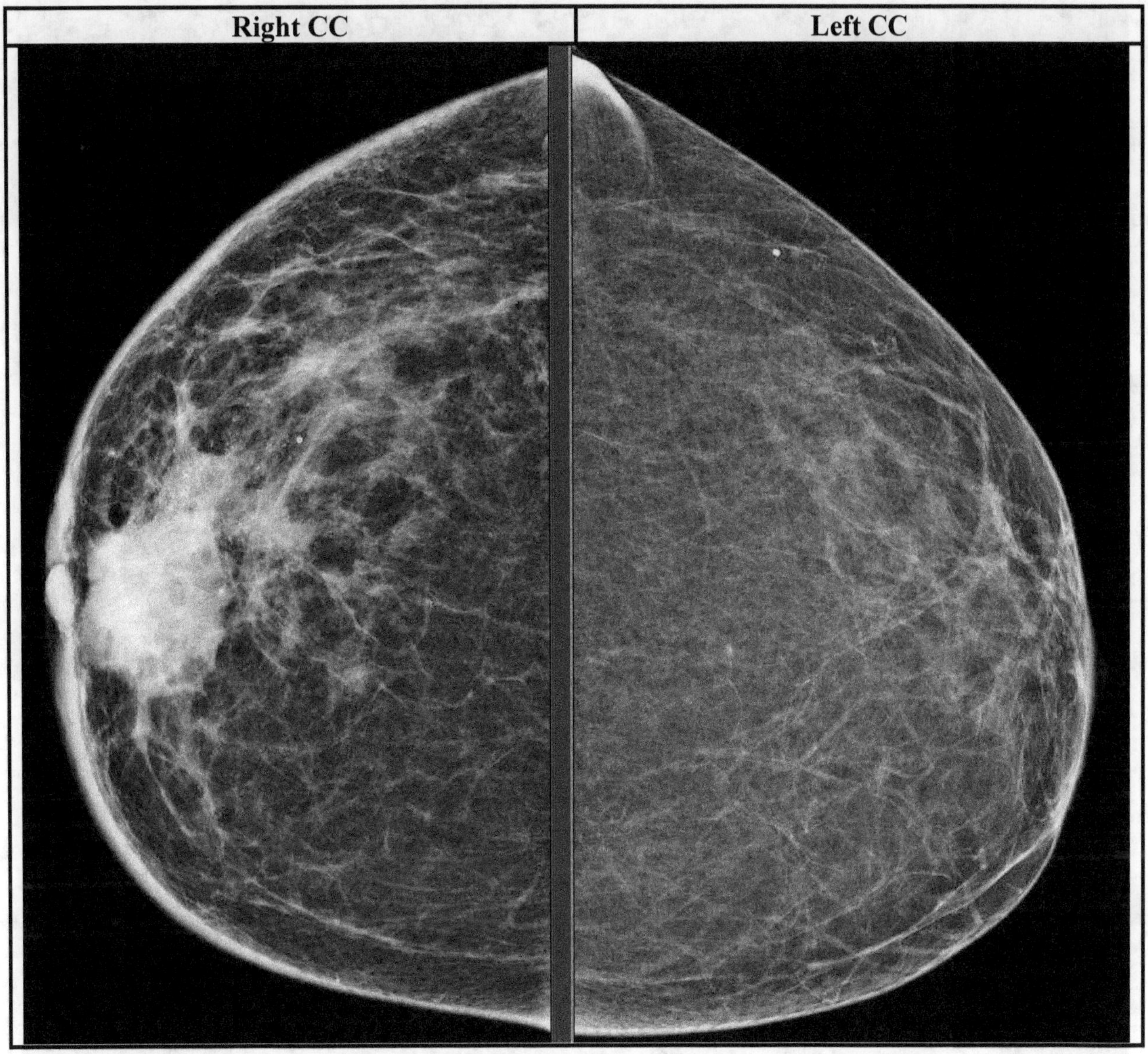
Right CC
Left CC

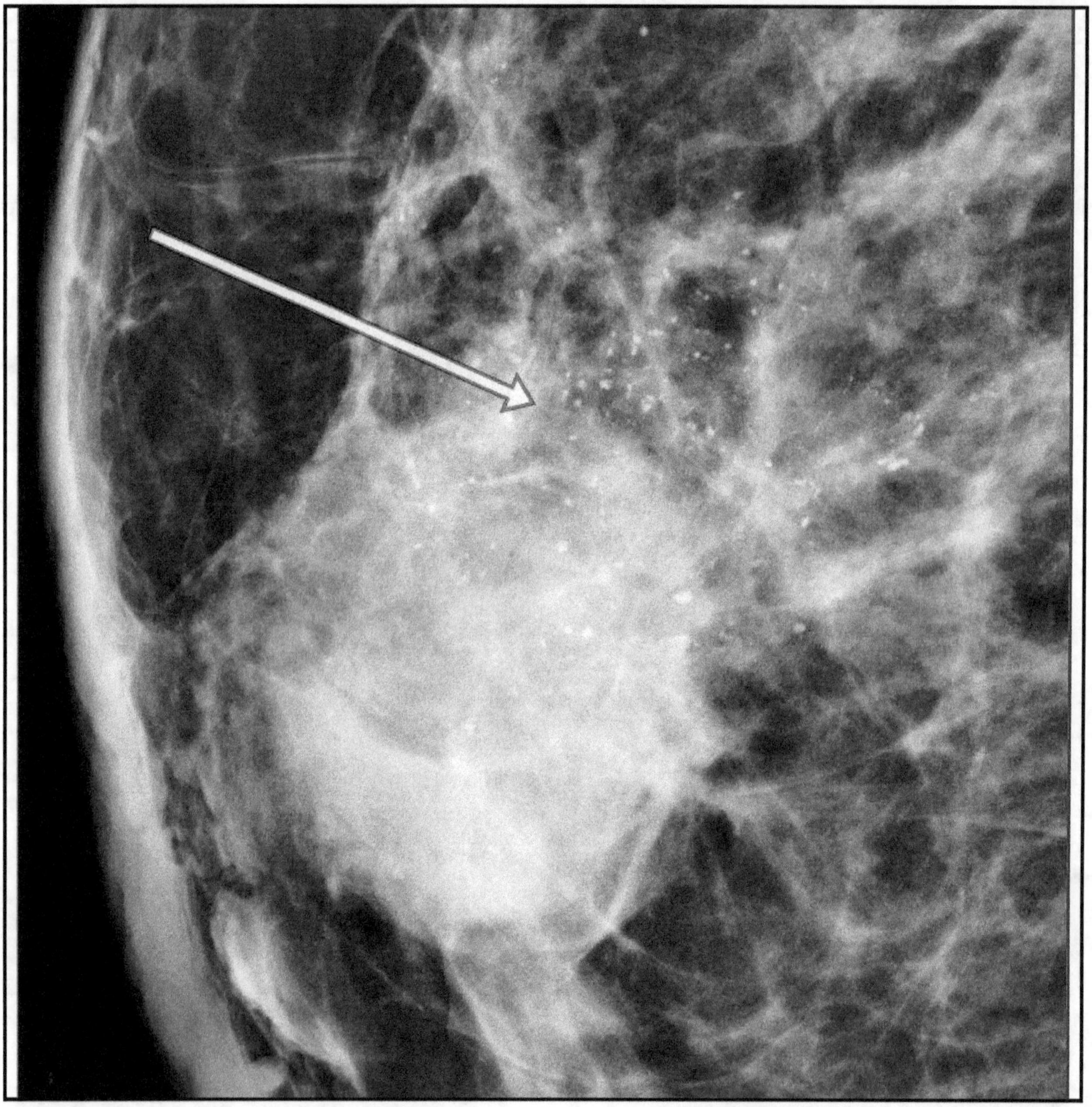

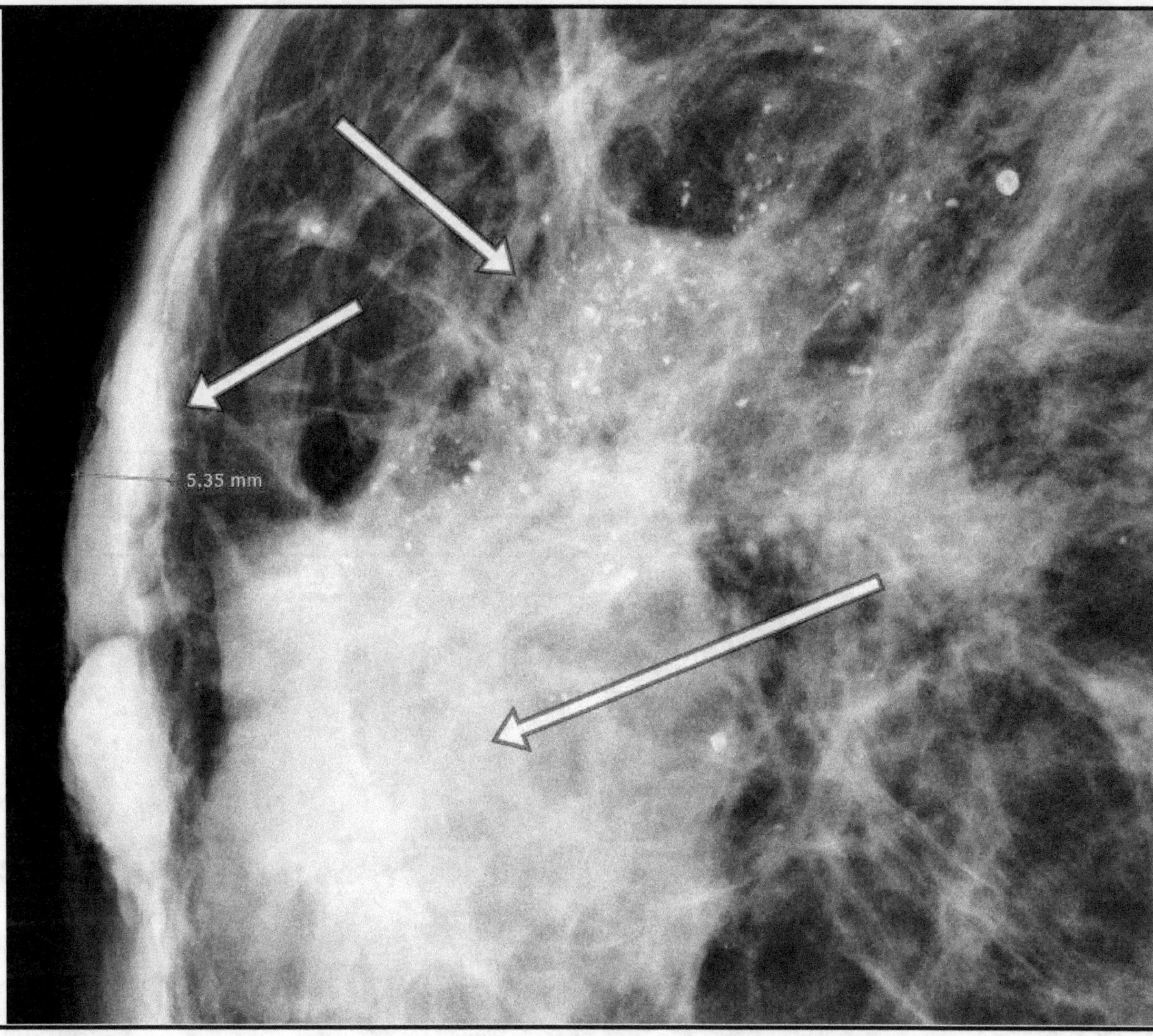

RIGHT BREAST	
Breast Parenchymal Density	***Scattered areas of fibroglandular density (ACR B)***
Focal Mass	***Upper central (12 o'clock) irregular indistinct mass lesion associated with fine pleomorphic suspicious micro-calcification /Trabecular edema***
Asymmetric Density	None
Parenchymal Distortion	None
Calcification	***fine pleomorphic suspicious micro-calcification***
Skin Thickening	Positive
Axillary Nodes	None

LEFT BREAST	
Breast Parenchymal Density	***Scattered areas of fibroglandular density (ACR B)***
Focal Mass	None
Asymmetric Density	None
Parenchymal Distortion	None
Calcification	None
Skin Thickening	None
Axillary Nodes	None

IMPRESSION:

RIGHT BREAST: (BI-RADS 5)
LEFT BREAST: (BI-RADS 1)

RECOMMENDATION: Histopathological Correlation

CASE 56: 41-year-old female/ Diagnostic

Right MLO	Left MLO

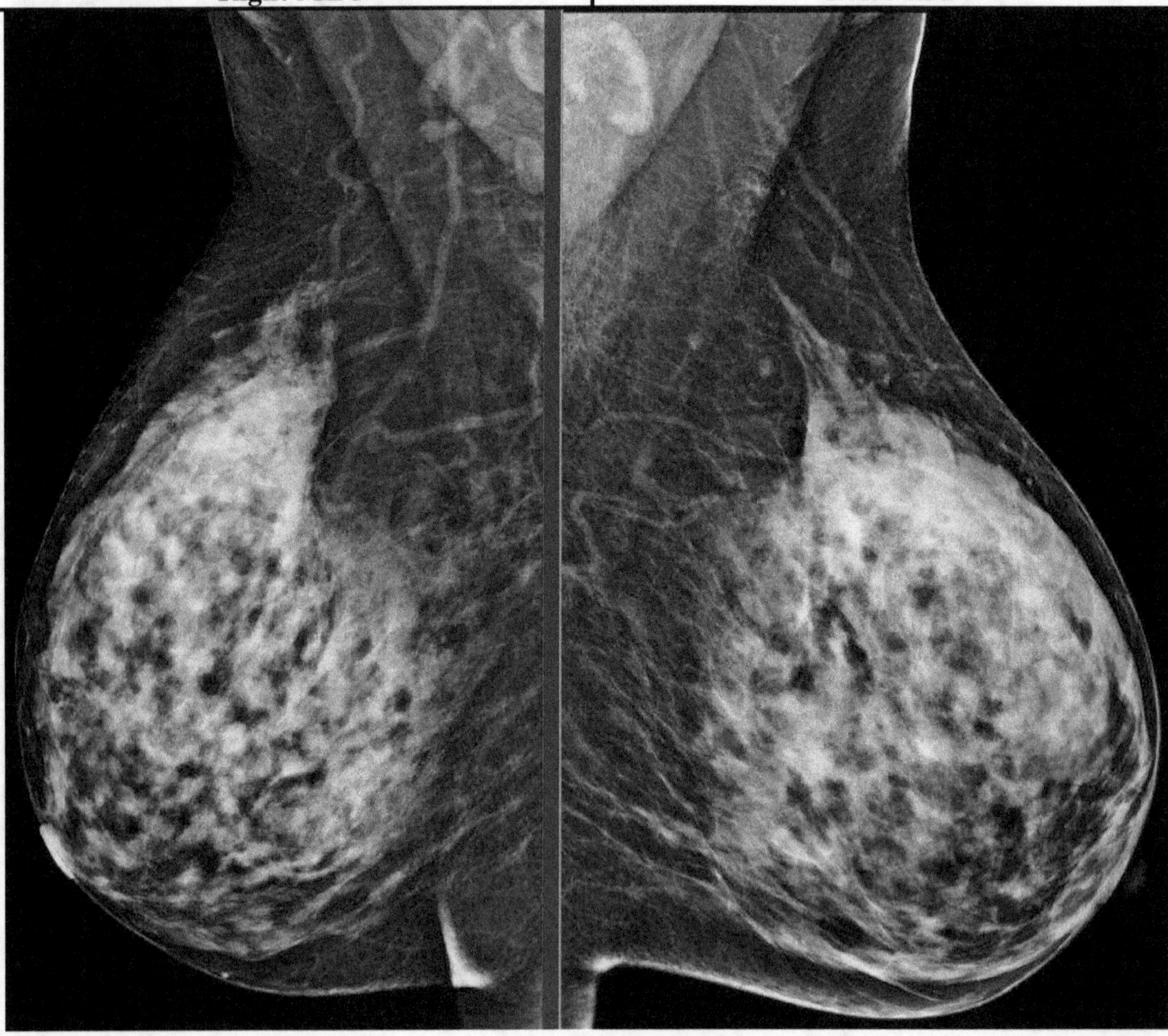

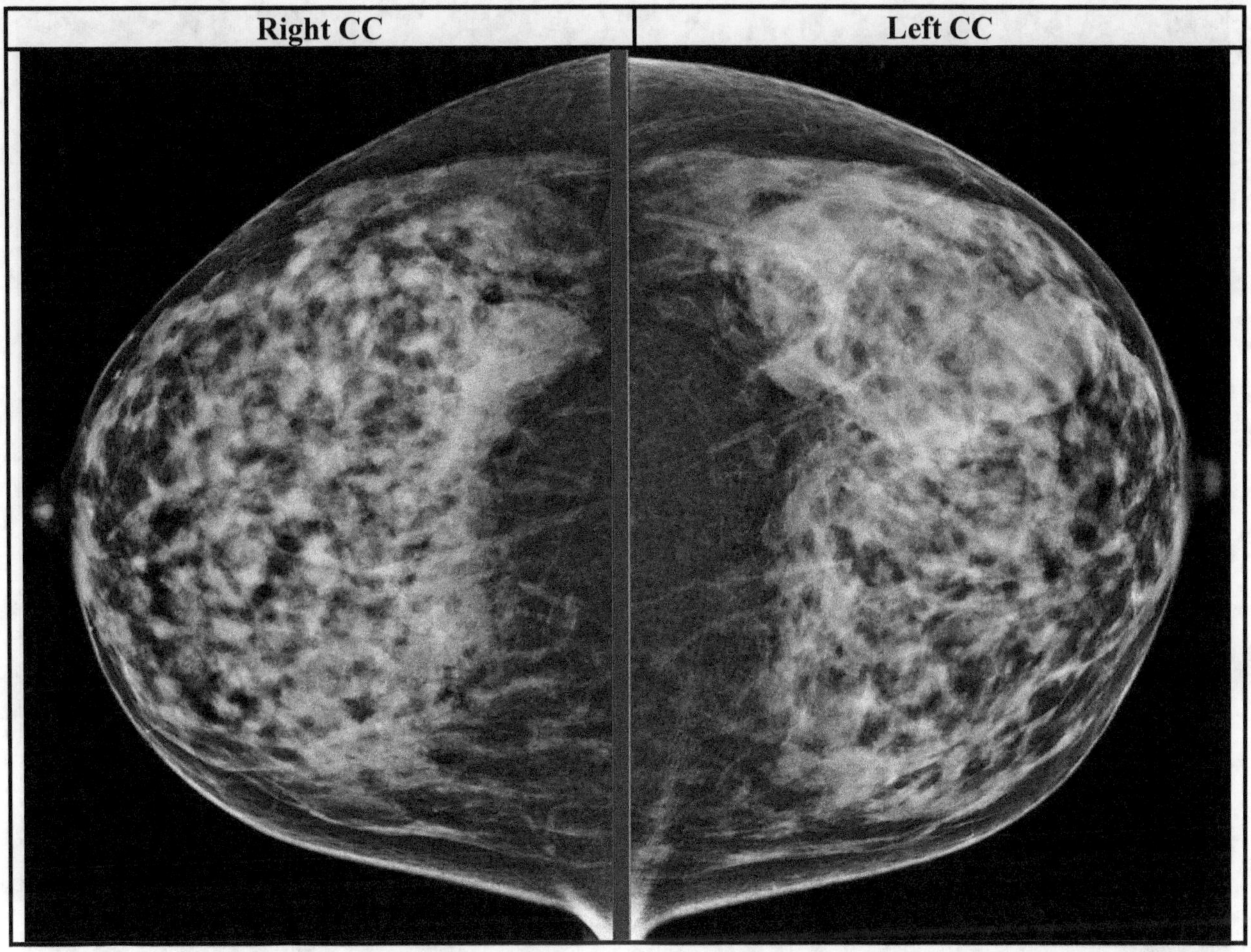
Right CC
Left CC

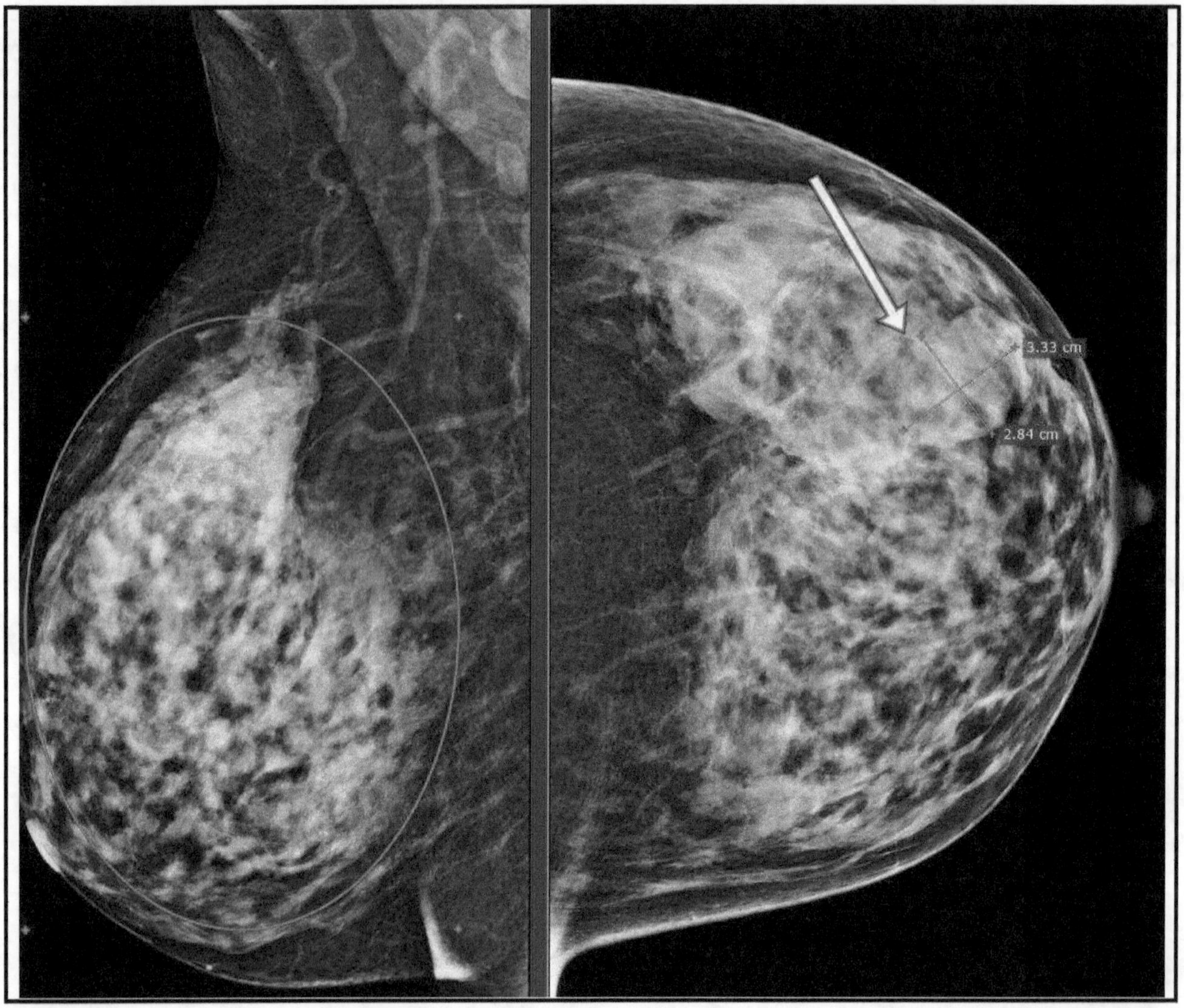

3.33 cm
2.84 cm

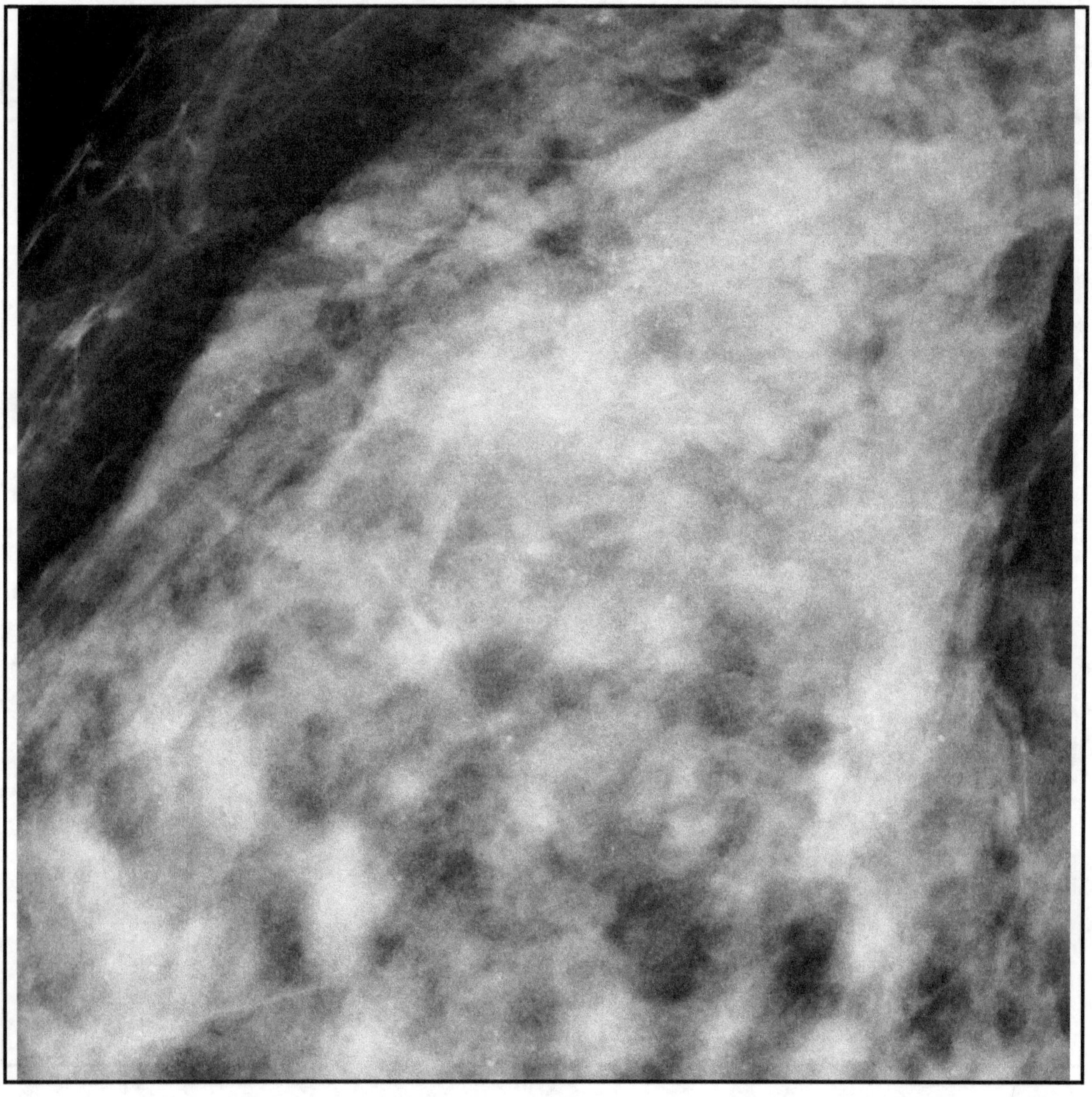

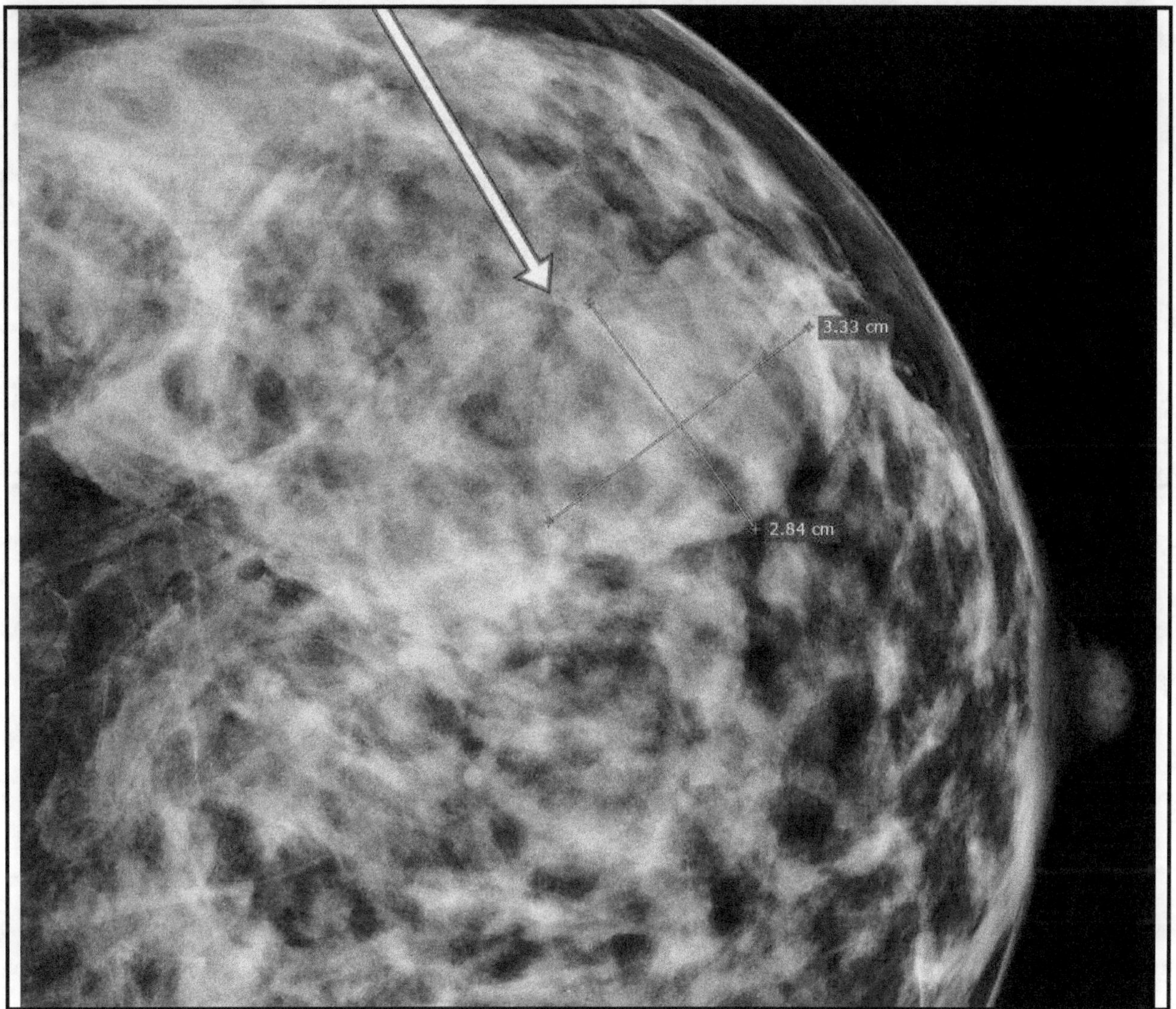

RIGHT BREAST	
Breast Parenchymal Density	***Extremely dense, which lowers the sensitivity of mammography (ACR D)***
Focal Mass	None
Asymmetric Density	None
Parenchymal Distortion	None
Calcification	***Diffuse Amorphous Suspicious Micro-Calcifications***
Skin Thickening	None
Axillary Nodes	None

LEFT BREAST	
Breast Parenchymal Density	***Extremely dense, which lowers the sensitivity of mammography (ACR D)***
Focal Mass	***UOQ oval circumscribed mass lesion***
Asymmetric Density	None
Parenchymal Distortion	None
Calcification	None
Skin Thickening	None
Axillary Nodes	None

IMPRESSION:

RIGHT BREAST: (BI-RADS 4b)
LEFT BREAST: (BI-RADS 0)

RECOMMENDATION: US Correlation/ Histopathological Correlation

Pathological proven right diffuse ductal carcinoma insitu (DCIS)

CASE 57: 47-year-old female/ Diagnostic	
Right MLO	Left MLO
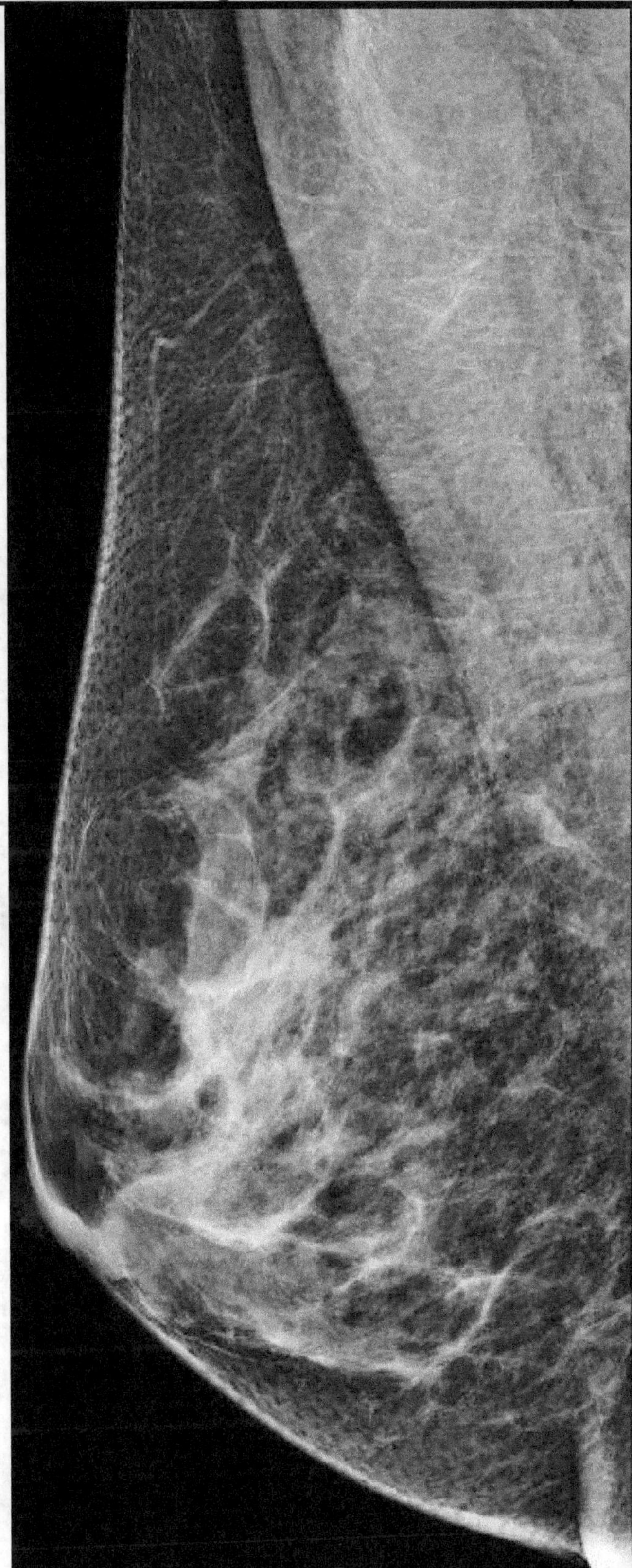	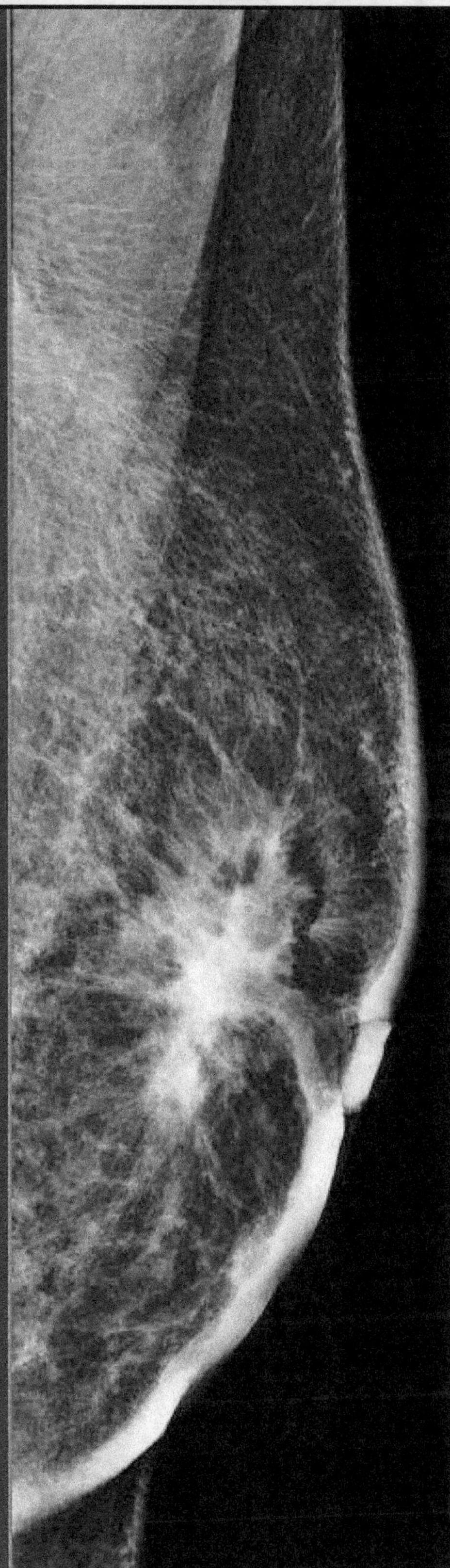

Right CC | **Left CC**

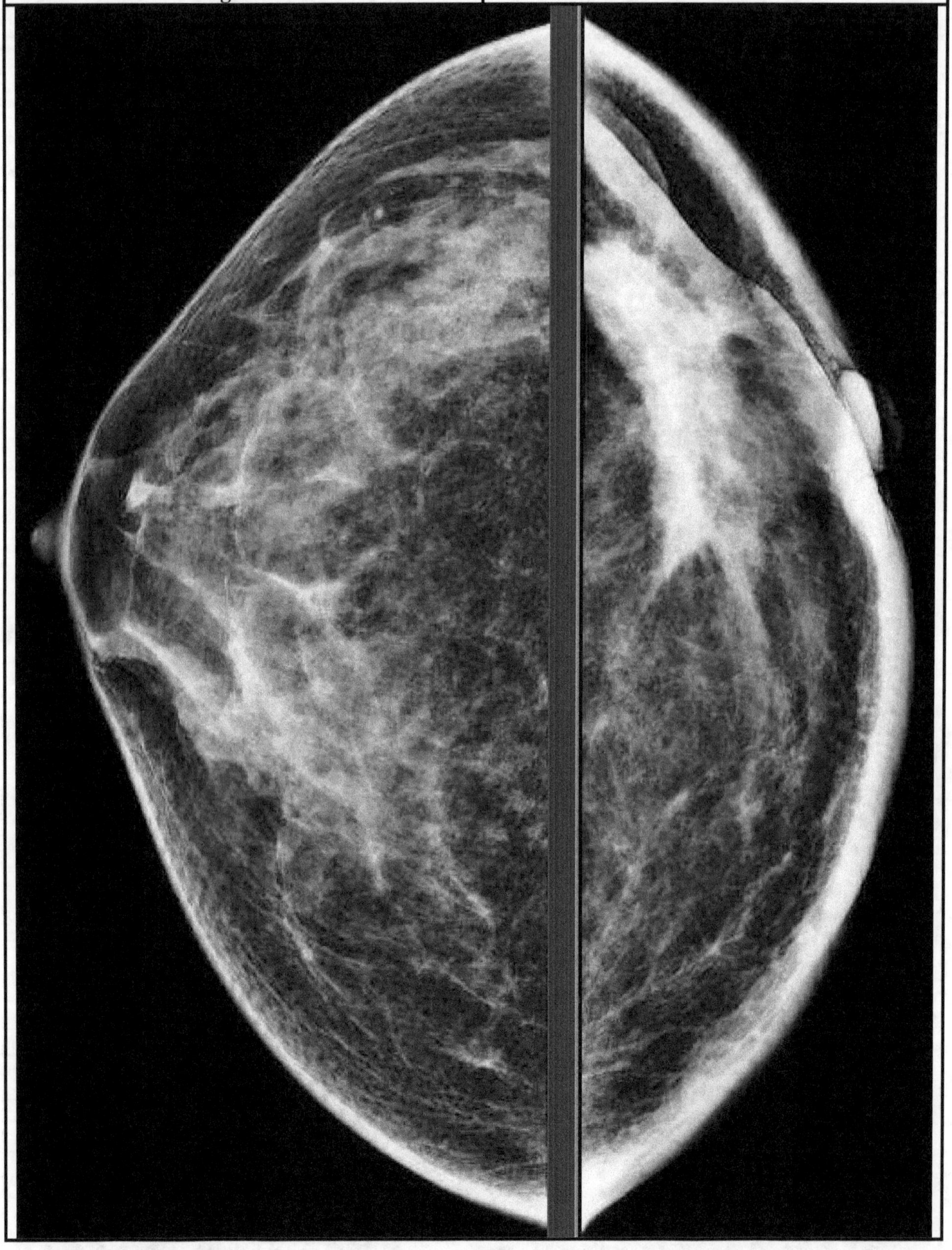

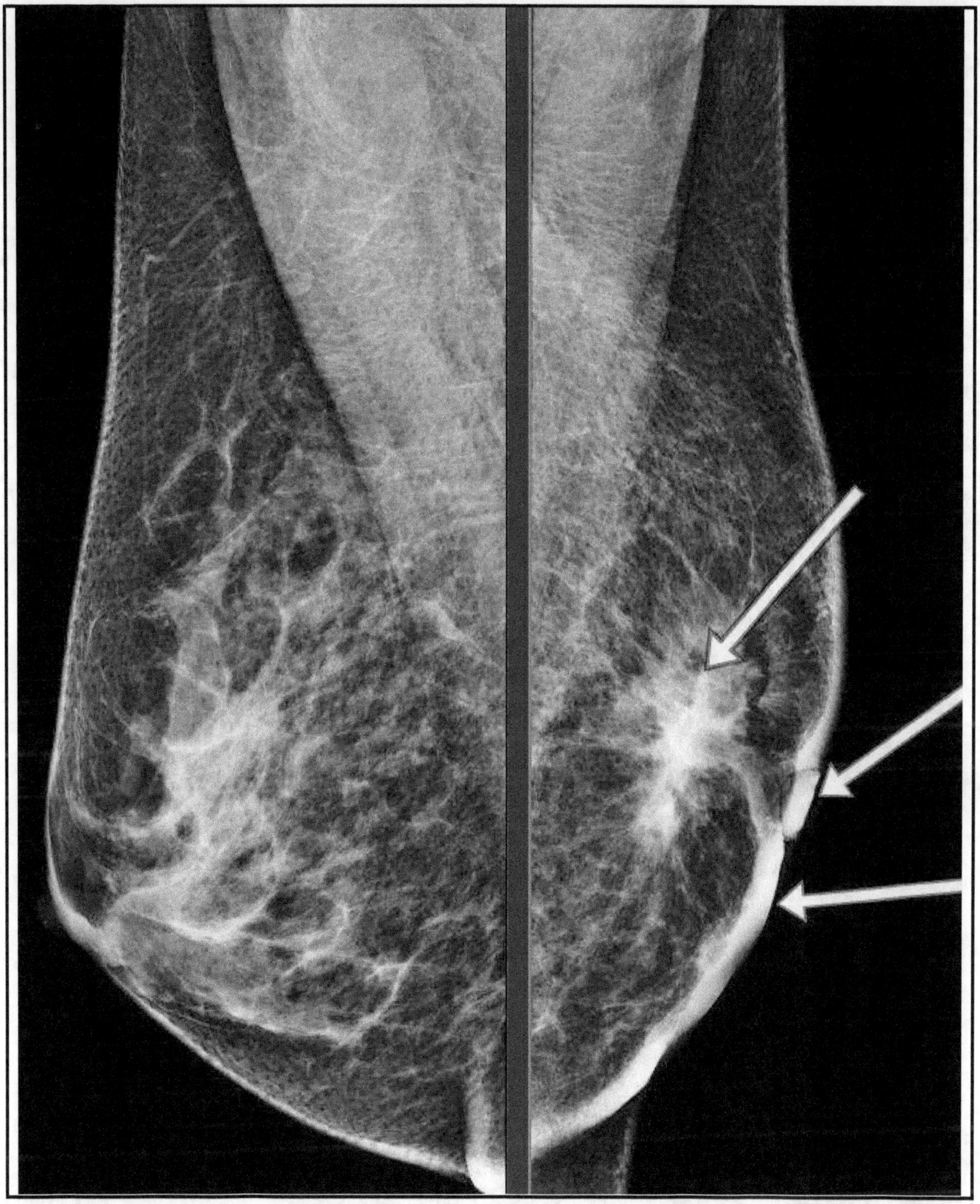

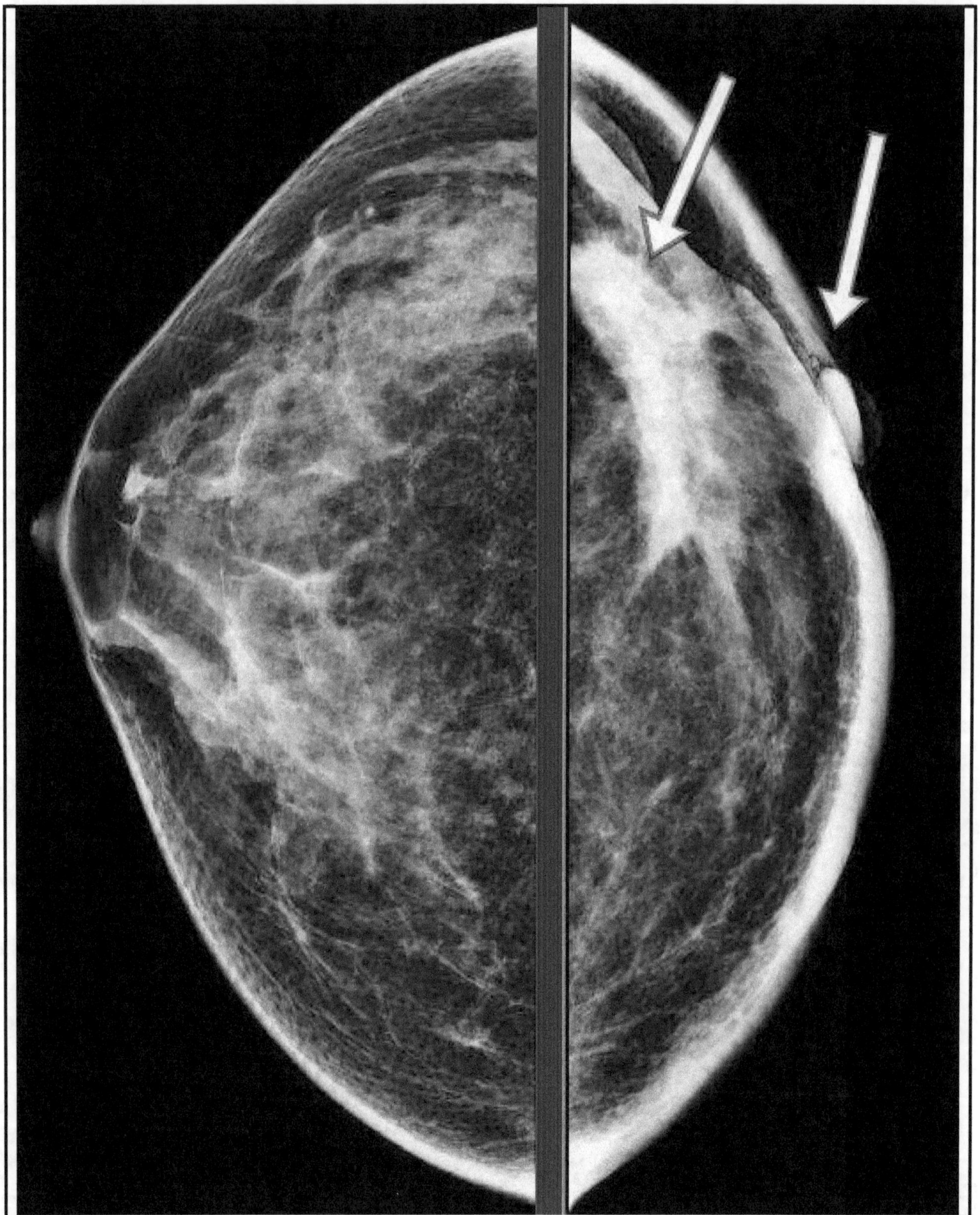

RIGHT BREAST	
Breast Parenchymal Density	***Heterogeneously dense, may obscure small masses (ACR C)***
Focal Mass	None
Asymmetric Density	None
Parenchymal Distortion	None
Calcification	None
Skin Thickening	None
Axillary Nodes	None

LEFT BREAST	
Breast Parenchymal Density	***Heterogeneously dense, may obscure small masses (ACR C)***
Focal Mass	***Retro-areolar irregular spiculated mass lesion***
Asymmetric Density	None
Parenchymal Distortion	None
Calcification	None
Skin Thickening	***Positive + skin and nipple retraction***
Axillary Nodes	None

IMPRESSION:

RIGHT BREAST: (BI-RADS 1)
LEFT BREAST: (BI-RADS 5)

RECOMMENDATION: Histopathological Correlation

CASE 58: 31-year-old female/screening	
Right MLO	Left MLO

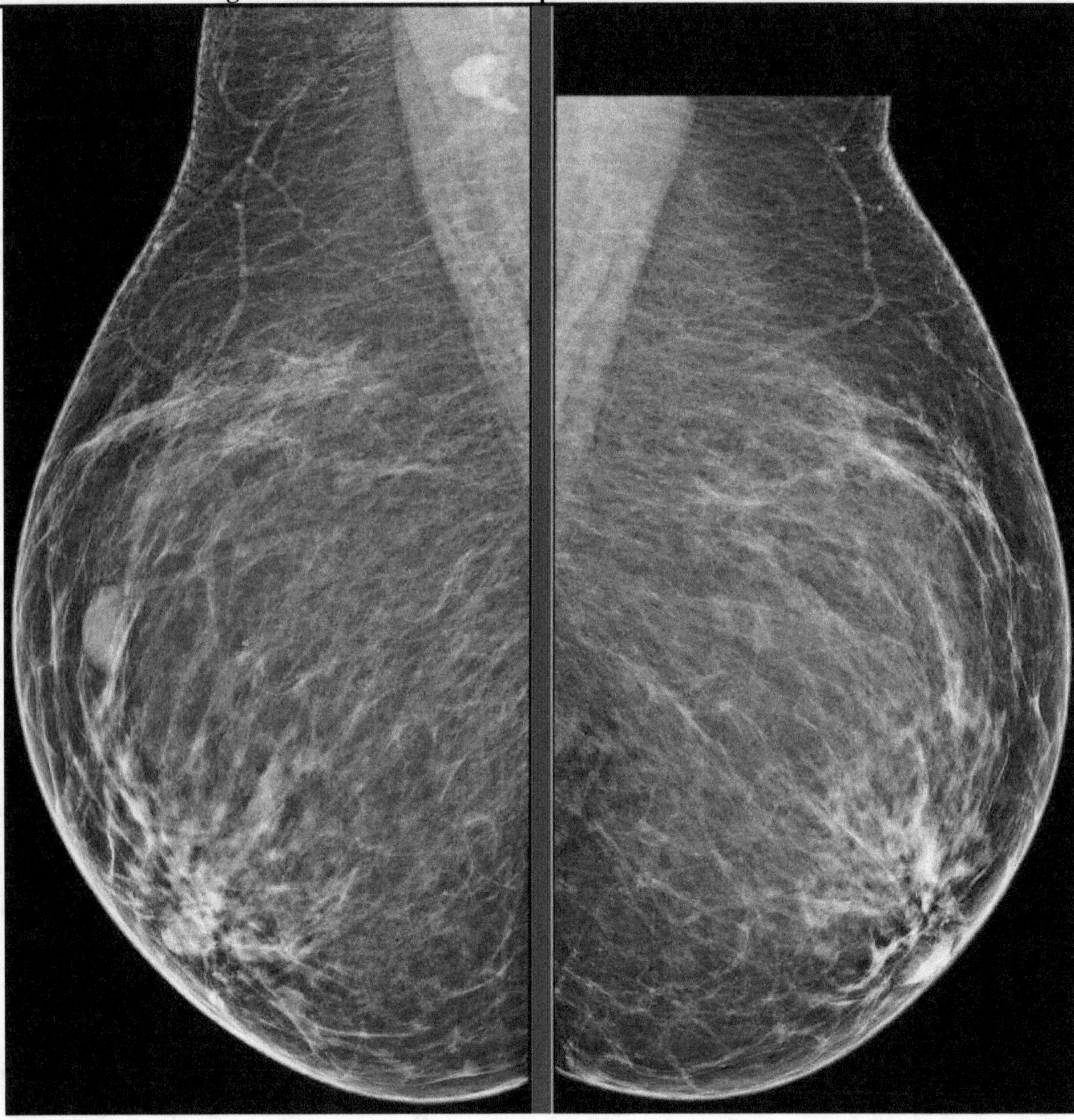

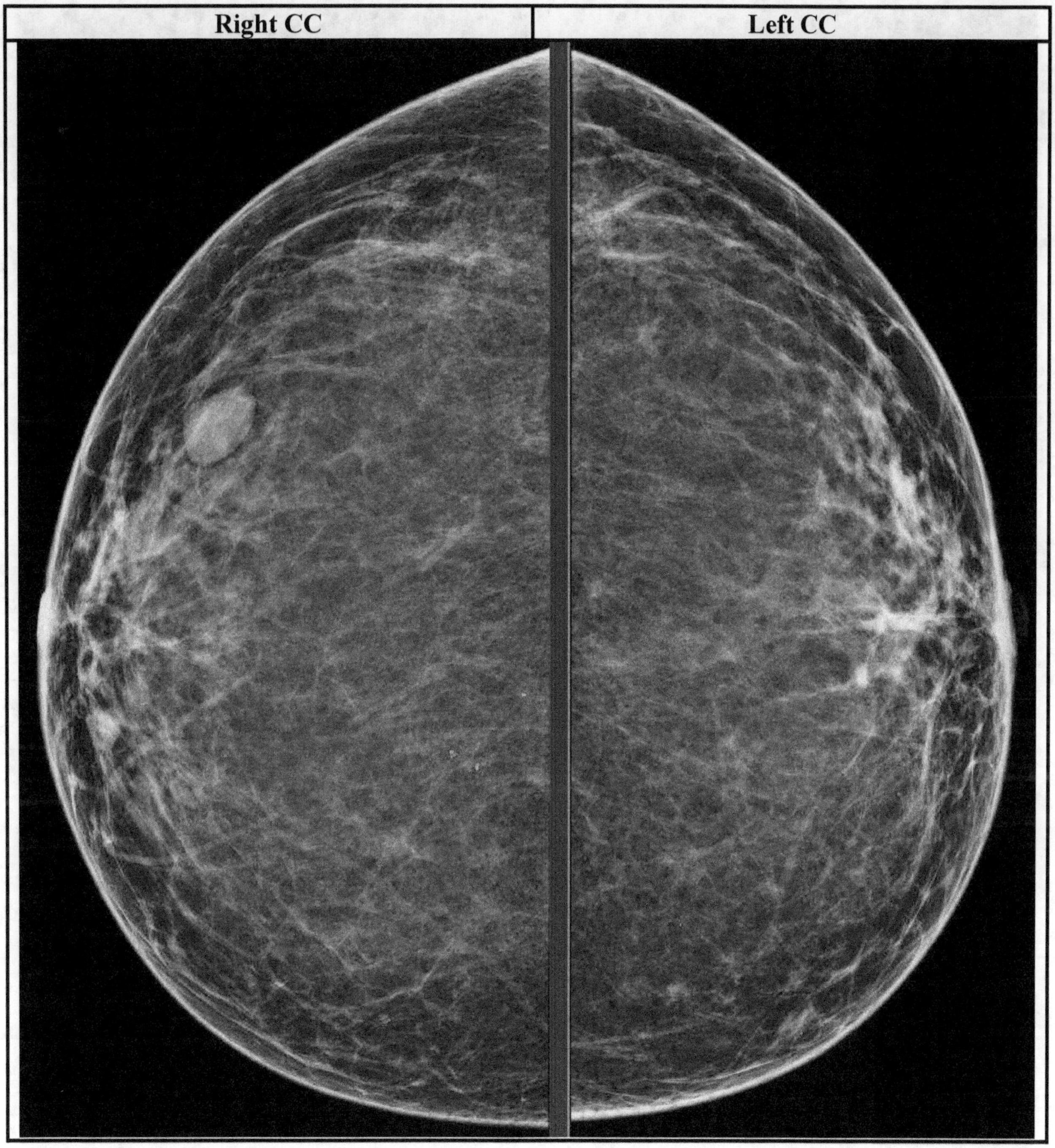
Right CC
Left CC

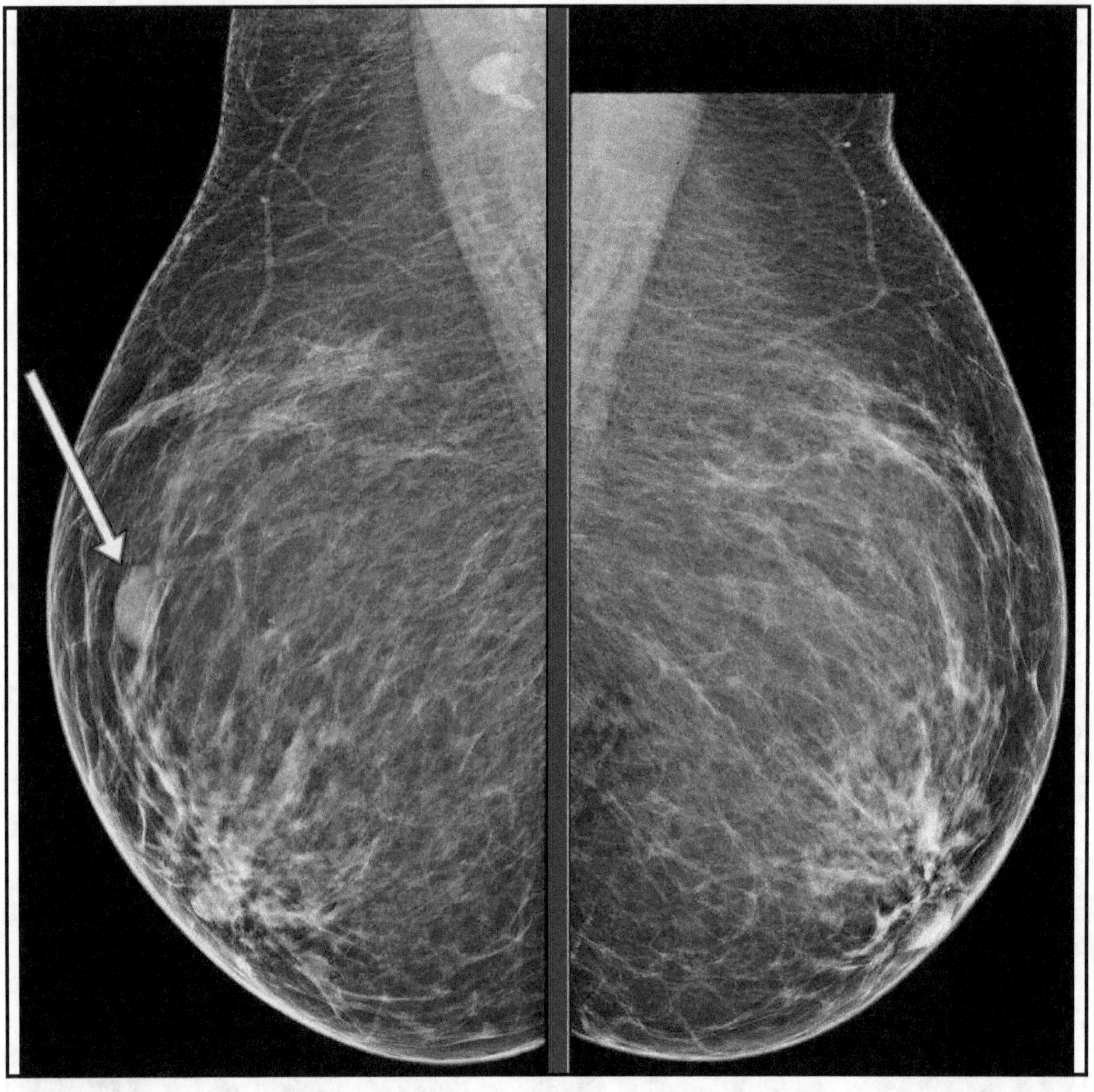

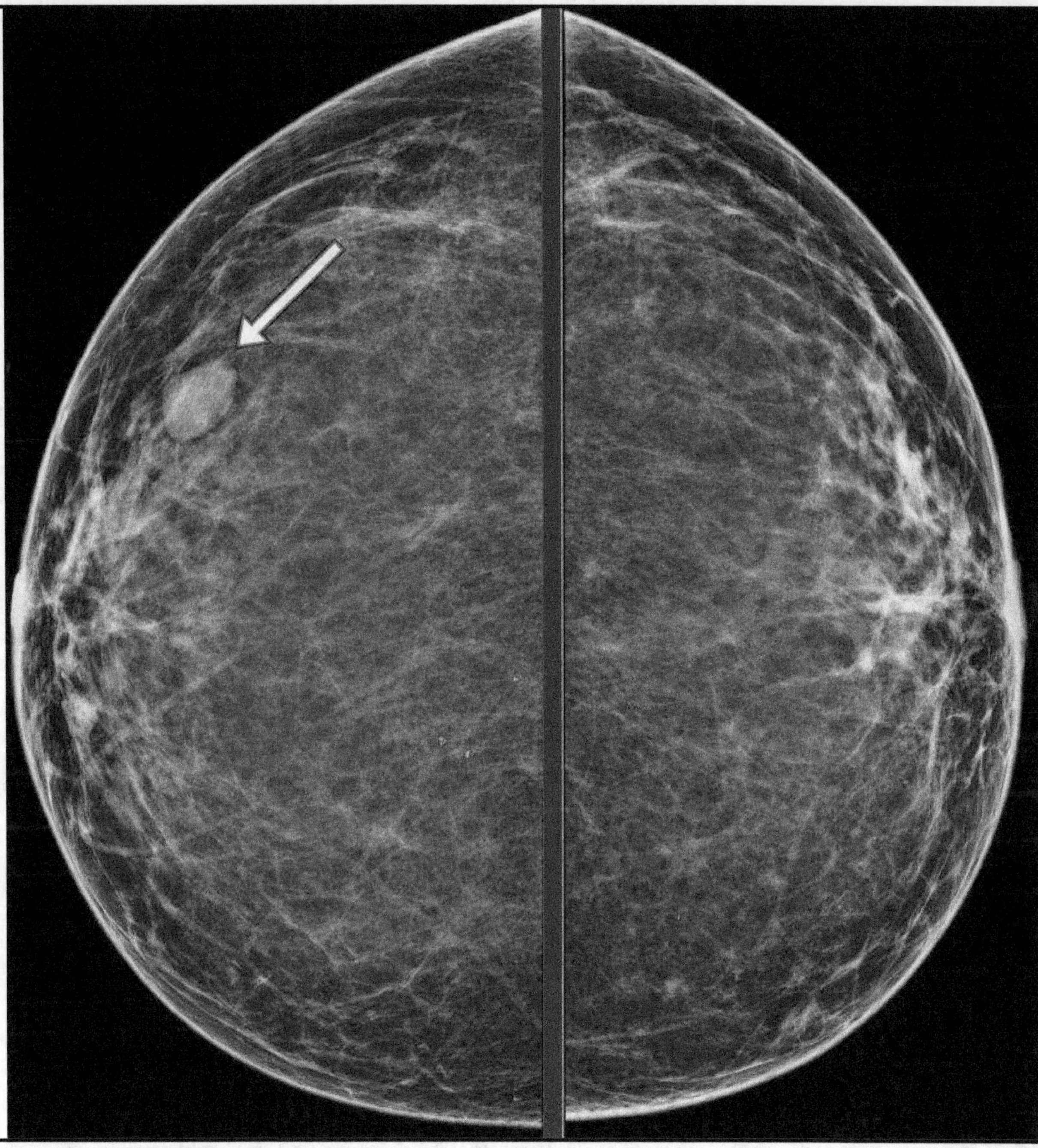

RIGHT BREAST	
Breast Parenchymal Density	***Scattered areas of fibroglandular density (ACR B)***
Focal Mass	***UOQ oval circumscribed mass lesion***
Asymmetric Density	None
Parenchymal Distortion	None
Calcification	None
Skin Thickening	None
Axillary Nodes	None

LEFT BREAST	
Breast Parenchymal Density	***Scattered areas of fibroglandular density (ACR B)***
Focal Mass	None
Asymmetric Density	None
Parenchymal Distortion	None
Calcification	None
Skin Thickening	None
Axillary Nodes	None

IMPRESSION:

RIGHT BREAST: (BI-RADS 0)
LEFT BREAST: (BI-RADS 1)

RECOMMENDATION: US Correlation

CASE 59: 48-year-old female/ Diagnostic

Right MLO	Left MLO

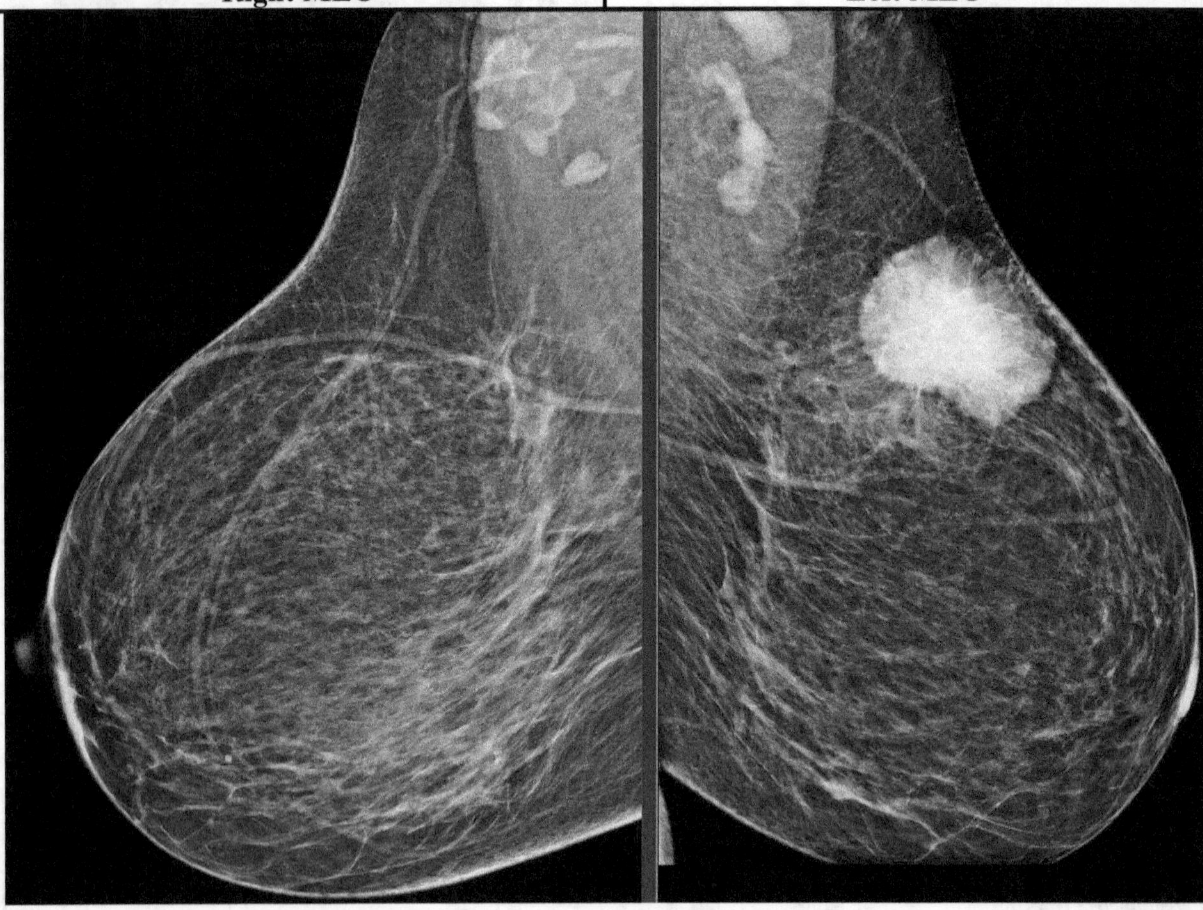

Right CC	Left CC

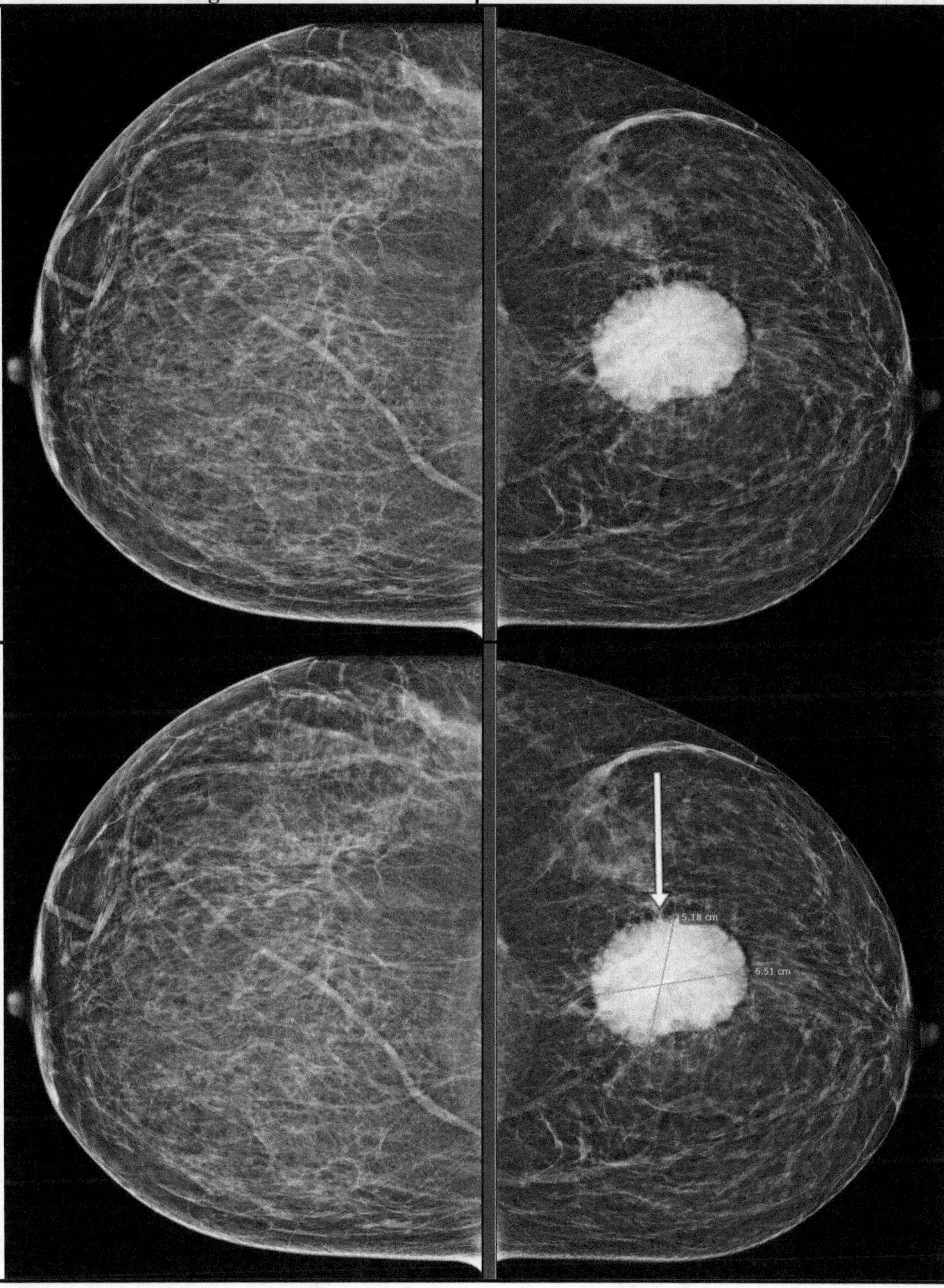

RIGHT BREAST	
Breast Parenchymal Density	***Scattered areas of fibroglandular density (ACR B)***
Focal Mass	None
Asymmetric Density	None
Parenchymal Distortion	None
Calcification	None
Skin Thickening	None
Axillary Nodes	None

LEFT BREAST	
Breast Parenchymal Density	***Scattered areas of fibroglandular density (ACR B)***
Focal Mass	***Upper central (12 o'clock) oval lobulated mass lesion measures (x)***
Asymmetric Density	None
Parenchymal Distortion	None
Calcification	None
Skin Thickening	None
Axillary Nodes	None

IMPRESSION:
RIGHT BREAST: (BI-RADS 1)
LEFT BREAST: (BI-RADS 4B)

RECOMMENDATION: Histopathological Correlation

CASE 60: 44 -year-old female complaining from skin erythema /pain

Right MLO	Left MLO
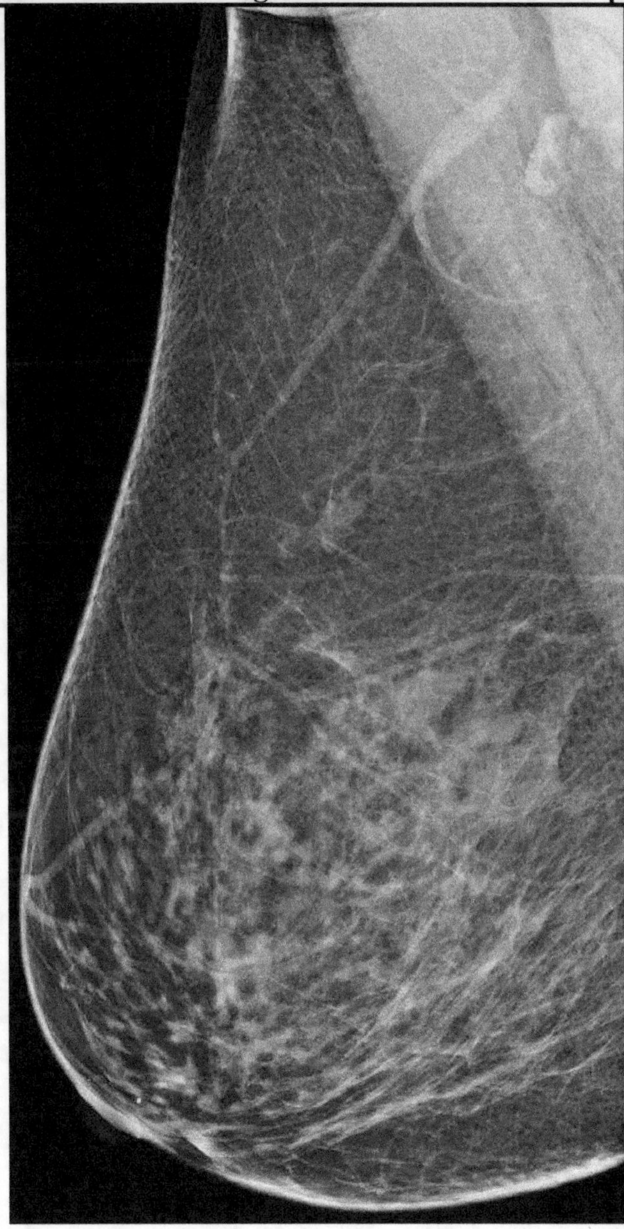	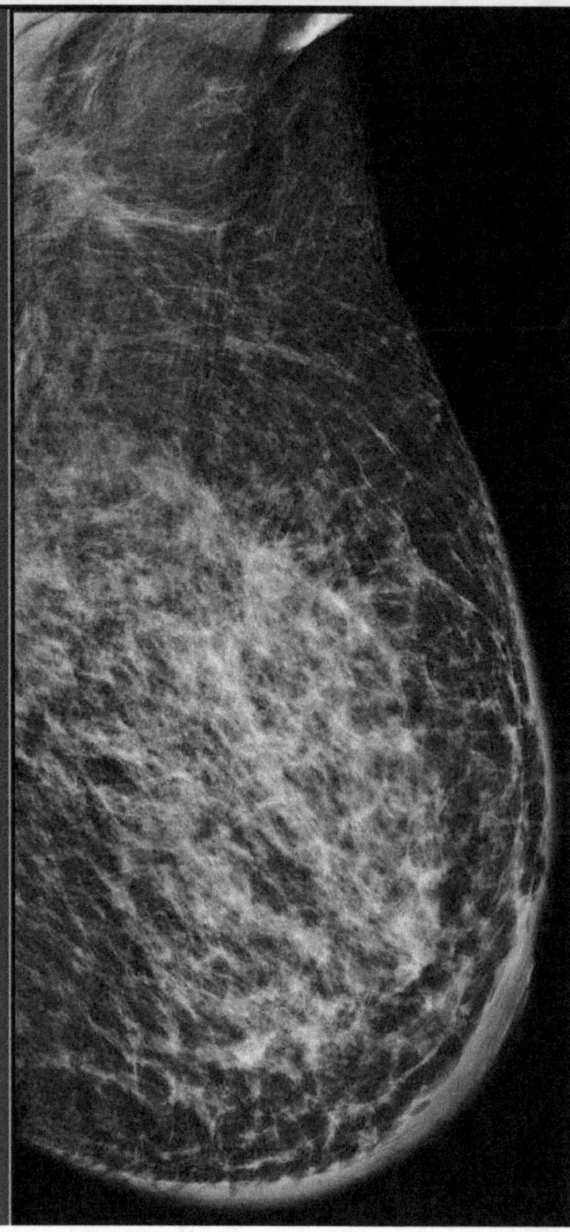

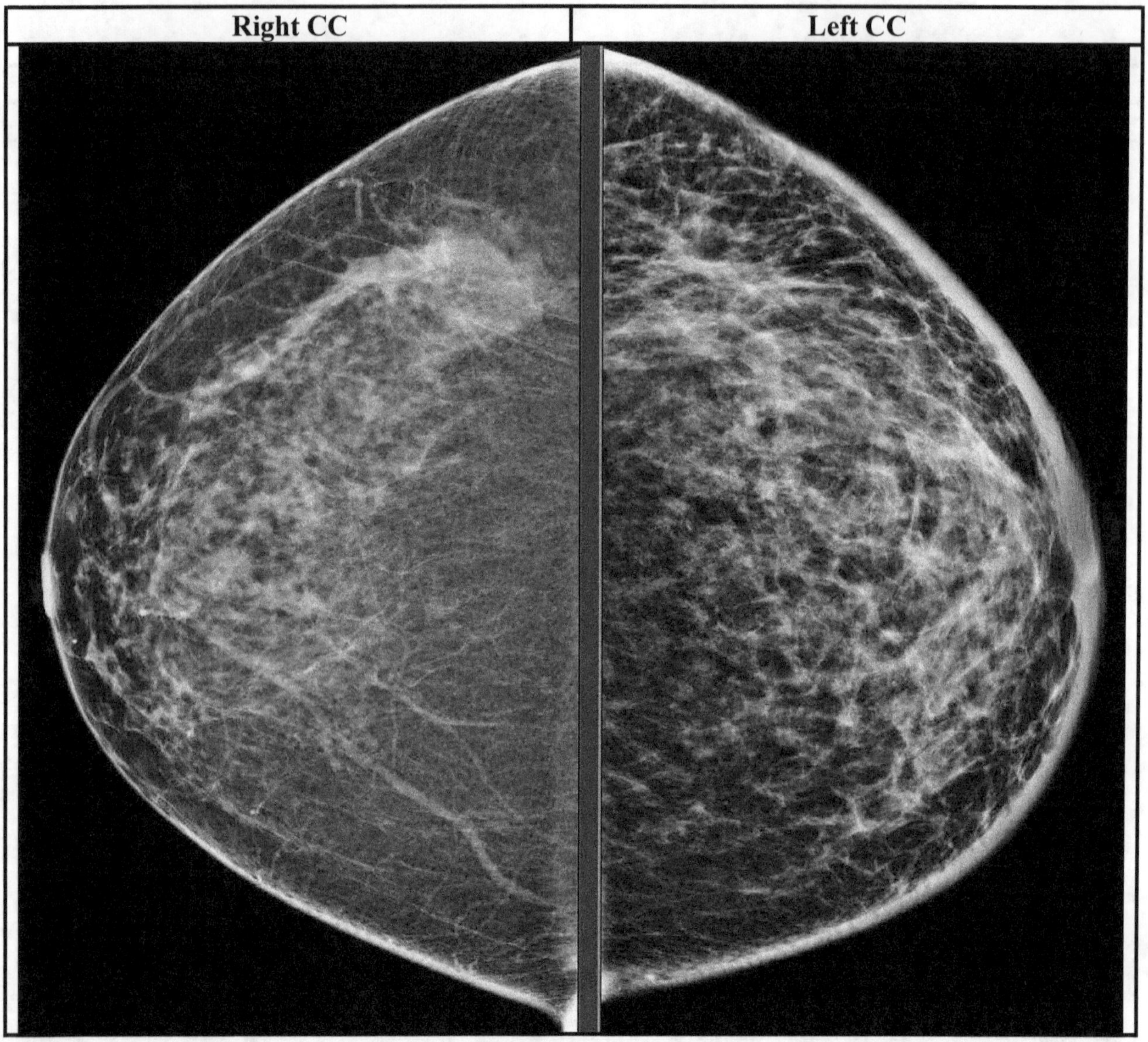
Right CC
Left CC

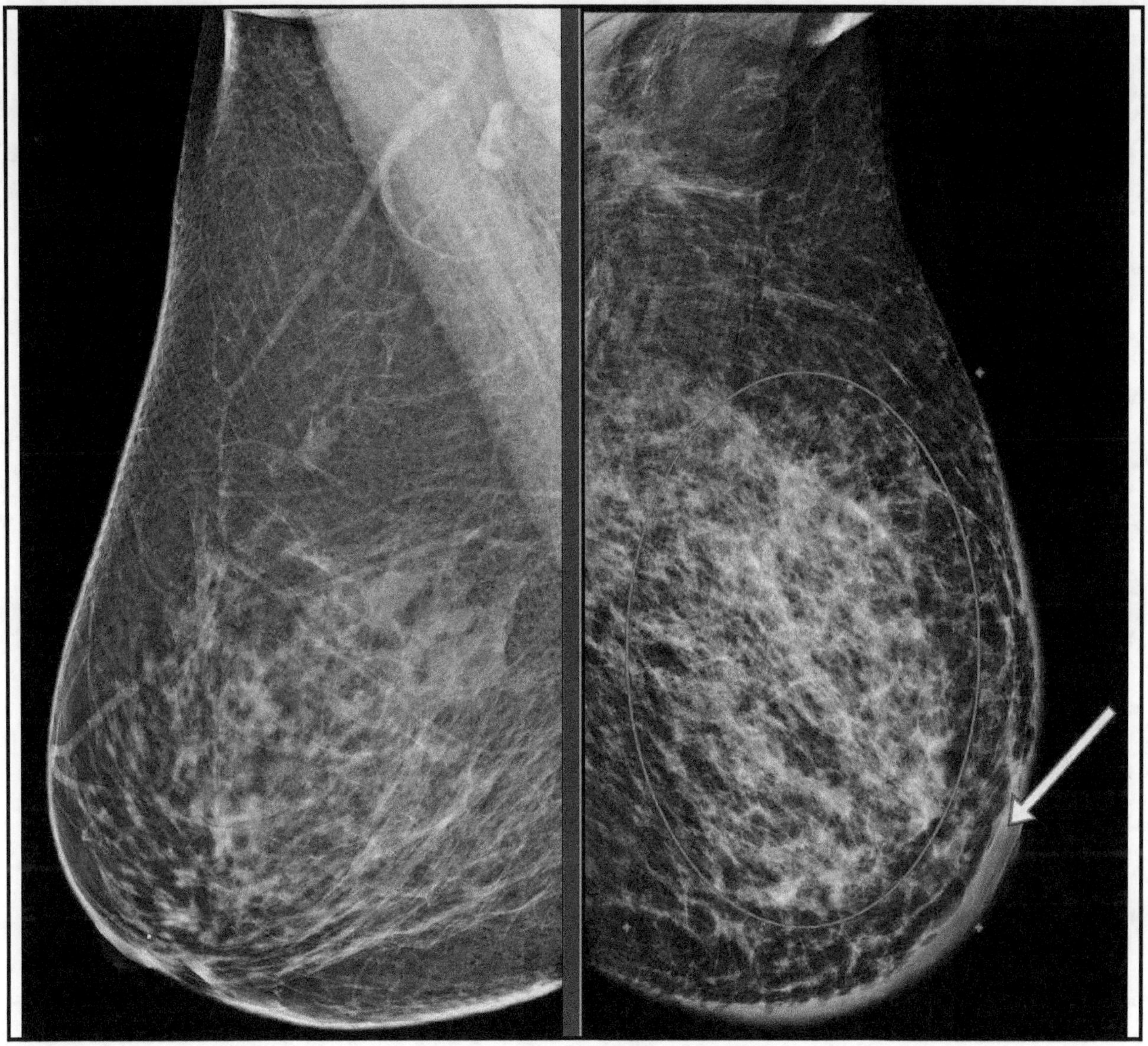

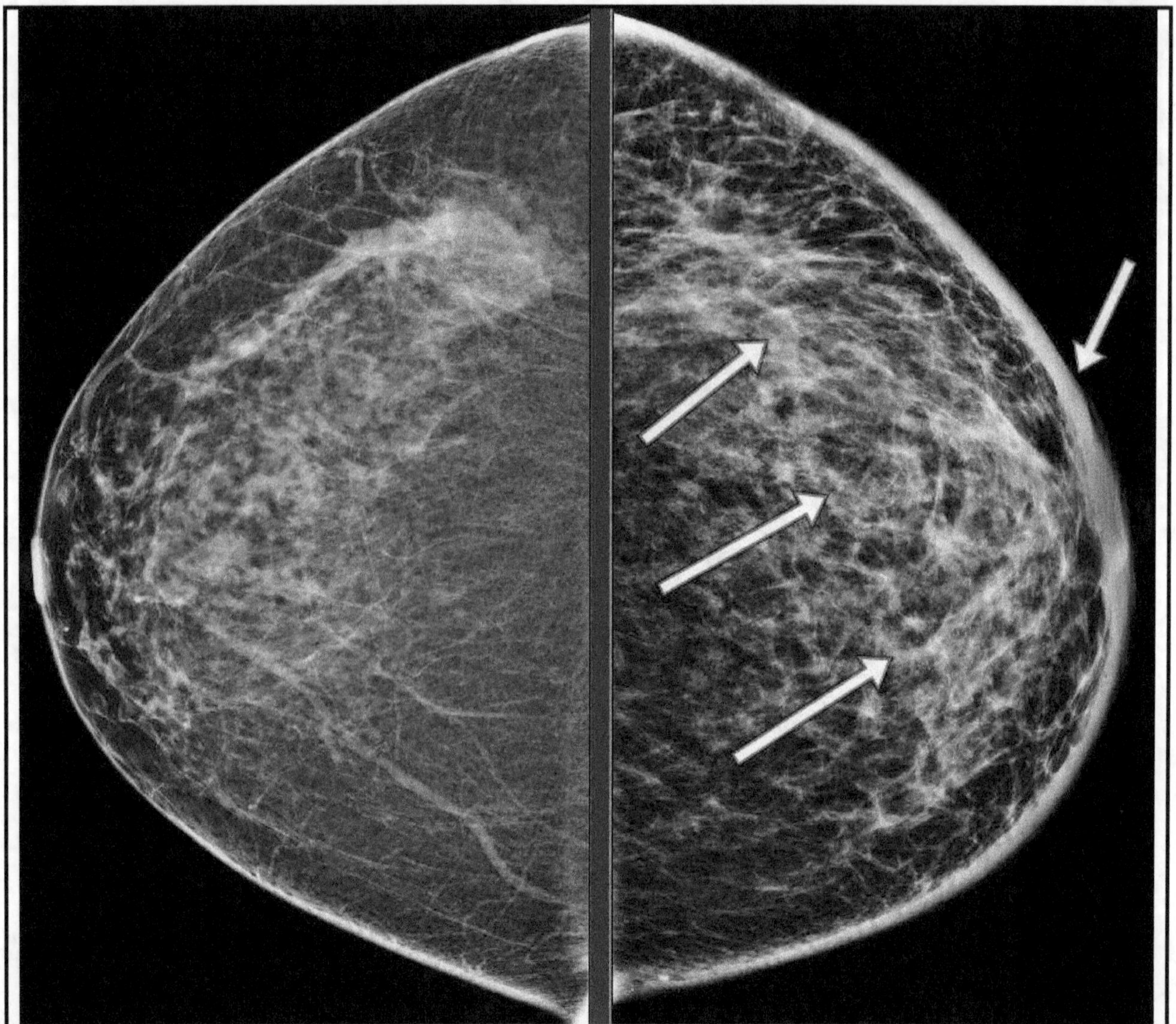

RIGHT BREAST	
Breast Parenchymal Density	***Scattered areas of fibroglandular density (ACR B)***
Focal Mass	None
Asymmetric Density	None
Parenchymal Distortion	None
Calcification	None
Skin Thickening	None
Axillary Nodes	None

LEFT BREAST	
Breast Parenchymal Density	***Scattered areas of fibroglandular density (ACR B) /Trabecular Edema***
Focal Mass	None
Asymmetric Density	None
Parenchymal Distortion	None
Calcification	None
Skin Thickening	***Positive***
Axillary Nodes	None

IMPRESSION:

RIGHT BREAST: (BI-RADS 1)
LEFT BREAST: (BI-RADS 4)

RECOMMENDATION: Histopathological Correlation (Punch Biopsy)

Pathological proven Inflammatory Breast Carcinoma (IBC)

CASE 61: 42 -year-old female/ Diagnostic	
Right MLO	Left MLO

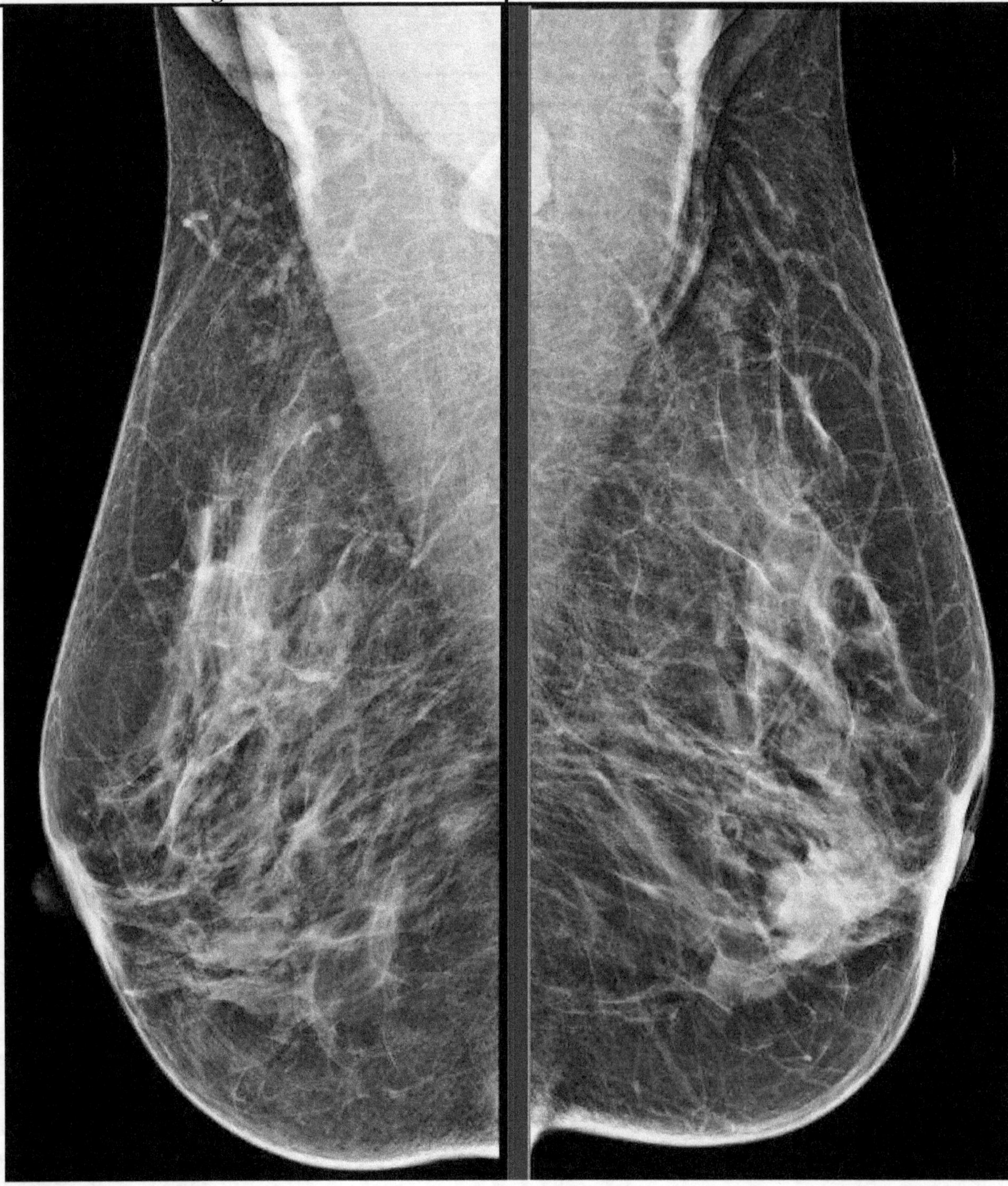

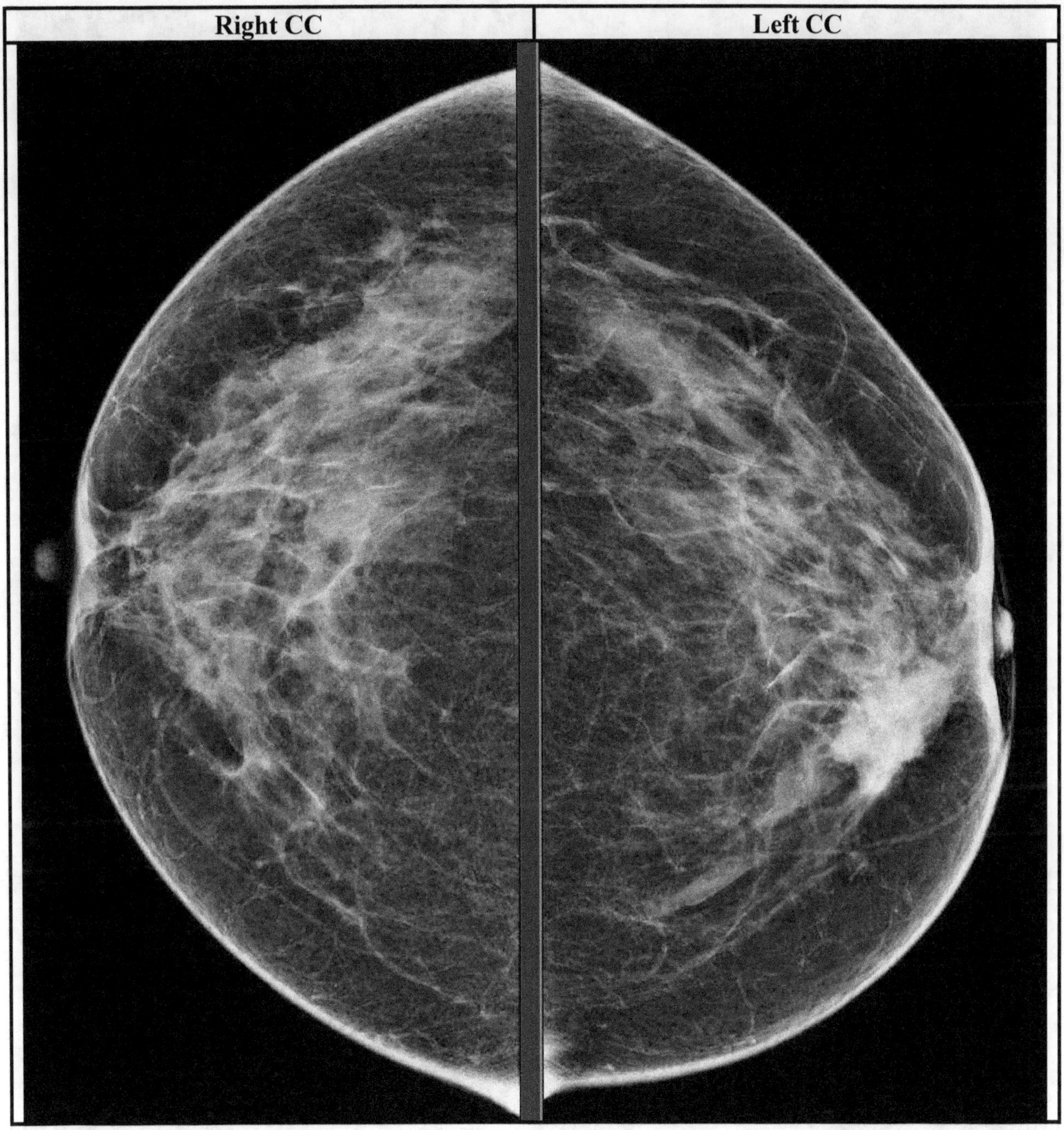
Right CC
Left CC

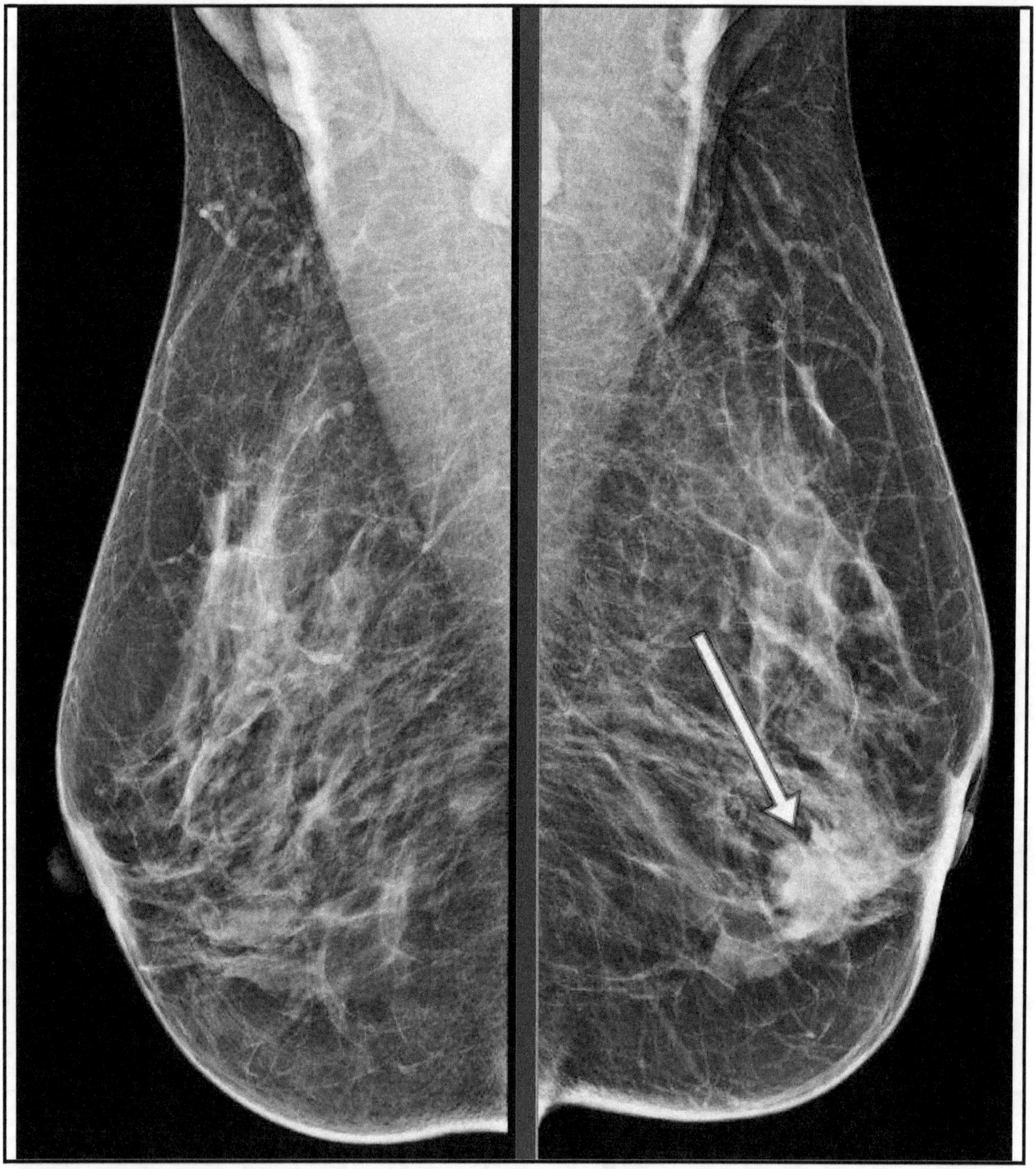

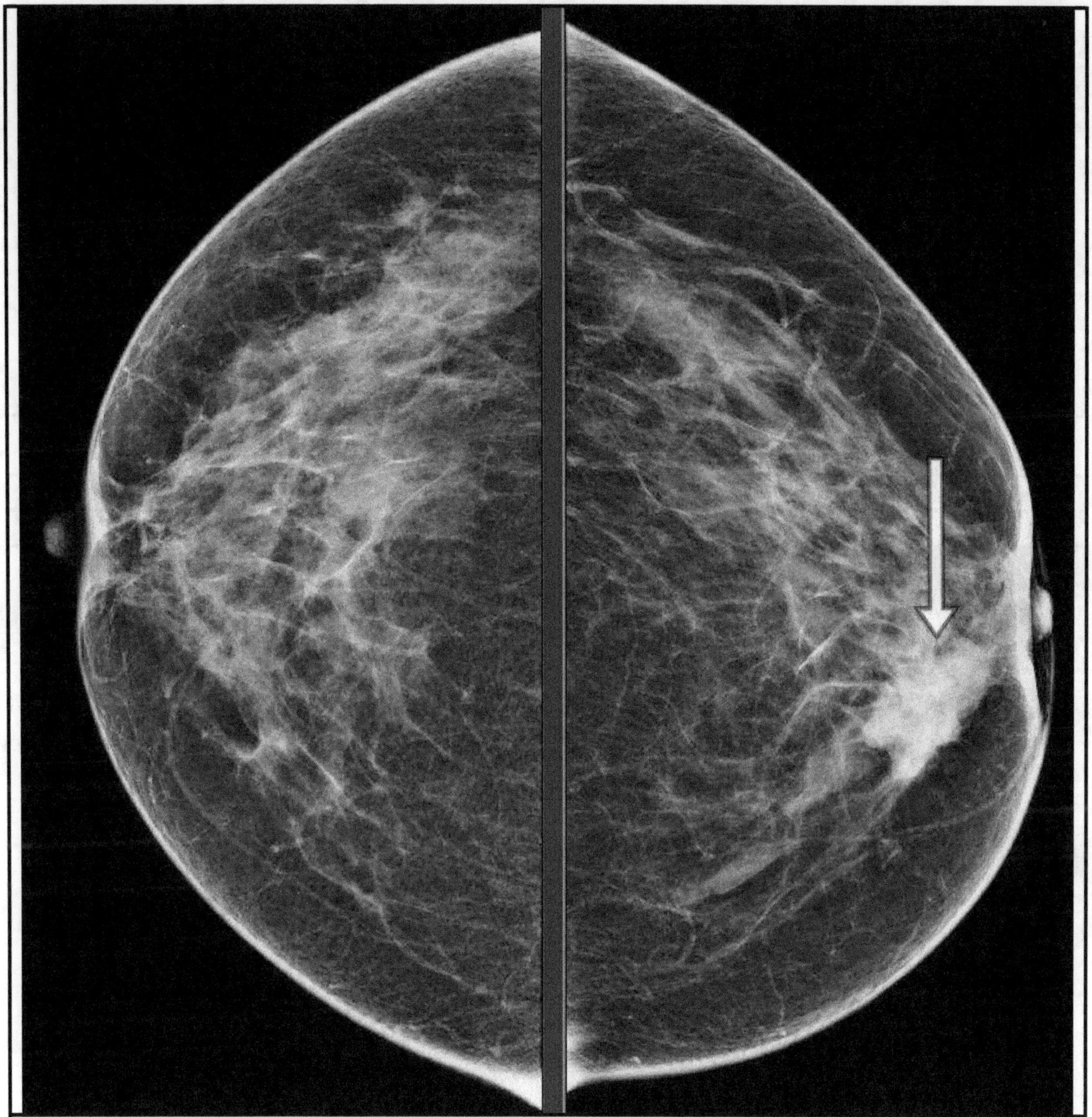

RIGHT BREAST	
Breast Parenchymal Density	***Heterogeneously dense, may obscure small masses (ACR C)***
Focal Mass	None
Asymmetric Density	None
Parenchymal Distortion	None
Calcification	None
Skin Thickening	None
Axillary Nodes	None

LEFT BREAST	
Breast Parenchymal Density	***Heterogeneously dense, may obscure small masses (ACR C)***
Focal Mass	***LIQ irregular indistinct mass lesion***
Asymmetric Density	None
Parenchymal Distortion	None
Calcification	None
Skin Thickening	None / ***Nipple Retraction***
Axillary Nodes	None

IMPRESSION:

RIGHT BREAST: (BI-RADS 1)

LEFT BREAST: (BI-RADS 5)

RECOMMENDATION: Histopathological Correlation

CASE 62: 53 -year-old female/diagnostic

Right MLO	**Left MLO**

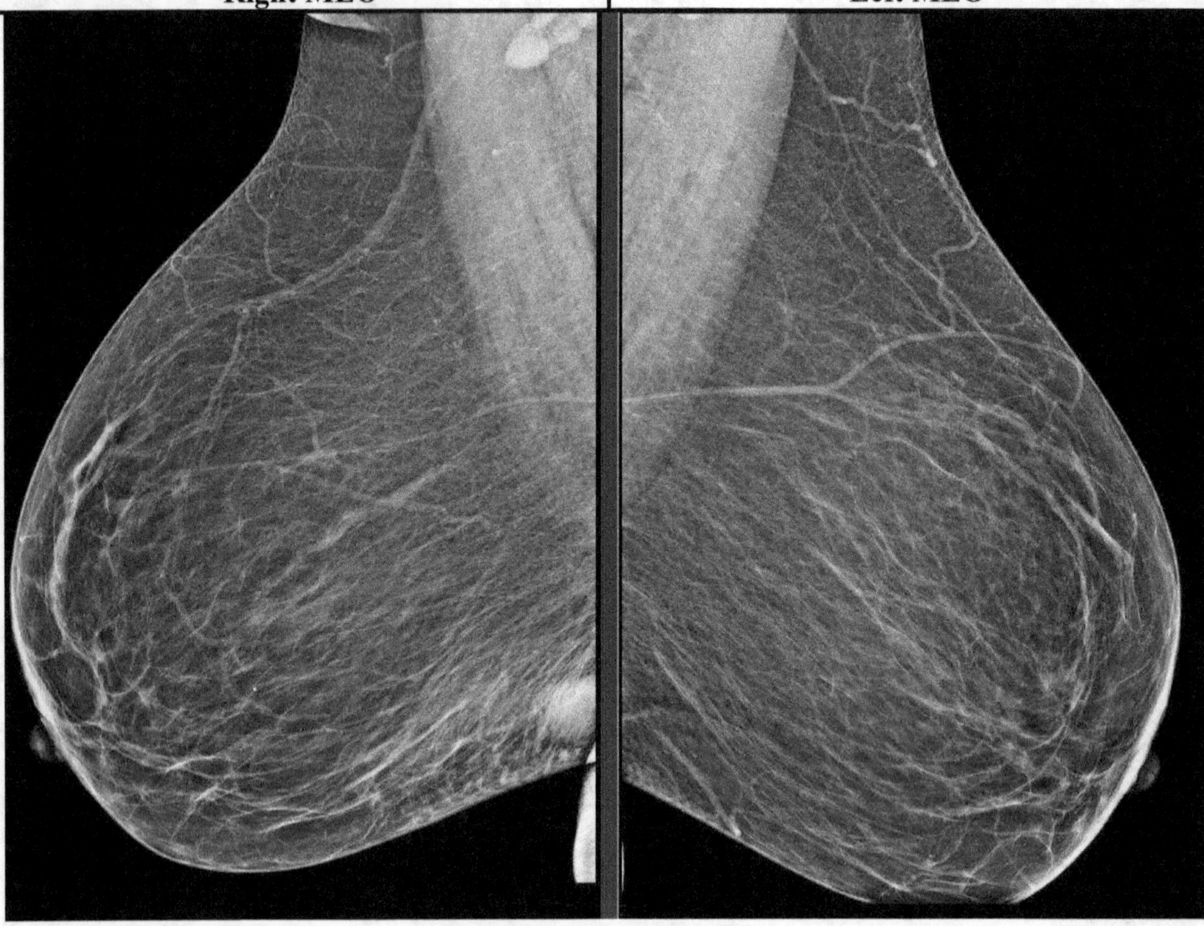

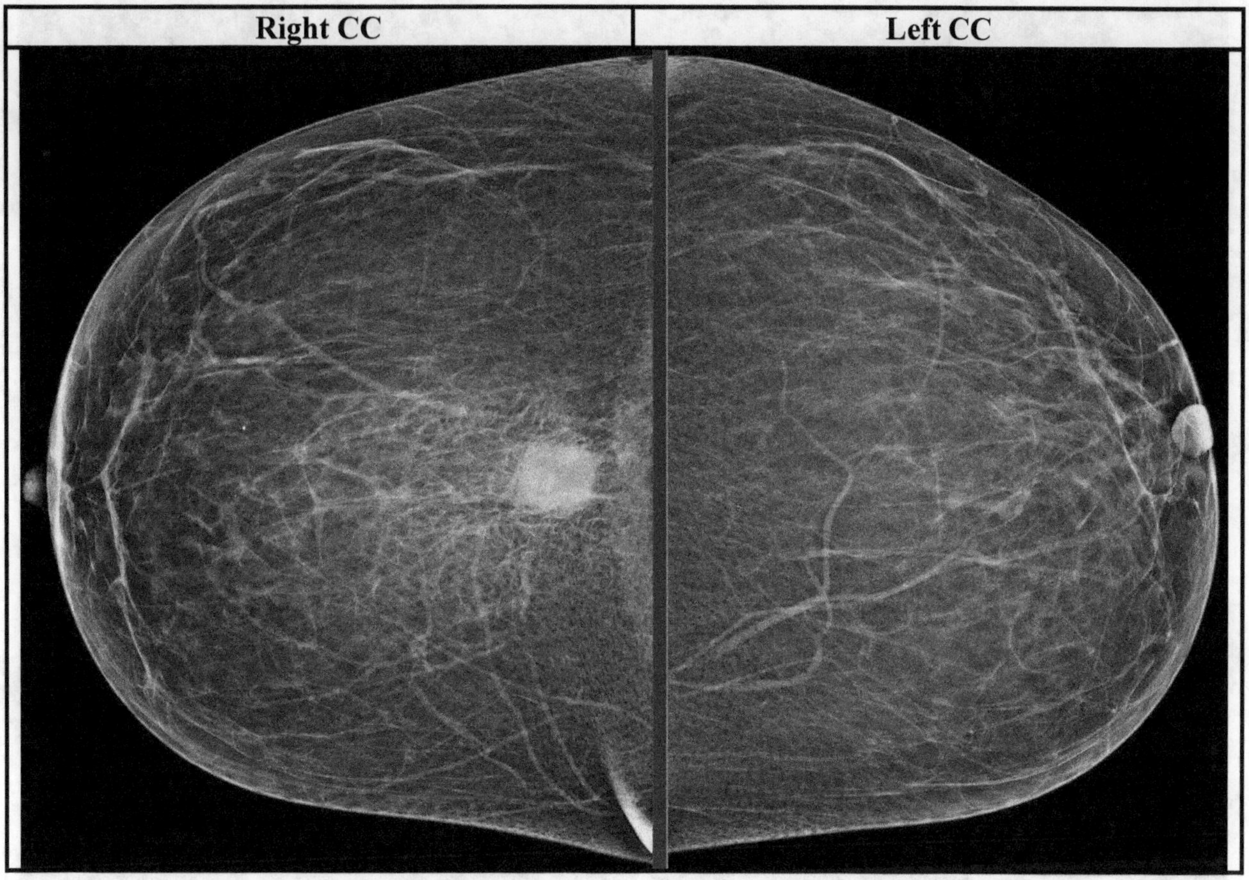
Right CC
Left CC

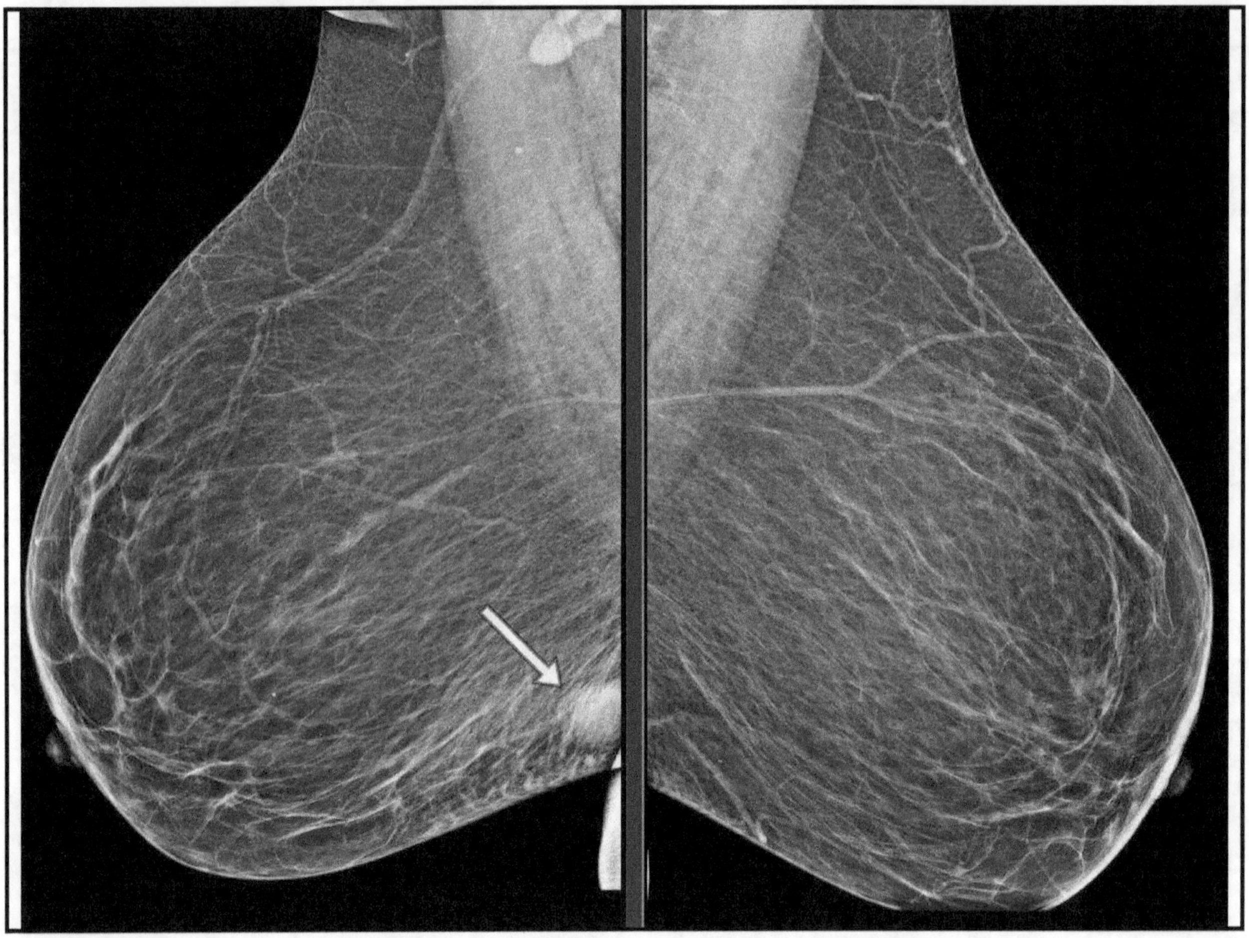

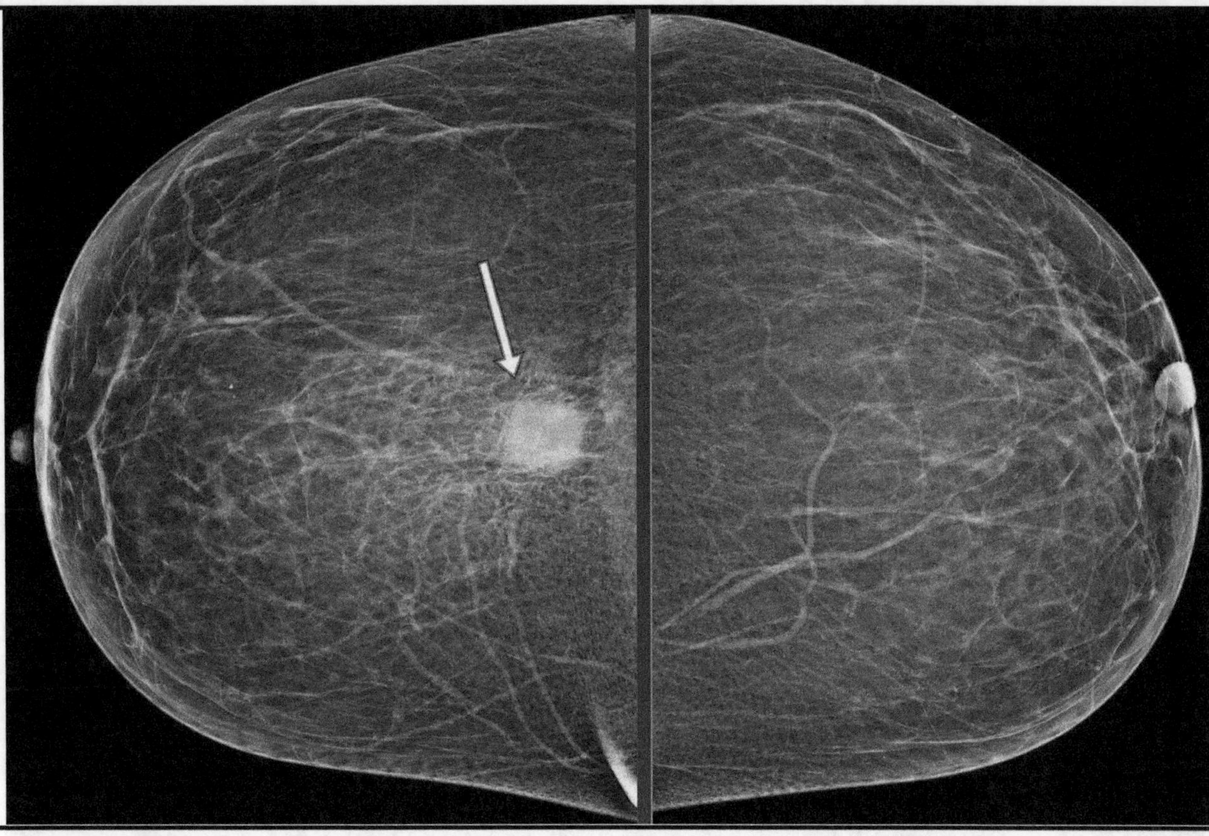

RIGHT BREAST	
Breast Parenchymal Density	***Almost entirely fatty (ACR A)***
Focal Mass	***Lower central (6 o'clock) round spiculated mass lesion touching the pectoralis major muscle***
Asymmetric Density	None
Parenchymal Distortion	None
Calcification	None
Skin Thickening	None
Axillary Nodes	None

LEFT BREAST	
Breast Parenchymal Density	***Almost entirely fatty (ACR A)***
Focal Mass	None
Asymmetric Density	None
Parenchymal Distortion	None
Calcification	None
Skin Thickening	None
Axillary Nodes	None

IMPRESSION:

RIGHT BREAST: (BI-RADS 5)
LEFT BREAST: (BI-RADS 1)

RECOMMENDATION: Histopathological Correlation
Breast MRI is indicated to exclude pectoralis muscle extension.

CASE 63: 44-year-old female/diagnostic	
Right MLO	**Left MLO**

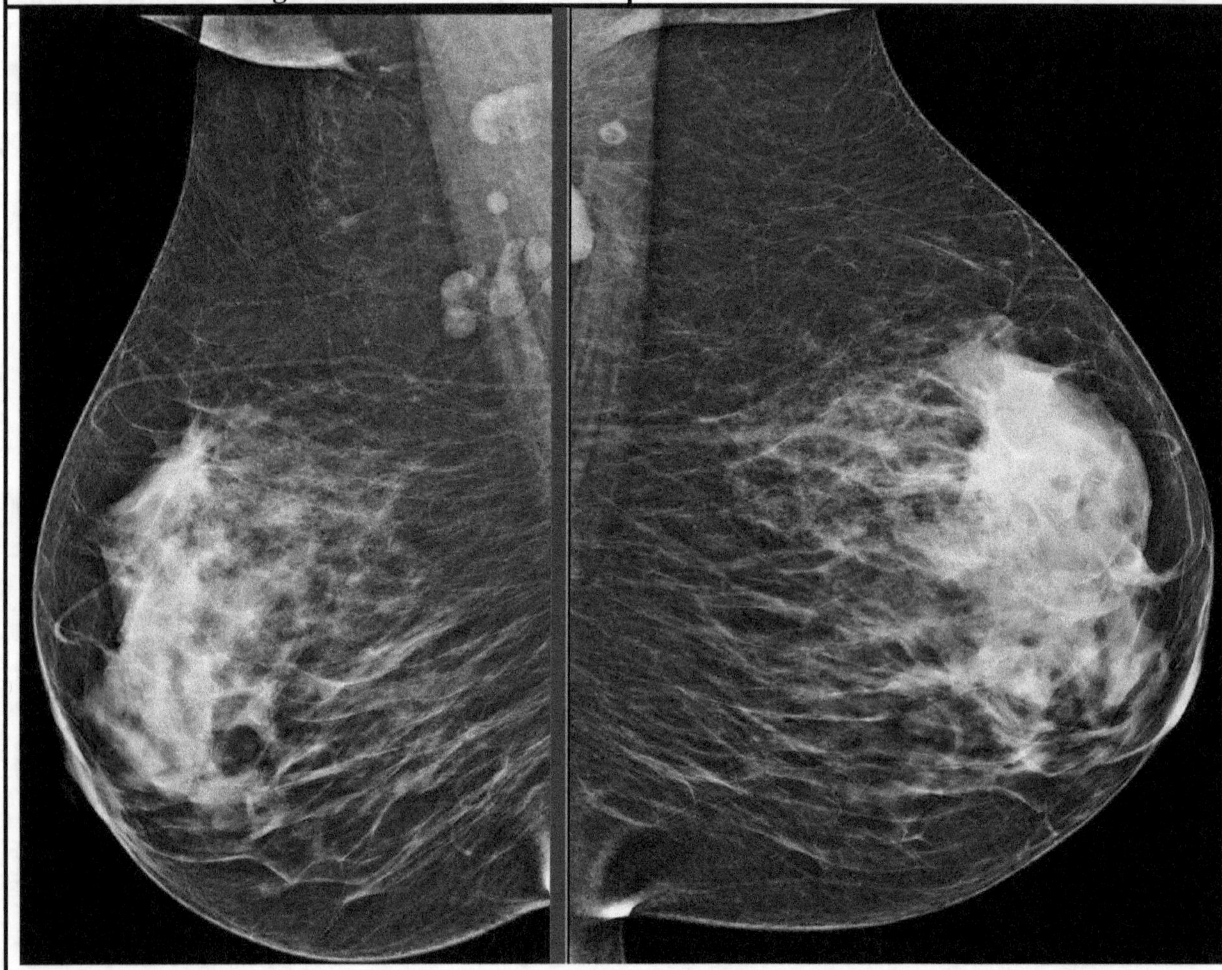

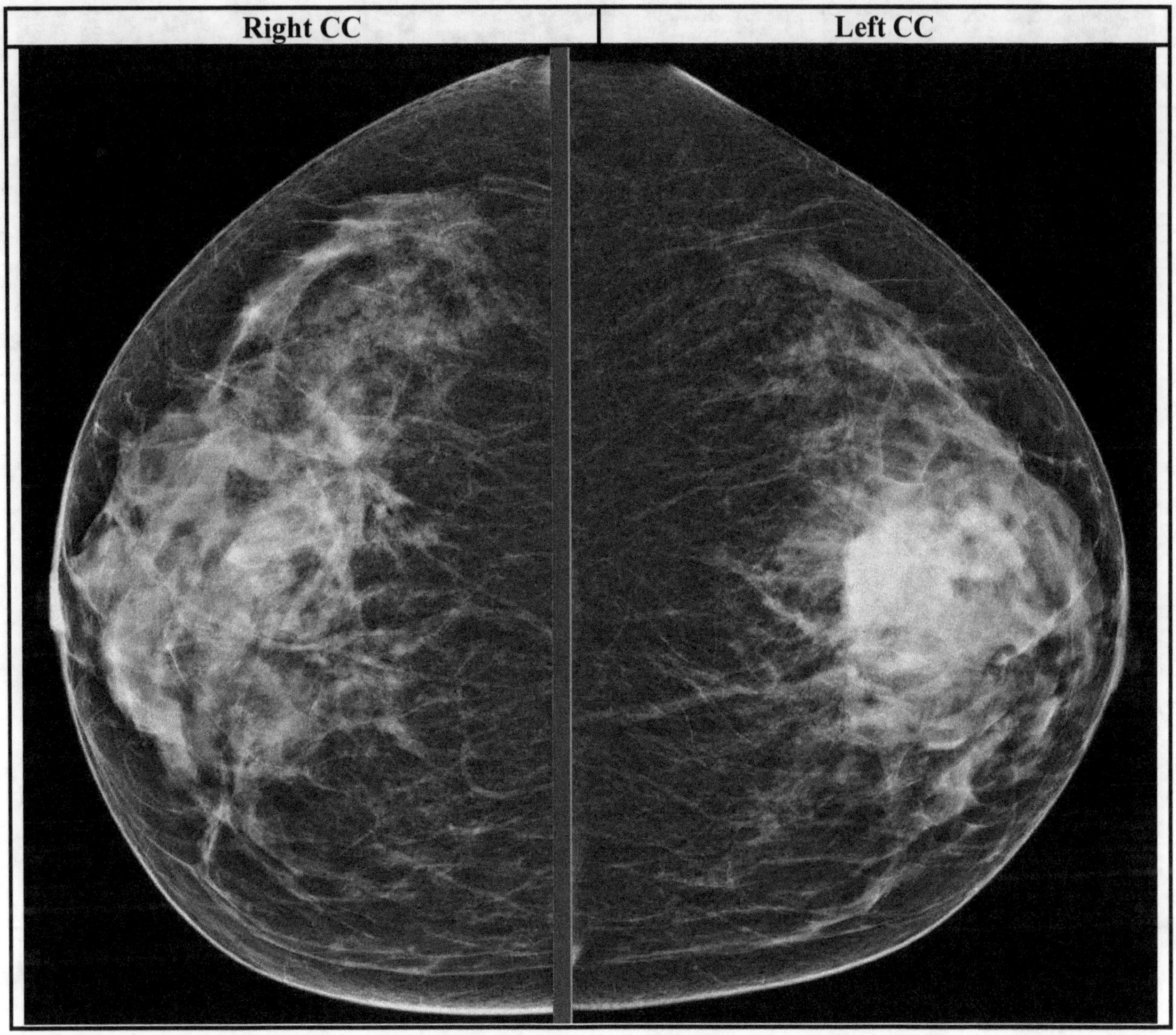
Right CC
Left CC

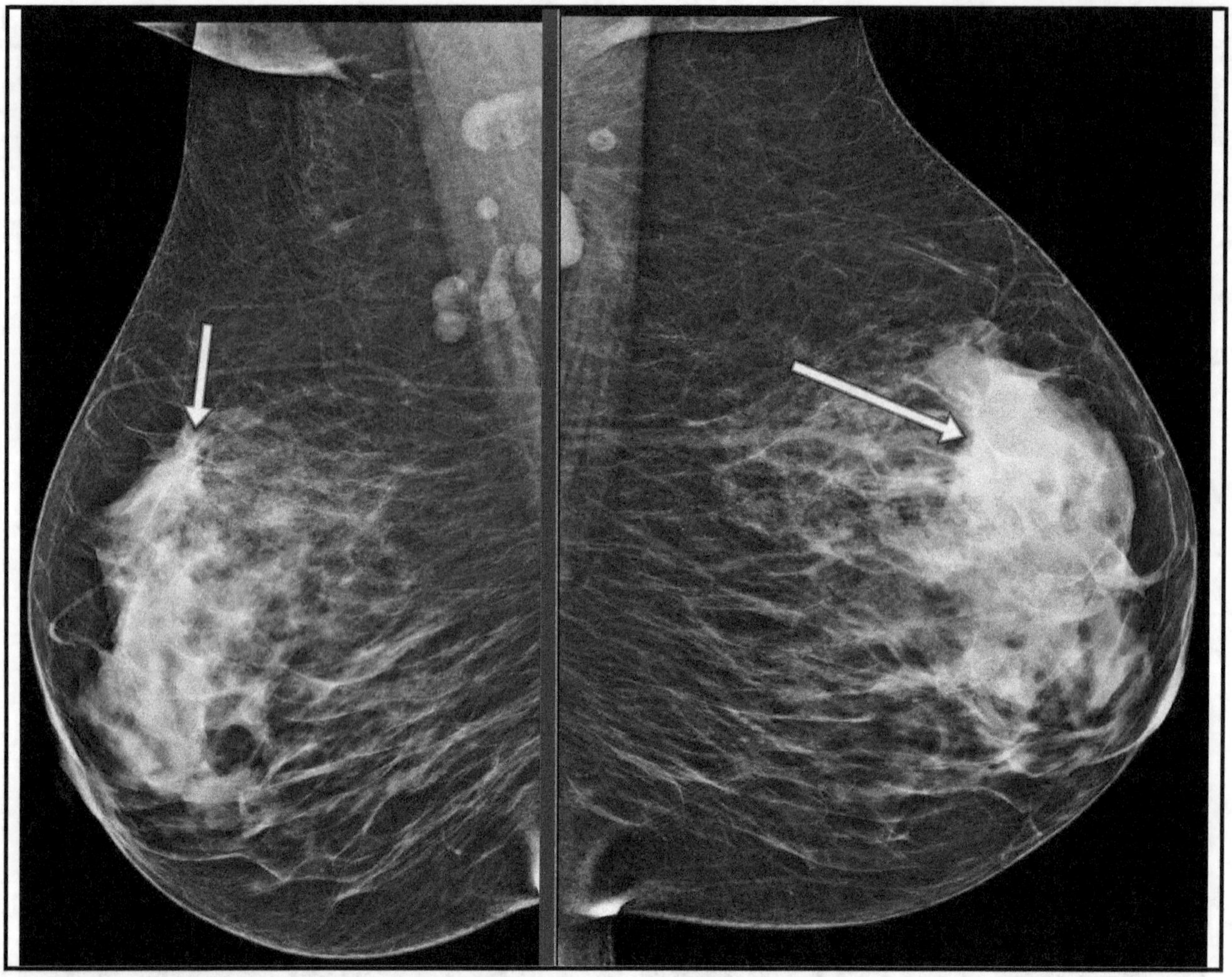

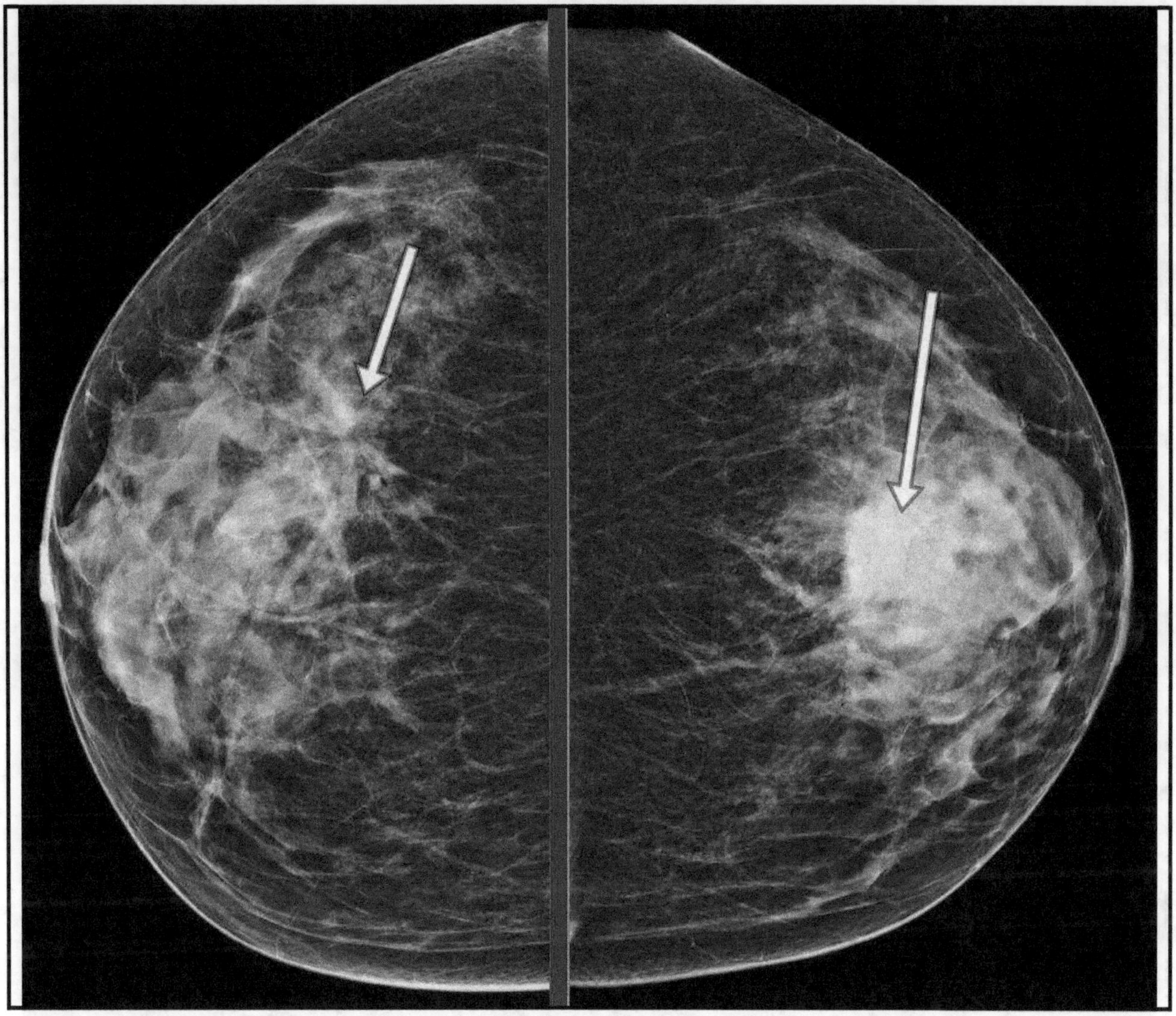

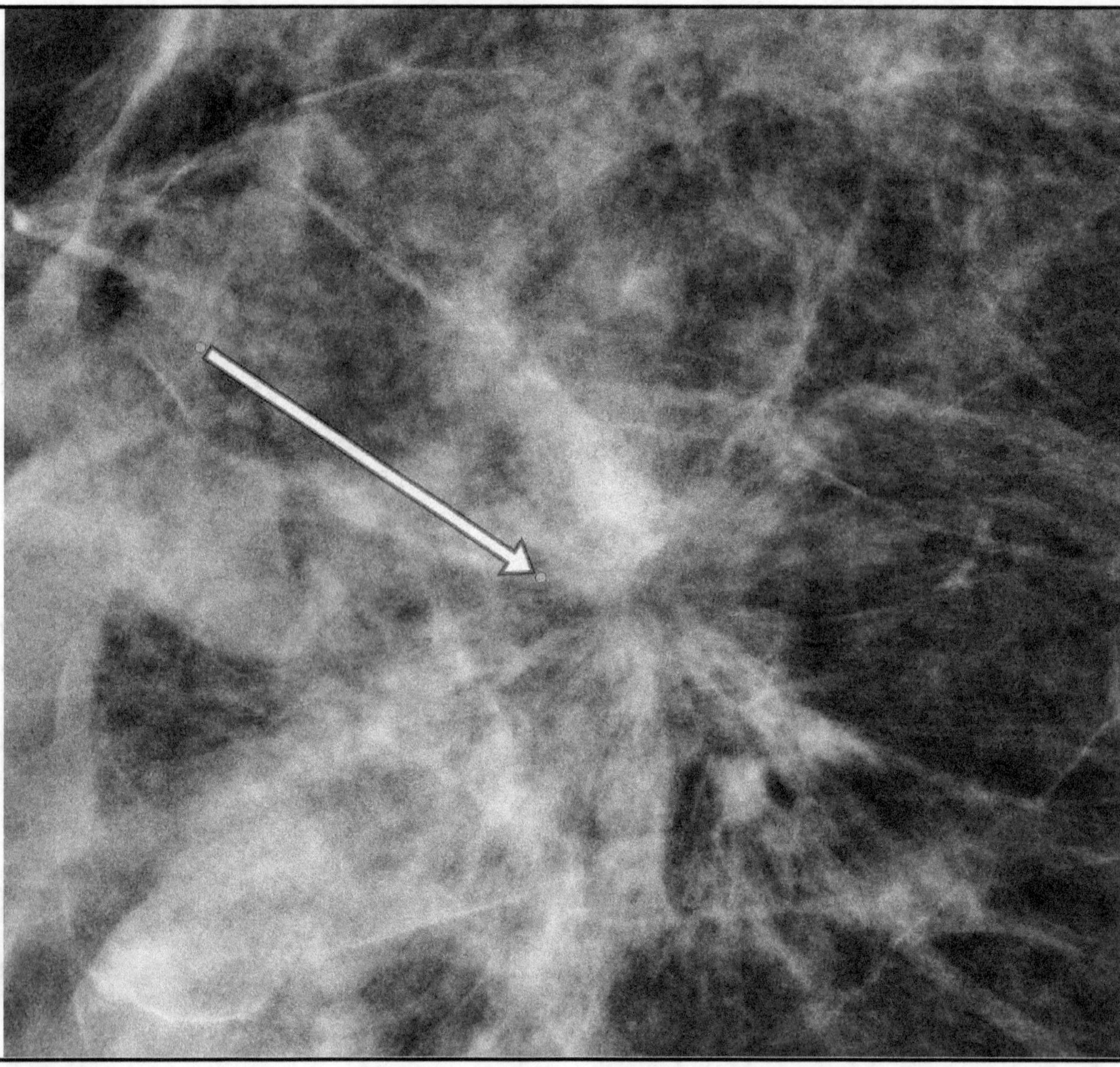

RIGHT BREAST	
Breast Parenchymal Density	***Heterogeneously dense, may obscure small masses (ACR C)***
Focal Mass	None
Asymmetric Density	None
Parenchymal Distortion	***UOQ area of Parenchymal Distortion***
Calcification	None
Skin Thickening	None
Axillary Nodes	None

LEFT BREAST	
Breast Parenchymal Density	***Heterogeneously dense, may obscure small masses (ACR C)***
Focal Mass	***Upper central (12 o'clock) oval obscured mass lesion***
Asymmetric Density	None
Parenchymal Distortion	None
Calcification	None
Skin Thickening	None
Axillary Nodes	None

IMPRESSION:

RIGHT BREAST:(BI-RADS 0)
LEFT BREAST: (BI-RADS 0)

RECOMMENDATION: US Correlation

CASE 64: 43-year-old female/screening

Right MLO	Left MLO

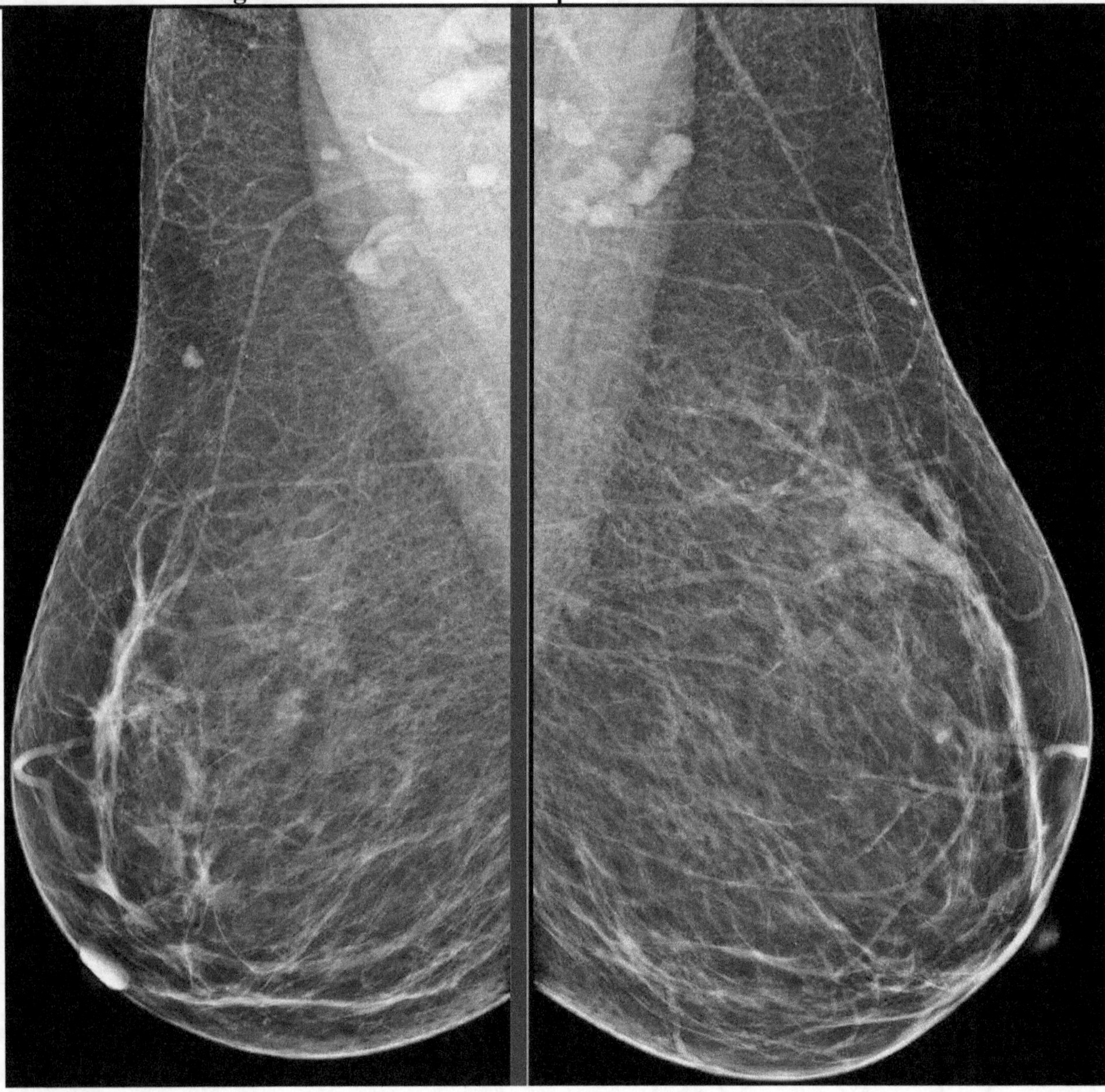

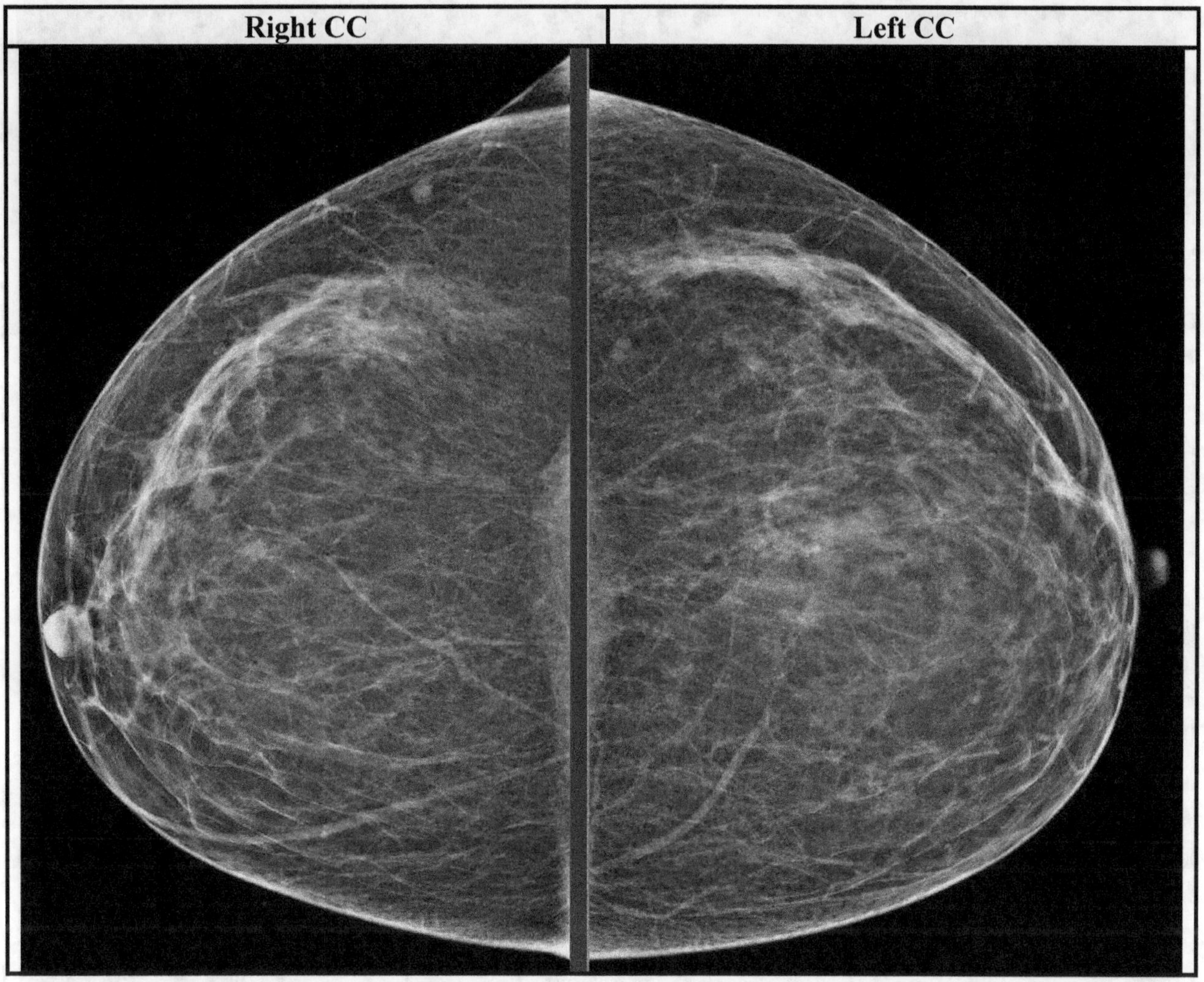
Right CC
Left CC

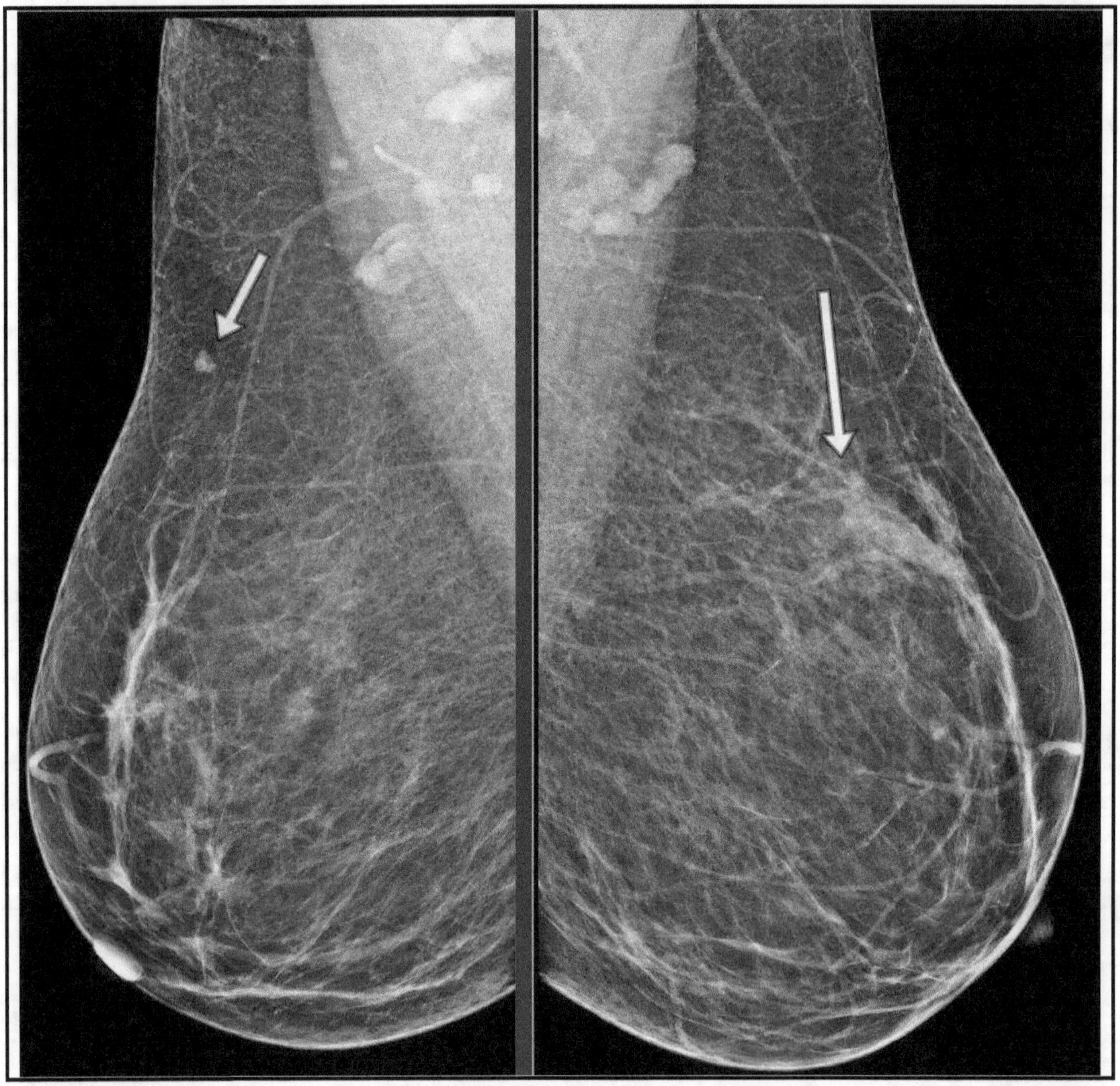

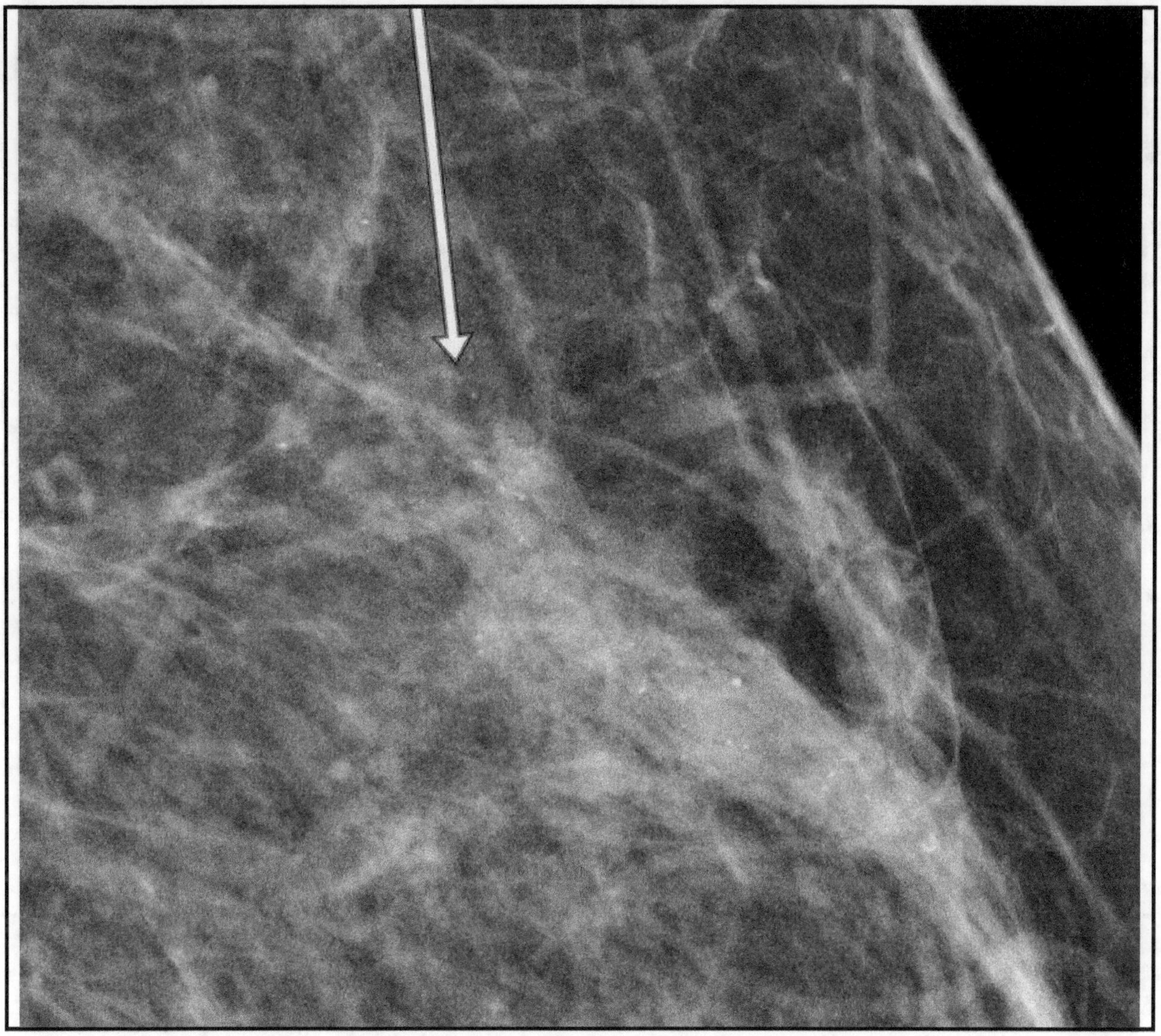

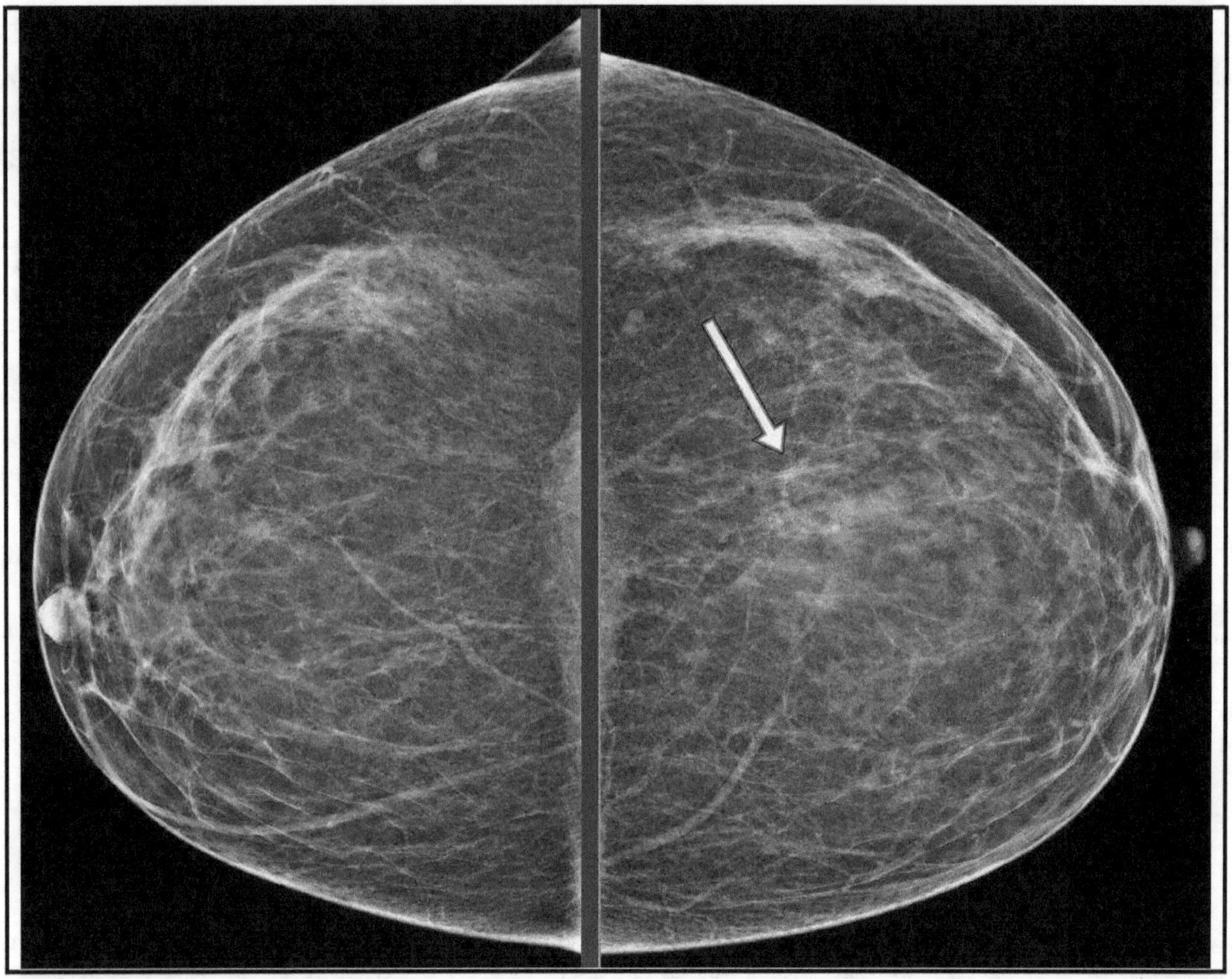

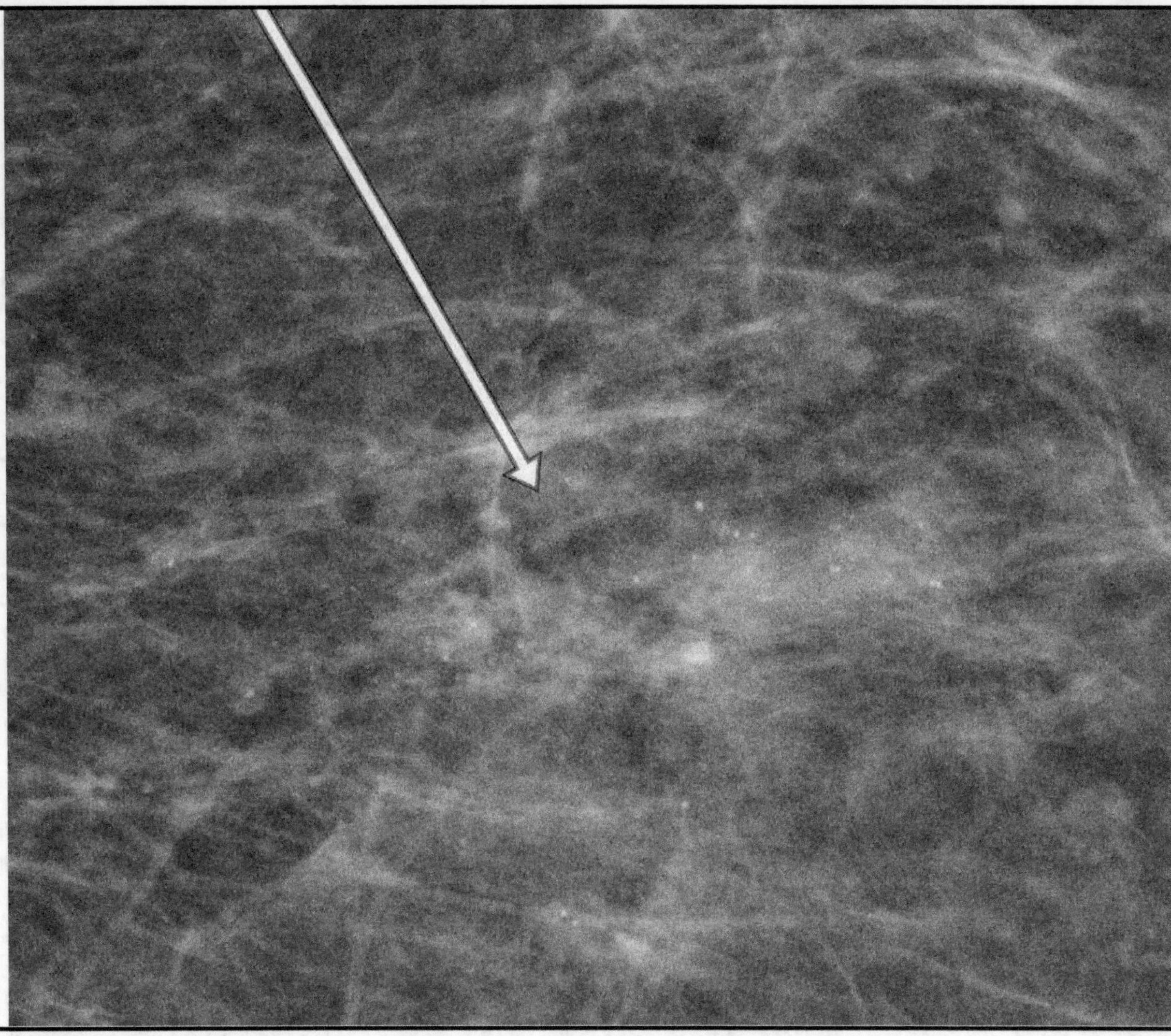

RIGHT BREAST	
Breast Parenchymal Density	***Scattered areas of fibroglandular density (ACR B)***
Focal Mass	None
Asymmetric Density	None
Parenchymal Distortion	None
Calcification	None
Skin Thickening	None
Axillary Nodes	None / ***IMLN***

LEFT BREAST	
Breast Parenchymal Density	***Scattered areas of fibroglandular density (ACR B)***
Focal Mass	None
Asymmetric Density	None
Parenchymal Distortion	None
Calcification	***Upper central area of suspicious amorphous micro-calcifications***
Skin Thickening	None
Axillary Nodes	None

IMPRESSION:

RIGHT BREAST: (BI-RADS 1)
LEFT BREAST: (BI-RADS 4B)

RECOMMENDATION: Histopathological Correlation

CASE 65: 46-year-old female/left conservative breast surgery	
Right MLO	**Left MLO**

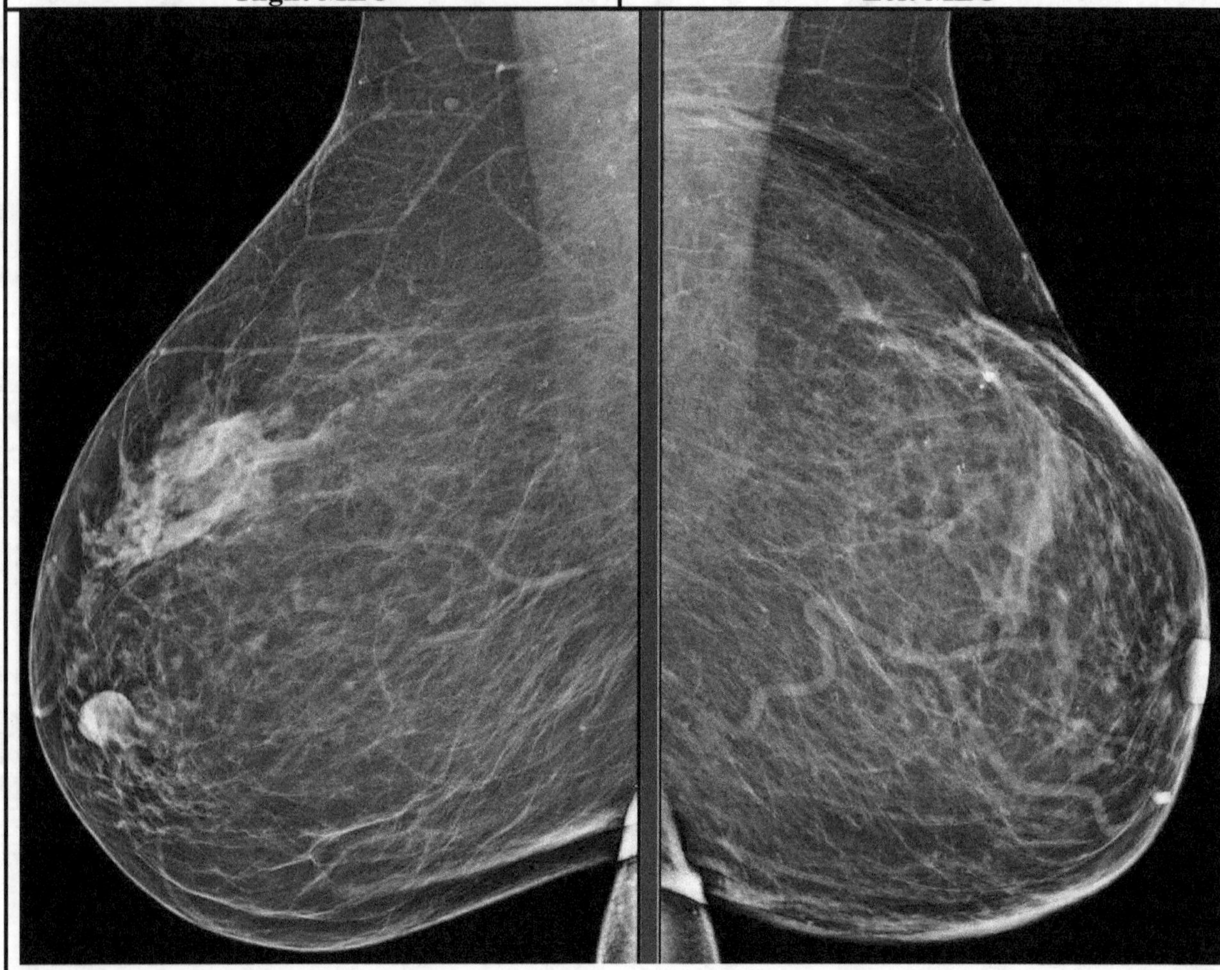

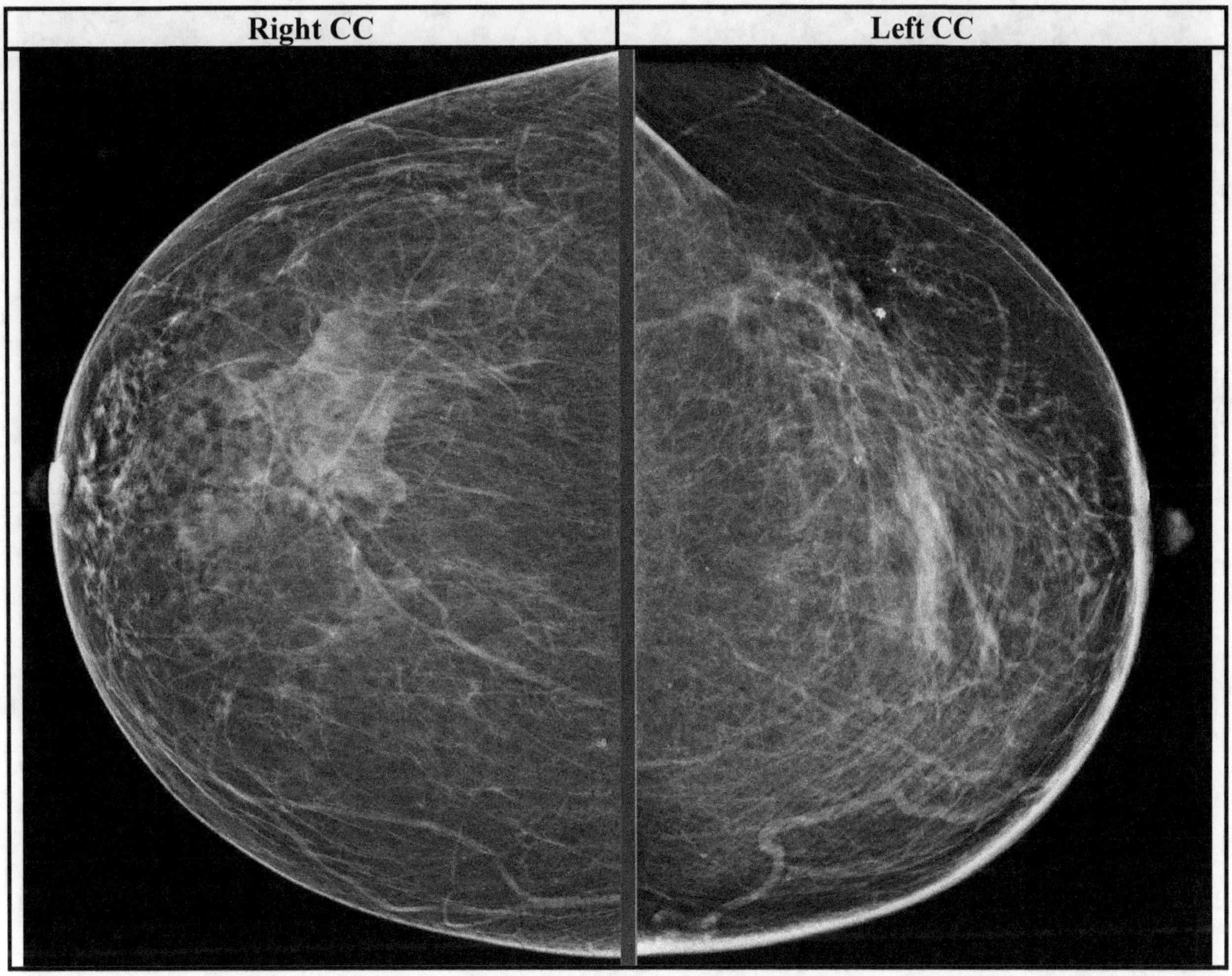

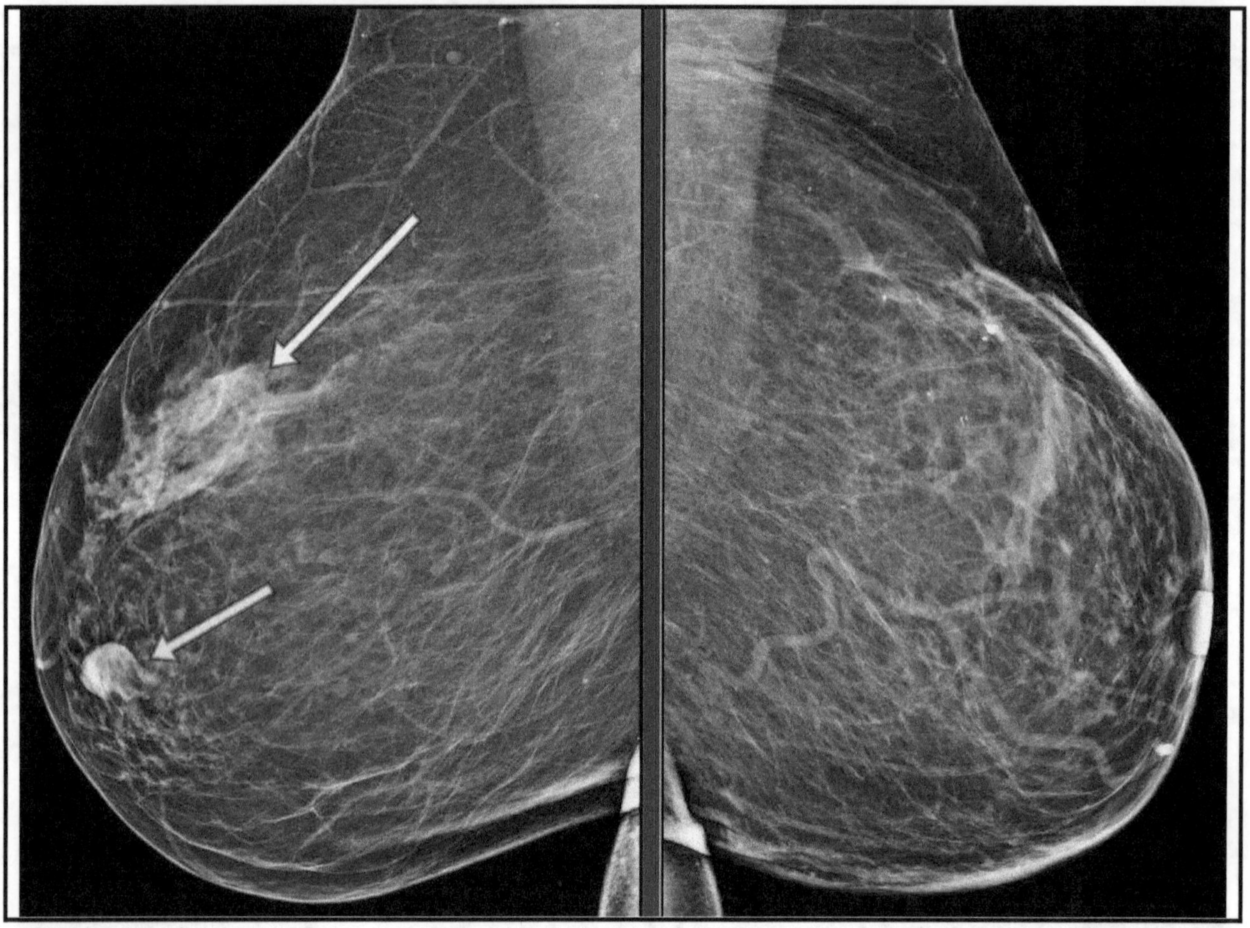

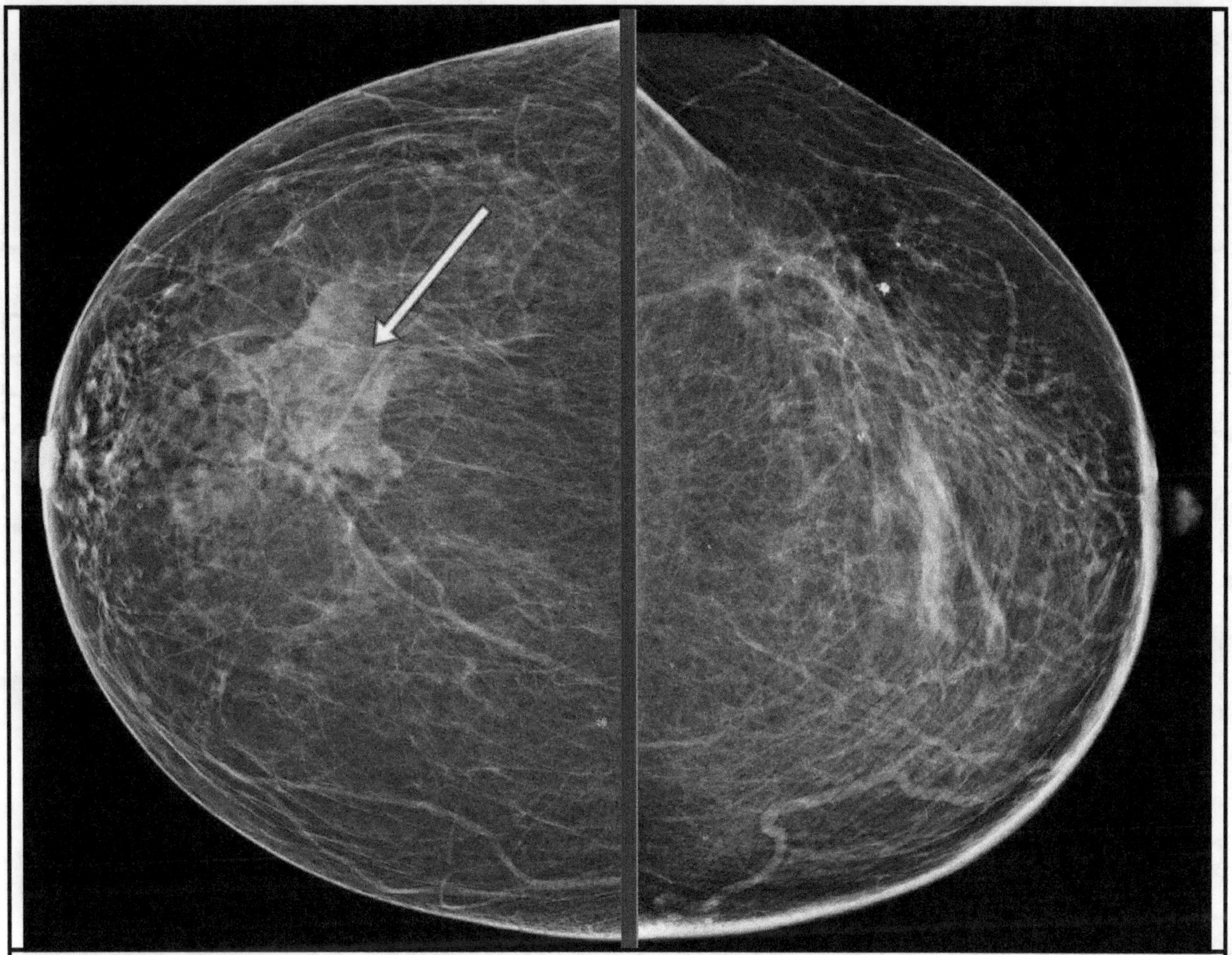

RIGHT BREAST	
Breast Parenchymal Density	***Scattered areas of fibroglandular density (ACR B)***
Focal Mass	None
Asymmetric Density	None
Parenchymal Distortion	None
Calcification	None
Skin Thickening	None
Axillary Nodes	None

LEFT BREAST	
Breast Parenchymal Density	***Scattered areas of fibroglandular density (ACR B)***
Focal Mass	None
Asymmetric Density	None
Parenchymal Distortion	None
Calcification	***UOQ dystrophic calcification***
Skin Thickening	None
Axillary Nodes	None

IMPRESSION:
RIGHT BREAST: (BI-RADS 1)
LEFT BREAST: (BI-RADS 2)

RECOMMENDATION: Routine Annual screening

The glandular component on the right breast is not considered as focal asymmetry it just due to remove the corresponding glandular tissue on the contralateral side (operated side)

CASE 66: 40-year-old female/diagnostic	
Right MLO	**Left MLO**

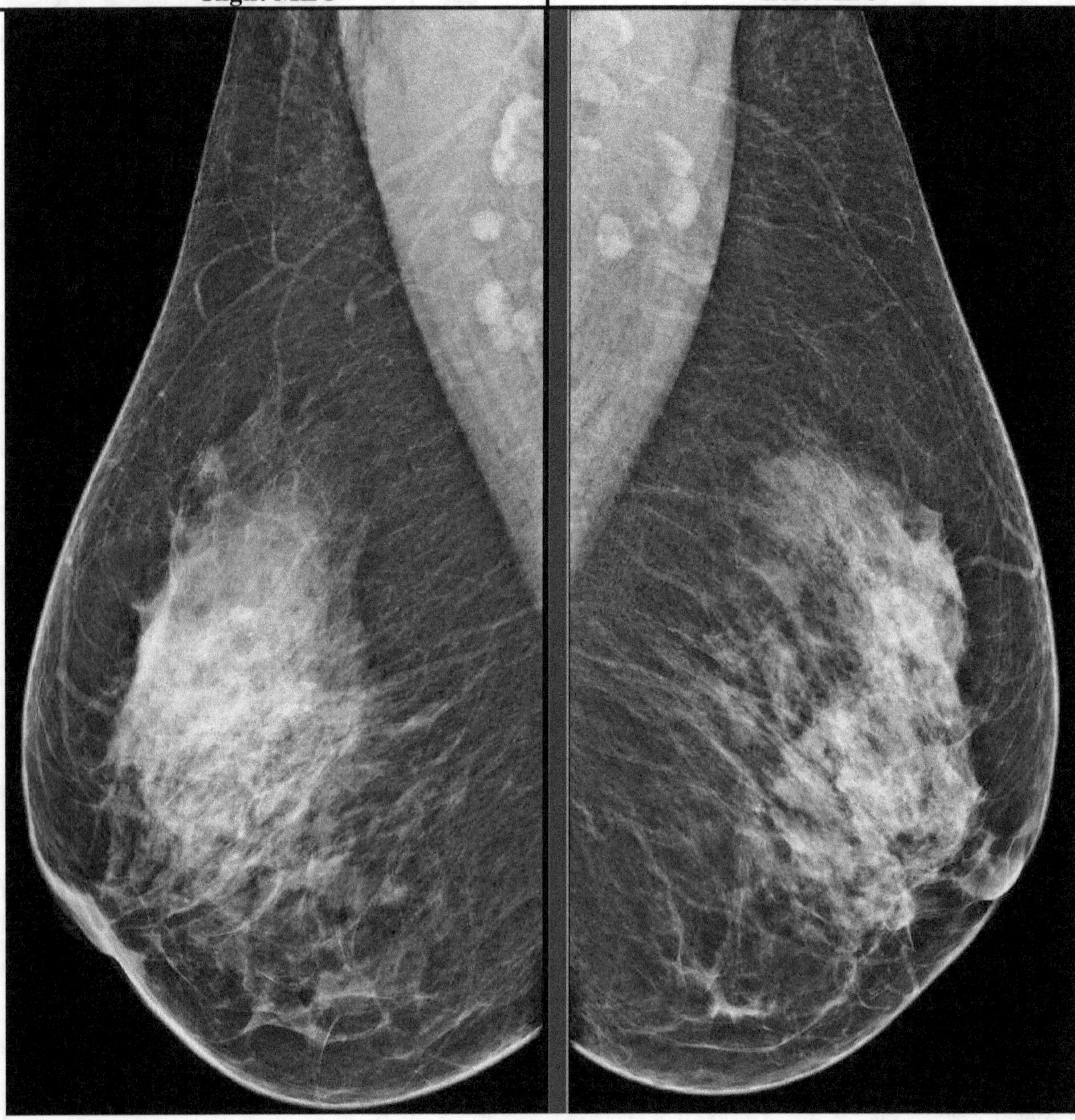

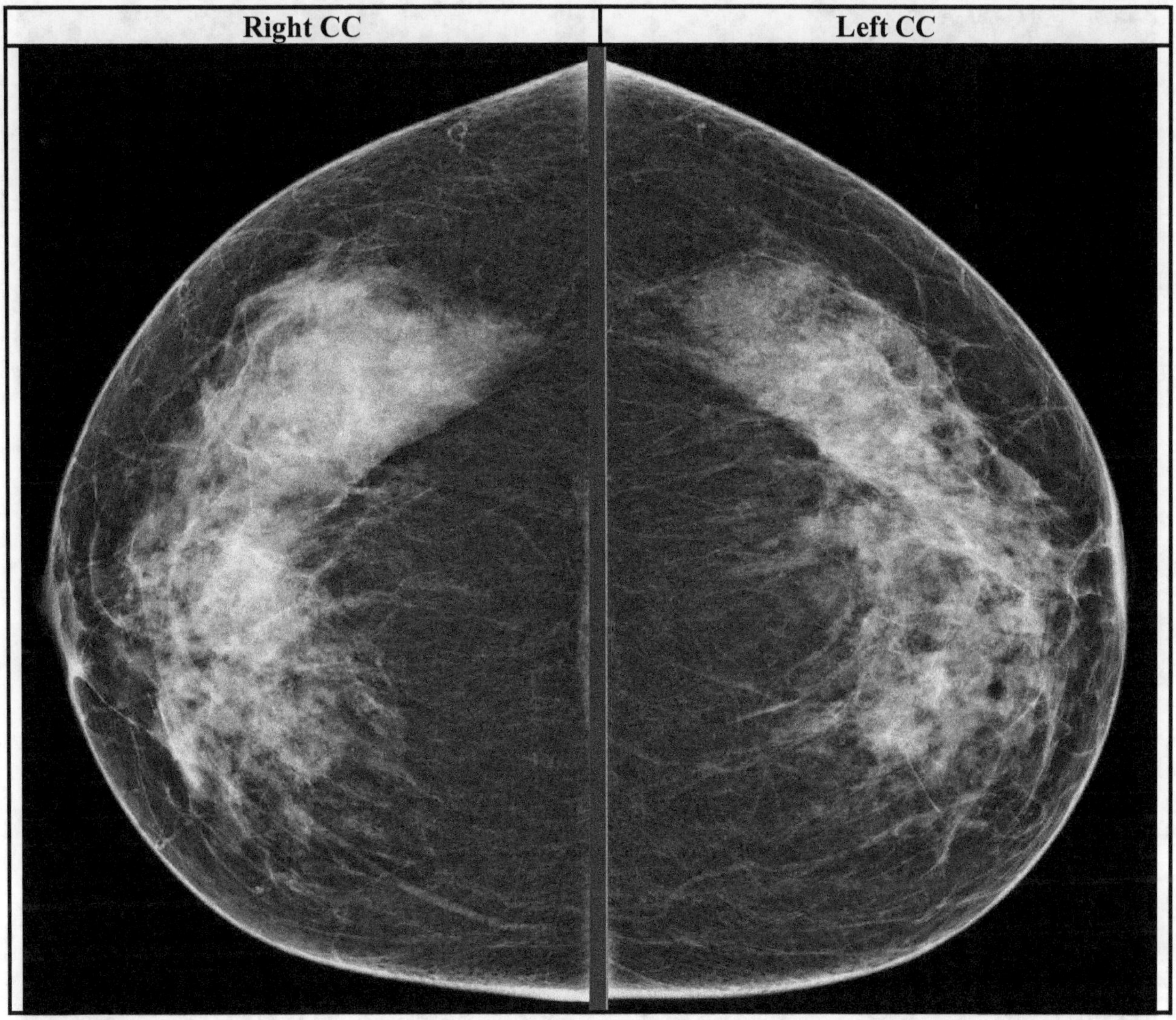
Right CC
Left CC

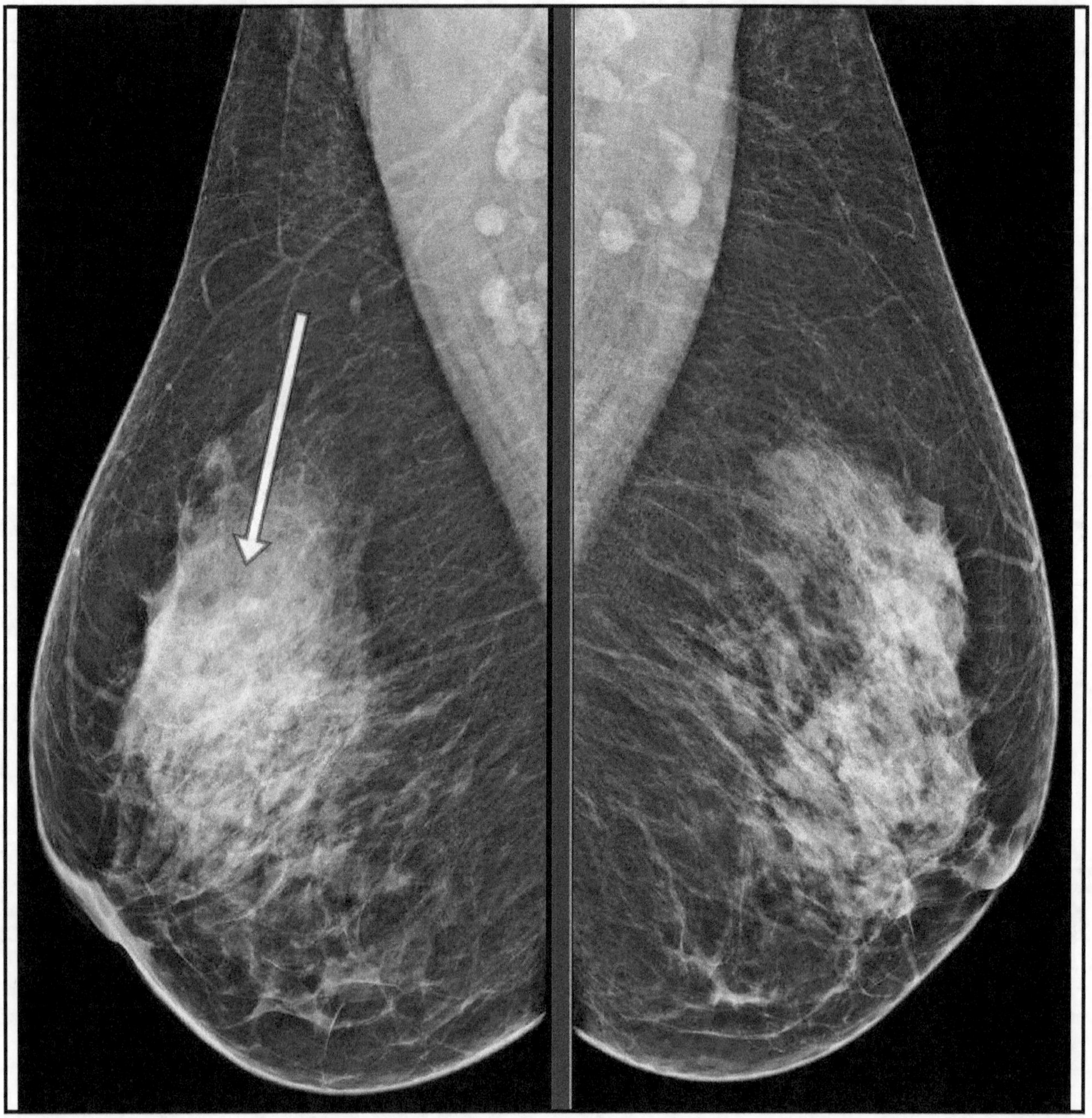

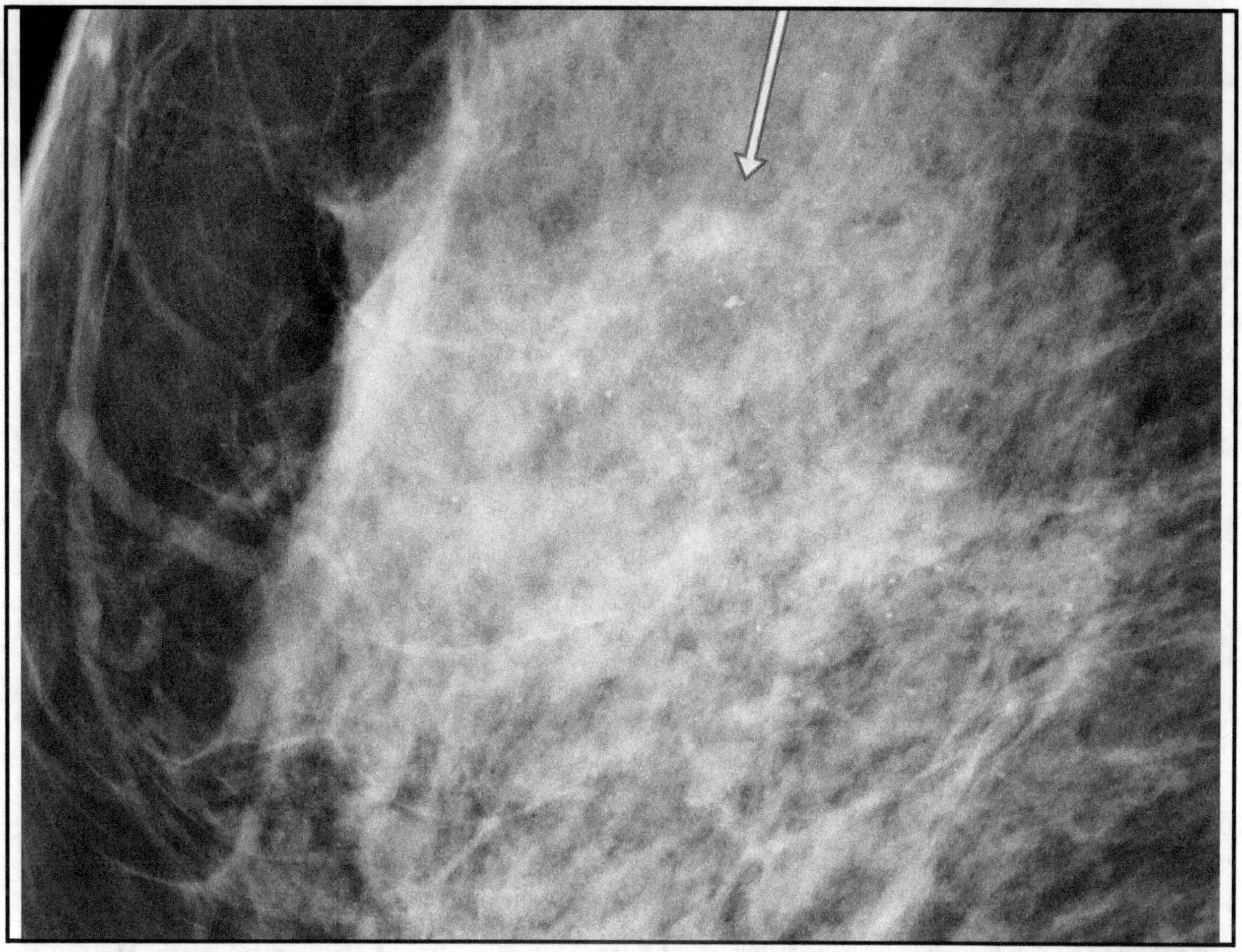

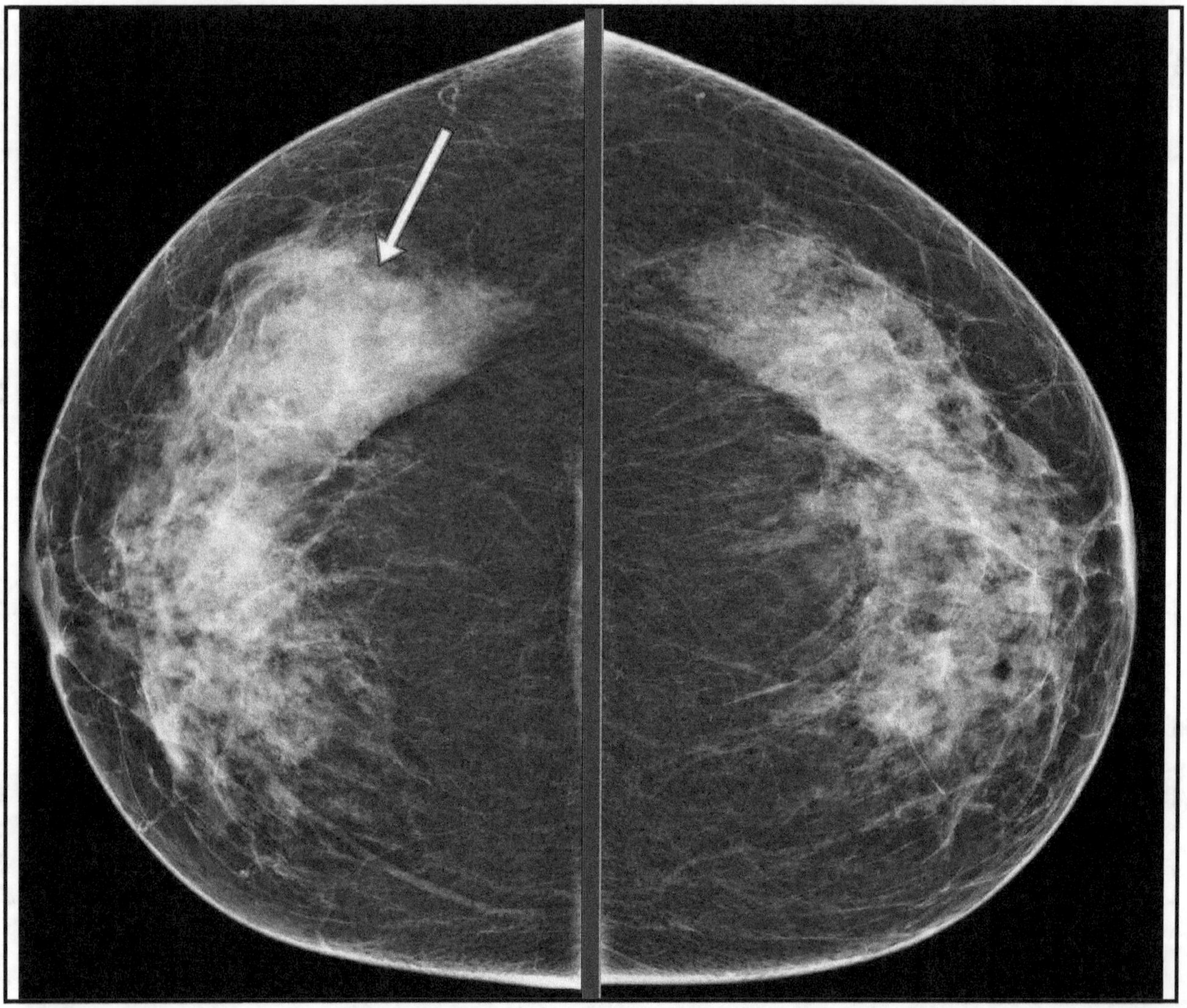

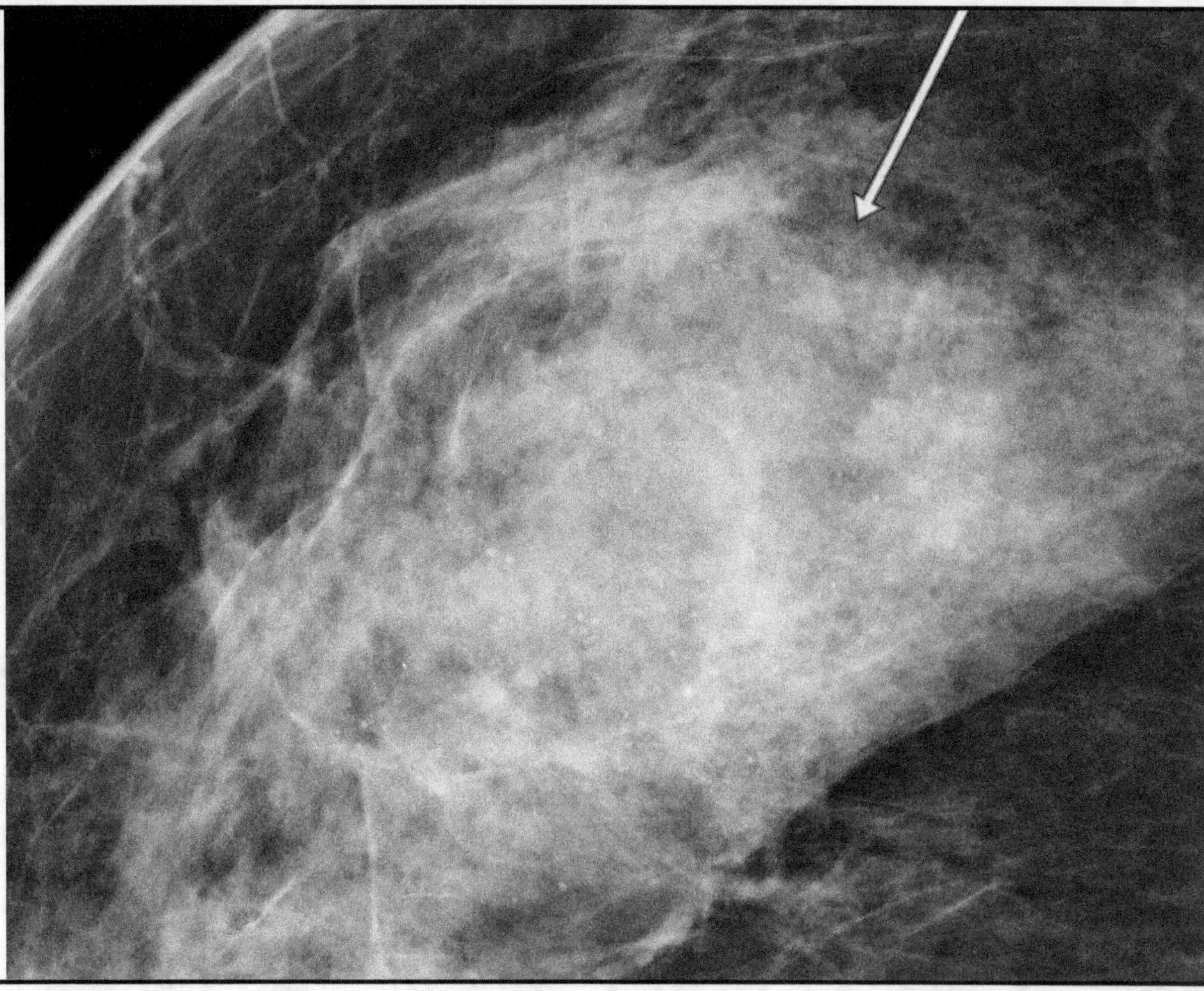

RIGHT BREAST	
Breast Parenchymal Density	***Heterogeneously dense, may obscure small masses (ACR C)***
Focal Mass	None
Asymmetric Density	None
Parenchymal Distortion	None
Calcification	***UOQ segmental are of suspicious amorphous micro-calcification***
Skin Thickening	None
Axillary Nodes	None

LEFT BREAST	
Breast Parenchymal Density	***Heterogeneously dense, may obscure small masses (ACR C)***
Focal Mass	None
Asymmetric Density	None
Parenchymal Distortion	None
Calcification	None
Skin Thickening	None
Axillary Nodes	None

IMPRESSION:
RIGHT BREAST: (BI-RADS 4b)
LEFT BREAST: (BI-RADS 1)

RECOMMENDATION: Histopathological Correlation

CASE 67: 38-year-old female/ diagnostic

Right MLO	Left MLO

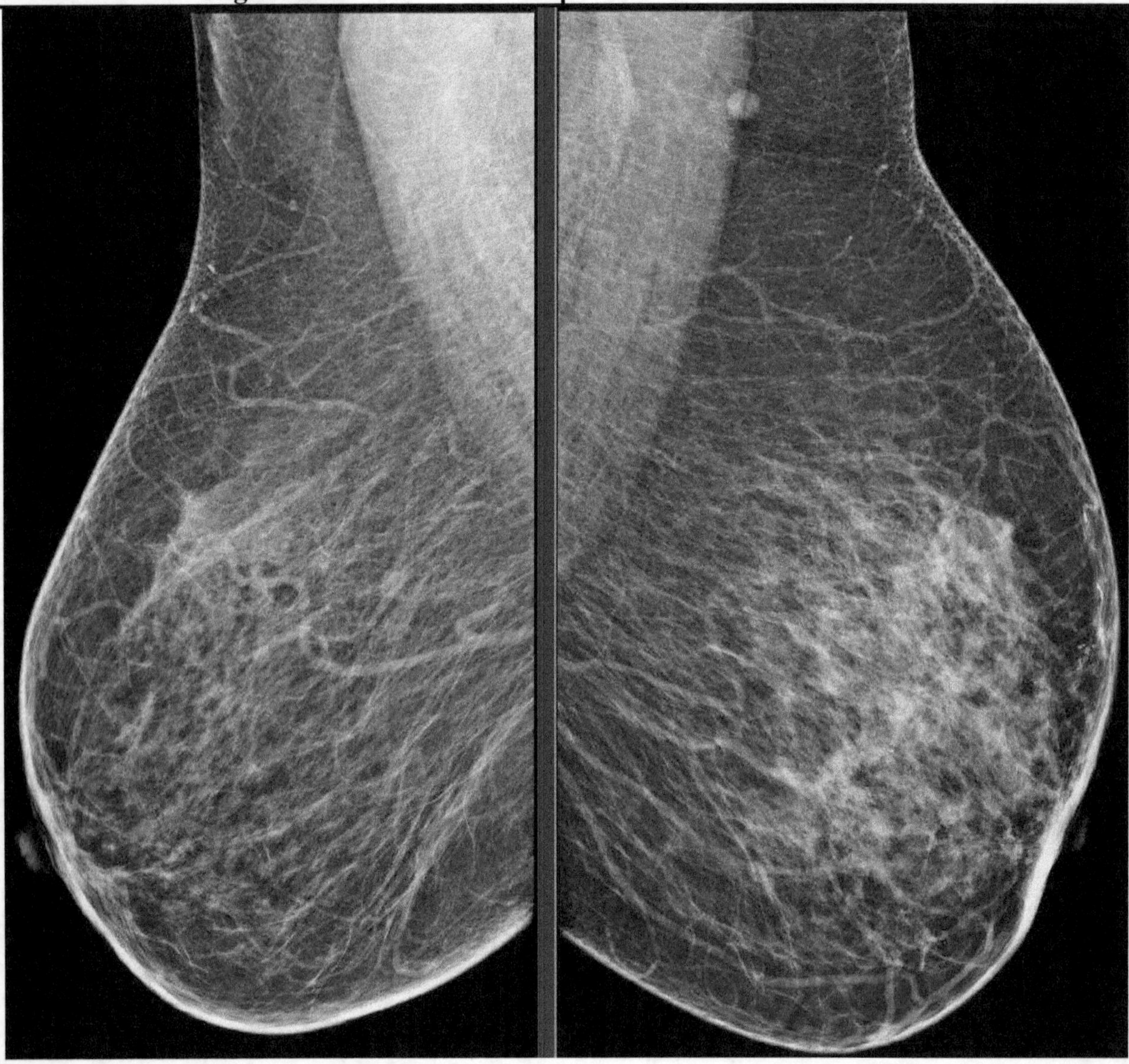

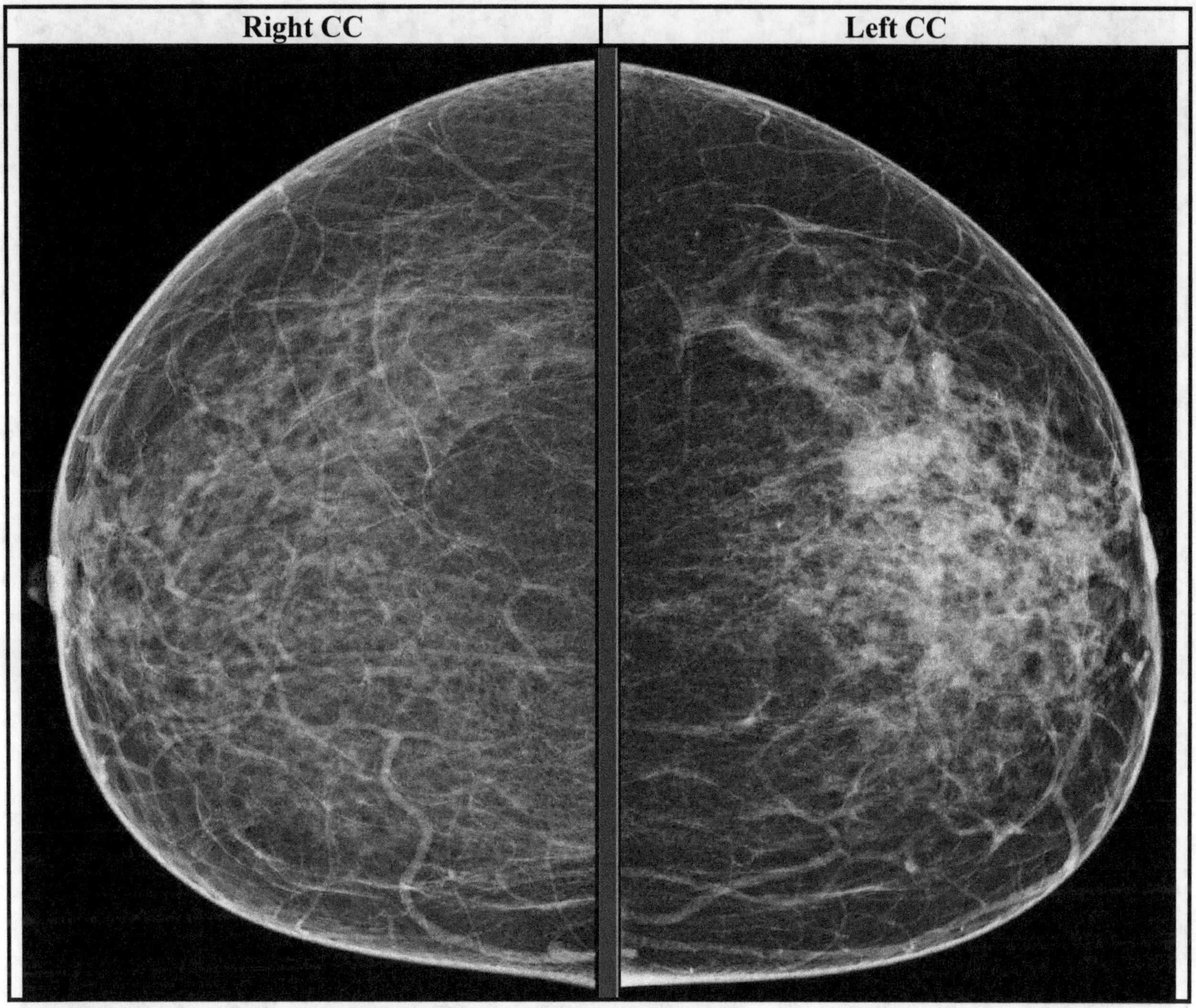
Right CC
Left CC

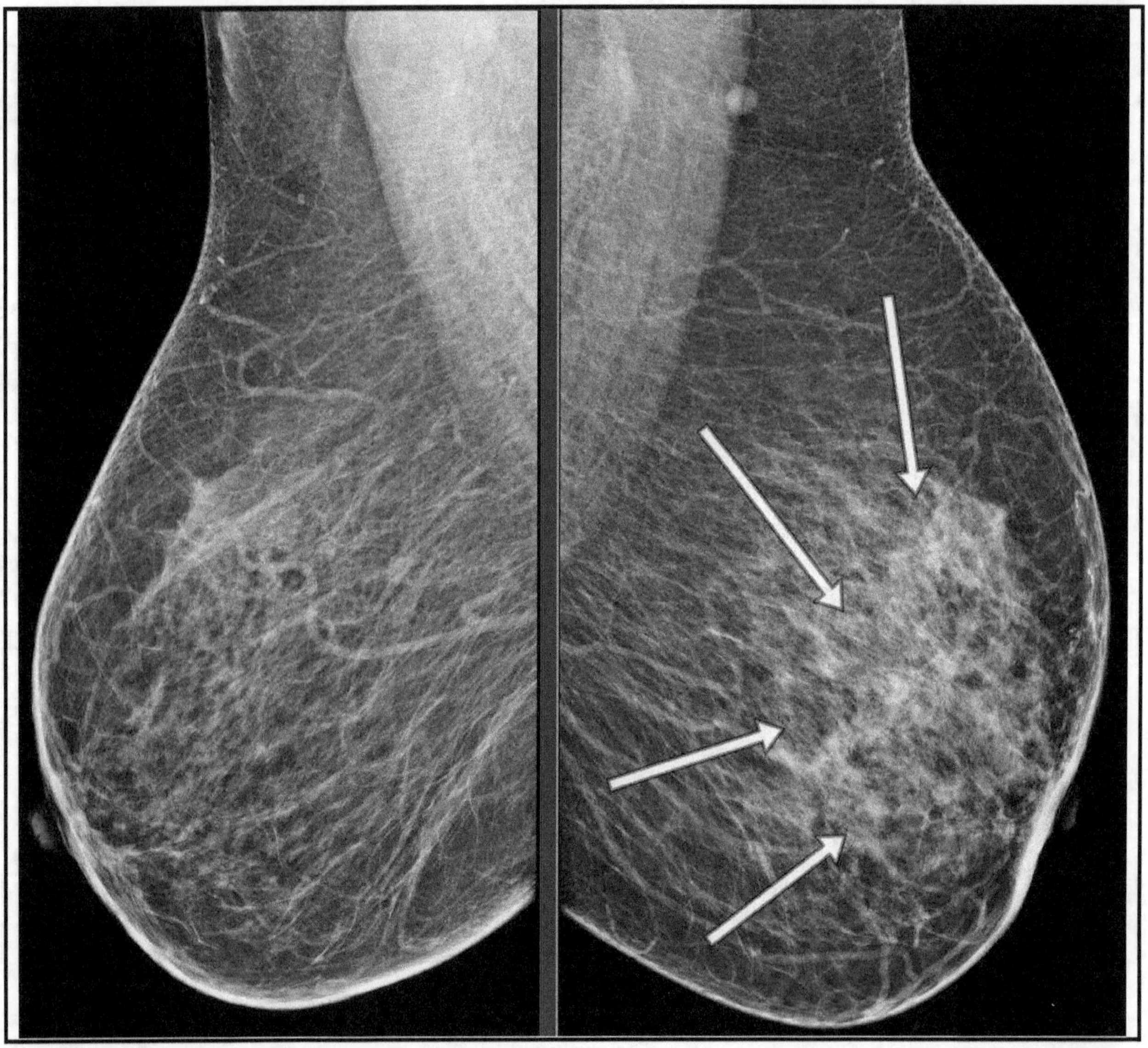

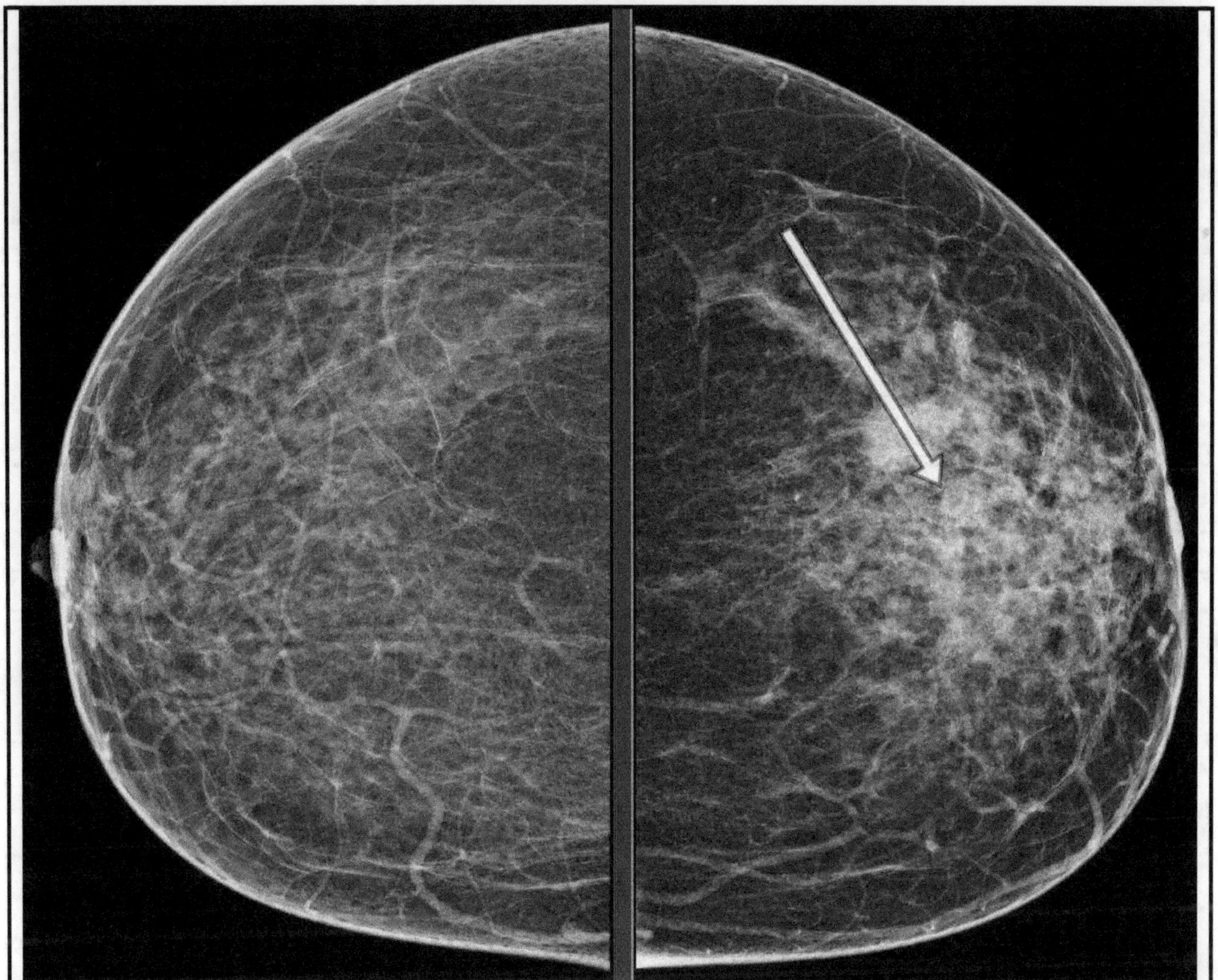

RIGHT BREAST	
Breast Parenchymal Density	***Scattered areas of fibroglandular density (ACR B)***
Focal Mass	None
Asymmetric Density	None
Parenchymal Distortion	None
Calcification	None
Skin Thickening	None
Axillary Nodes	None

LEFT BREAST	
Breast Parenchymal Density	***Scattered areas of fibroglandular density (ACR B)***
Focal Mass	None
Asymmetric Density	***Global Asymmetry***
Parenchymal Distortion	None
Calcification	None
Skin Thickening	None
Axillary Nodes	None

IMPRESSION:

RIGHT BREAST: (BI-RADS 1)
LEFT BREAST: (BI-RADS 2)

RECOMMENDATION: Routine Annual screening

CASE 68: 41-year-old female/ right conservative breast surgery

Right MLO	Left MLO

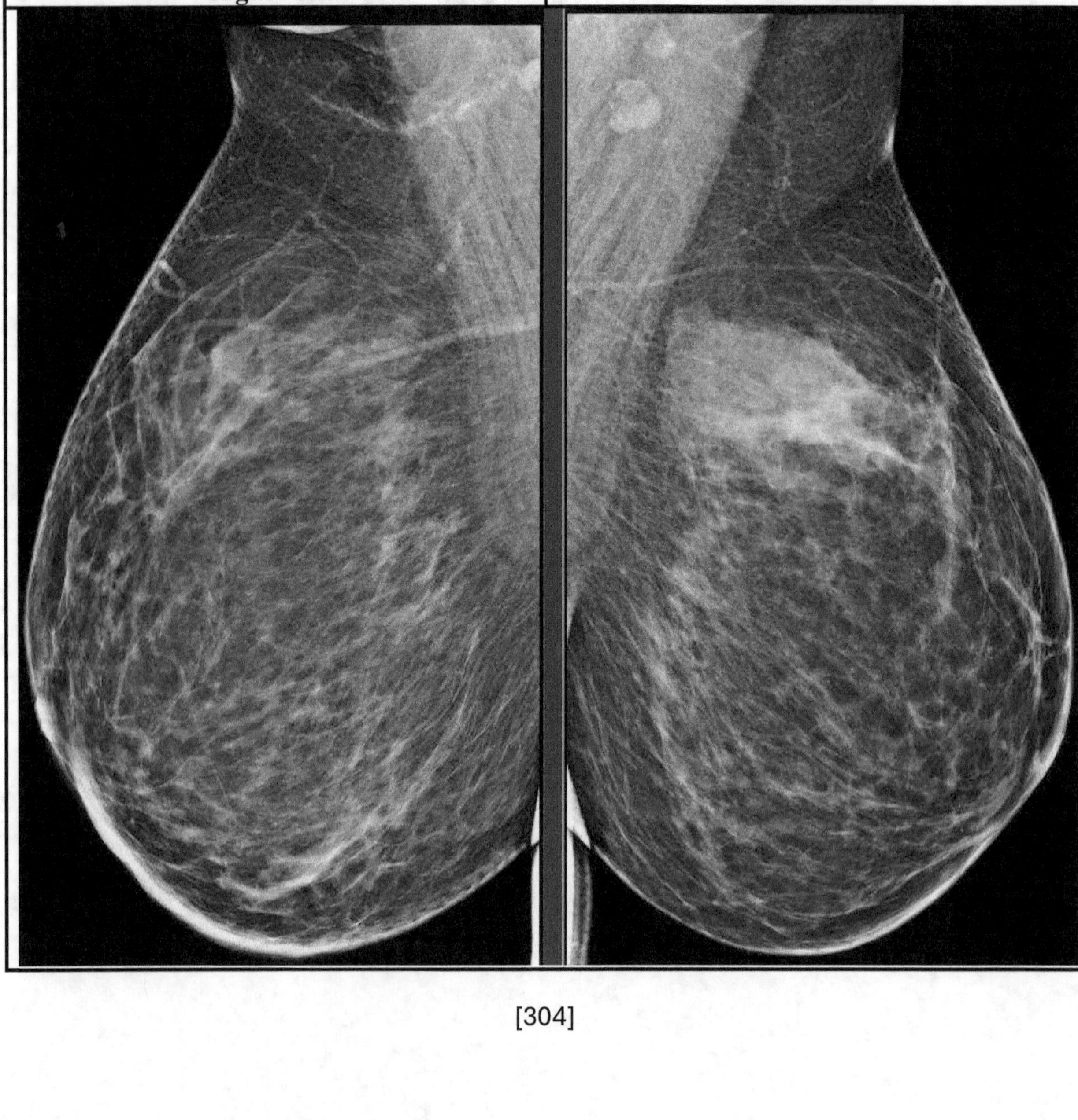

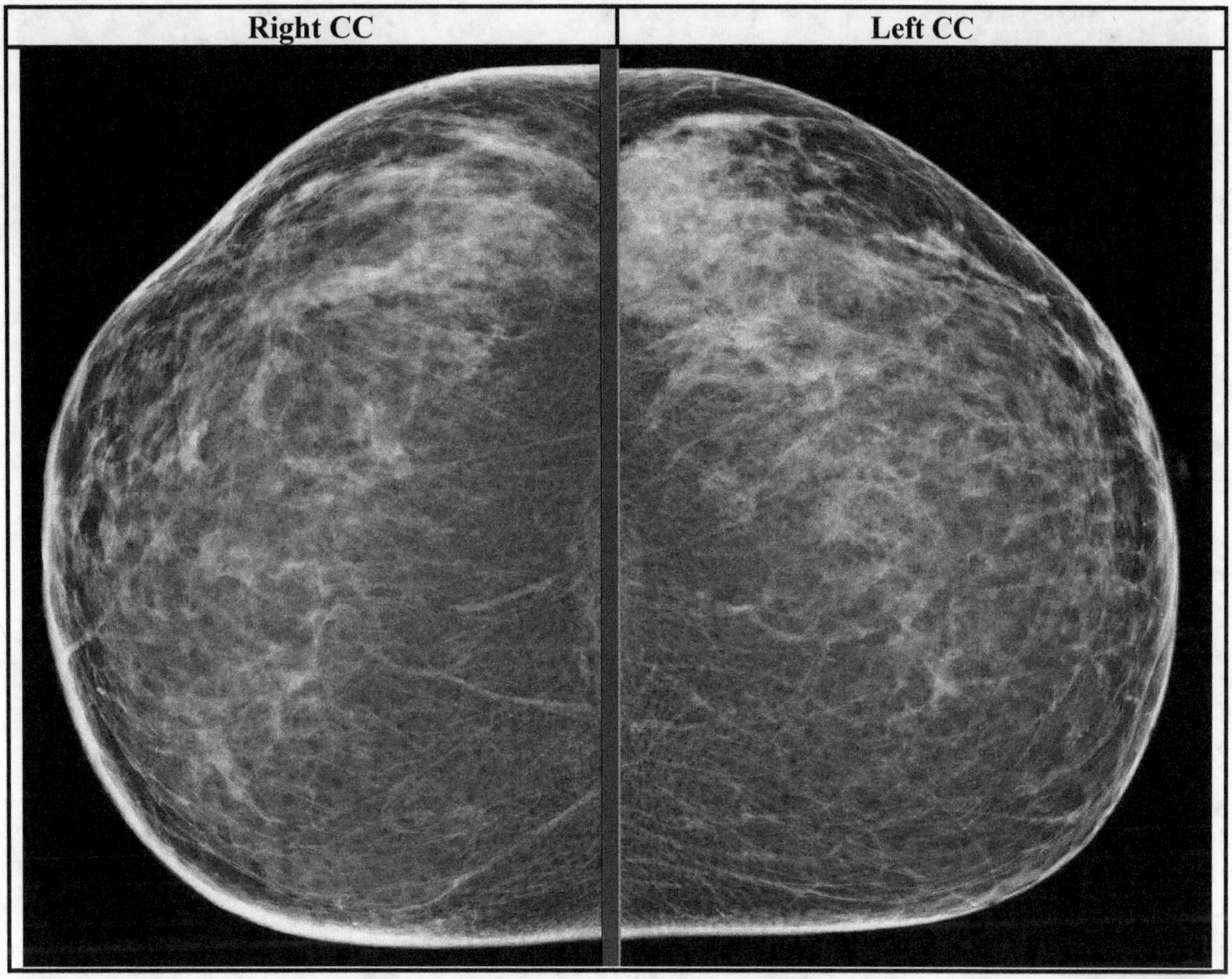
Right CC
Left CC

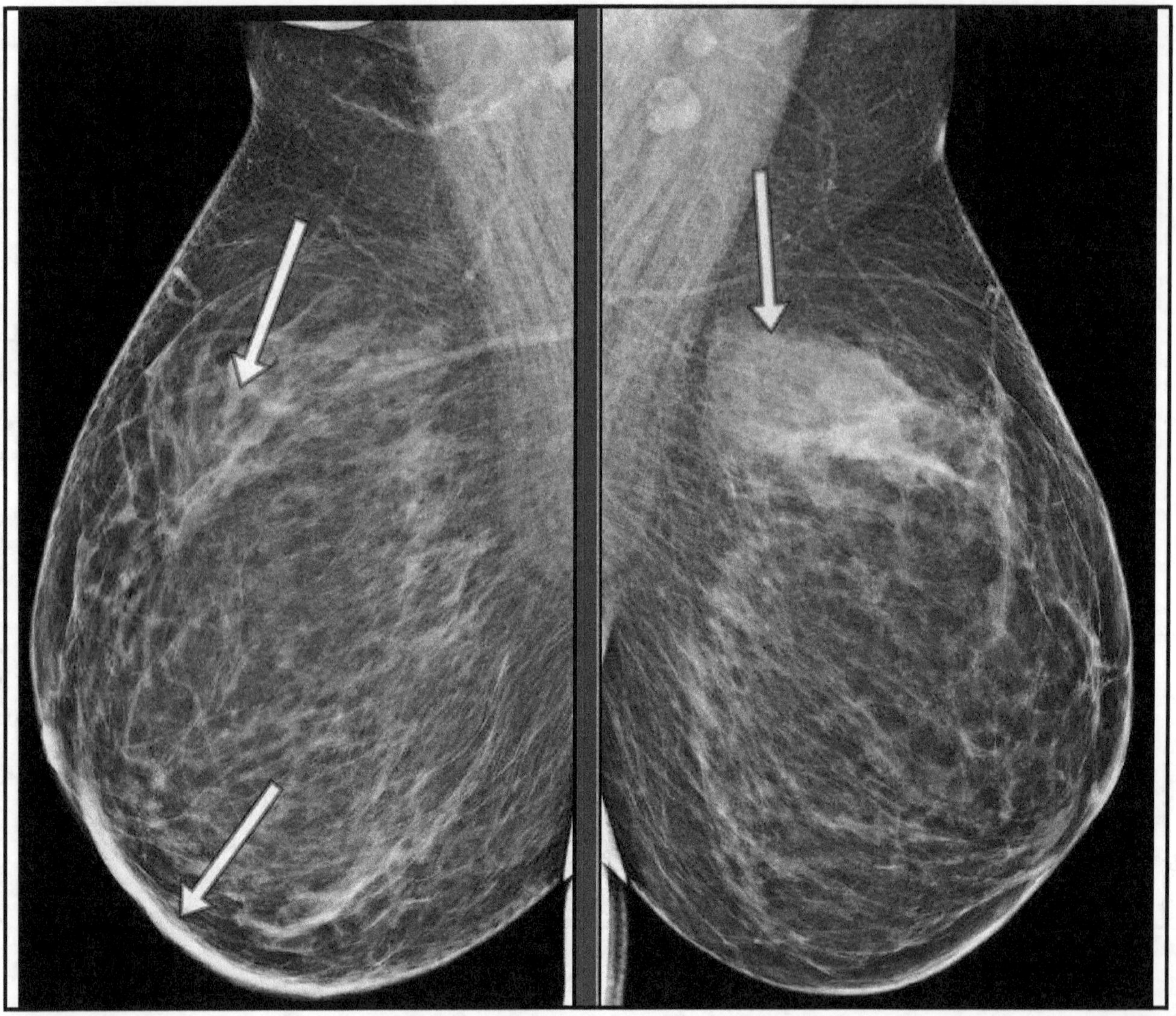

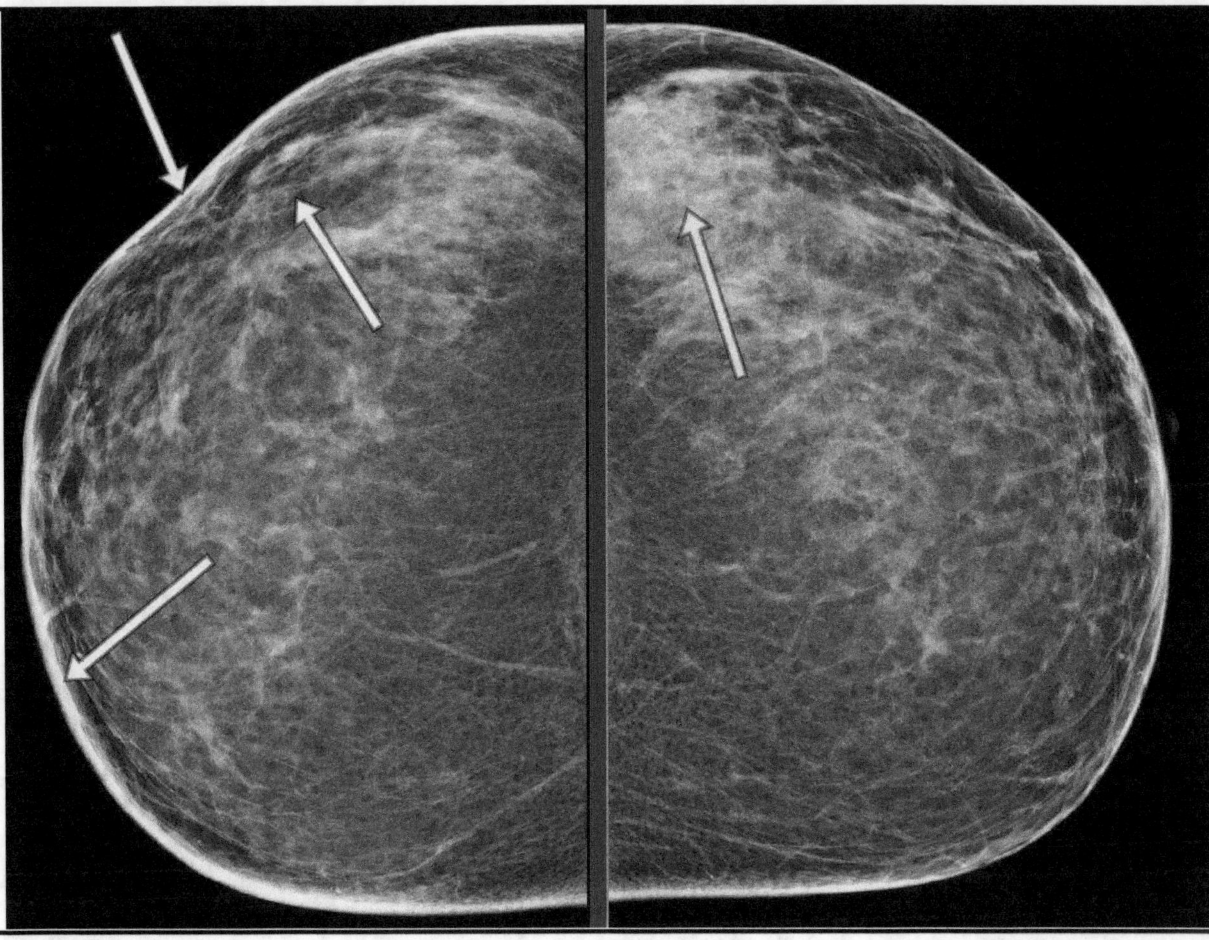

RIGHT BREAST	
Breast Parenchymal Density	***Scattered areas of fibroglandular density (ACR B)***
Focal Mass	None
Asymmetric Density	None
Parenchymal Distortion	None
Calcification	None
Skin Thickening	***Positive /UOQ skin retraction (operative site)***
Axillary Nodes	None

LEFT BREAST	
Breast Parenchymal Density	***Scattered areas of fibroglandular density (ACR B)***
Focal Mass	None
Asymmetric Density	None
Parenchymal Distortion	None
Calcification	None
Skin Thickening	None
Axillary Nodes	None

IMPRESSION:

RIGHT BREAST: (BI-RADS 2)
LEFT BREAST: (BI-RADS 1)

RECOMMENDATION: Routine Annual Follow-Up

See Case 65

CASE 69: 62-year-old female/screening

Right MLO	**Left MLO**
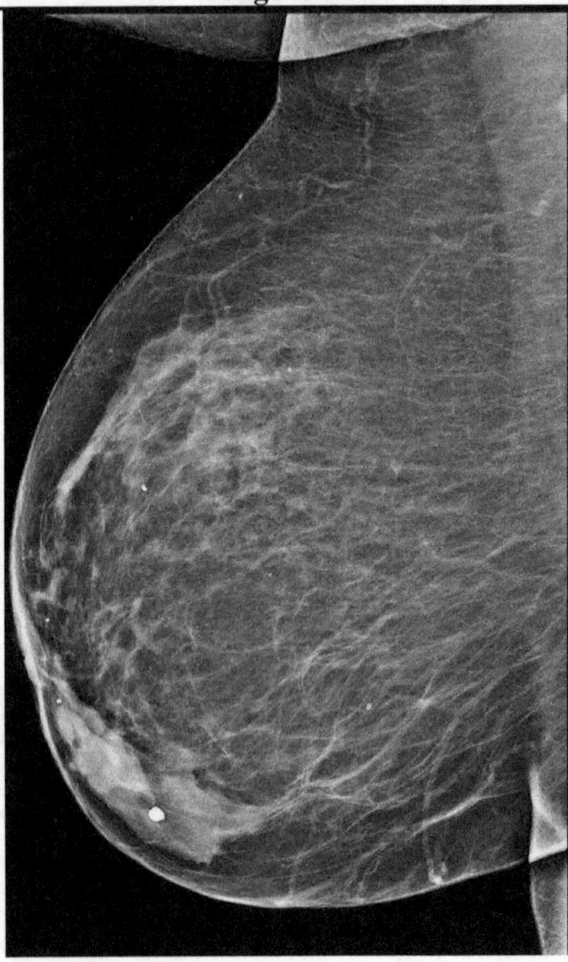	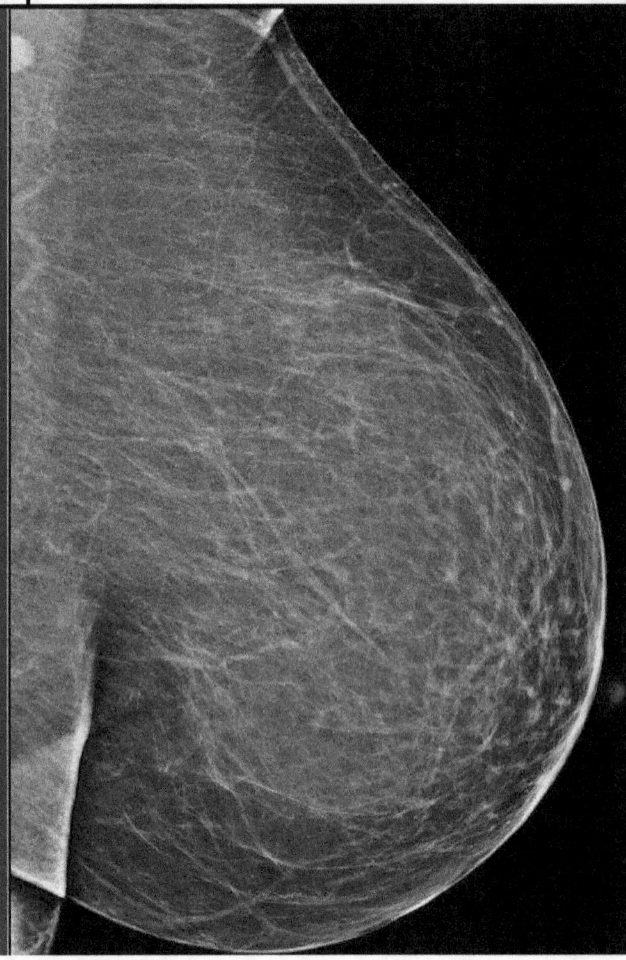

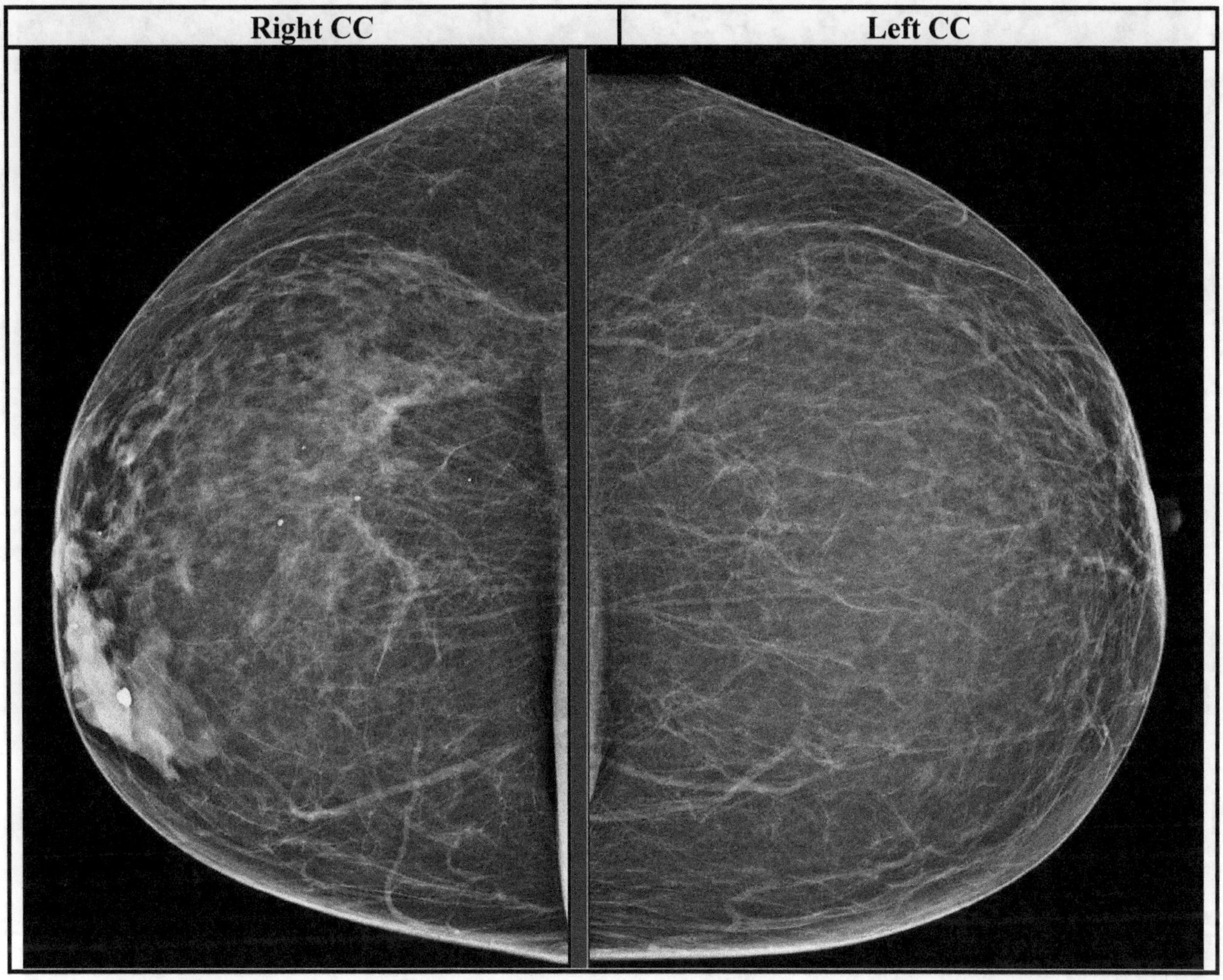
Right CC
Left CC

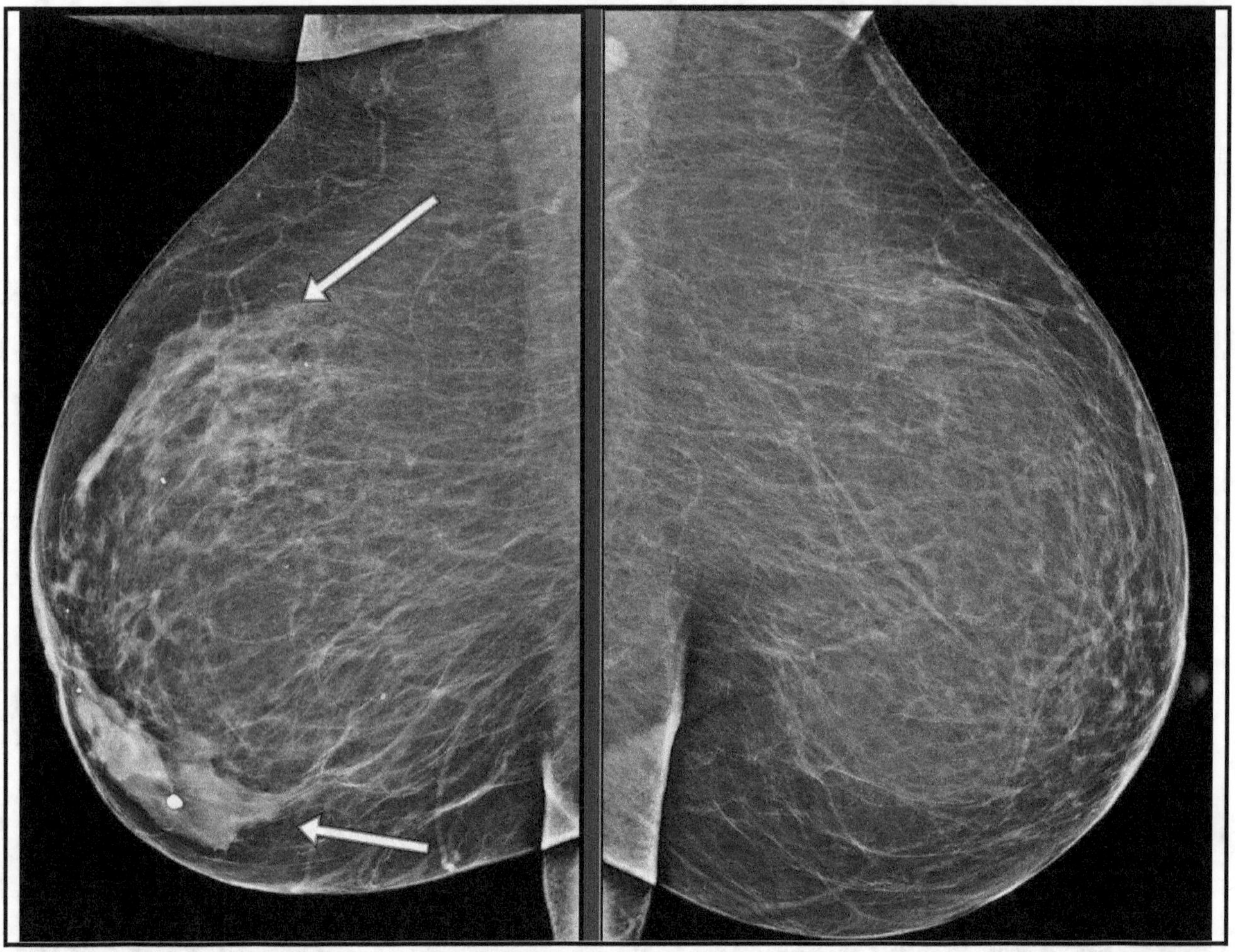

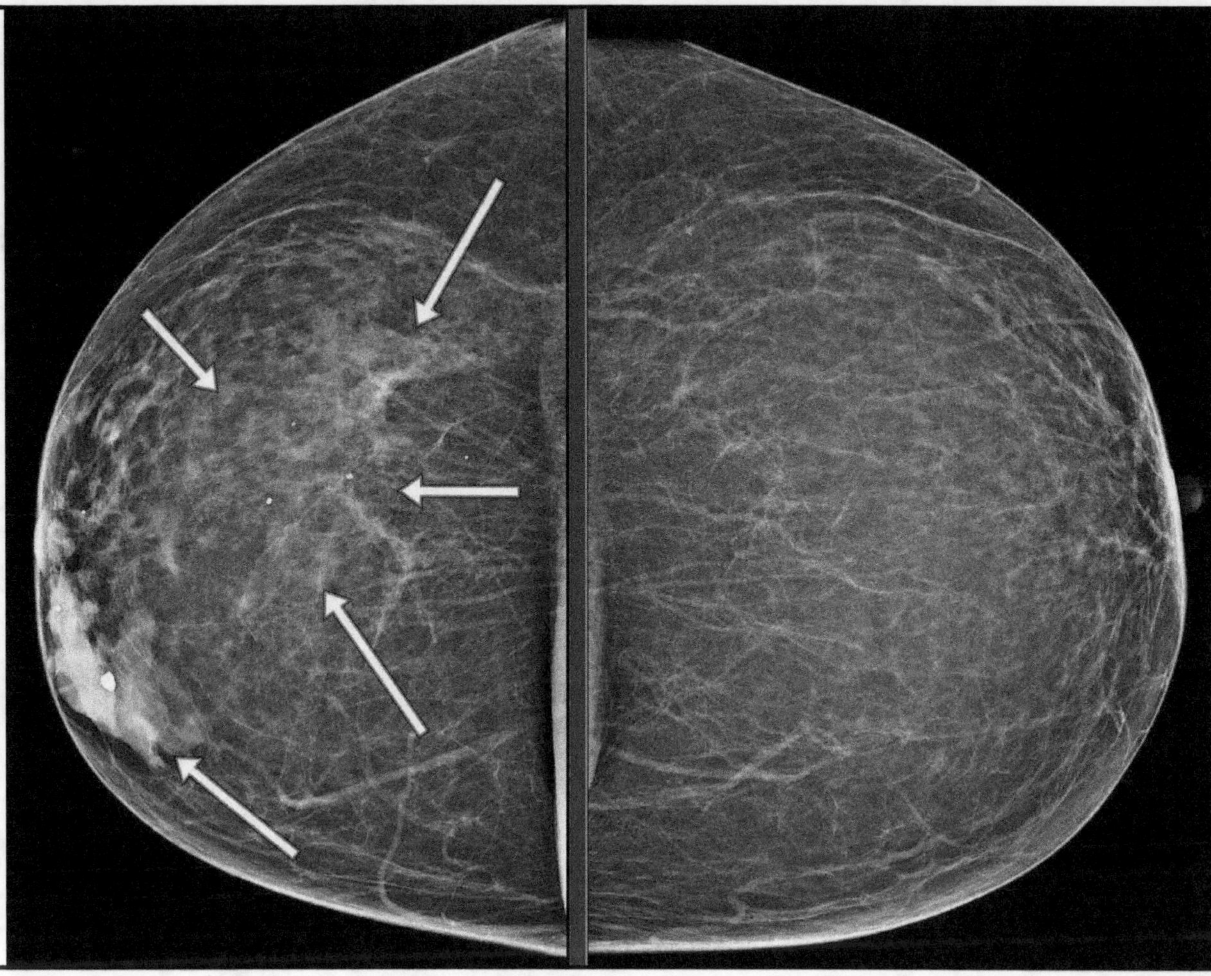

RIGHT BREAST	
Breast Parenchymal Density	***Scattered areas of fibroglandular density (ACR B)***
Focal Mass	None
Asymmetric Density	***UOQ/LIQ focal asymmetries***
Parenchymal Distortion	None
Calcification	***Skin / Coarse Calcification***
Skin Thickening	None
Axillary Nodes	None

LEFT BREAST	
Breast Parenchymal Density	***Almost entirely fatty (ACR A)***
Focal Mass	None
Asymmetric Density	None
Parenchymal Distortion	None
Calcification	None
Skin Thickening	None
Axillary Nodes	None

IMPRESSION:

RIGHT BREAST: (BI-RADS 0)
LEFT BREAST: (BI-RADS 1)

RECOMMENDATION: US Correlation

CASE 70: 35-year-old female/ diagnostic

Right MLO	Left MLO

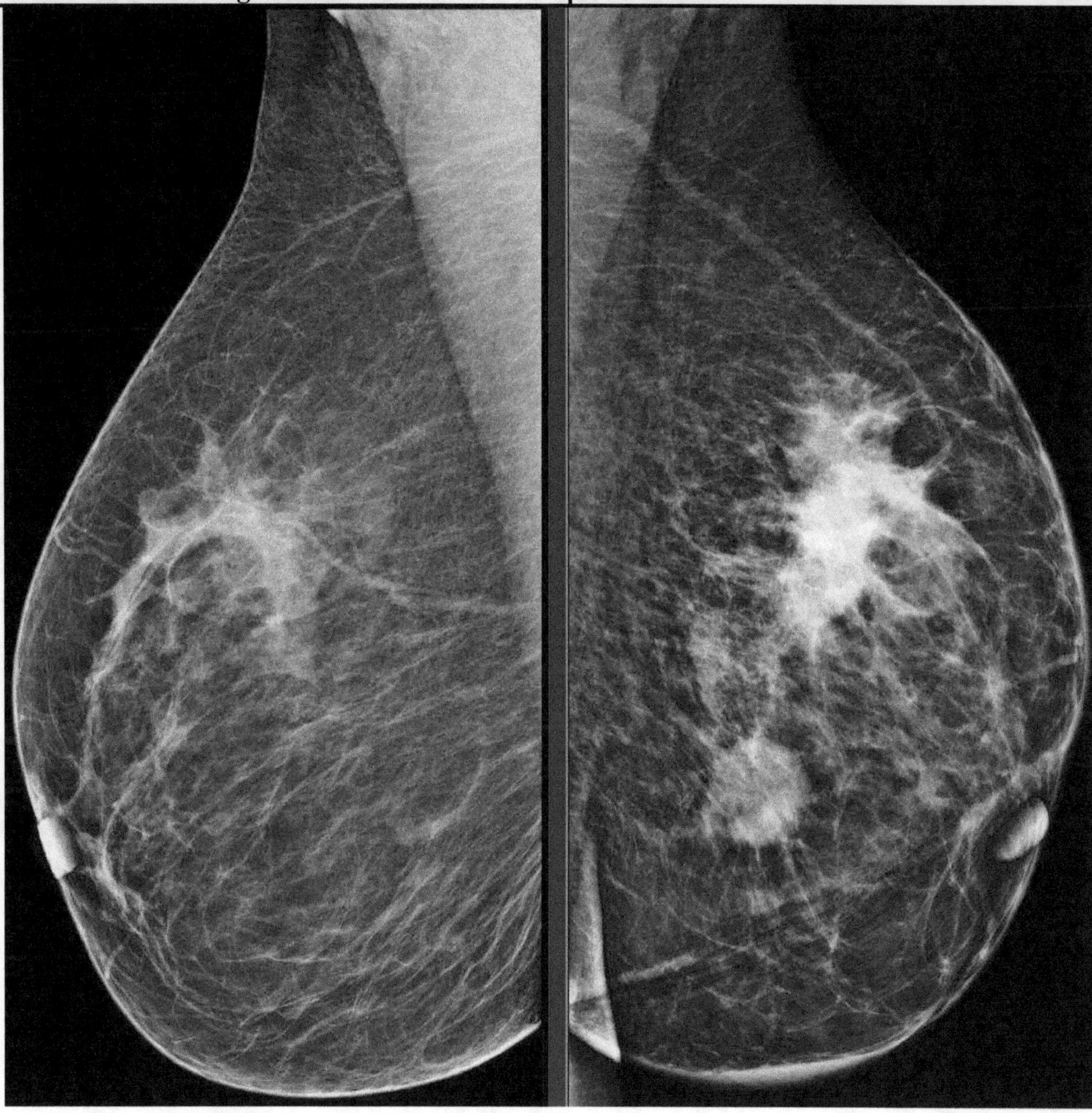

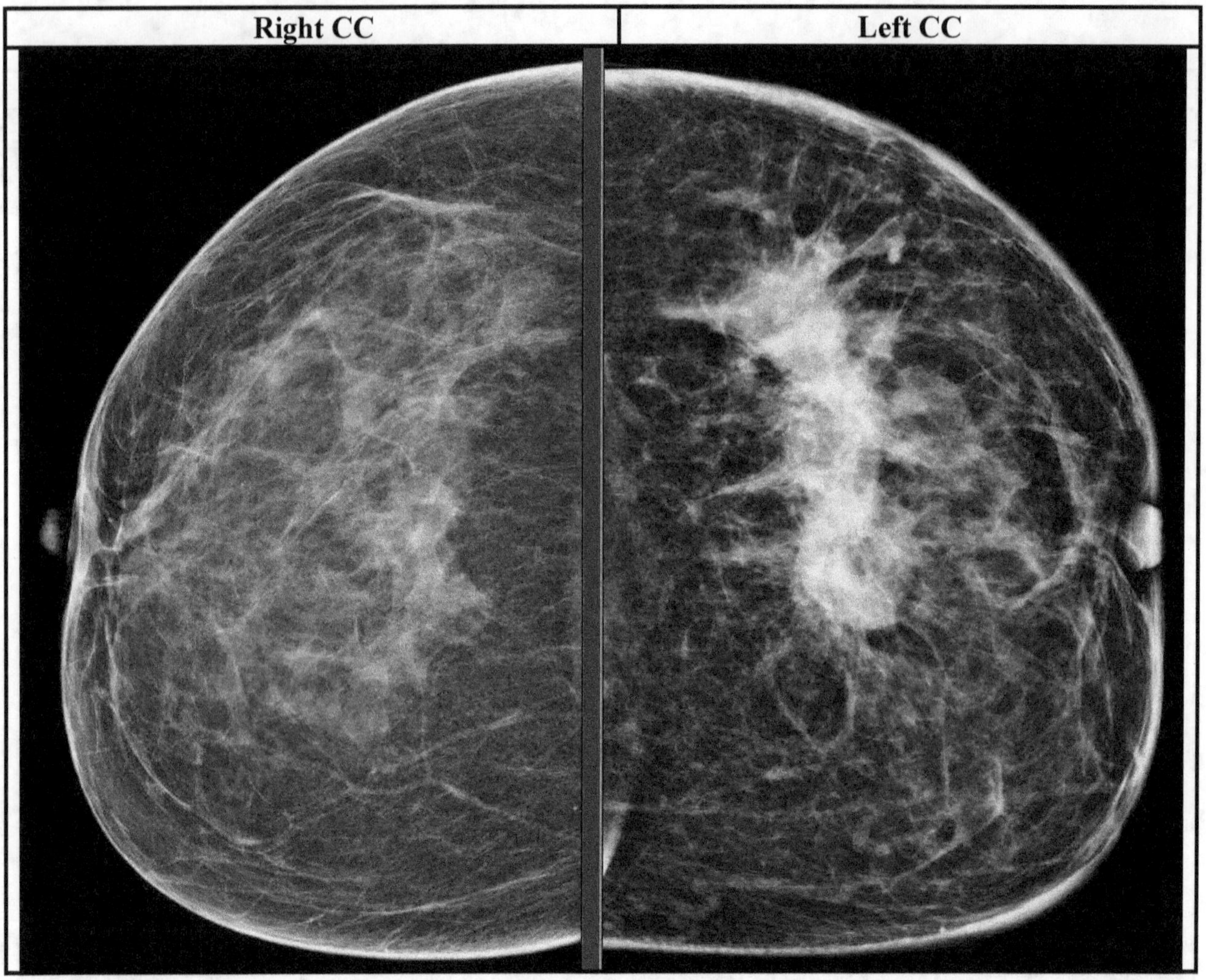
Right CC
Left CC

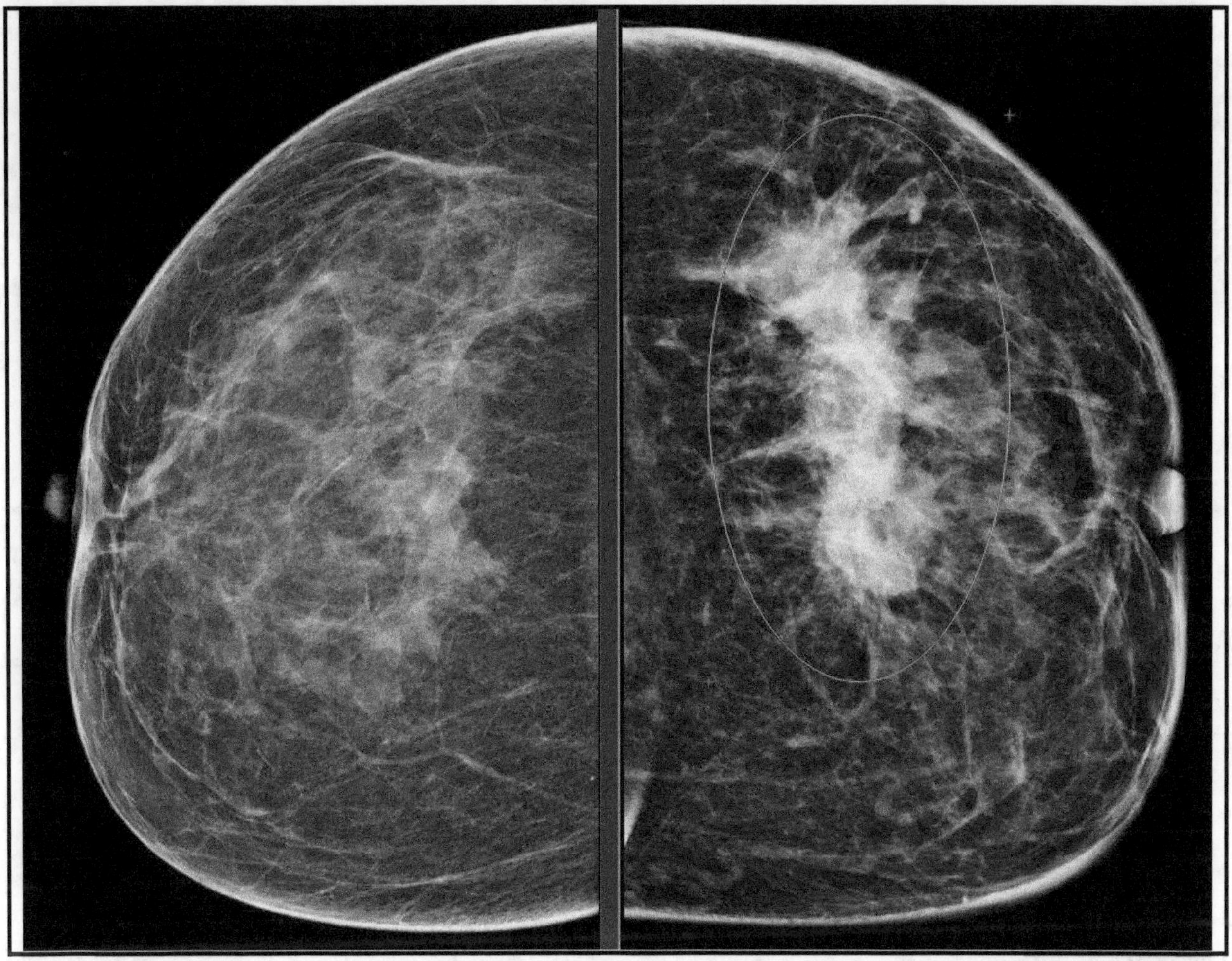

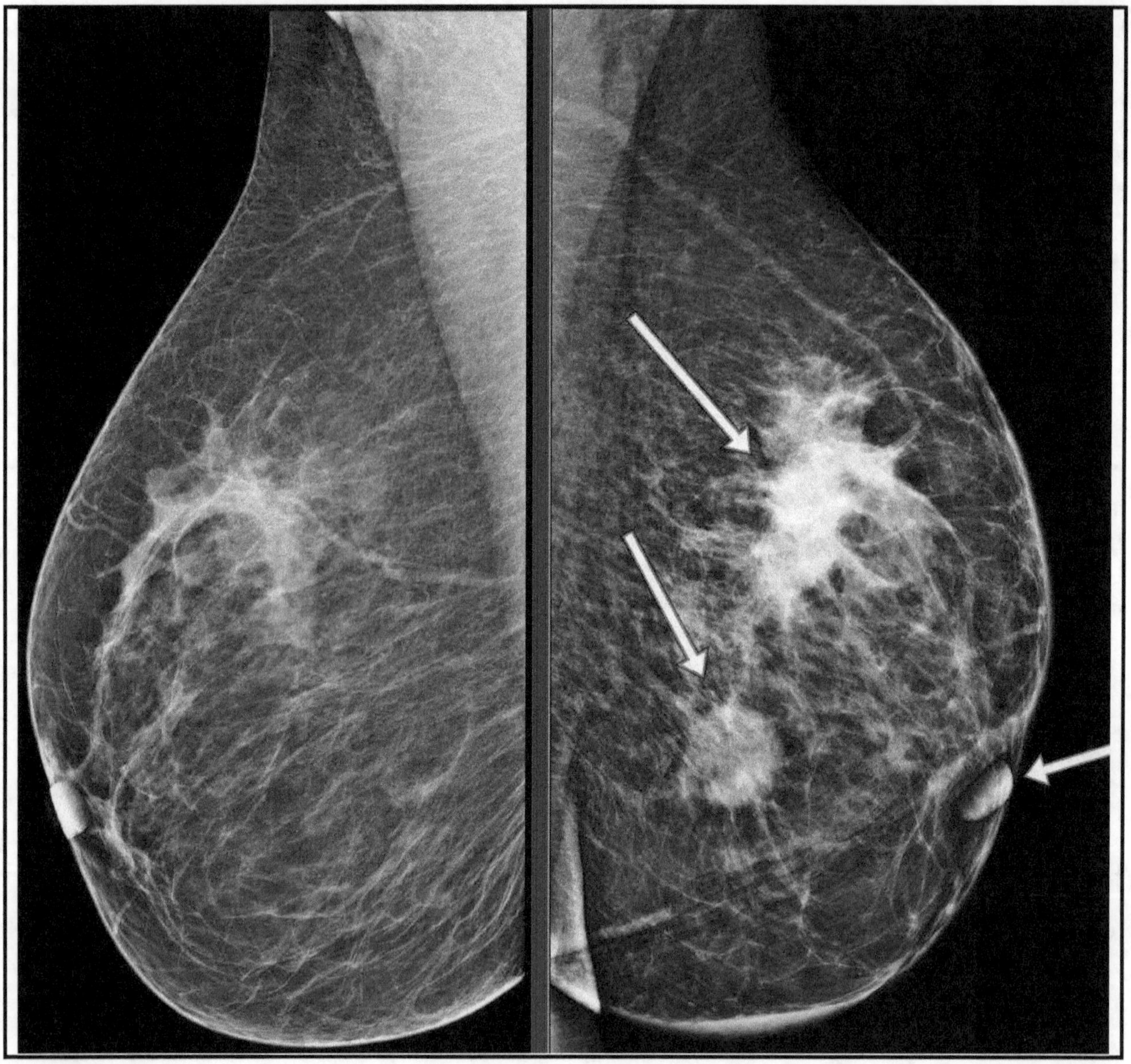

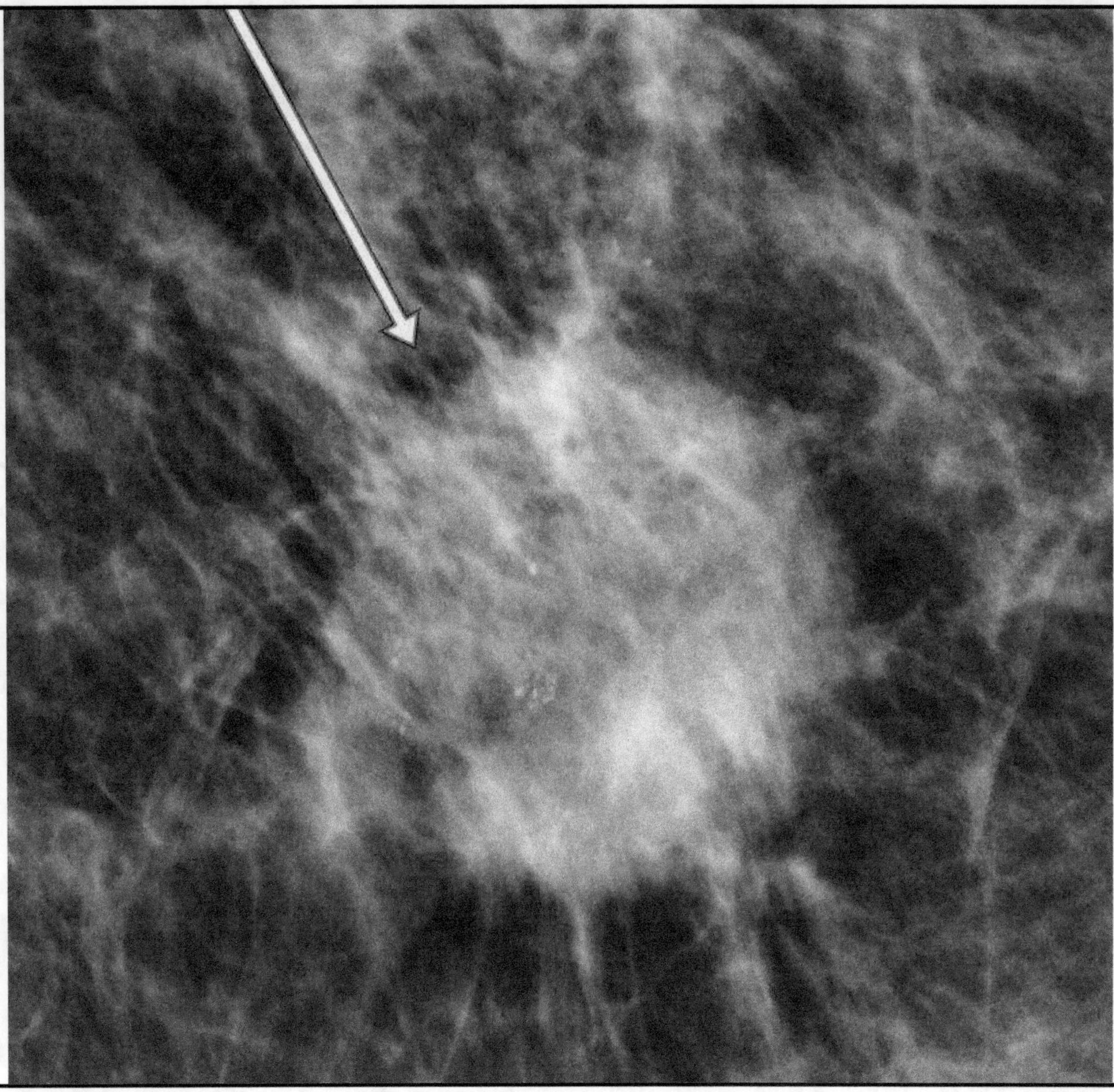

RIGHT BREAST	
Breast Parenchymal Density	***Scattered areas of fibroglandular density (ACR B)***
Focal Mass	None
Asymmetric Density	None
Parenchymal Distortion	None
Calcification	None
Skin Thickening	None
Axillary Nodes	None

LEFT BREAST	
Breast Parenchymal Density	***Scattered areas of fibroglandular density (ACR B)***
Focal Mass	***UOQ multifocal irregular /rounded indistinct /spiculated mass lesions associated amorphous microcalcification***
Asymmetric Density	None
Parenchymal Distortion	None
Calcification	None
Skin Thickening	None/ ***Nipple Retraction***
Axillary Nodes	None

IMPRESSION:

RIGHT BREAST: (BI-RADS 1)
LEFT BREAST: (BI-RADS 5)

RECOMMENDATION: Histopathological Correlation

CASE 71: 64-year-old female/left breast conservative surgery	
Right MLO	Left MLO
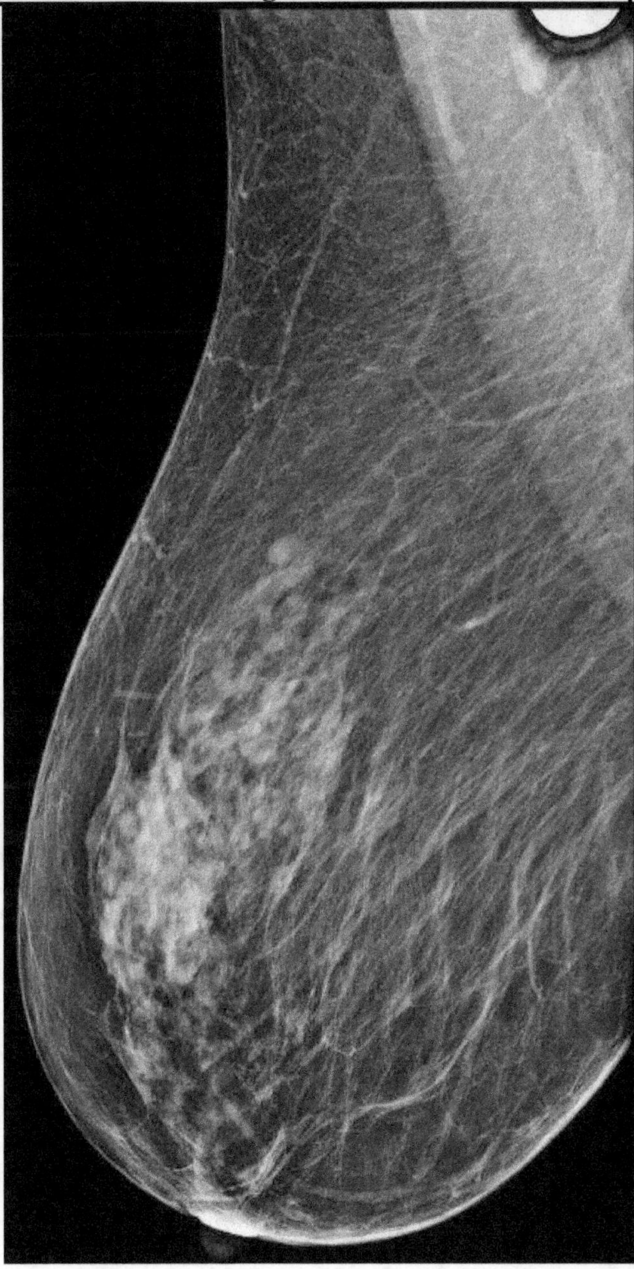	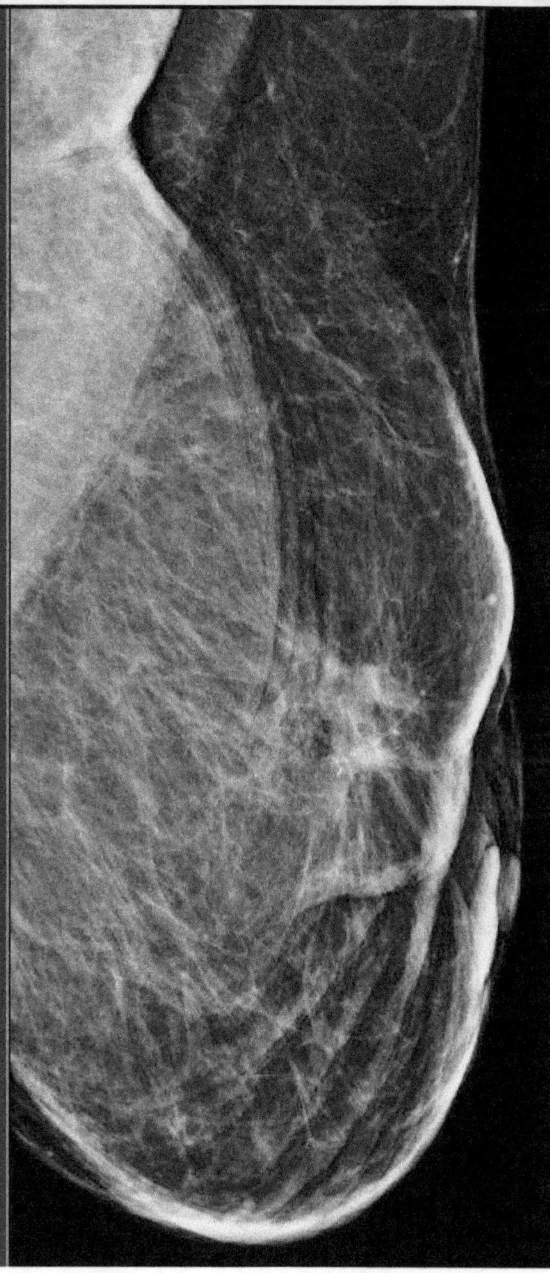

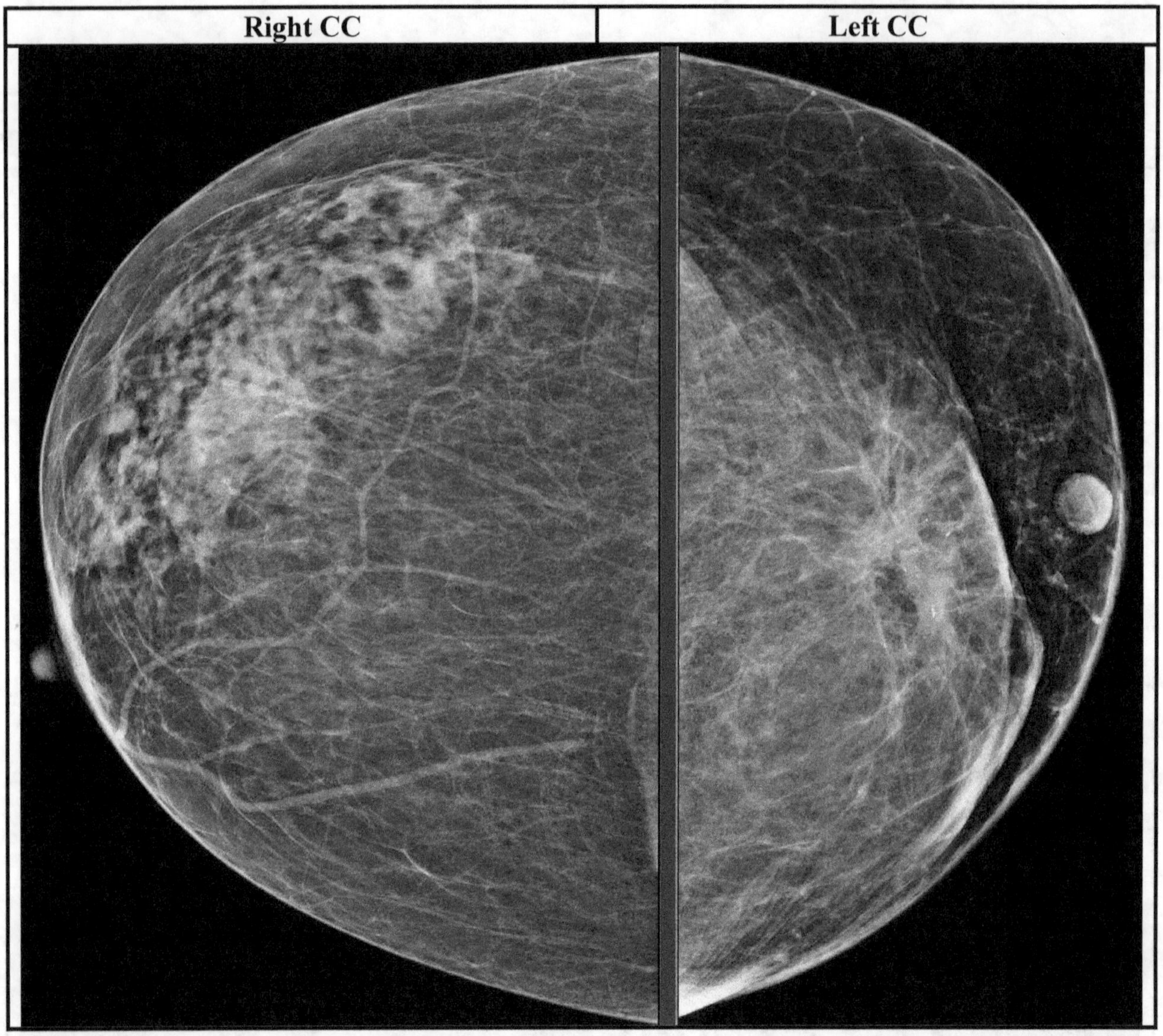
Right CC
Left CC

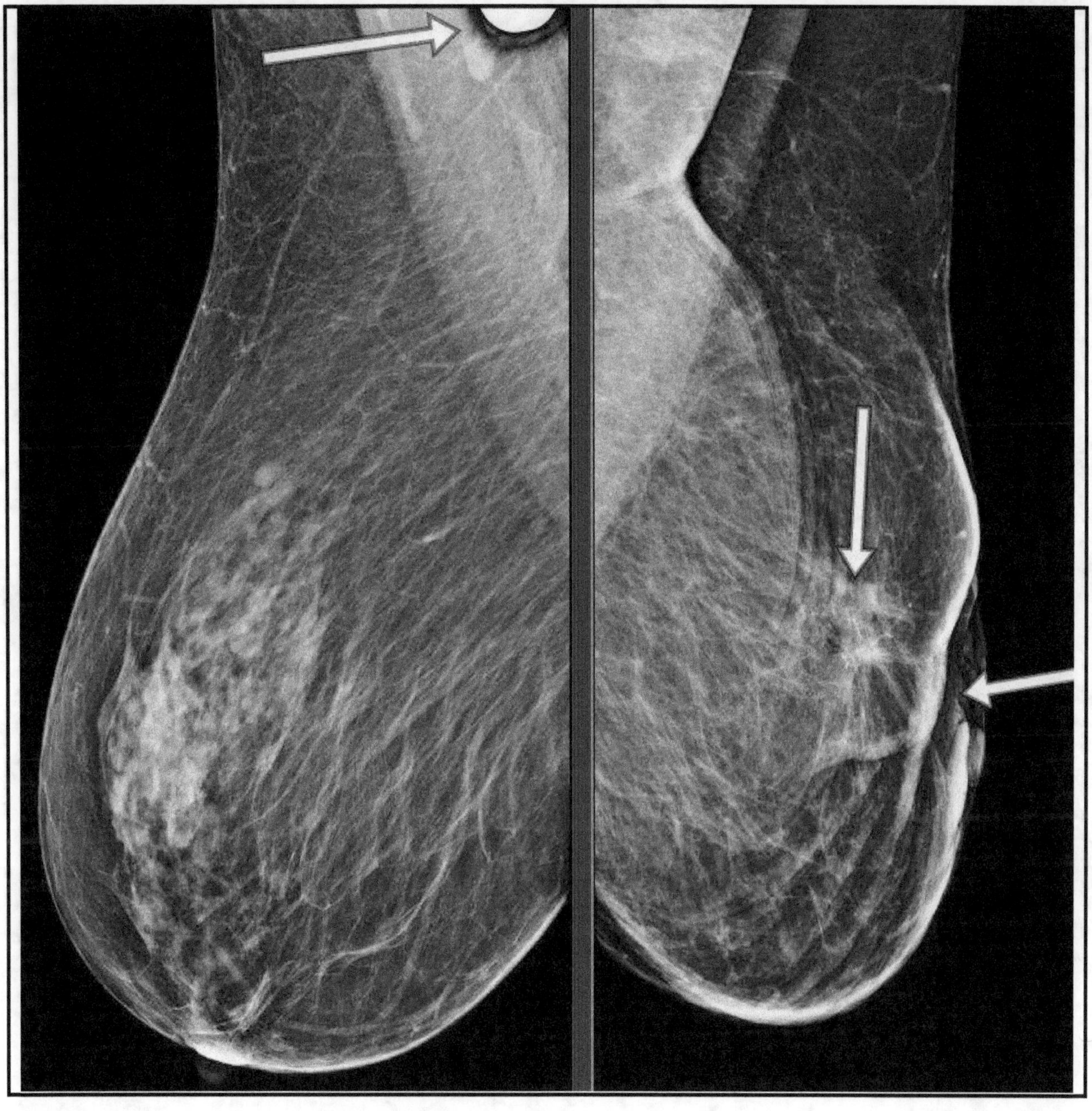

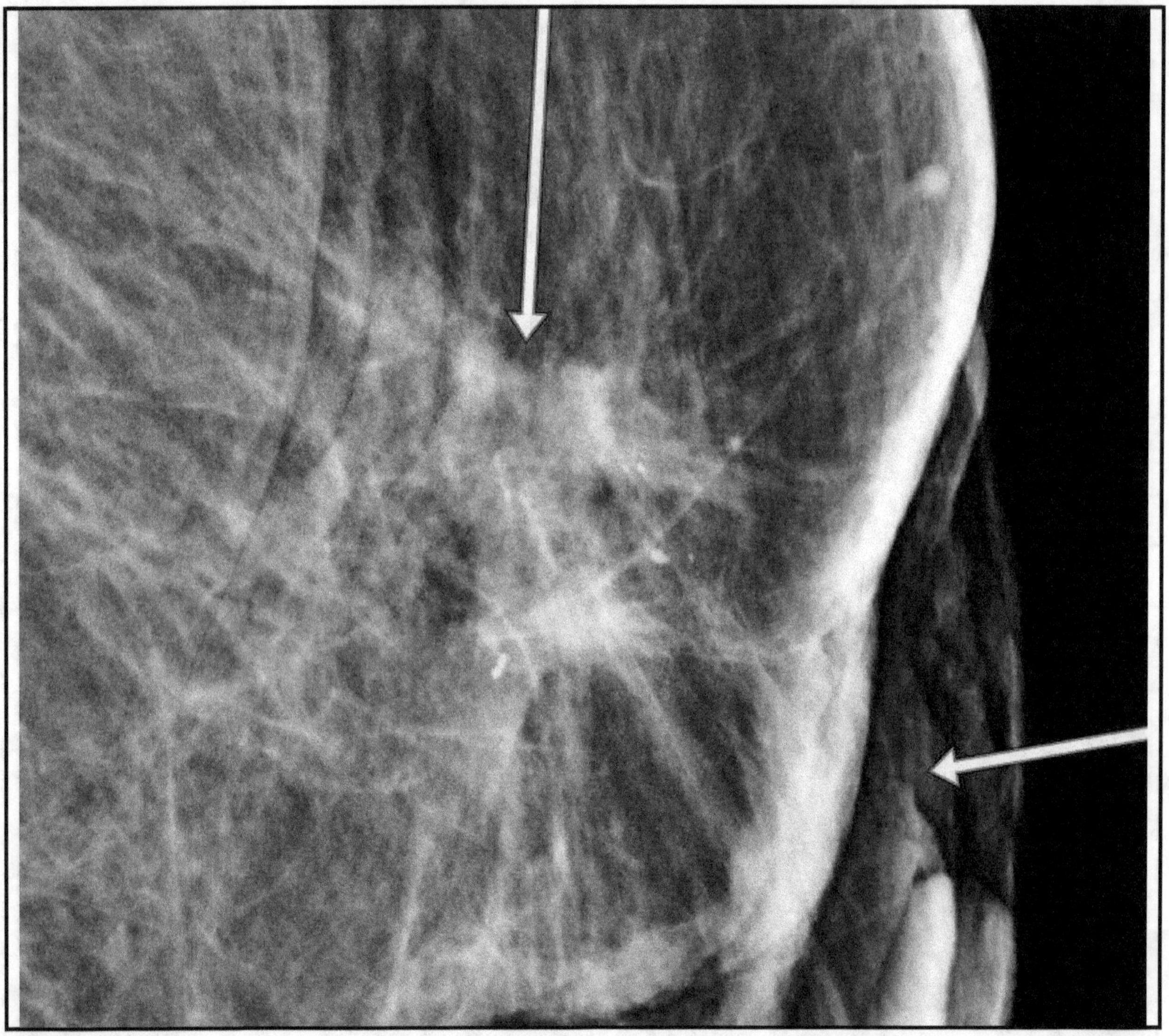

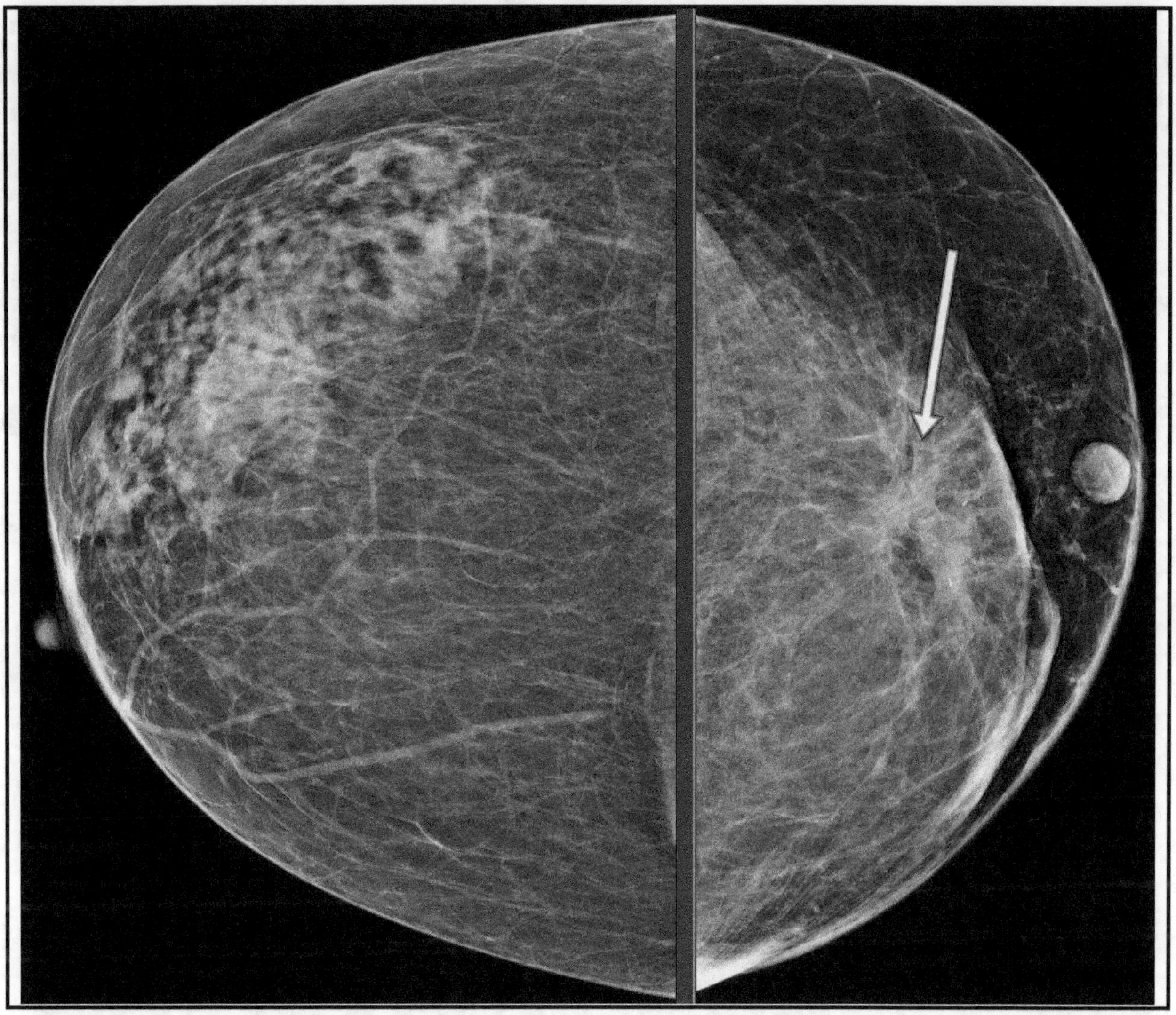

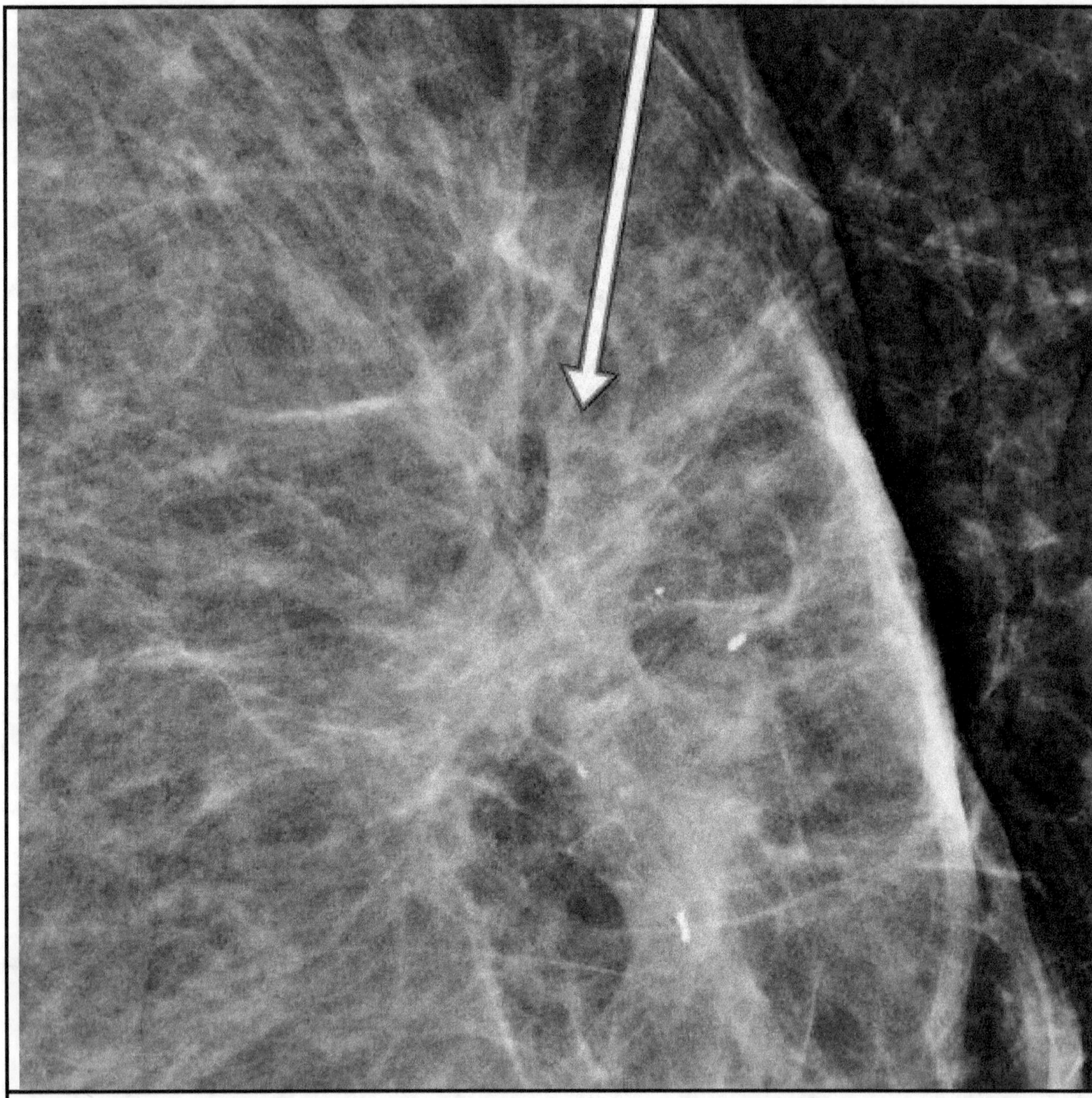

RIGHT BREAST	
Breast Parenchymal Density	***Scattered areas of fibroglandular density (ACR B)***
Focal Mass	None
Asymmetric Density	None
Parenchymal Distortion	None
Calcification	None
Skin Thickening	None
Axillary Nodes	None

LEFT BREAST	
Breast Parenchymal Density	***Scattered areas of fibroglandular density (ACR B)***
Focal Mass	None
Asymmetric Density	None
Parenchymal Distortion	***Upper central area of Parenchymal Distortion***
Calcification	None
Skin Thickening	None / ***Skin Retraction***
Axillary Nodes	None

IMPRESSION:

RIGHT BREAST: (BI-RADS 1)
LEFT BREAST: (BI-RADS 0)

RECOMMENDATION: US Correlation

Note Right Port -A-Cath

CASE 72: 52 -year-old female/diagnostic

Right MLO	Left MLO
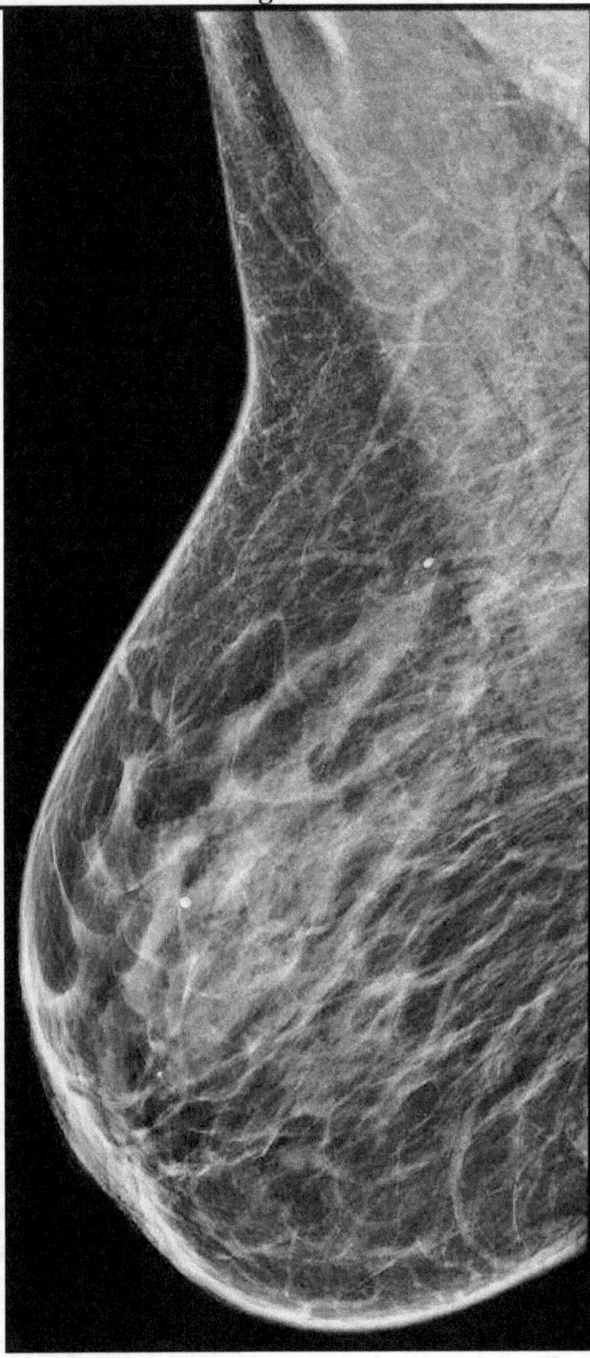	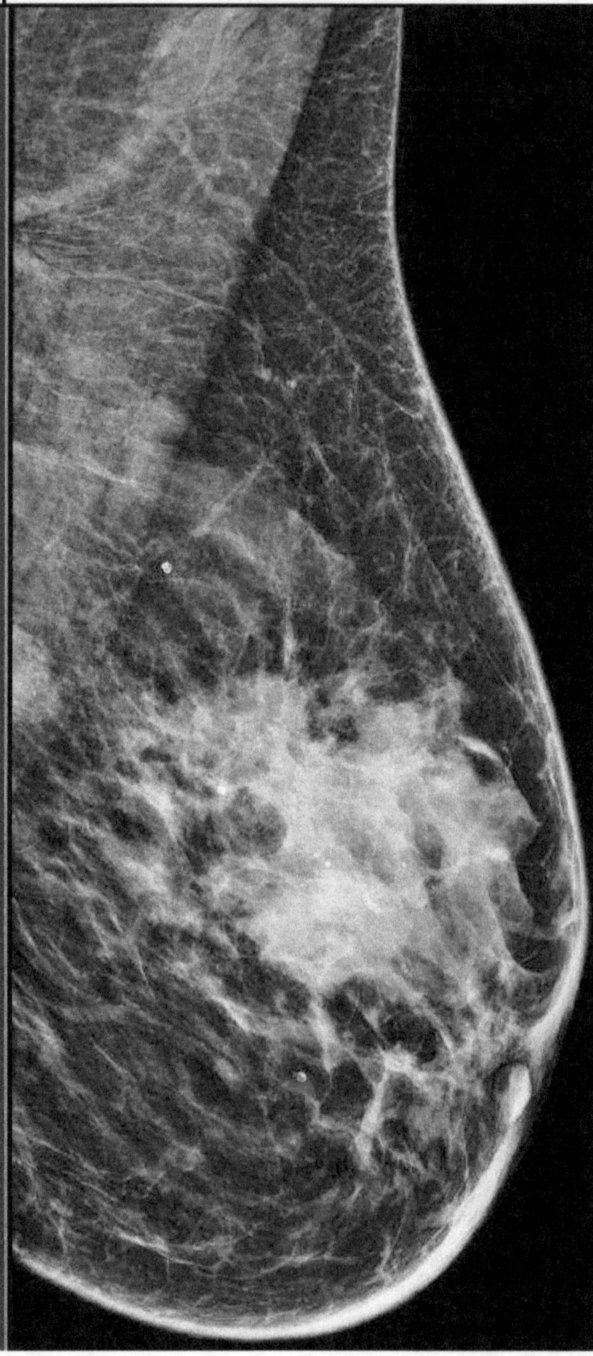

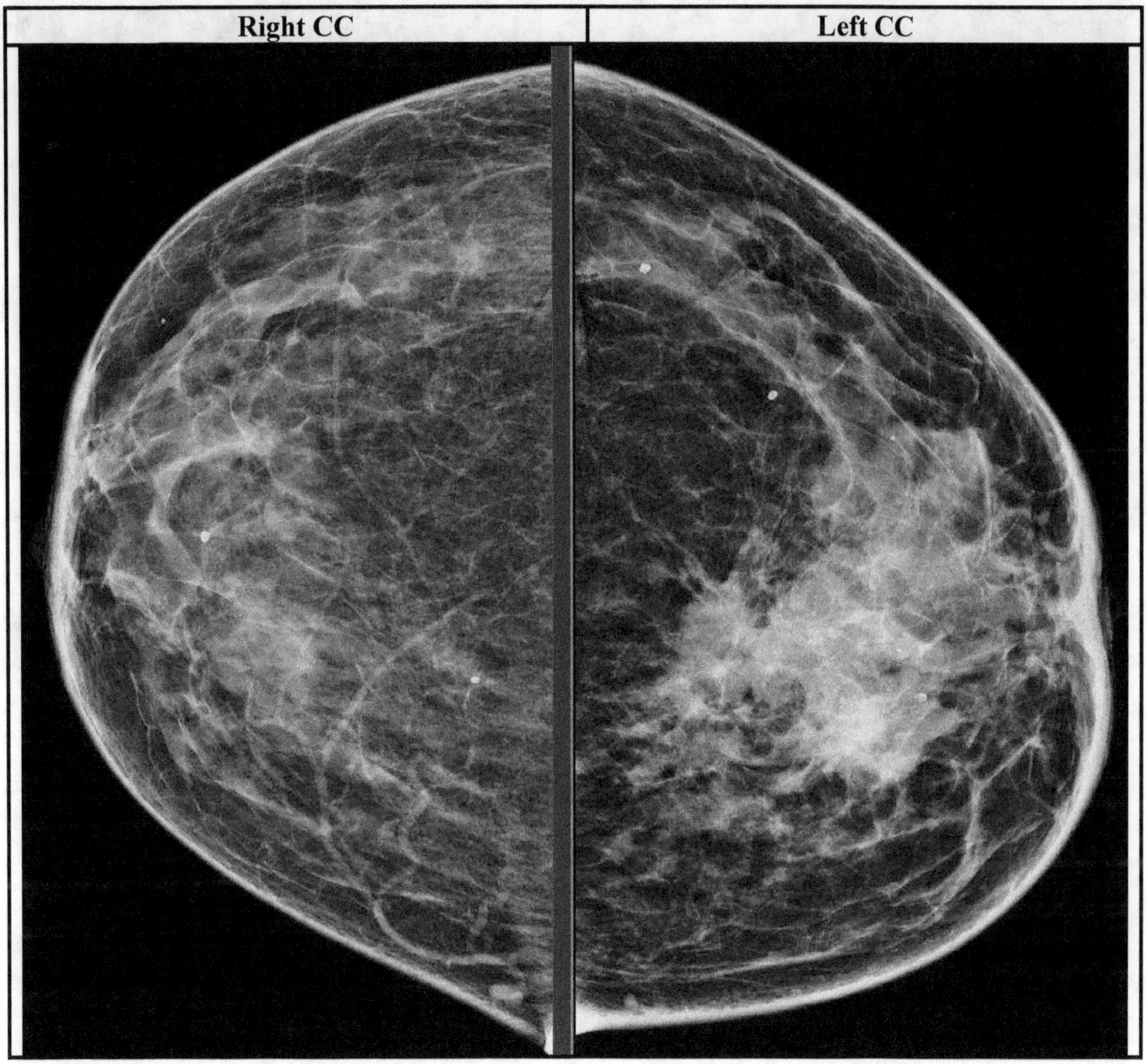
Right CC
Left CC

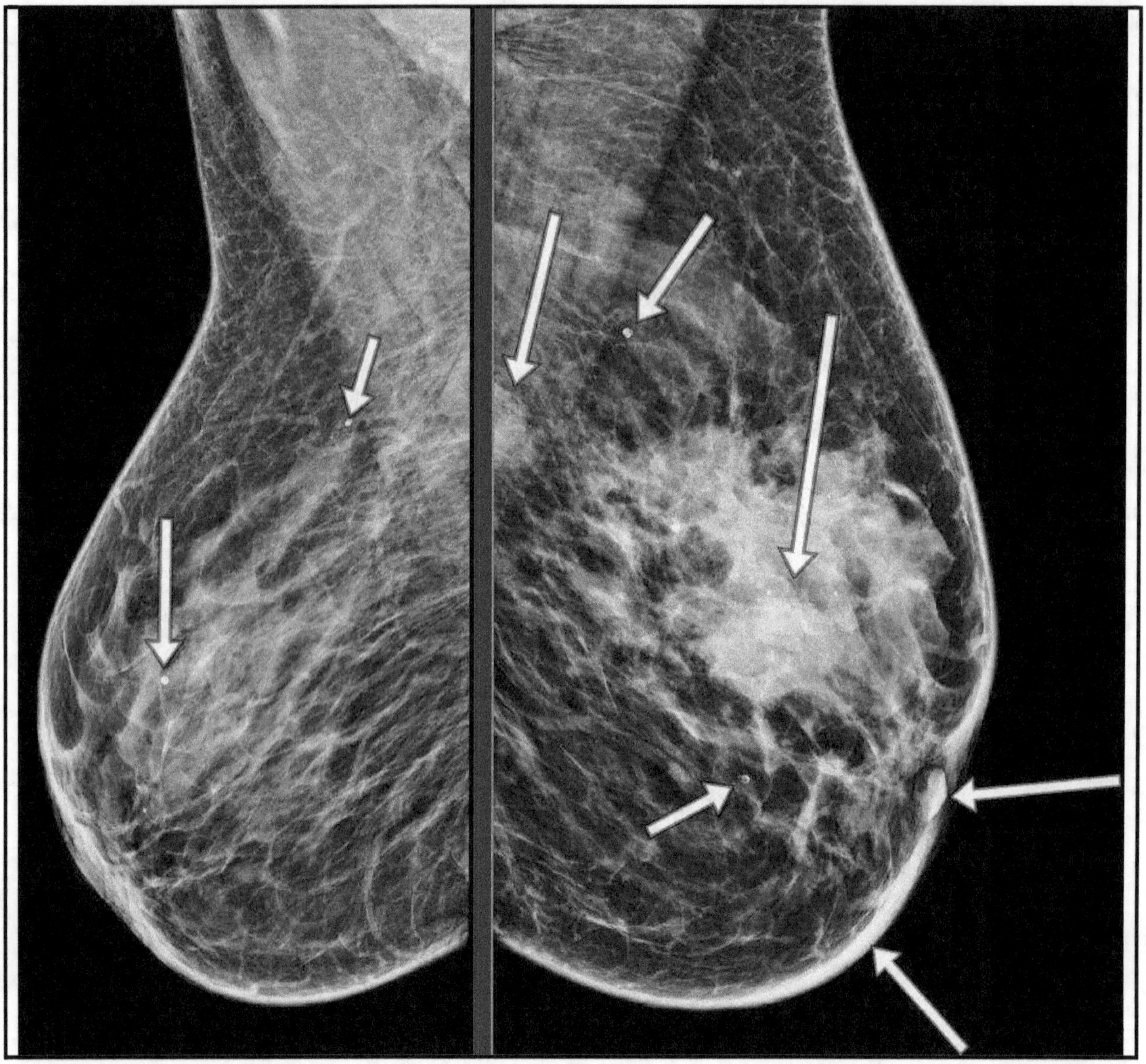

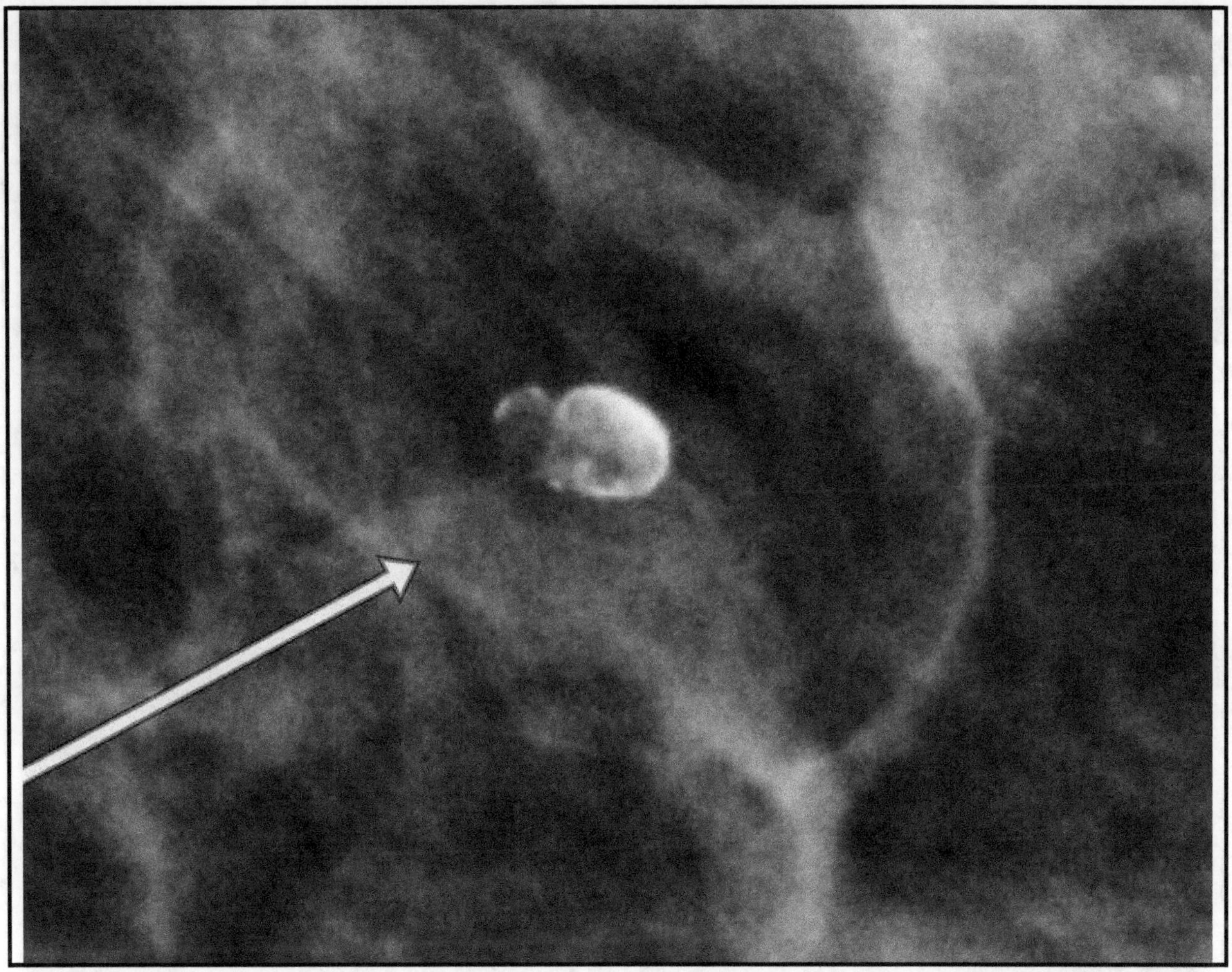

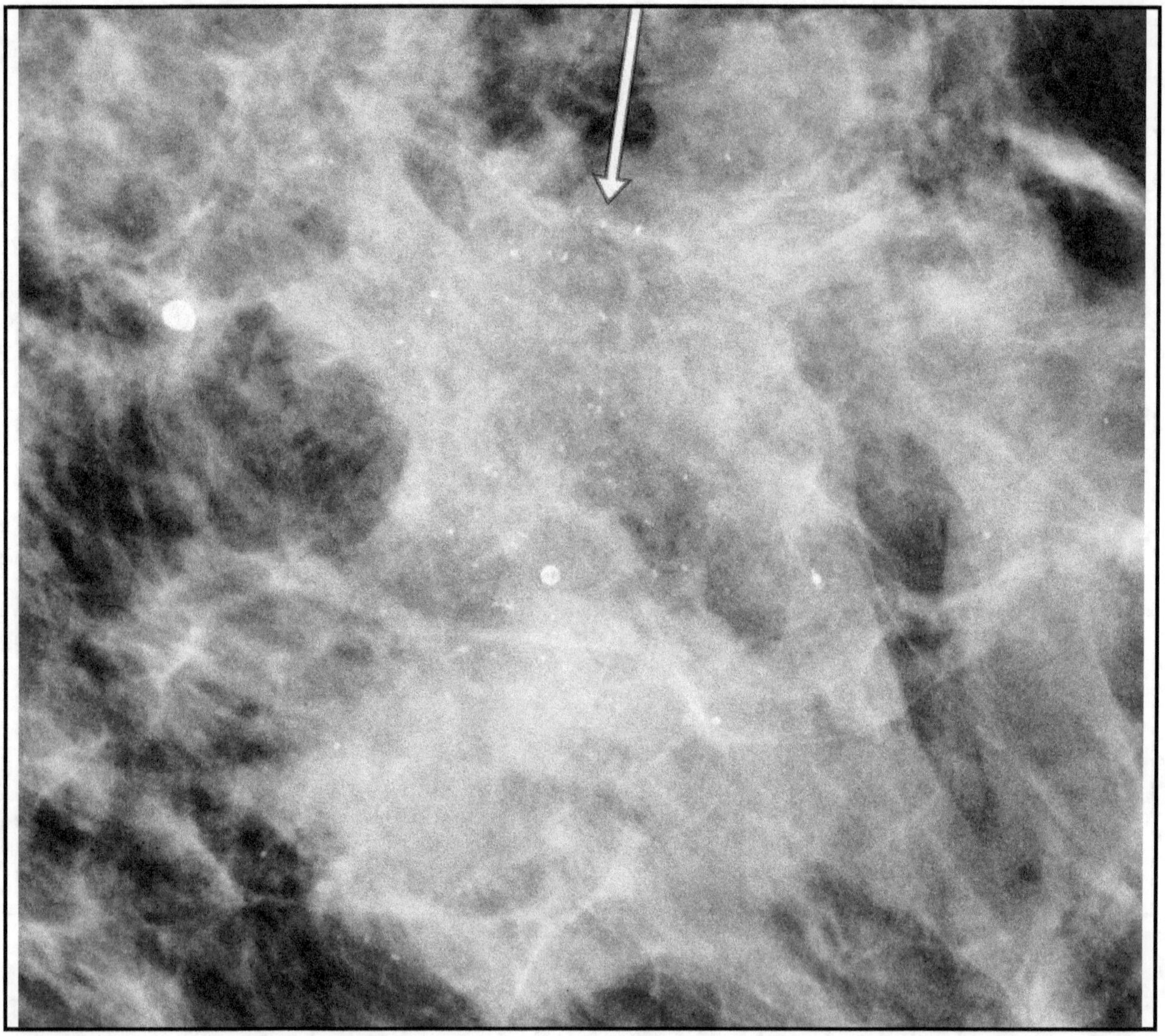

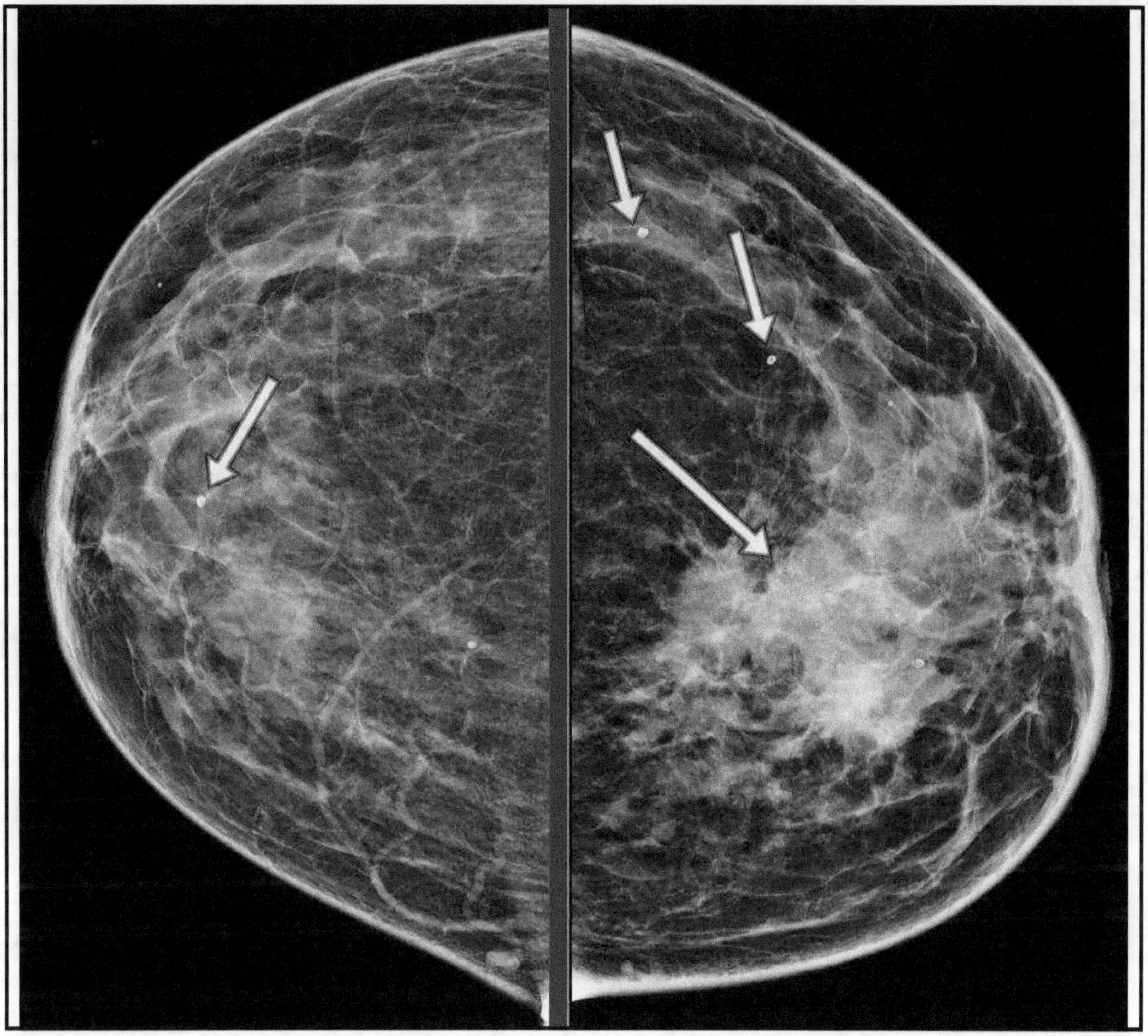

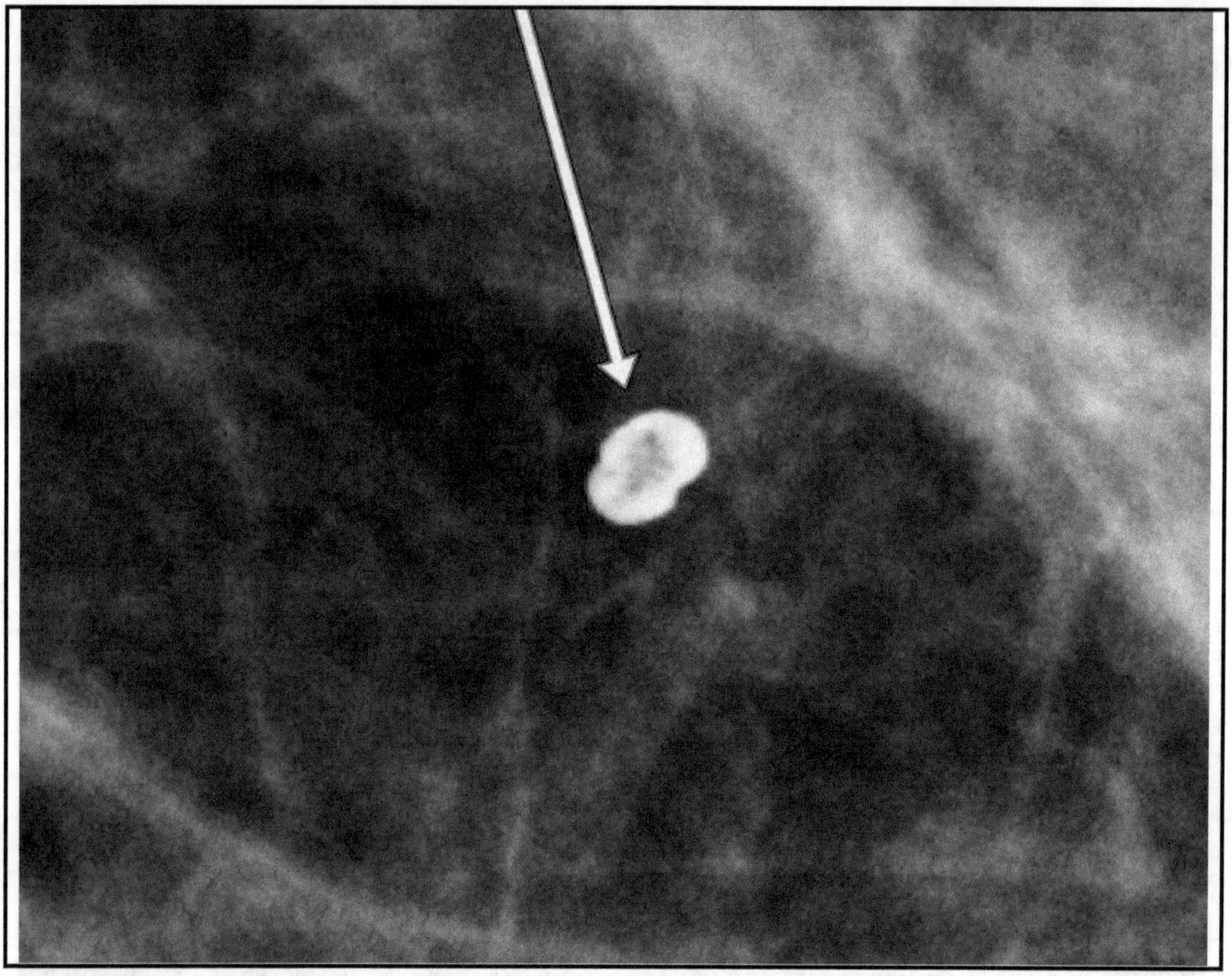

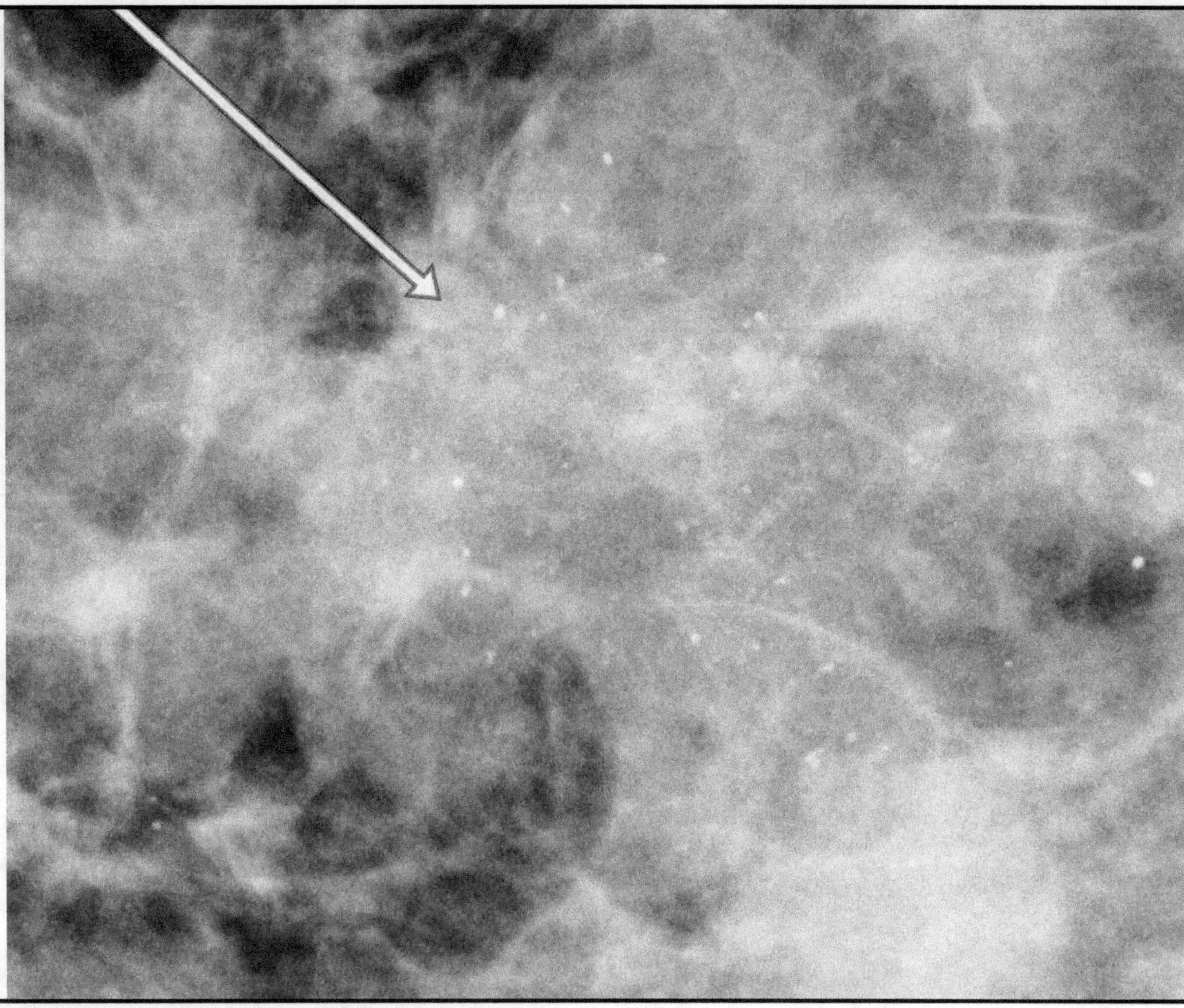

RIGHT BREAST	
Breast Parenchymal Density	***Heterogeneously dense, may obscure small masses (ACR C)***
Focal Mass	None
Asymmetric Density	None
Parenchymal Distortion	None
Calcification	***Skin calcification***
Skin Thickening	None
Axillary Nodes	None

LEFT BREAST	
Breast Parenchymal Density	***Heterogeneously dense, may obscure small masses (ACR C)***
Focal Mass	None
Asymmetric Density	***Upper central multifocal areas of focal asymmetries associated with amorphous micro-calcification***
Parenchymal Distortion	None
Calcification	***Amorphous Micro-Calcification / Skin Calcification***
Skin Thickening	***Positive /Nipple Retraction***
Axillary Nodes	None

IMPRESSION:

RIGHT BREAST: (BI-RADS 2)
LEFT BREAST: (BI-RADS 5)

RECOMMENDATION: Histopathological Correlation

CASE 73: 45 -year-old female /right conservative breast surgery	
Right MLO	Left MLO
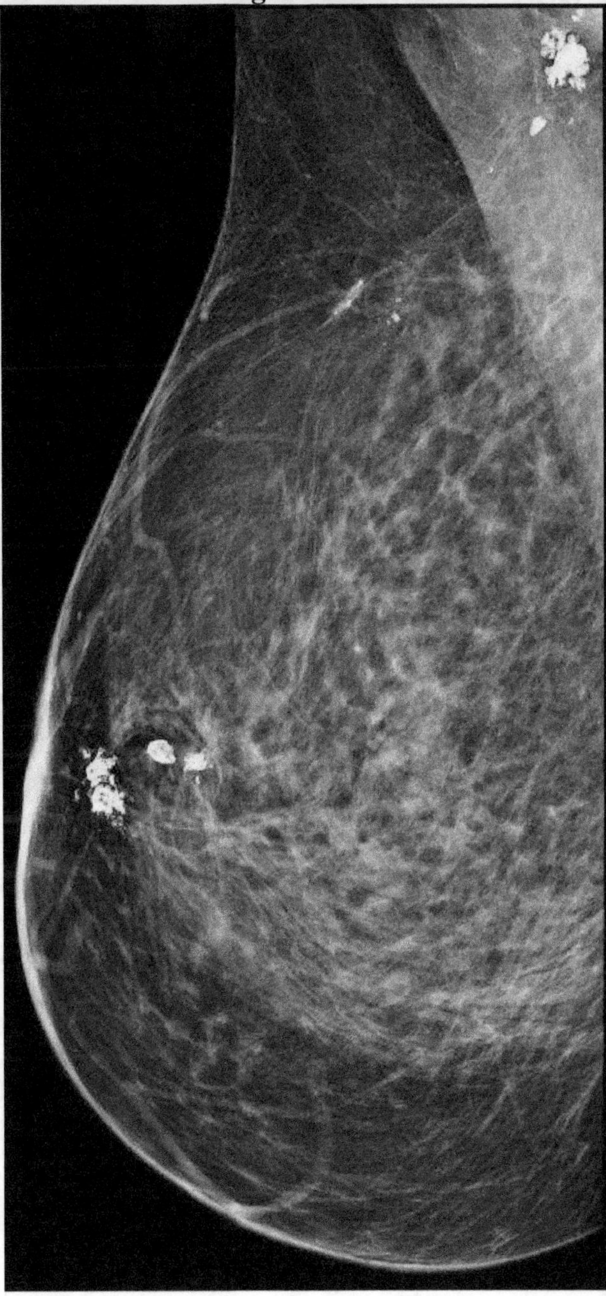	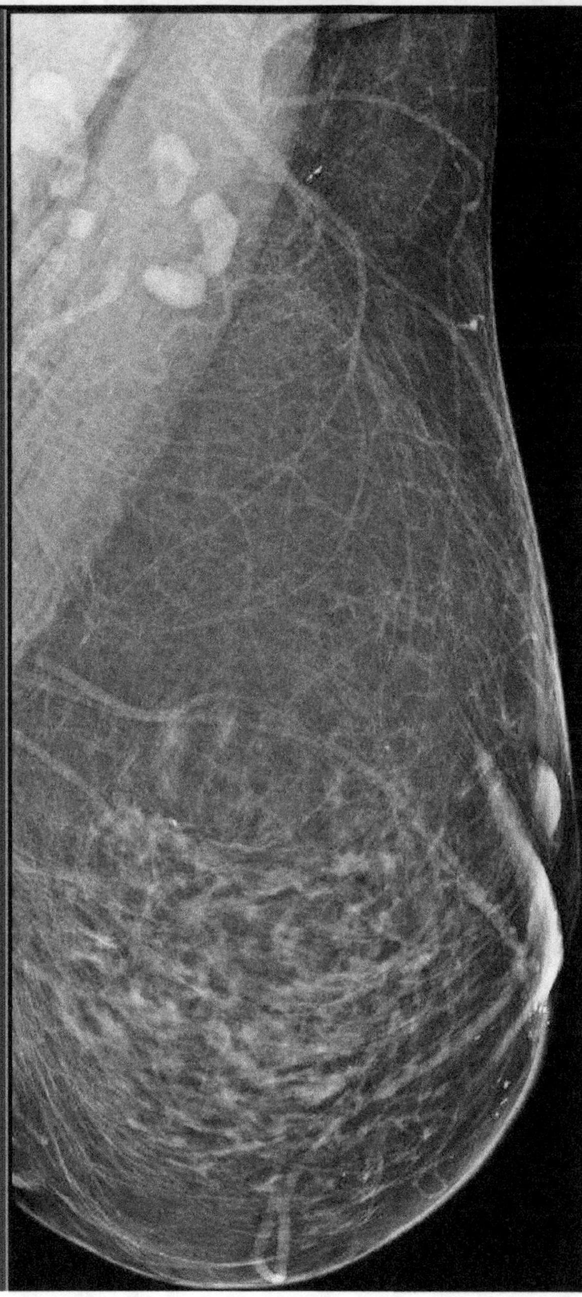

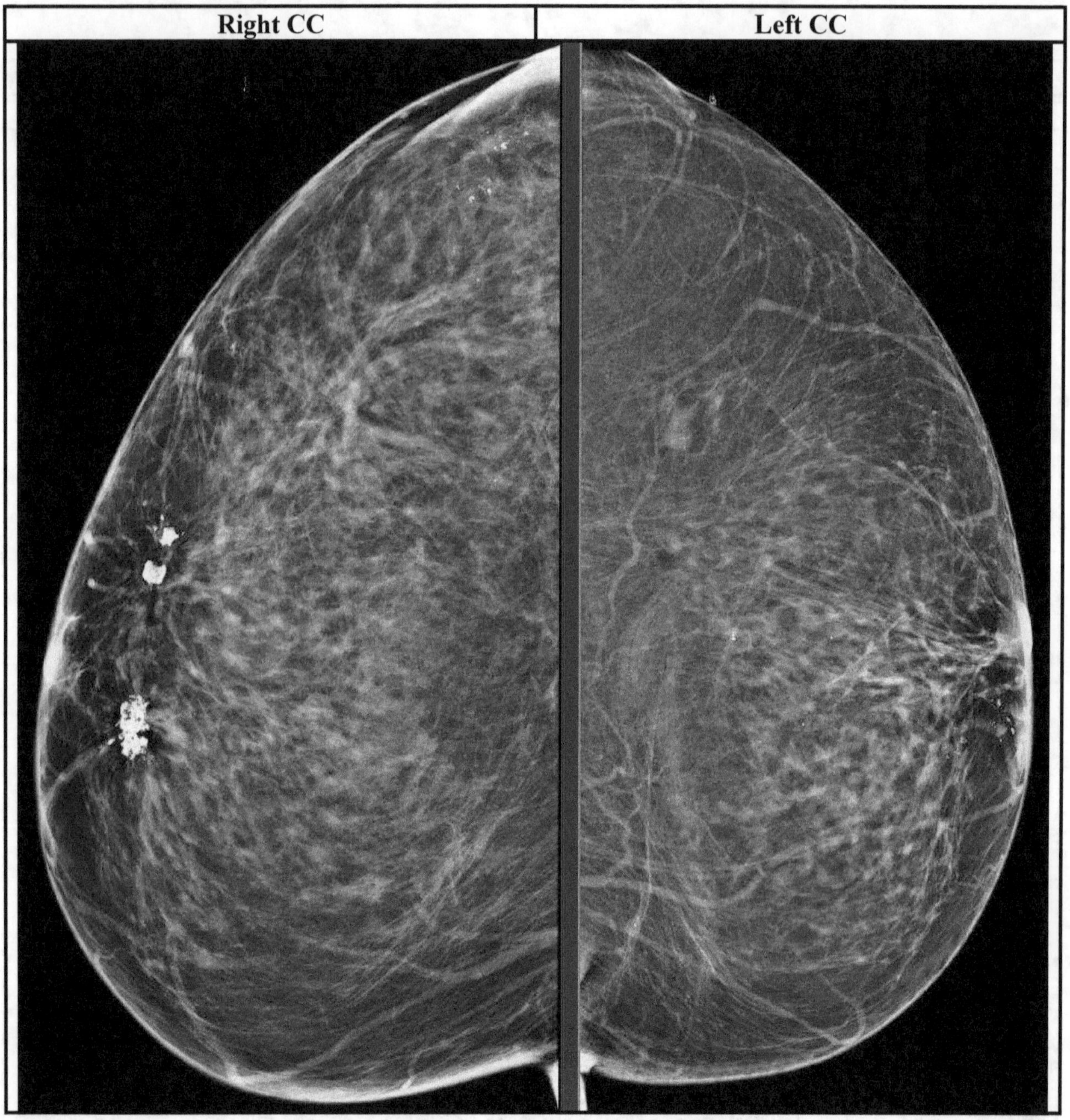
Right CC
Left CC

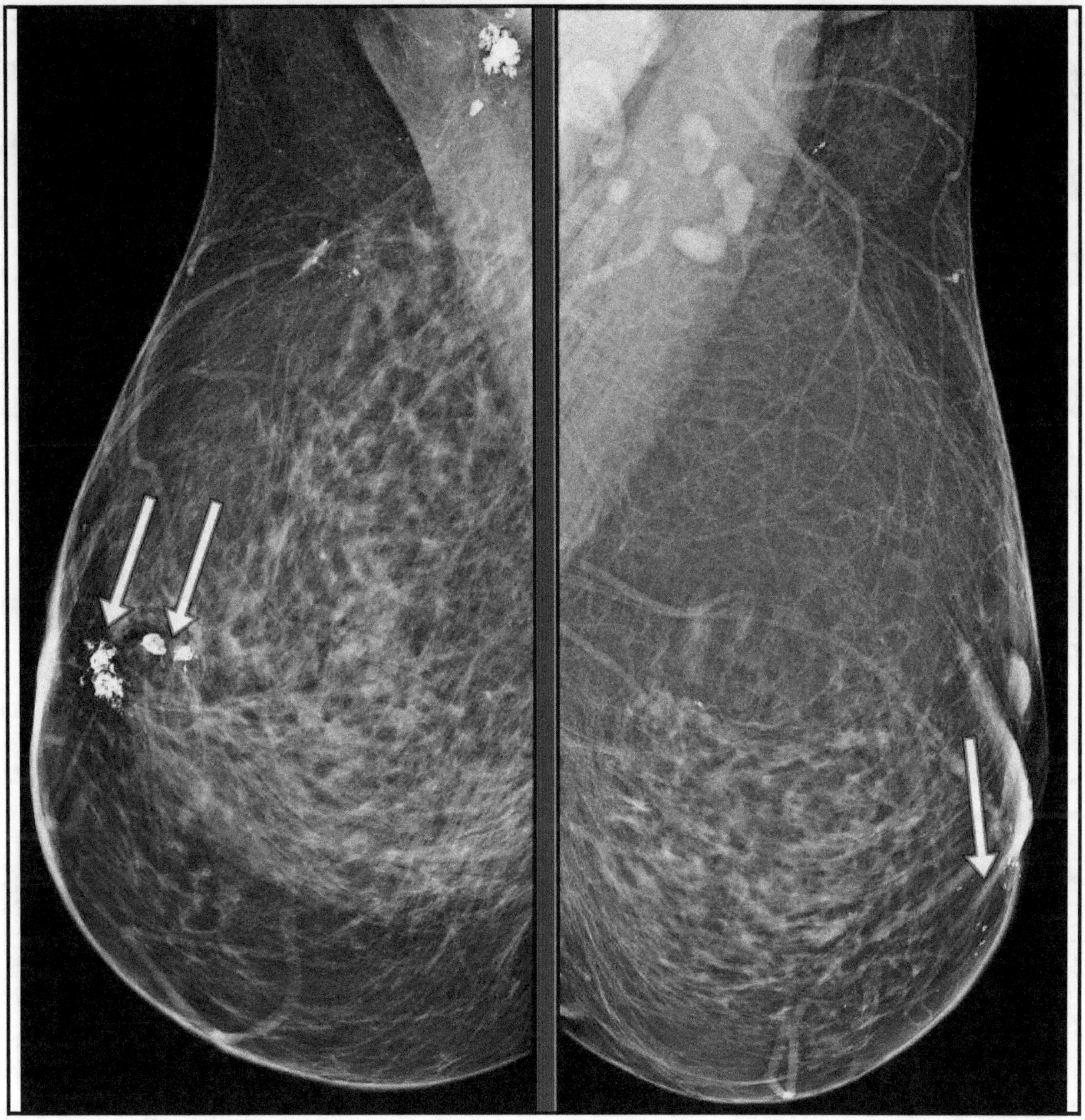

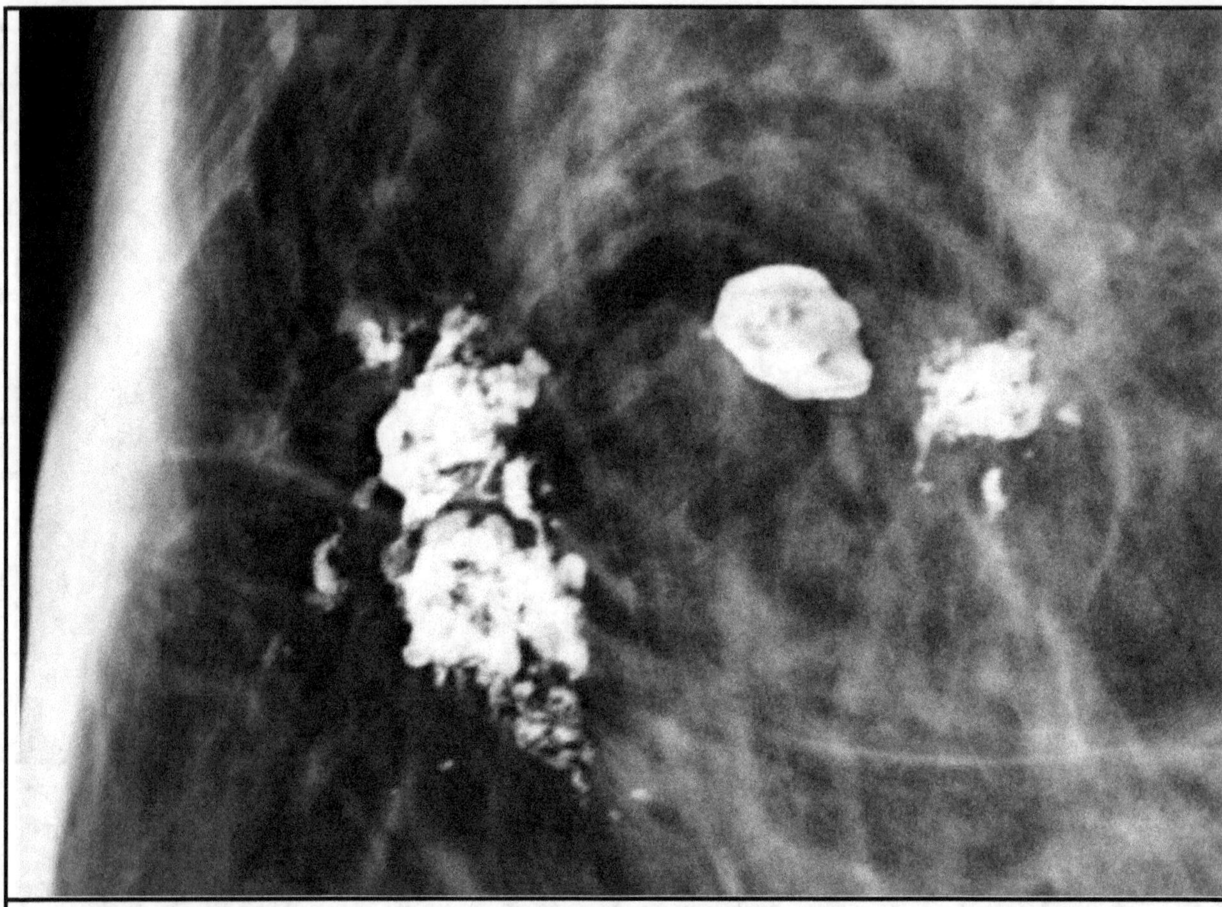

RIGHT BREAST	
Breast Parenchymal Density	***Scattered areas of fibroglandular density (ACR B)***
Focal Mass	None
Asymmetric Density	None
Parenchymal Distortion	None
Calcification	***Dystrophic calcification***
Skin Thickening	None
Axillary Nodes	None

LEFT BREAST	
Breast Parenchymal Density	***Scattered areas of fibroglandular density (ACR B)***
Focal Mass	None
Asymmetric Density	None
Parenchymal Distortion	None
Calcification	***Skin calcification***
Skin Thickening	None
Axillary Nodes	None

IMPRESSION:

RIGHT BREAST: (BI-RADS 2)

LEFT BREAST: (BI-RADS 2)
RECOMMENDATION: Routine Annual Follow-Up

CASE 74: 47-year-old female /screening

Right MLO	Left MLO

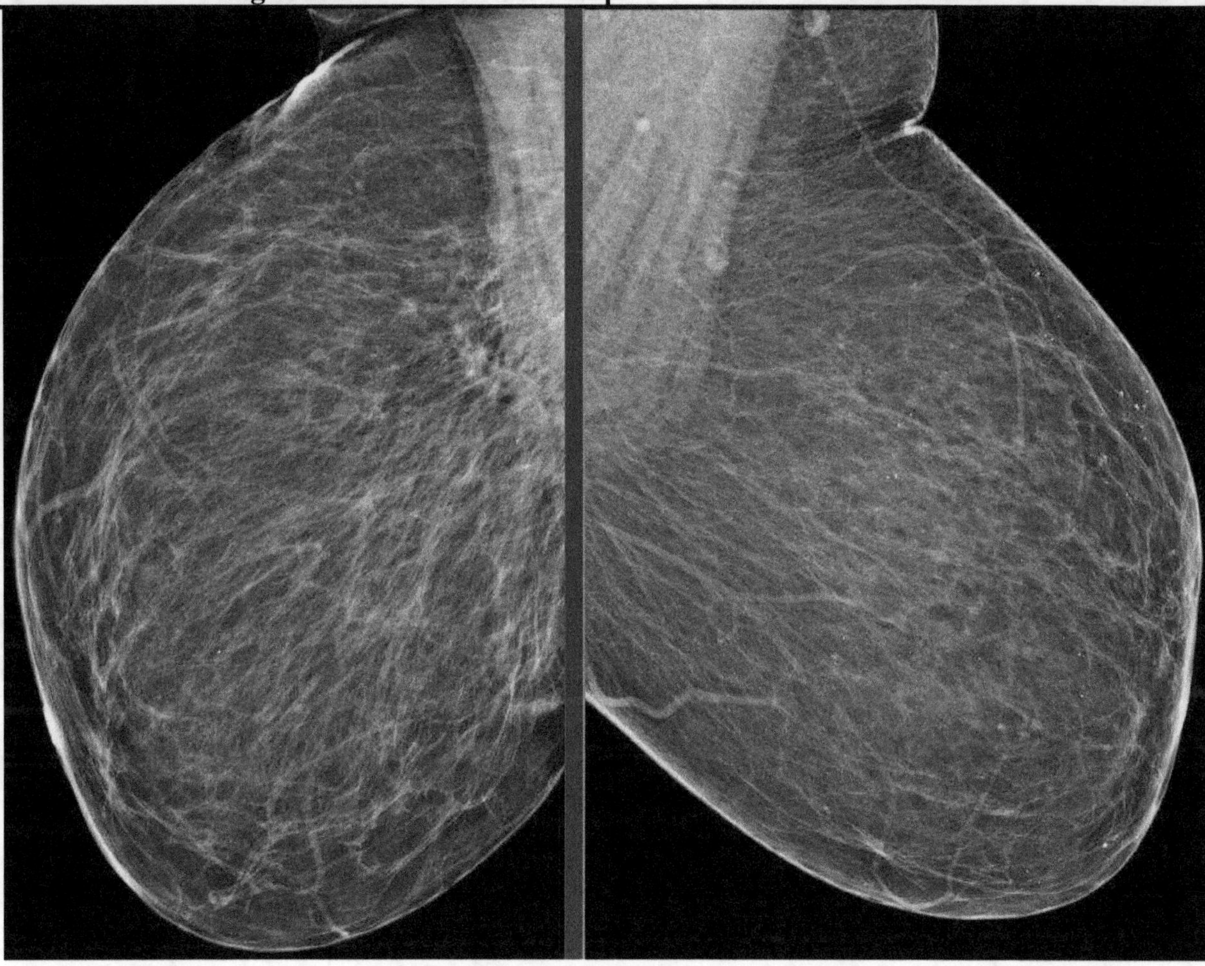

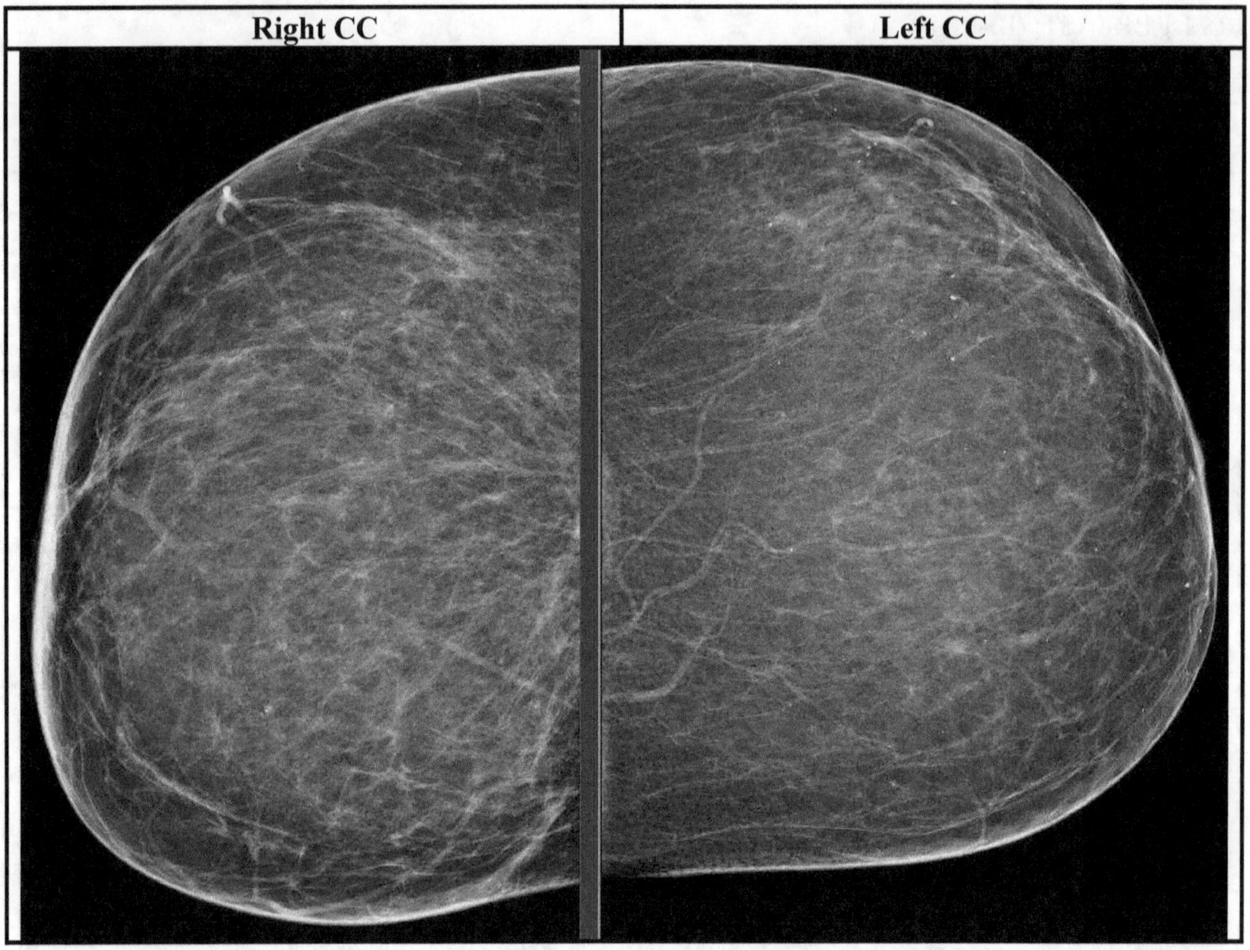
Right CC
Left CC

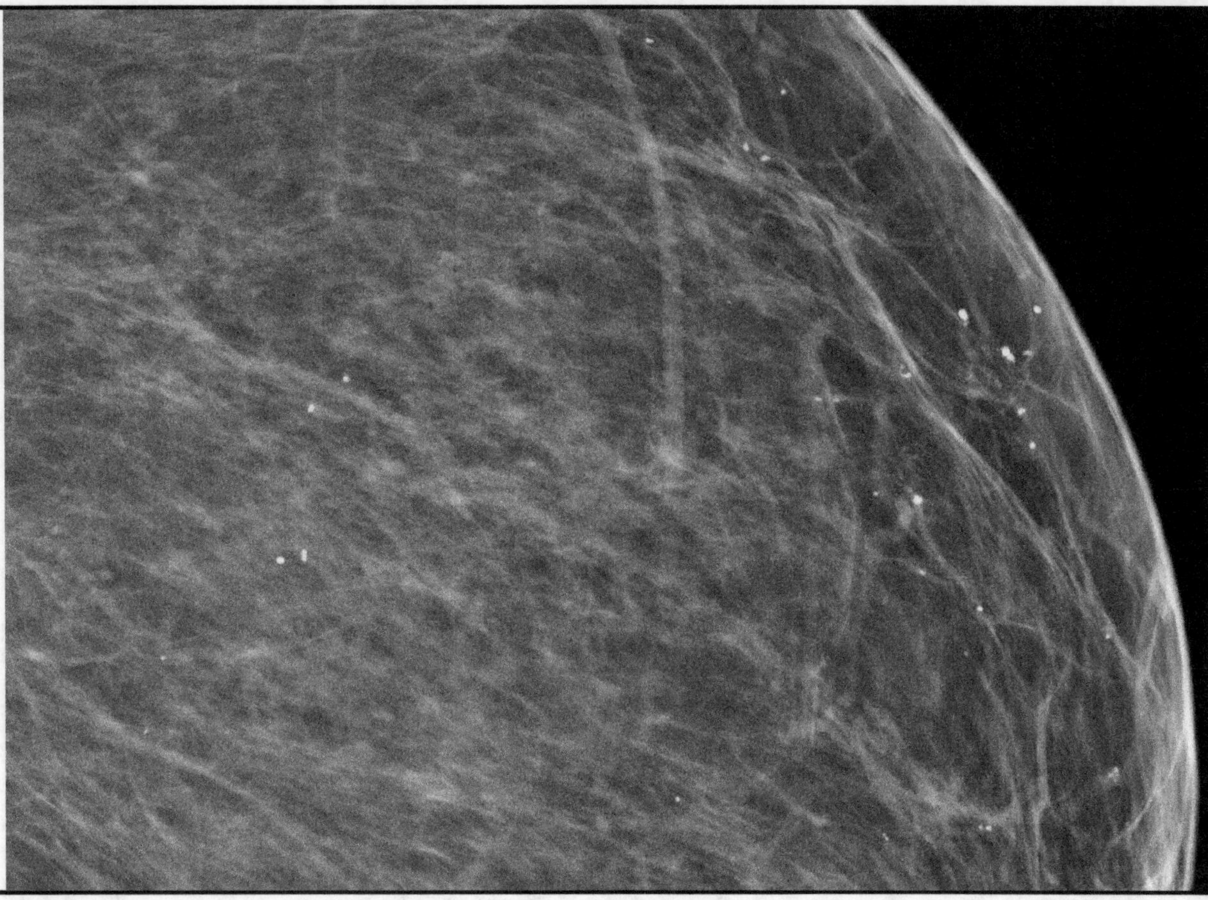

RIGHT BREAST	
Breast Parenchymal Density	***Scattered areas of fibroglandular density (ACR B)***
Focal Mass	None
Asymmetric Density	None
Parenchymal Distortion	None
Calcification	***Skin calcification***
Skin Thickening	None
Axillary Nodes	None

LEFT BREAST	
Breast Parenchymal Density	***Almost entirely fatty (ACR A)***
Focal Mass	None
Asymmetric Density	None
Parenchymal Distortion	None
Calcification	***Diffuse skin calcification***
Skin Thickening	None
Axillary Nodes	None

<u>IMPRESSION:</u>

RIGHT BREAST: (BI-RADS 2)

LEFT BREAST: (BI-RADS 2)
RECOMMENDATION: Routine Annual screening

CASE 75: 53-year-old female /screening	
Right MLO	**Left MLO**

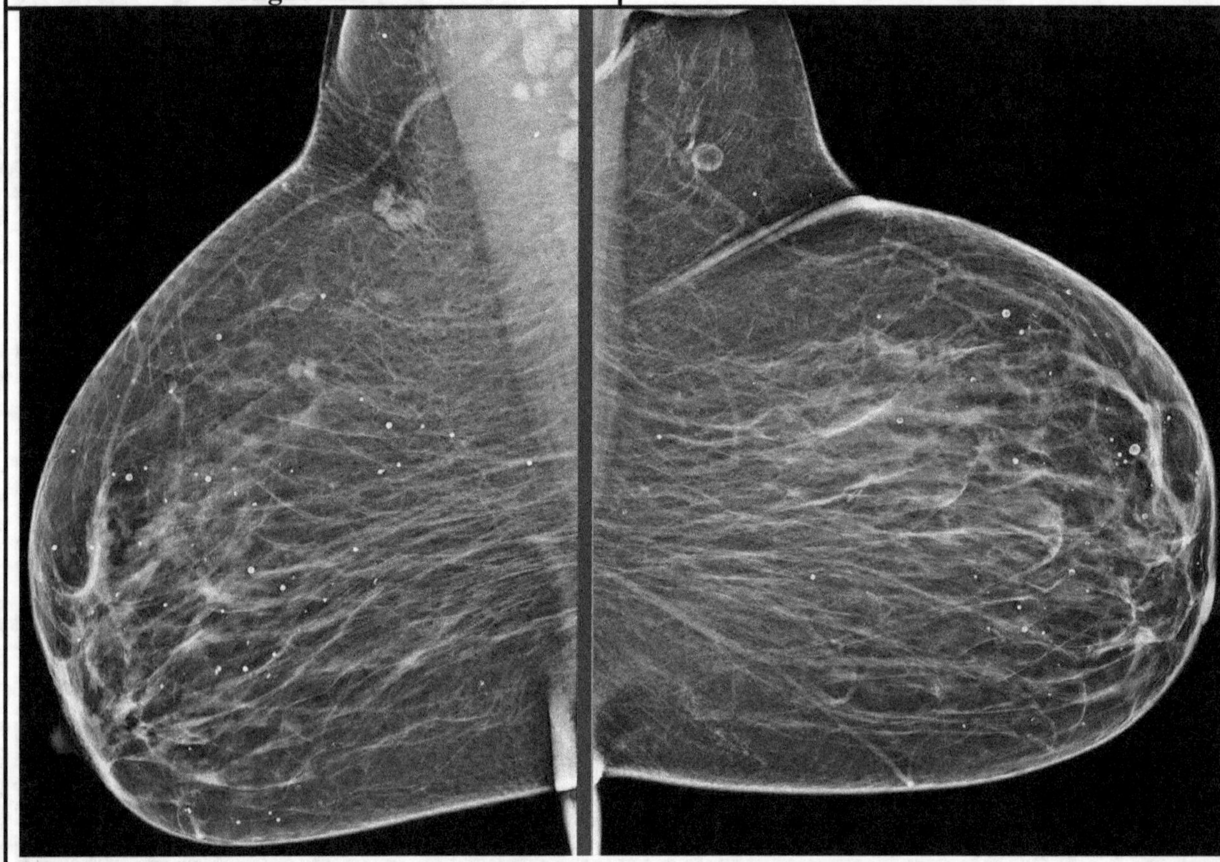

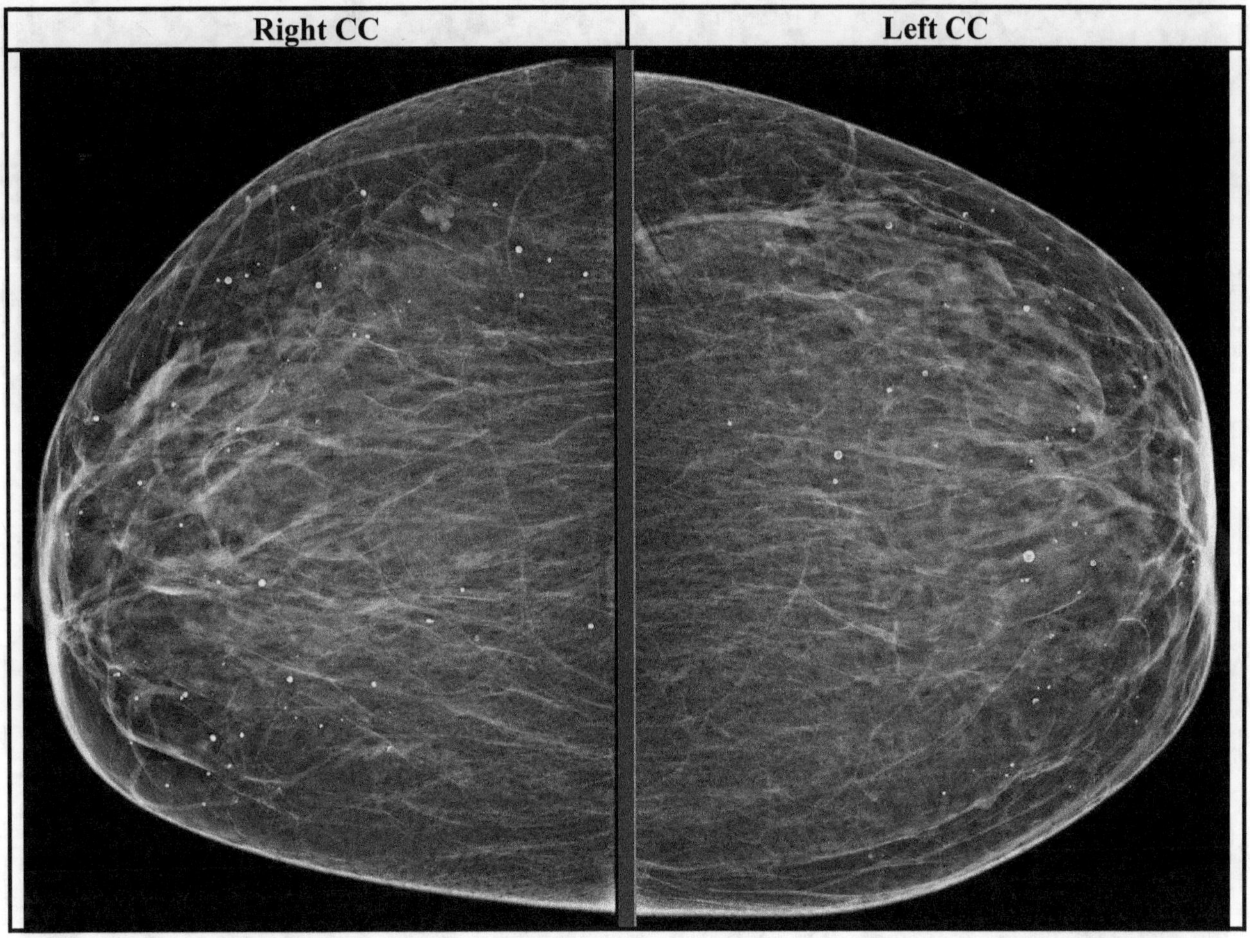
Right CC
Left CC

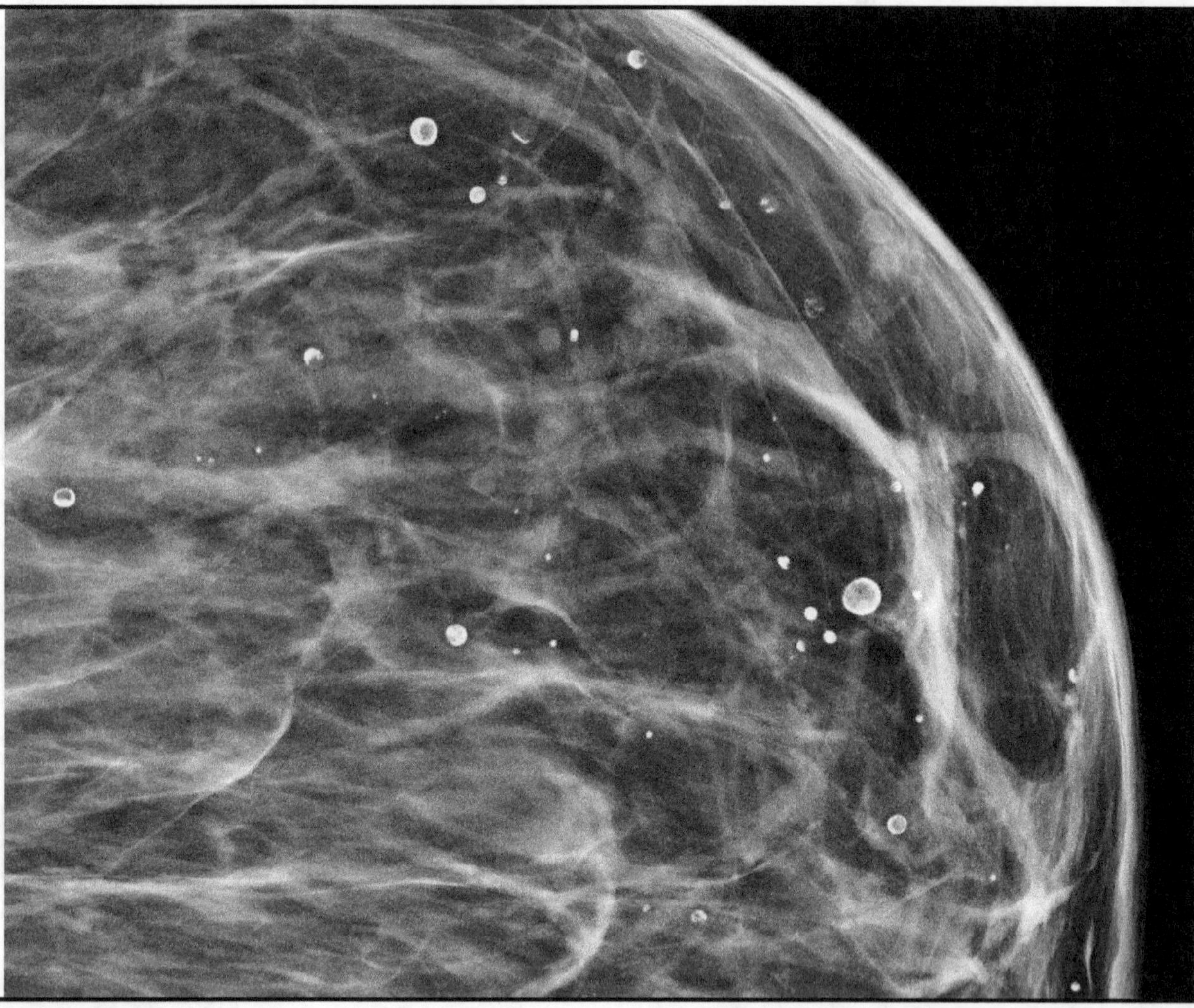

RIGHT BREAST	
Breast Parenchymal Density	***Scattered areas of fibroglandular density (ACR B)***
Focal Mass	None
Asymmetric Density	None
Parenchymal Distortion	None
Calcification	***Diffuse skin calcification***
Skin Thickening	None
Axillary Nodes	None

LEFT BREAST	
Breast Parenchymal Density	***Scattered areas of fibroglandular density (ACR B)***
Focal Mass	None
Asymmetric Density	None
Parenchymal Distortion	None
Calcification	***Diffuse skin calcification***
Skin Thickening	None
Axillary Nodes	None

IMPRESSION:

RIGHT BREAST: (BI-RADS 2)
LEFT BREAST: (BI-RADS 2)

RECOMMENDATION: Routine Annual screening

CASE 76: 54-year-old female /screening

Right MLO	Left MLO

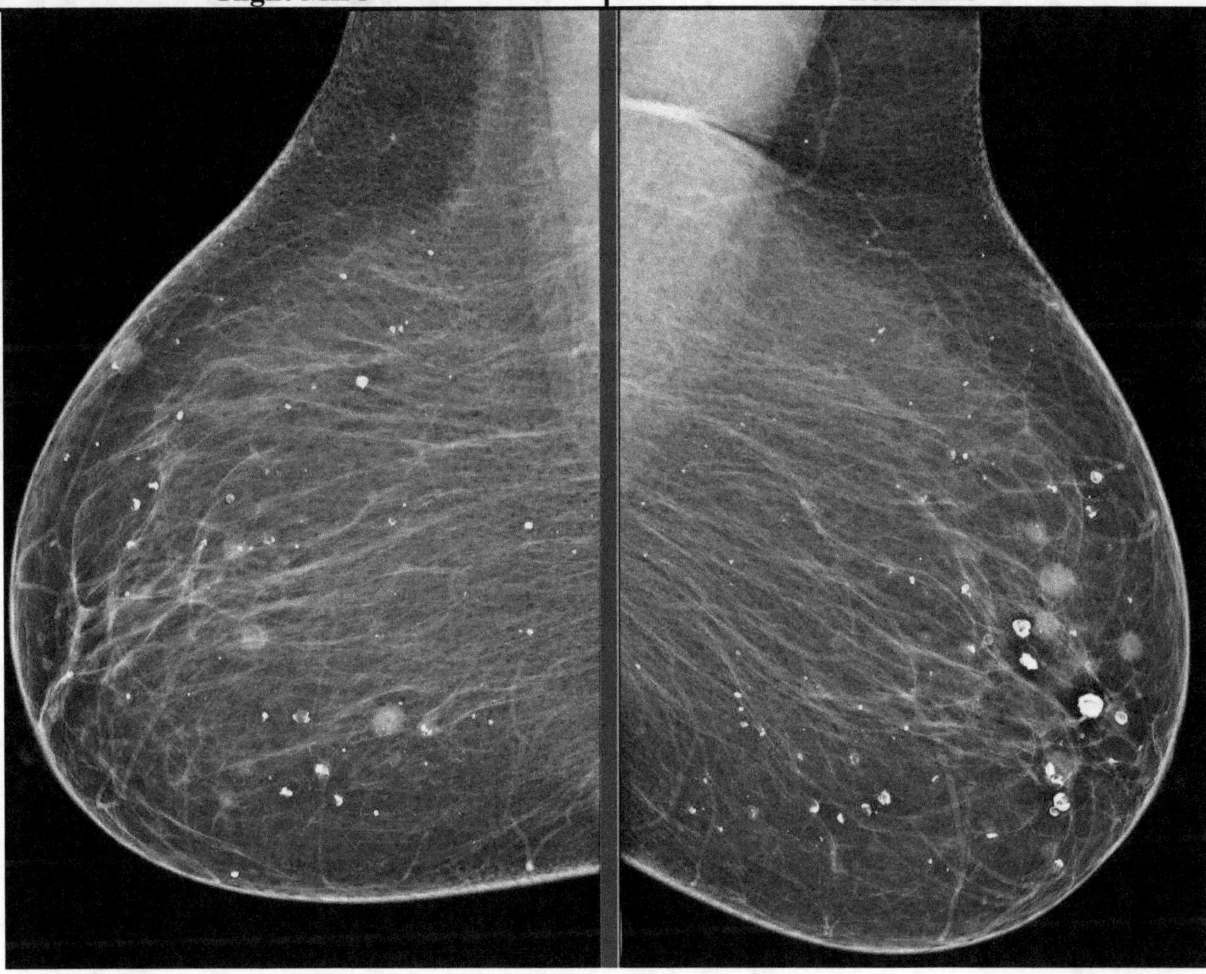

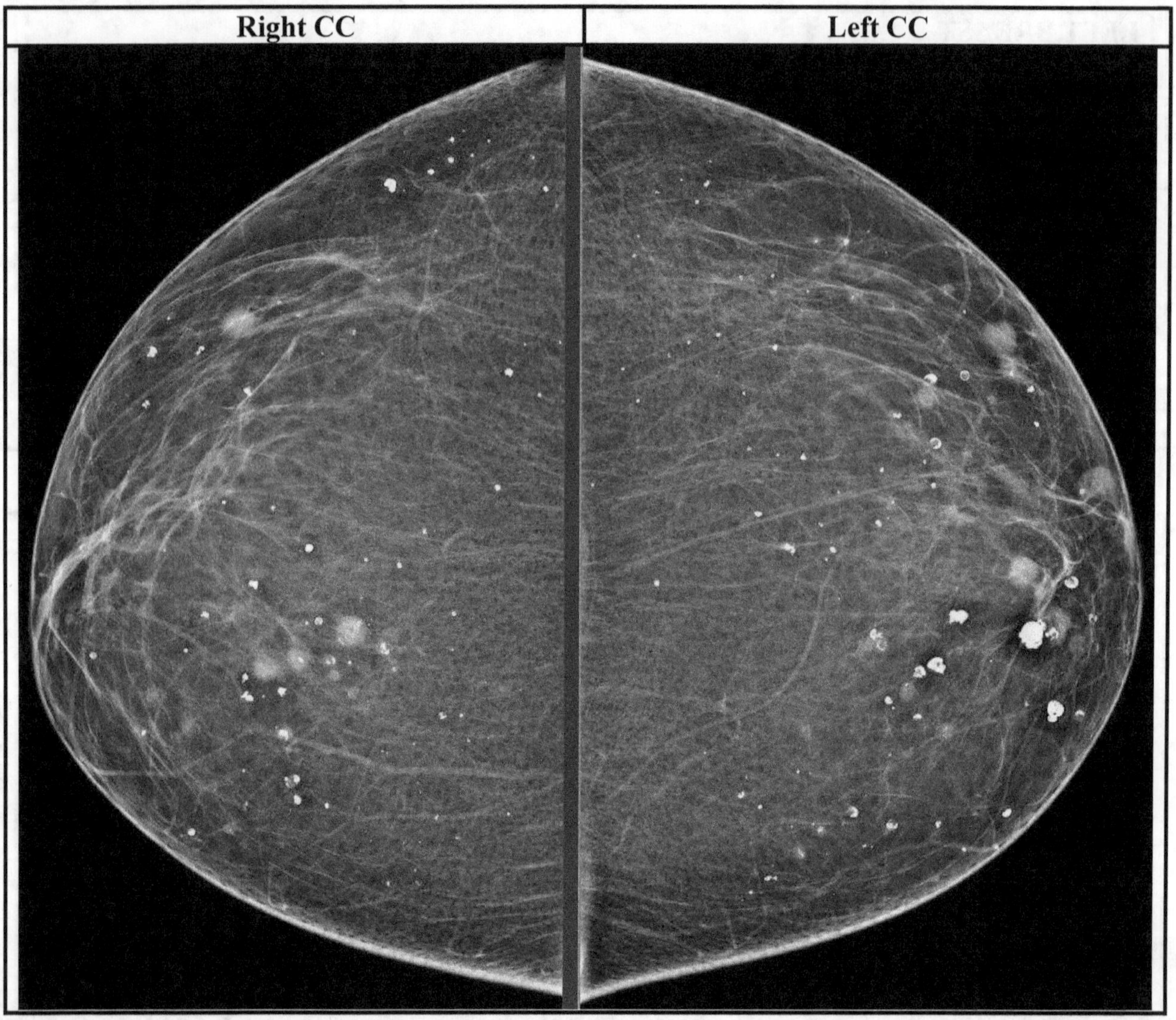
Right CC
Left CC

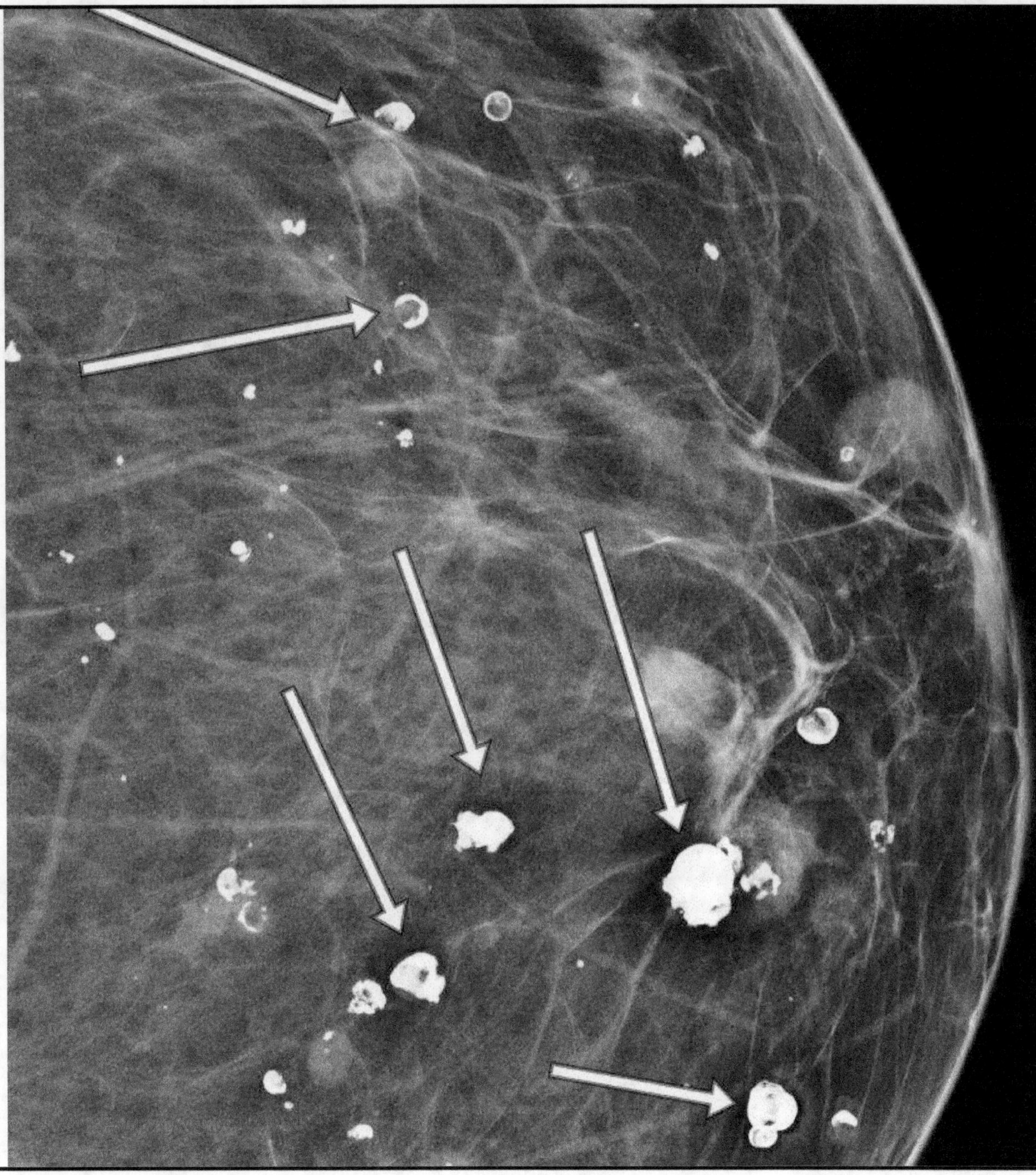

RIGHT BREAST	
Breast Parenchymal Density	***Scattered areas of fibroglandular density (ACR B)***
Focal Mass	***Involuted fibroadenomas***
Asymmetric Density	None
Parenchymal Distortion	None
Calcification	***Diffuse skin and coarse calcification***
Skin Thickening	None
Axillary Nodes	None

LEFT BREAST	
Breast Parenchymal Density	***Scattered areas of fibroglandular density (ACR B)***
Focal Mass	***Involuted fibroadenomas***
Asymmetric Density	None
Parenchymal Distortion	None
Calcification	***Diffuse skin and coarse calcification***
Skin Thickening	None
Axillary Nodes	None

IMPRESSION:
RIGHT BREAST: (BI-RADS 2)
LEFT BREAST: (BI-RADS 2)

RECOMMENDATION: Routine Annual screening

CASE 77: 68-year-old female / diagnostic	
Right MLO	Left MLO

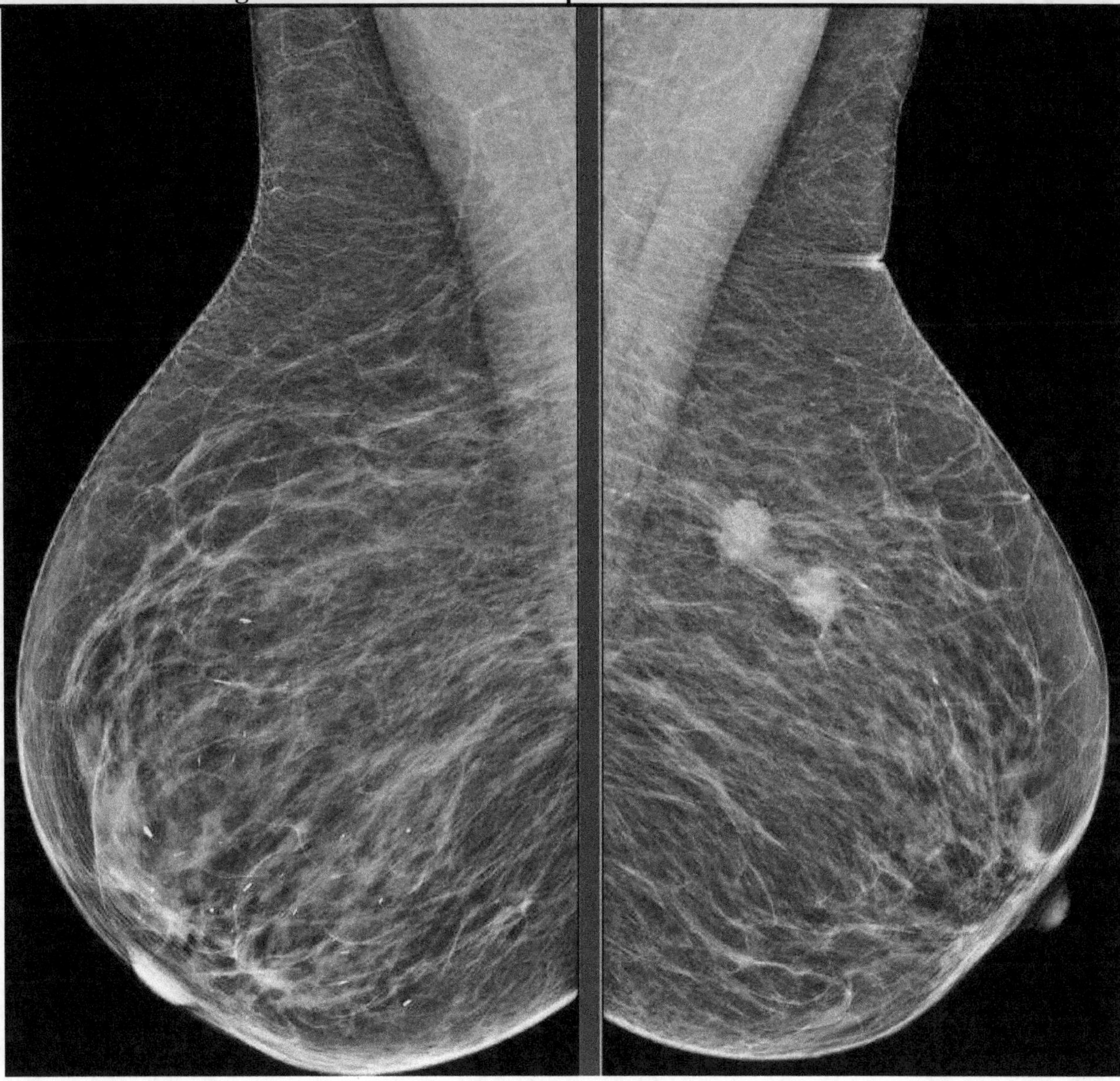

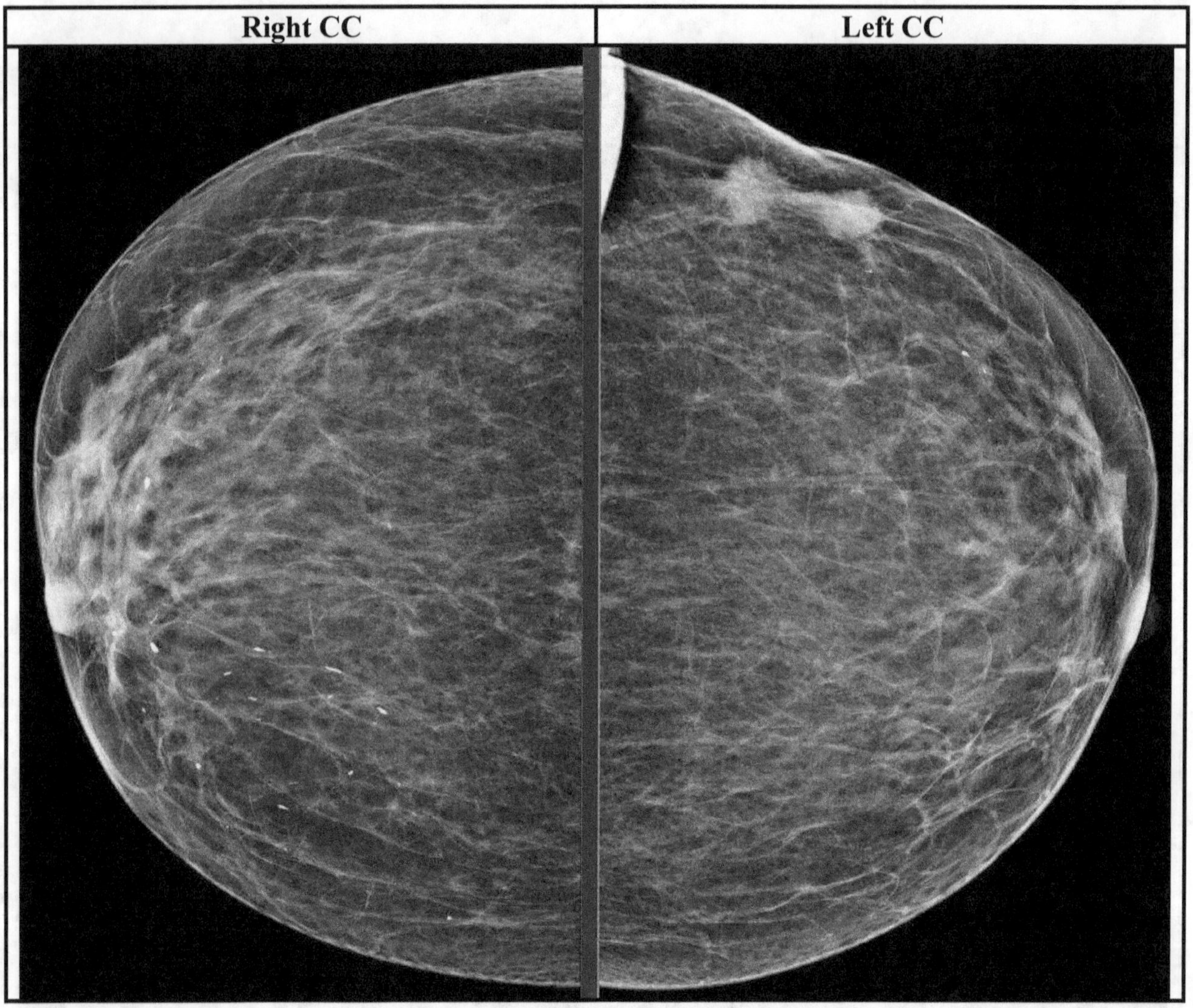
Right CC
Left CC

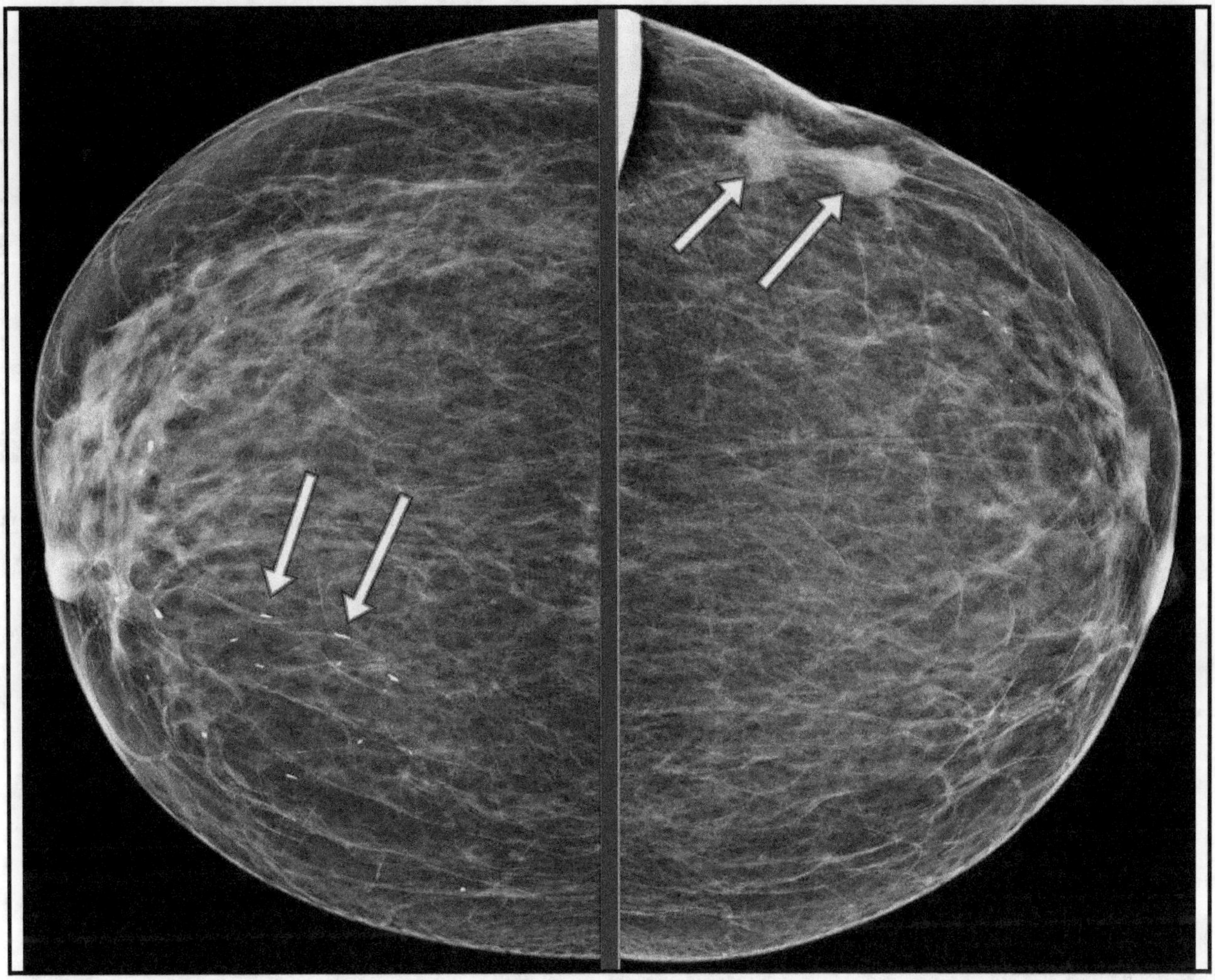

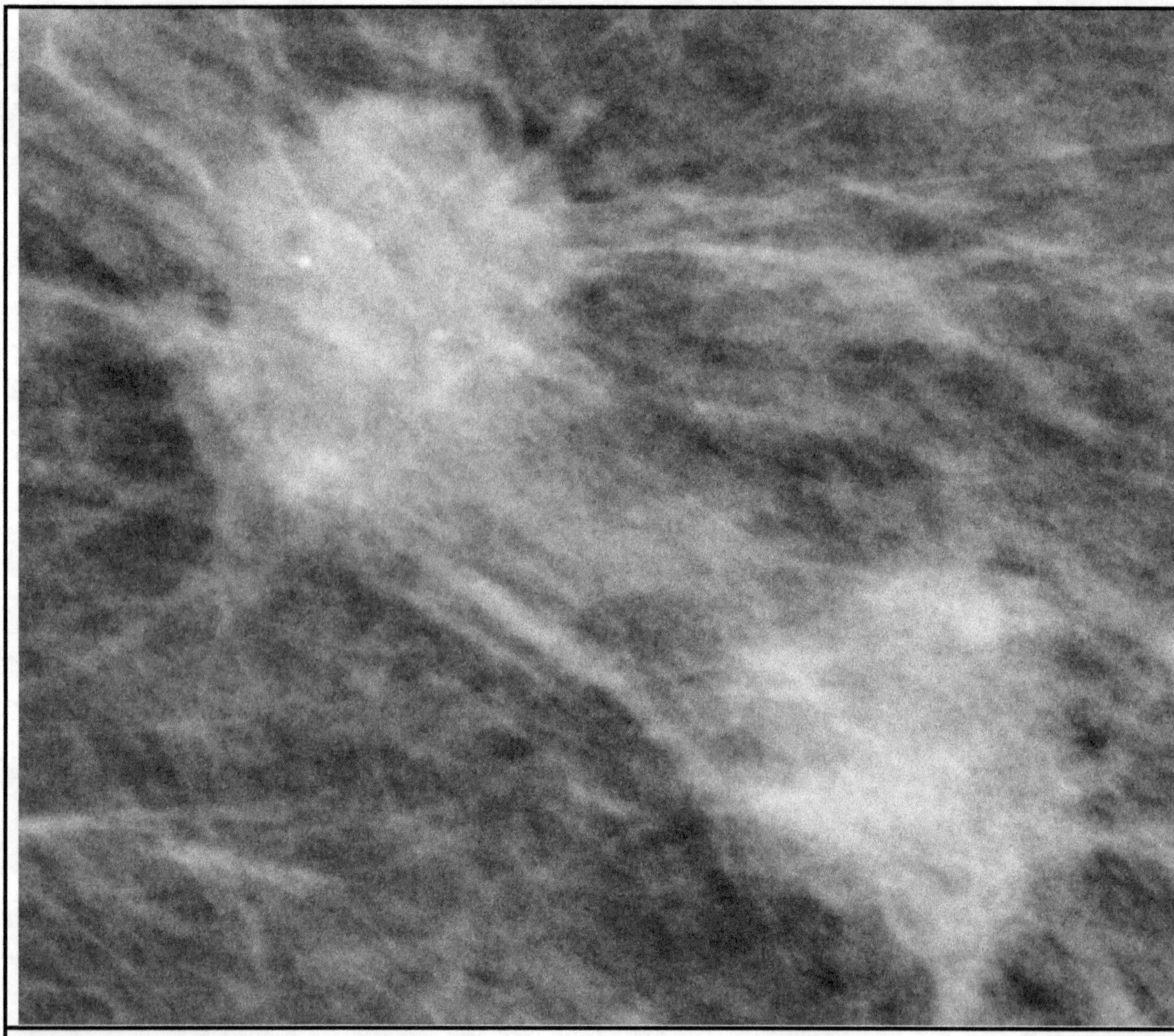

RIGHT BREAST	
Breast Parenchymal Density	***Scattered areas of fibroglandular density (ACR B)***
Focal Mass	None
Asymmetric Density	None
Parenchymal Distortion	None
Calcification	***Rod Like / Skin Calcification***
Skin Thickening	None
Axillary Nodes	None

LEFT BREAST	
Breast Parenchymal Density	***Scattered areas of fibroglandular density (ACR B)***
Focal Mass	***UOQ multifocal round spiculated mass lesions with associated amorphous micro-calcifications***
Asymmetric Density	None
Parenchymal Distortion	None
Calcification	***amorphous micro-calcifications***
Skin Thickening	None / ***Skin Retraction***
Axillary Nodes	None

IMPRESSION:

RIGHT BREAST: (BI-RADS 2)
LEFT BREAST: (BI-RADS 5)

RECOMMENDATION: Histopathological Correlation

CASE 78: 64-year-old female /screening

Right MLO	Left MLO

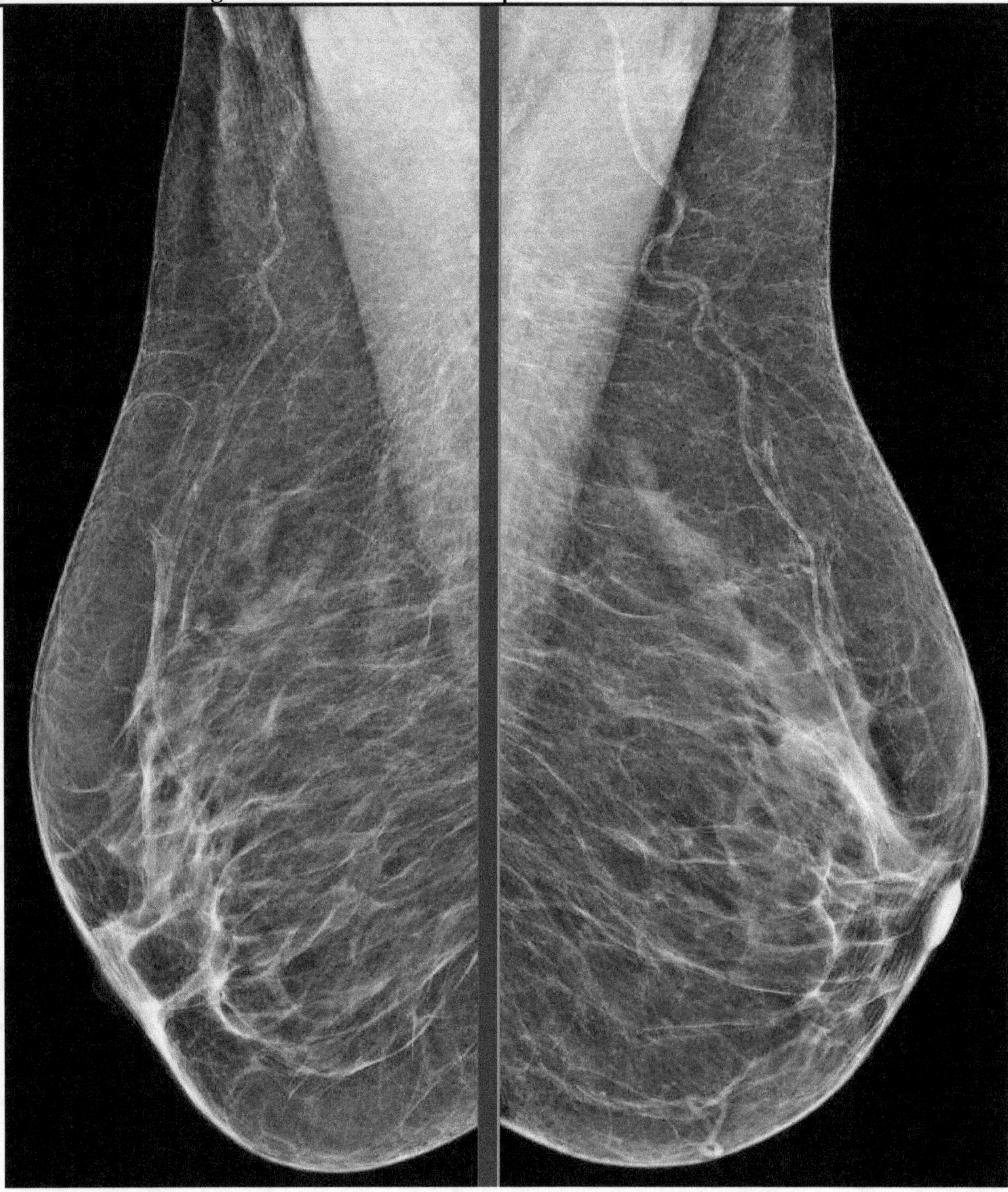

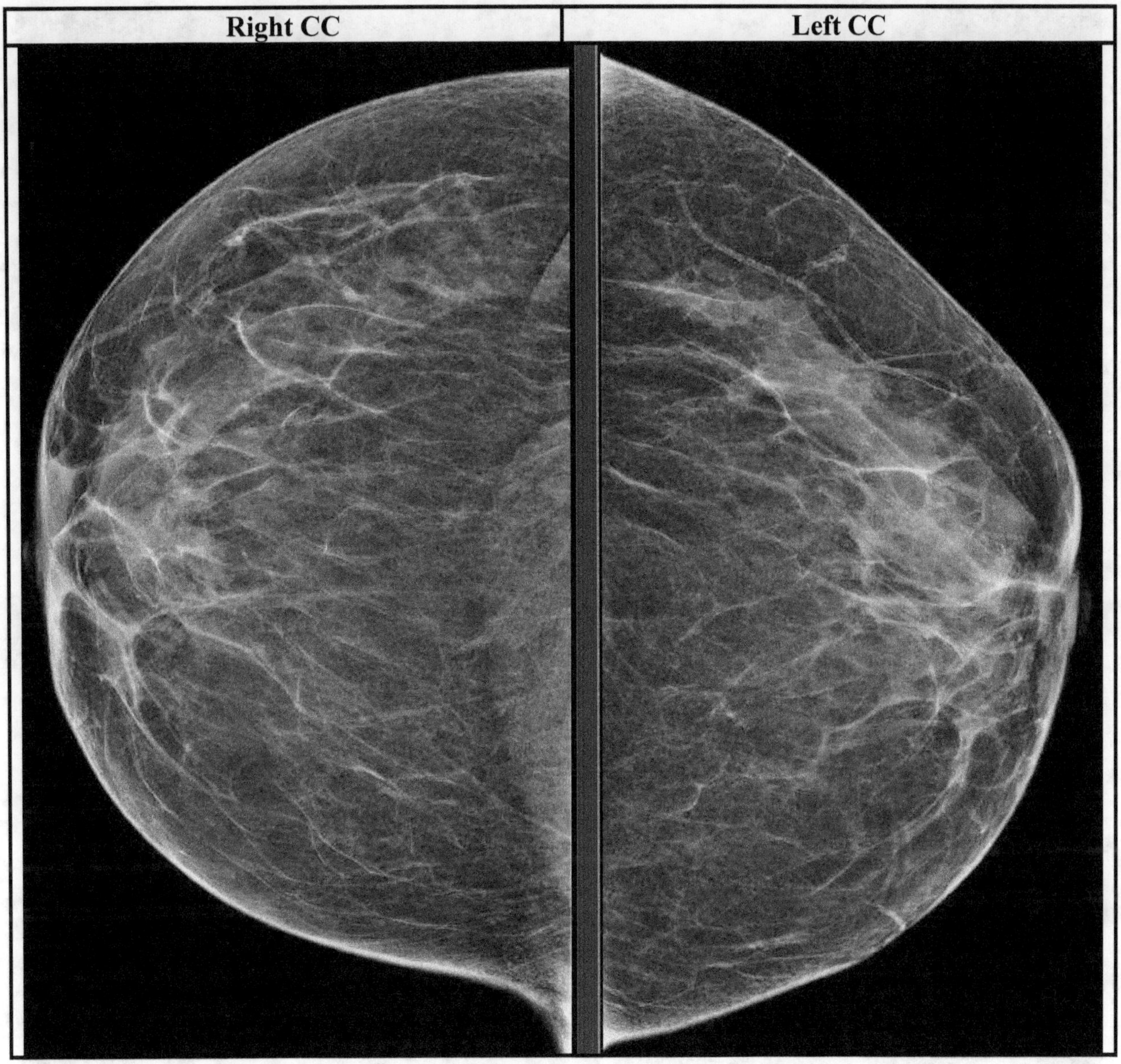
Right CC
Left CC

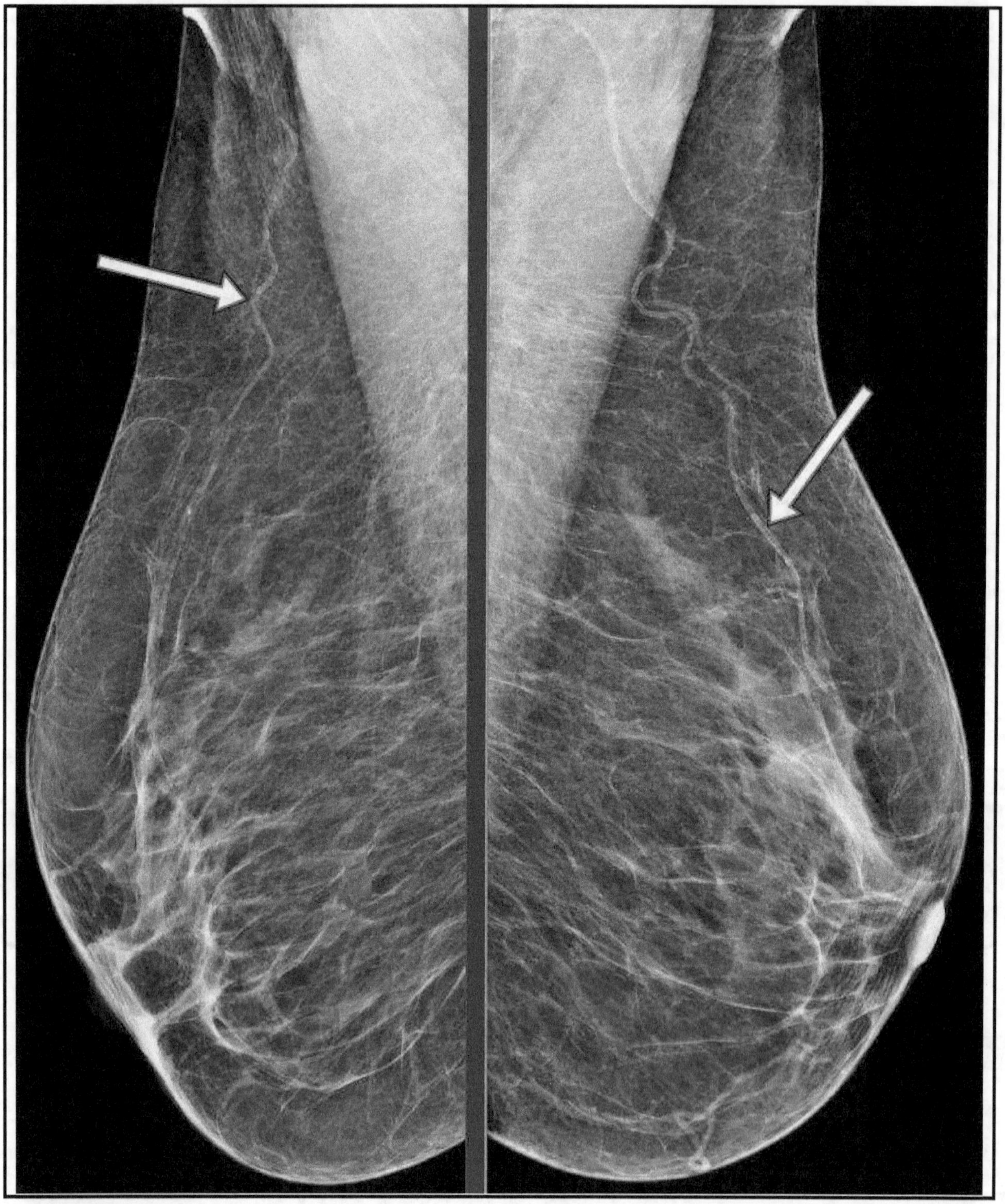

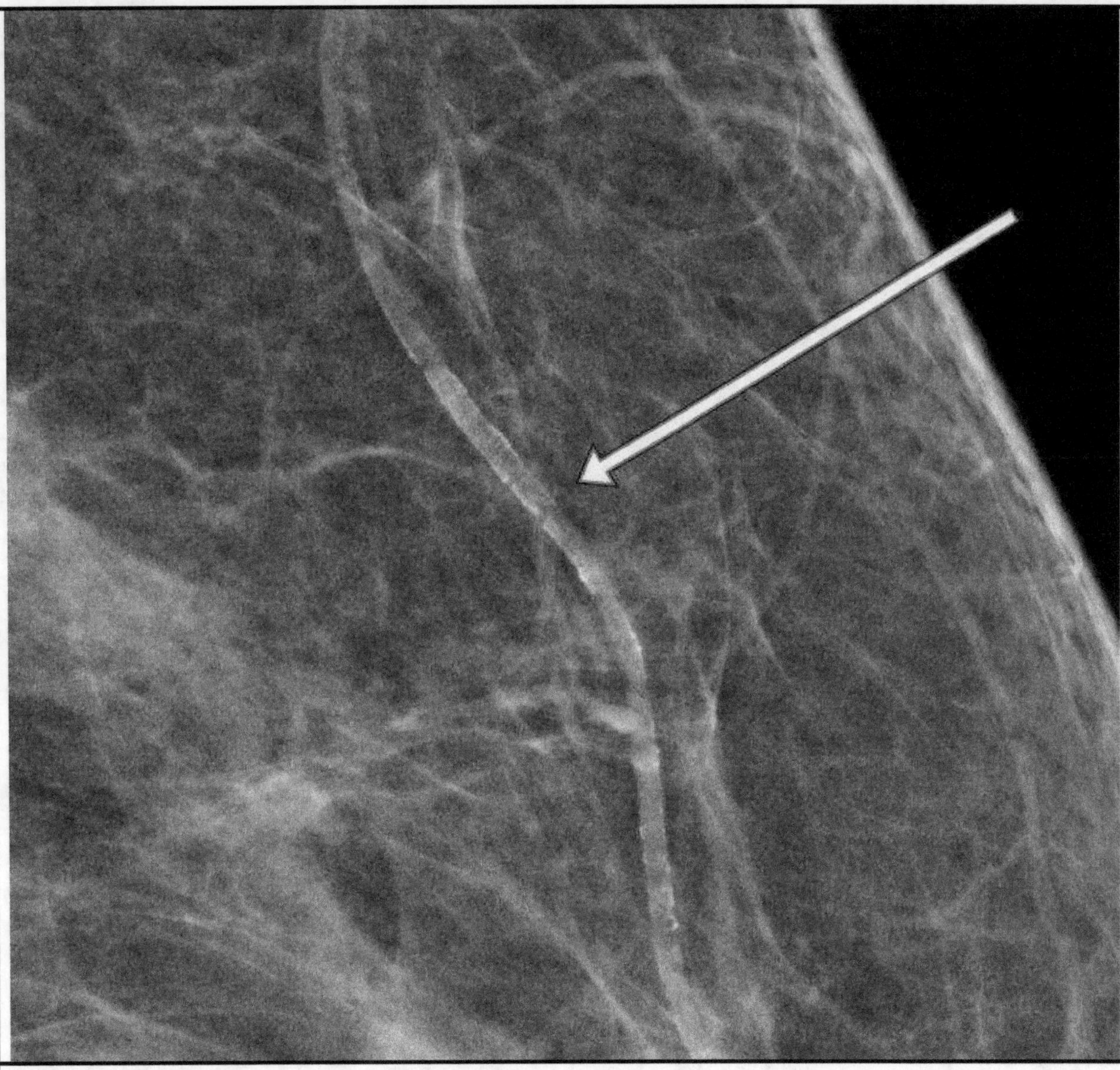

RIGHT BREAST	
Breast Parenchymal Density	***Scattered areas of fibroglandular density (ACR B)***
Focal Mass	None
Asymmetric Density	None
Parenchymal Distortion	None
Calcification	***Vascular calcification***
Skin Thickening	None
Axillary Nodes	None

LEFT BREAST	
Breast Parenchymal Density	***Scattered areas of fibroglandular density (ACR B)***
Focal Mass	None
Asymmetric Density	None
Parenchymal Distortion	None
Calcification	***Vascular calcification***
Skin Thickening	None
Axillary Nodes	None

IMPRESSION:

RIGHT BREAST: (BI-RADS 2)
LEFT BREAST: (BI-RADS 2)

RECOMMENDATION: Routine Annual screening

CASE 79: 53-year-old female /screening

Right MLO	Left MLO

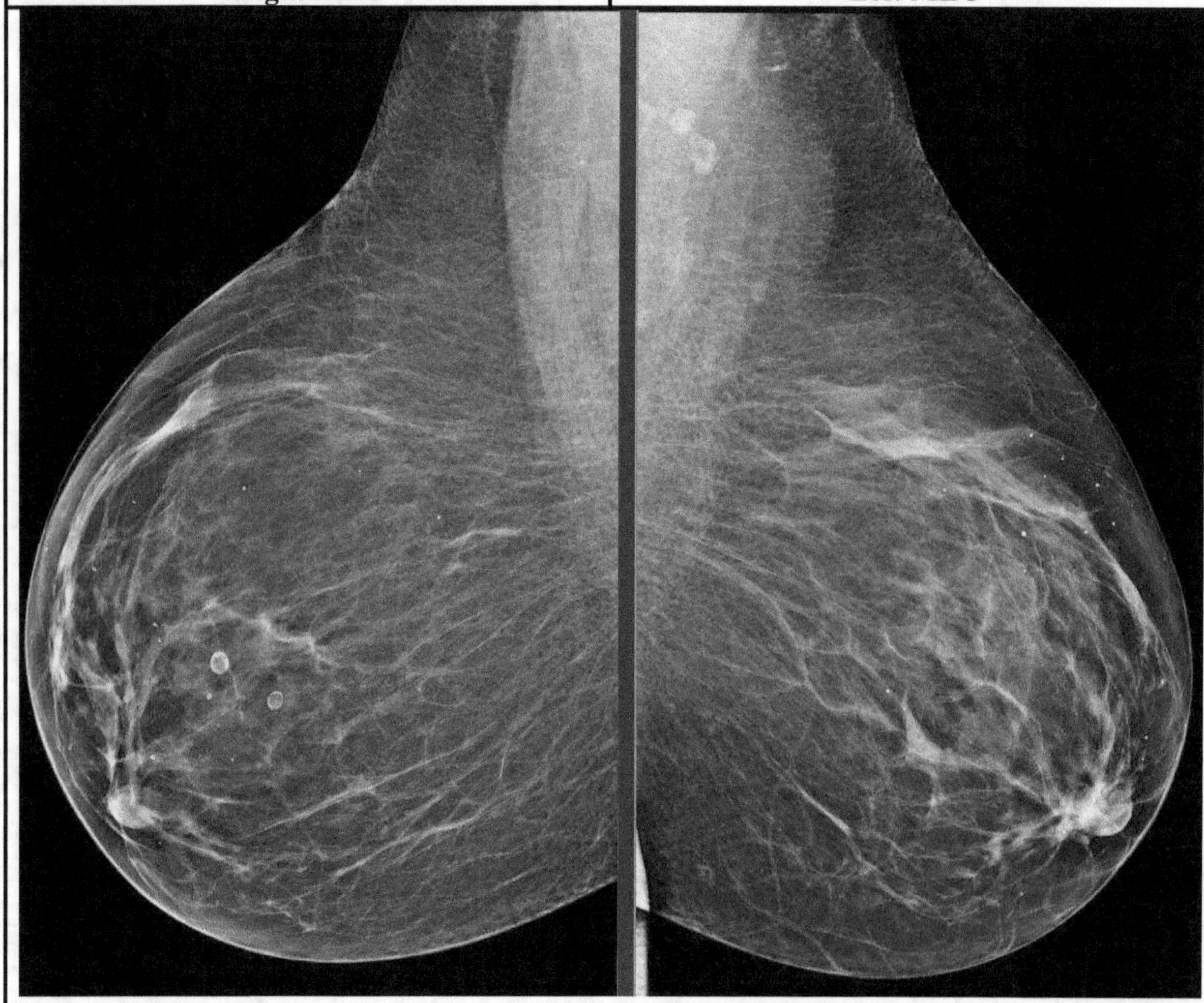

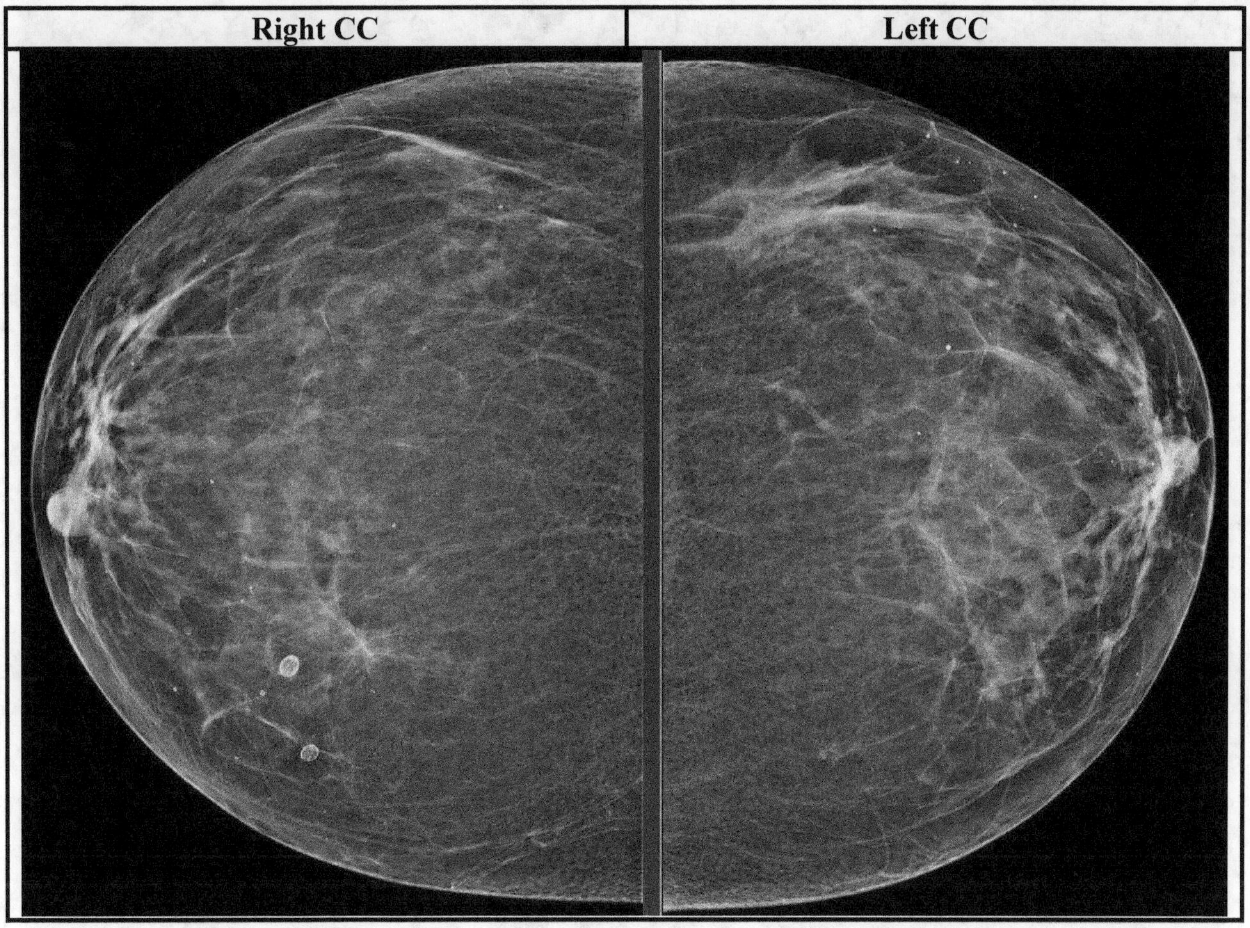
Right CC
Left CC

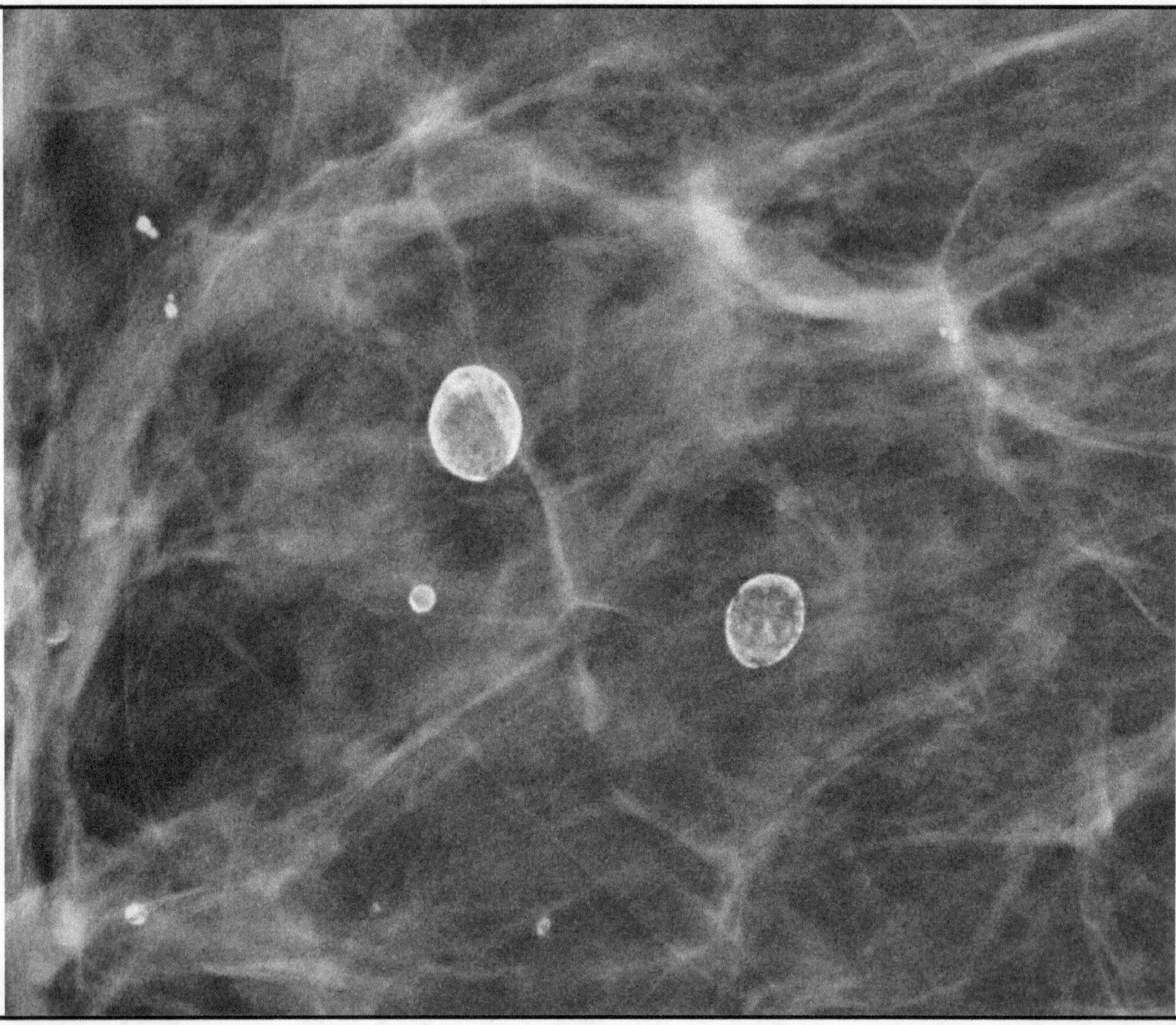

RIGHT BREAST	
Breast Parenchymal Density	***Scattered areas of fibroglandular density (ACR B)***
Focal Mass	None
Asymmetric Density	None
Parenchymal Distortion	None
Calcification	***Rim /Vascular Calcification***
Skin Thickening	None
Axillary Nodes	None

LEFT BREAST	
Breast Parenchymal Density	***Scattered areas of fibroglandular density (ACR B)***
Focal Mass	None
Asymmetric Density	None
Parenchymal Distortion	None
Calcification	***Vascular Calcification***
Skin Thickening	None
Axillary Nodes	None

IMPRESSION:

RIGHT BREAST: (BI-RADS 2)
LEFT BREAST: (BI-RADS 2)

RECOMMENDATION: Routine Annual screening

CASE 80: 52-year-old female / diagnostic

Right MLO	Left MLO

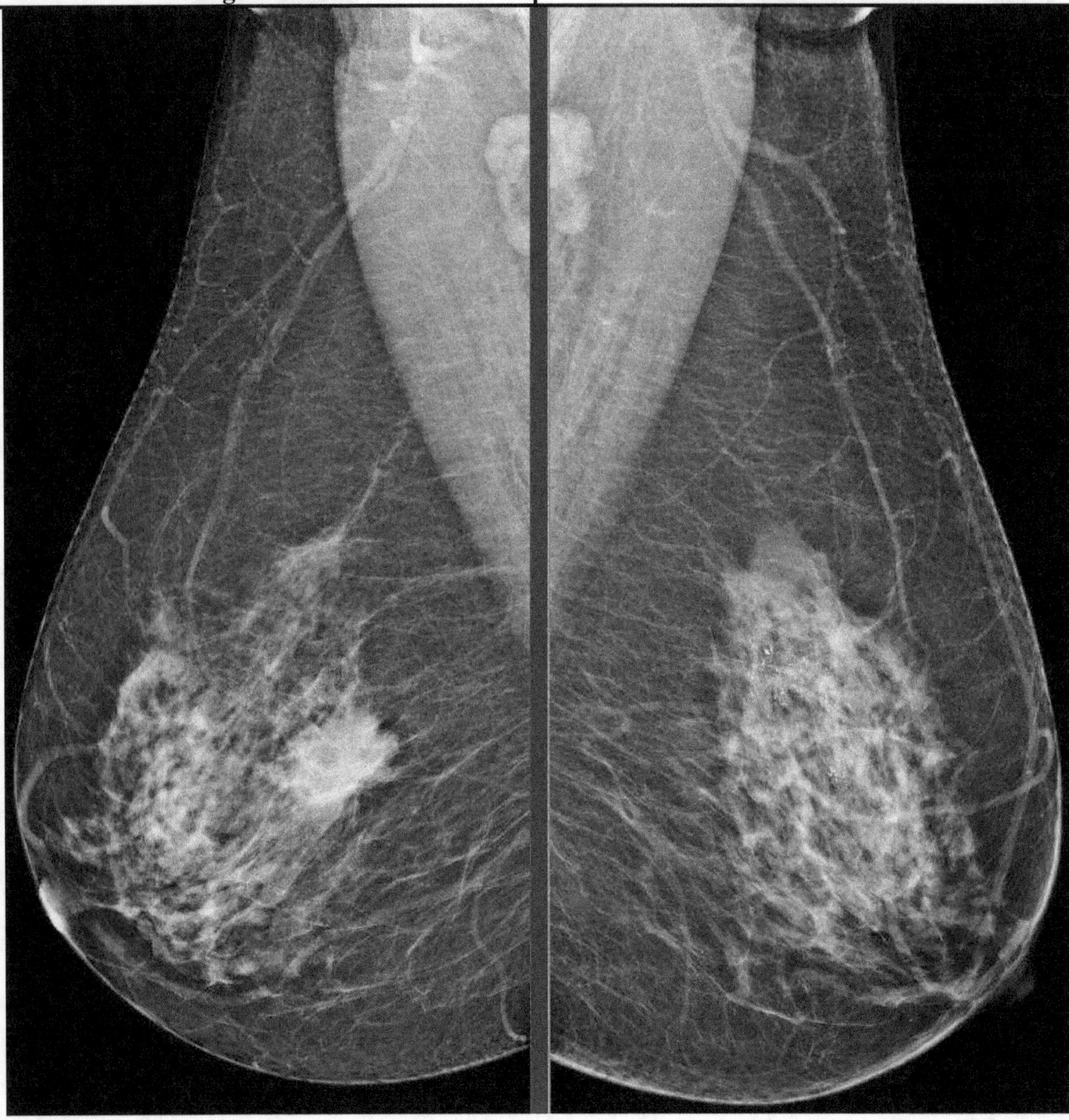

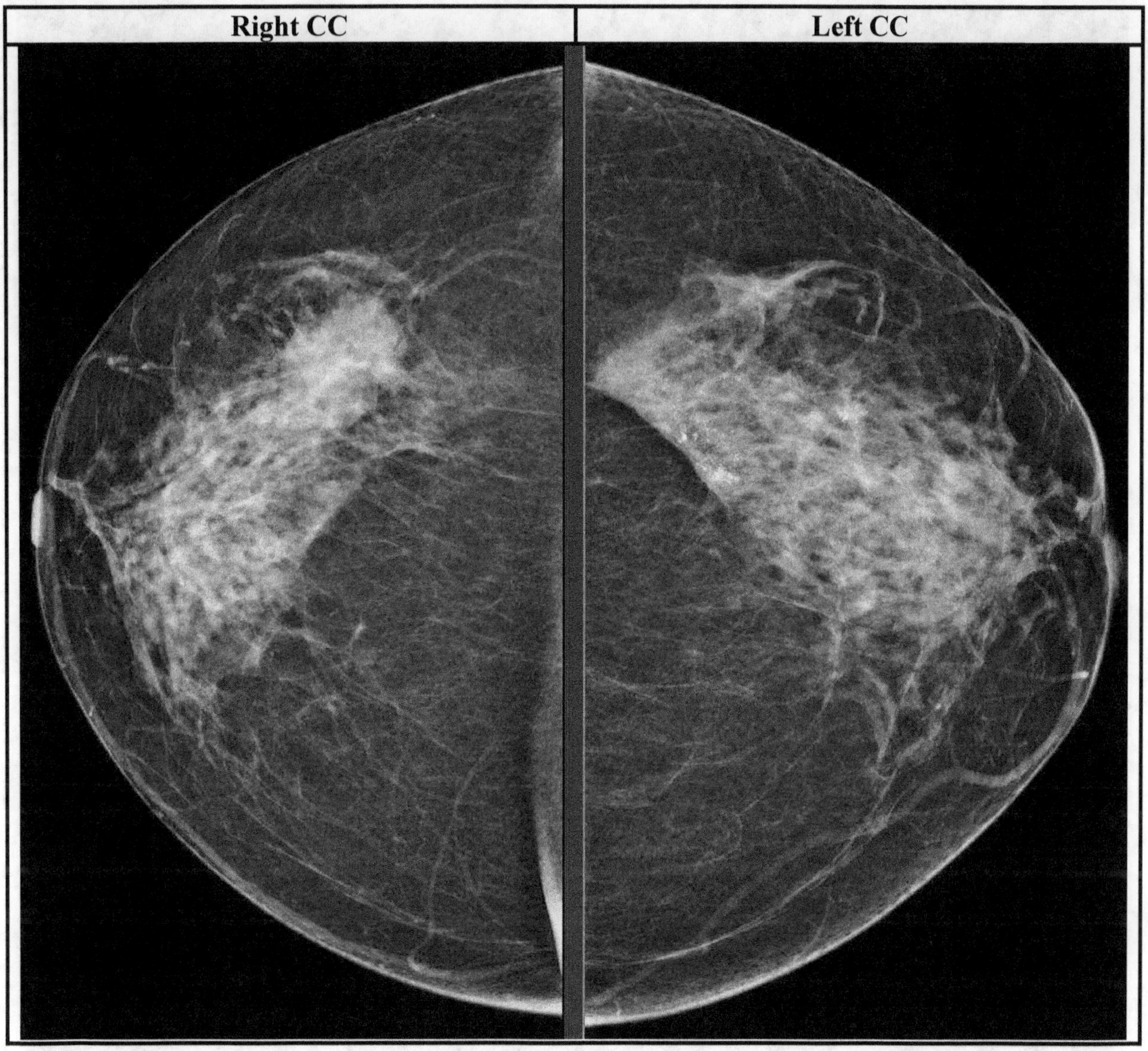
Right CC
Left CC

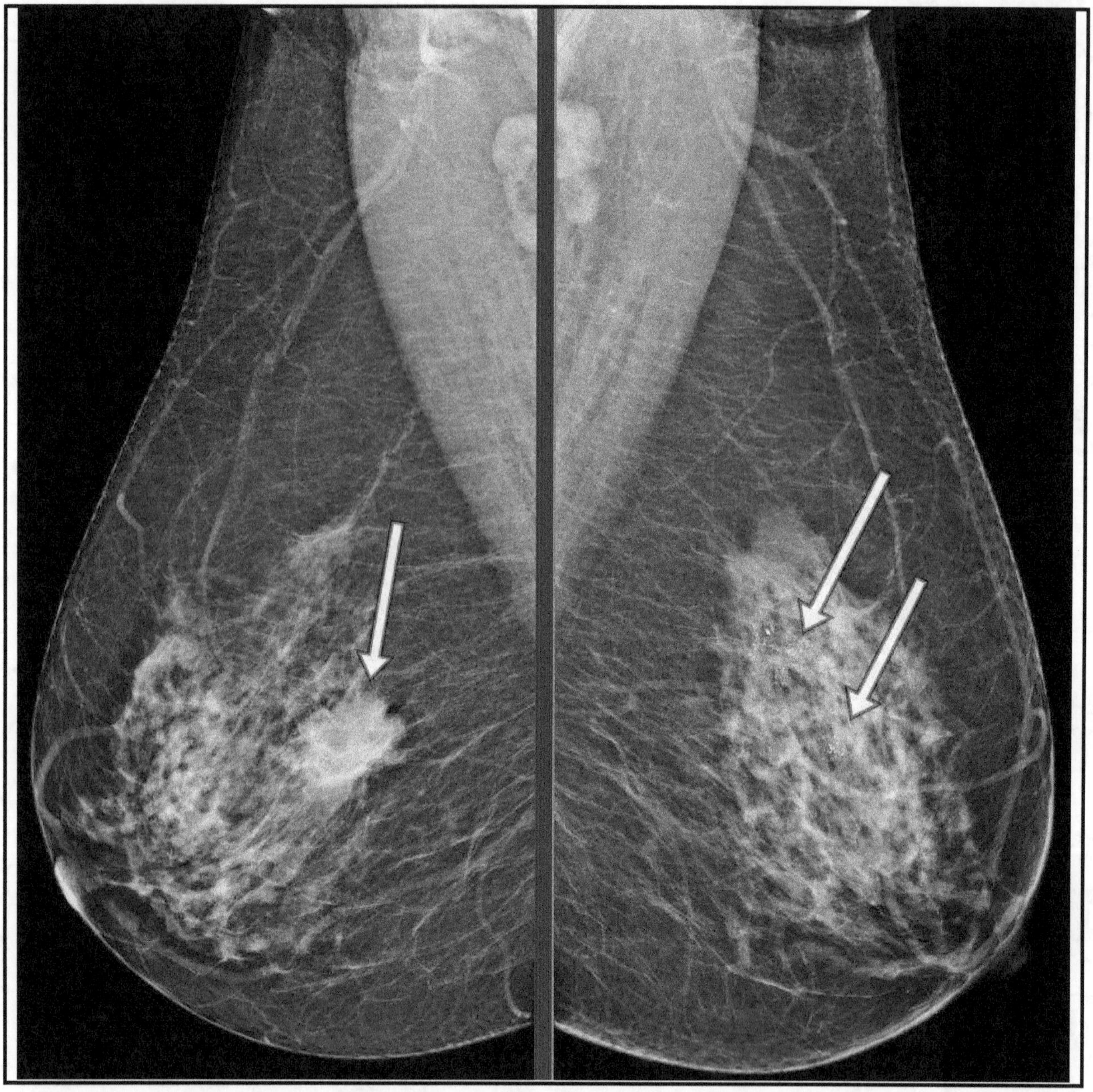

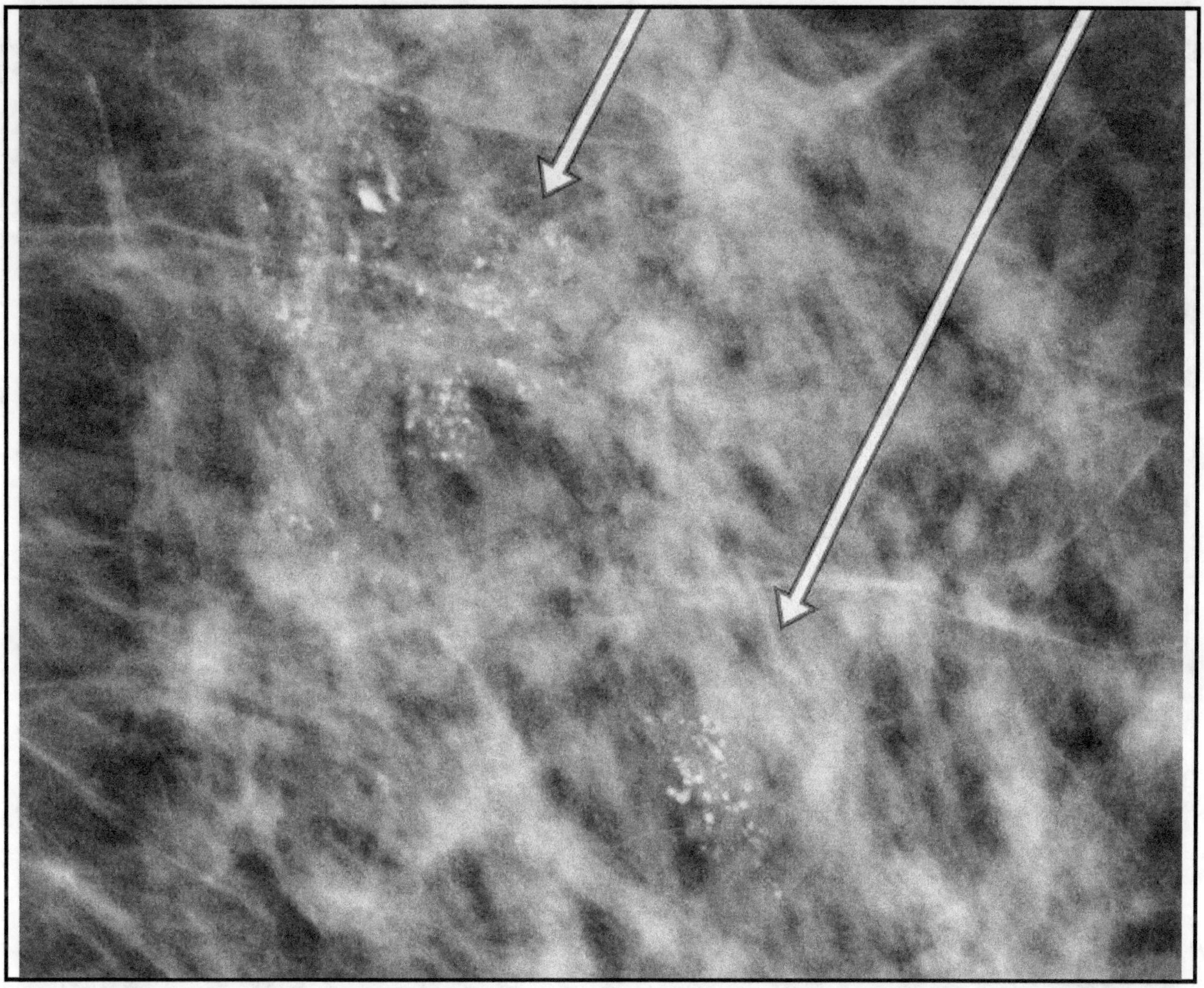

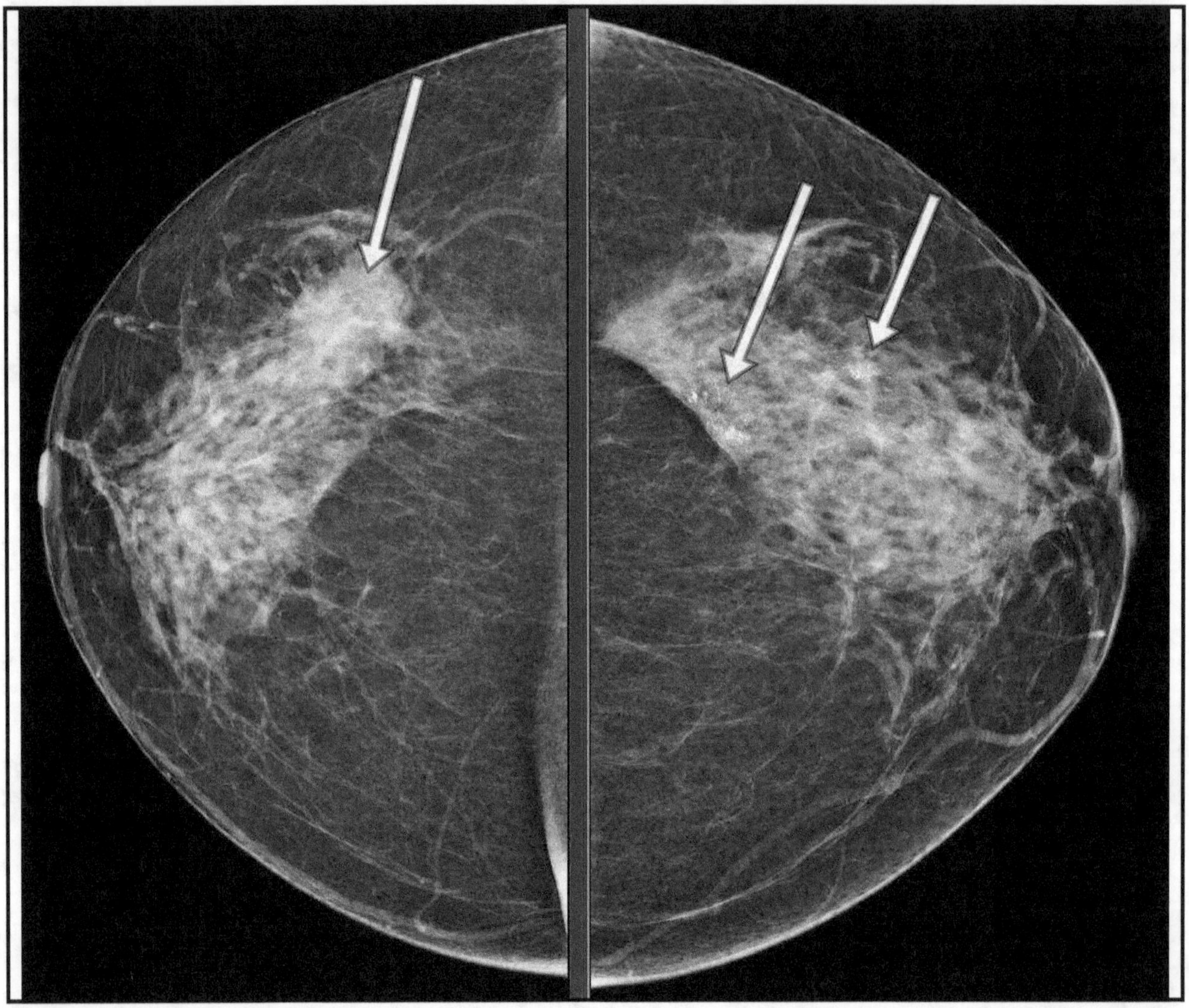

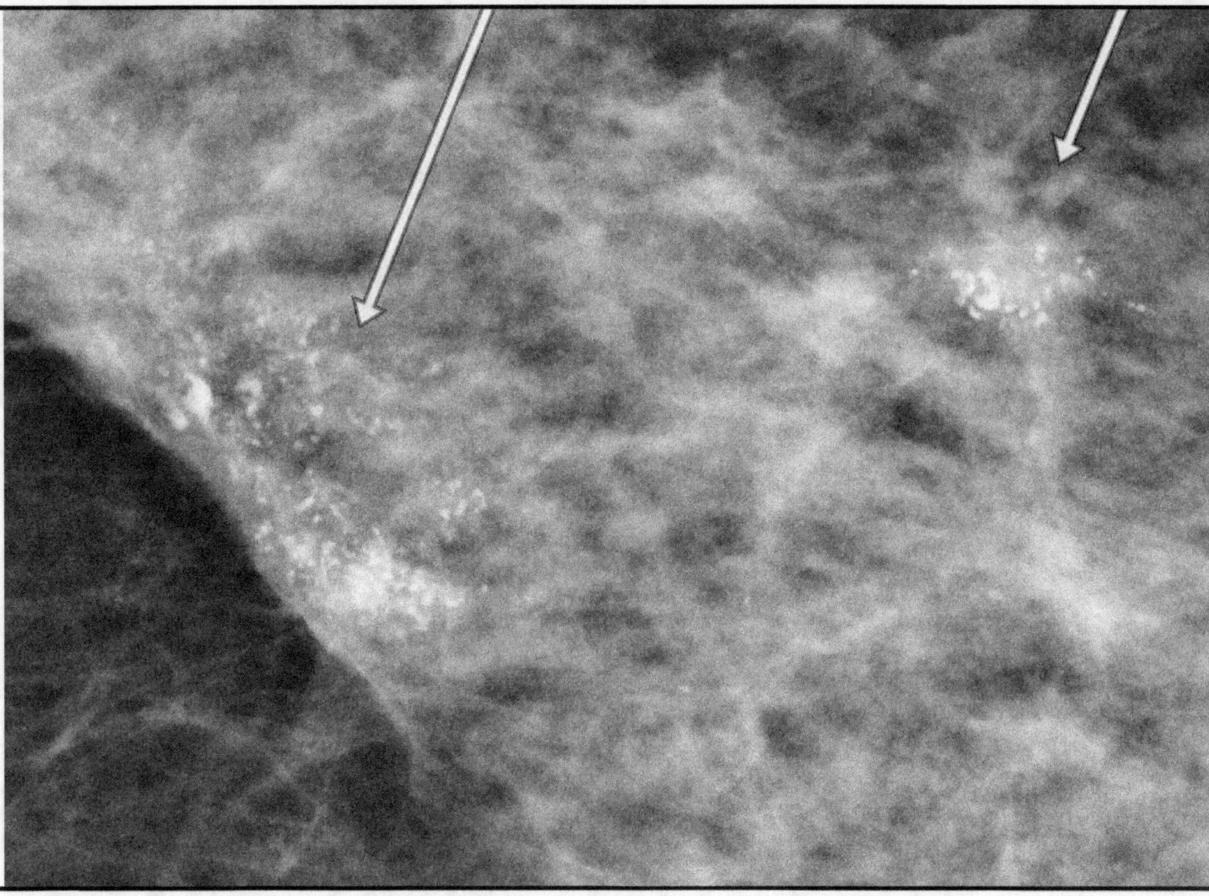

RIGHT BREAST	
Breast Parenchymal Density	***Heterogeneously dense, may obscure small masses (ACR C)***
Focal Mass	***UOQ irregular spiculated mass lesion***
Asymmetric Density	None
Parenchymal Distortion	None
Calcification	None
Skin Thickening	None
Axillary Nodes	None

LEFT BREAST	
Breast Parenchymal Density	***Heterogeneously dense, may obscure small masses (ACR C)***
Focal Mass	None
Asymmetric Density	None
Parenchymal Distortion	None
Calcification	***UOQ grouped areas of fine pleomorphic calcification***
Skin Thickening	None
Axillary Nodes	None

IMPRESSION:
RIGHT BREAST: (BI-RADS 5)

LEFT BREAST: (BI-RADS 4C)

RECOMMENDATION: Histopathological Correlation

CASE 81: 43-year-old female / diagnostic

Right MLO	**Left MLO**

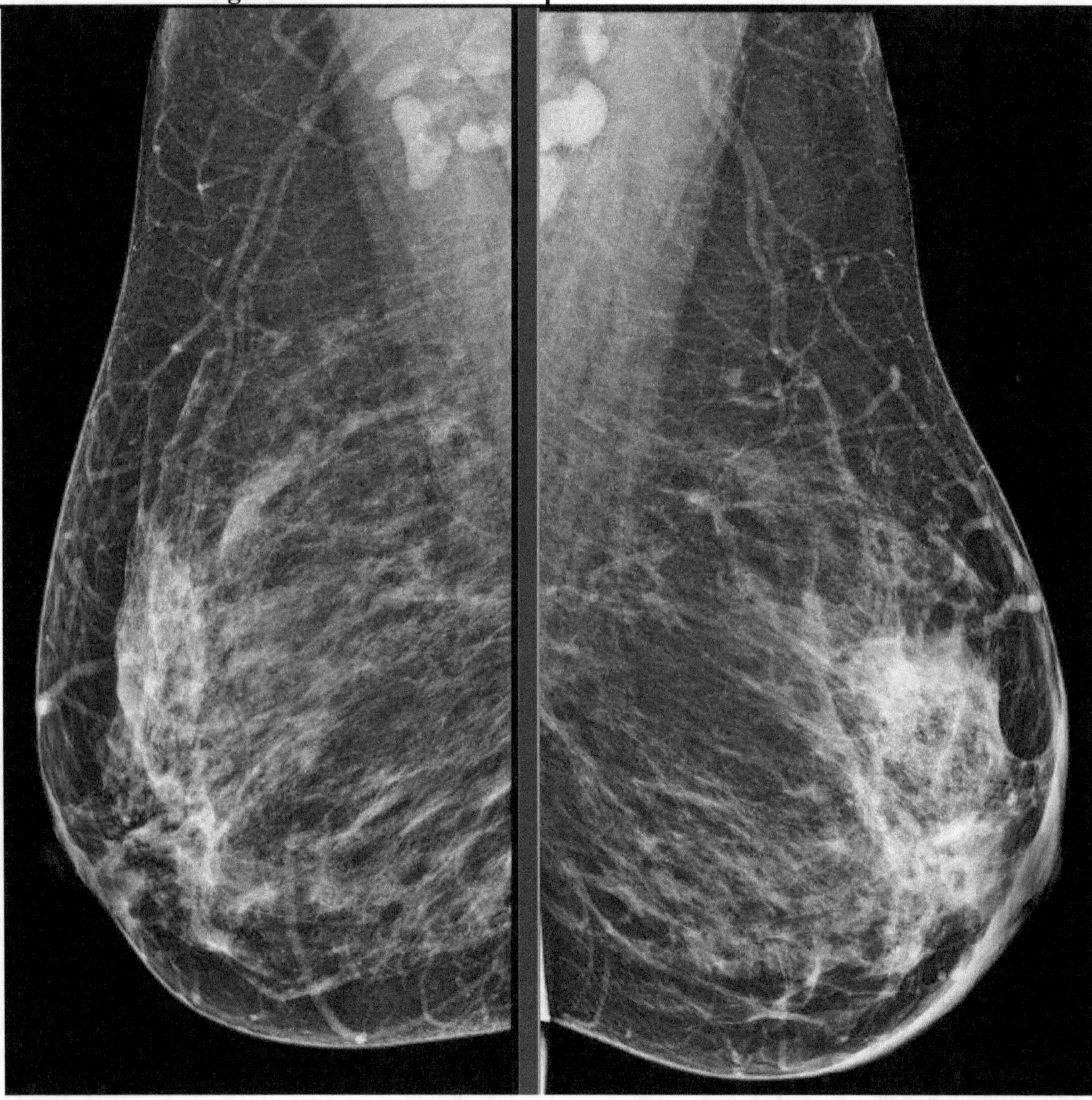

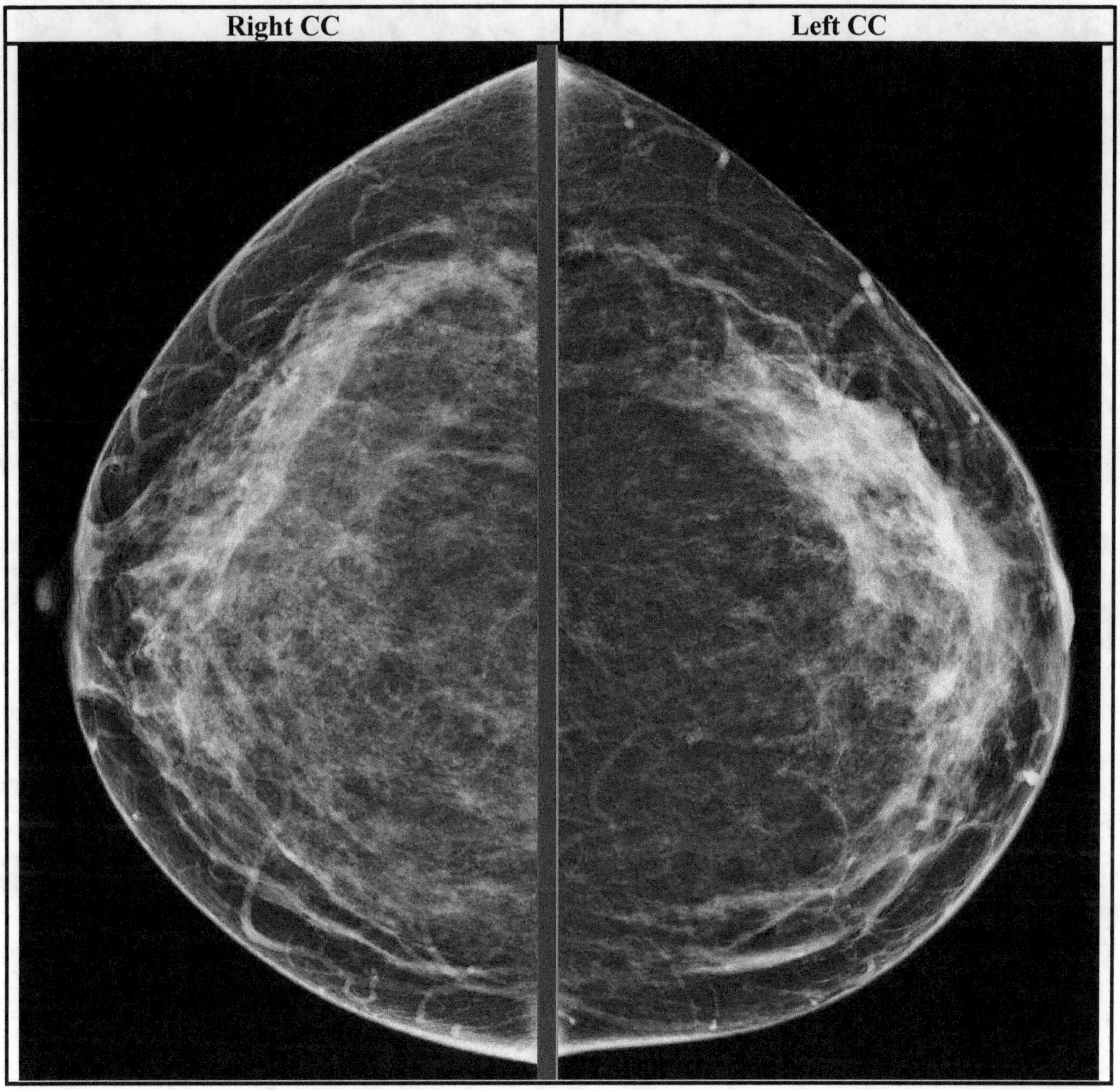
Right CC
Left CC

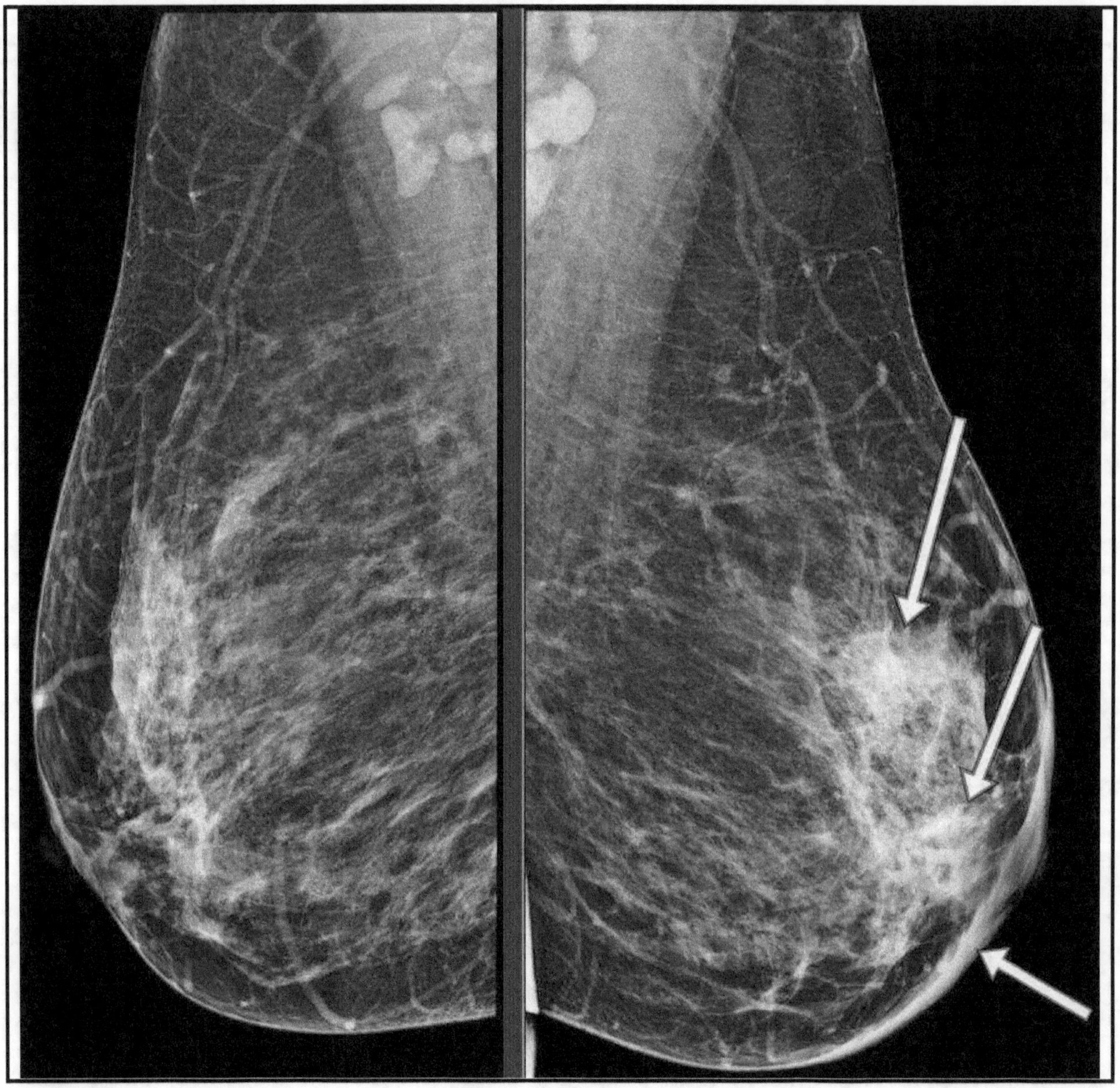

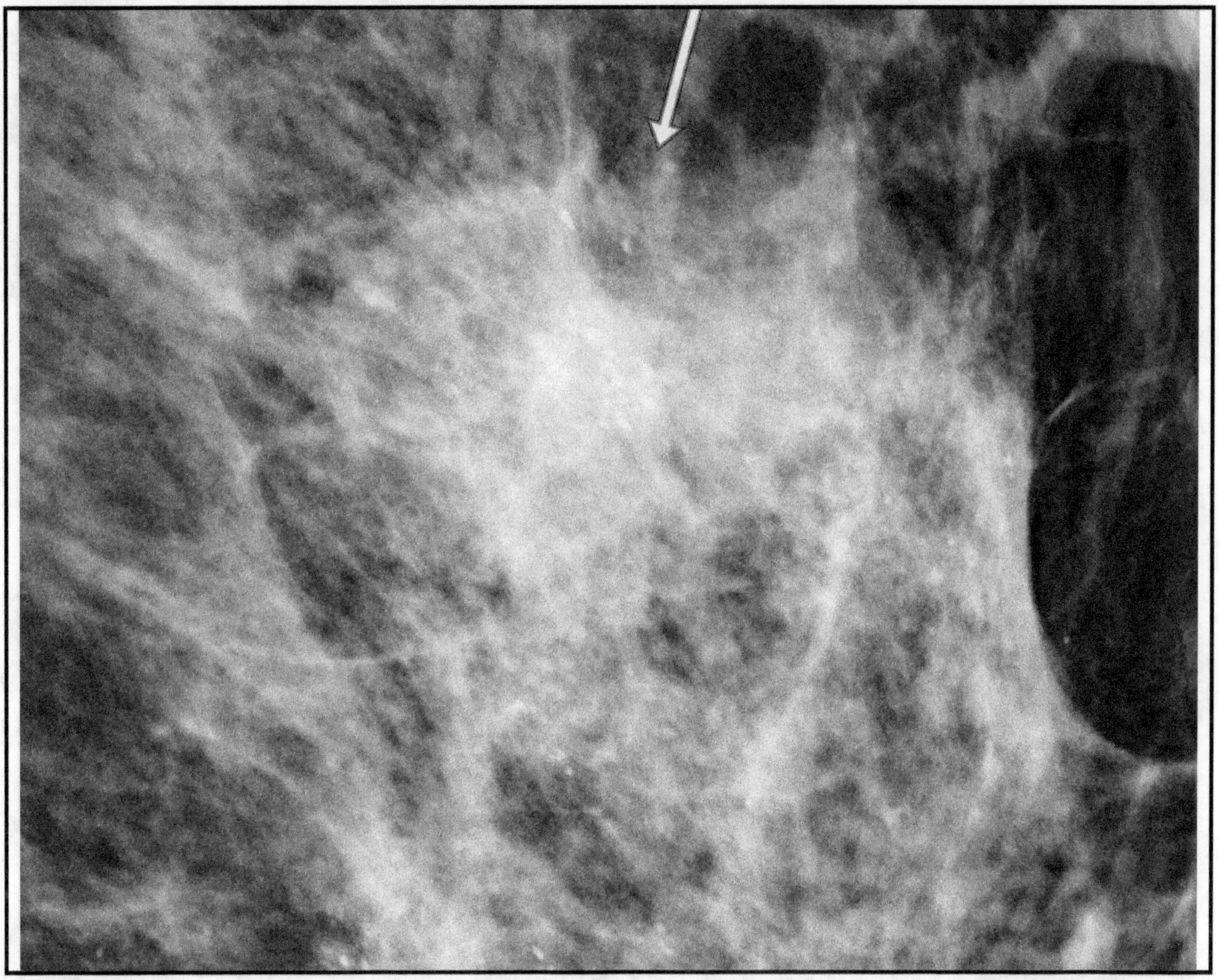

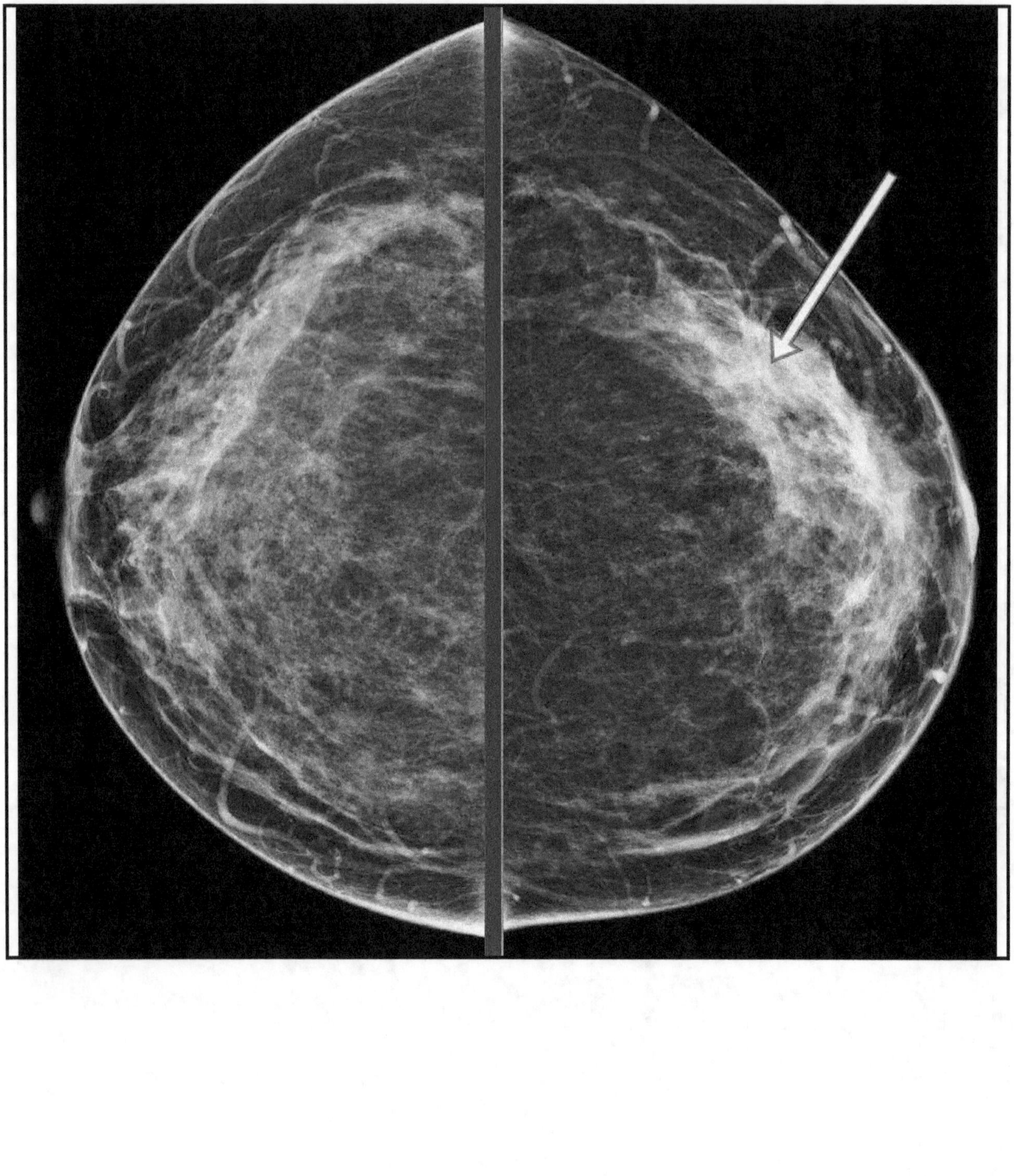

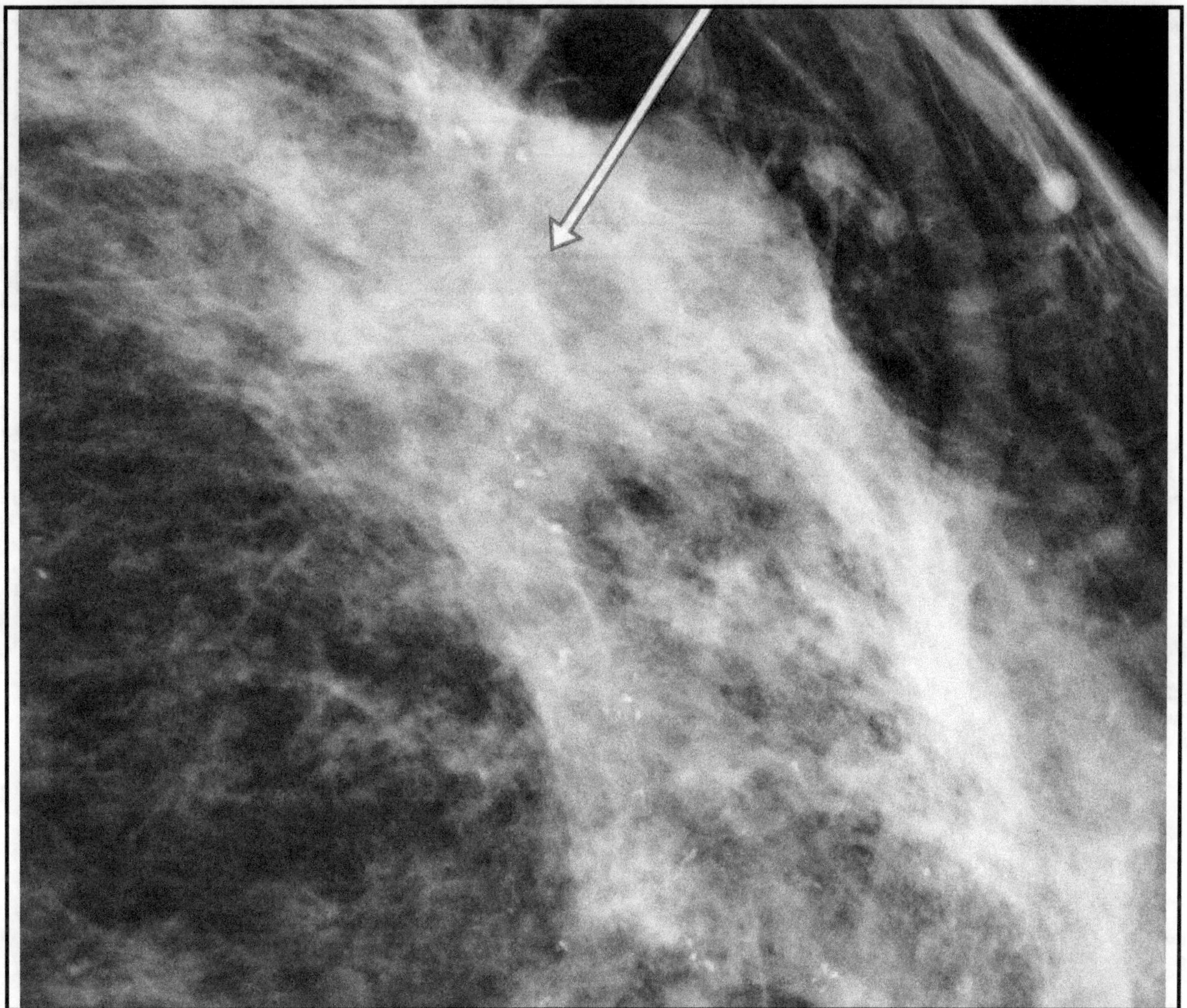

RIGHT BREAST	
Breast Parenchymal Density	***Heterogeneously dense, may obscure small masses (ACR C)***
Focal Mass	None
Asymmetric Density	None
Parenchymal Distortion	None
Calcification	None
Skin Thickening	None
Axillary Nodes	None

LEFT BREAST	
Breast Parenchymal Density	***Heterogeneously dense, may obscure small masses (ACR C)***
Focal Mass	None
Asymmetric Density	None
Parenchymal Distortion	None
Calcification	***UOQ segmental area of amorphous micro-calcification***
Skin Thickening	None
Axillary Nodes	None

IMPRESSION:

RIGHT BREAST: (BI-RADS 1)
LEFT BREAST: (BI-RADS 4B)

RECOMMENDATION: Histopathological Correlation

CASE 82: 90-year-old female / diagnostic

Right MLO	Left MLO

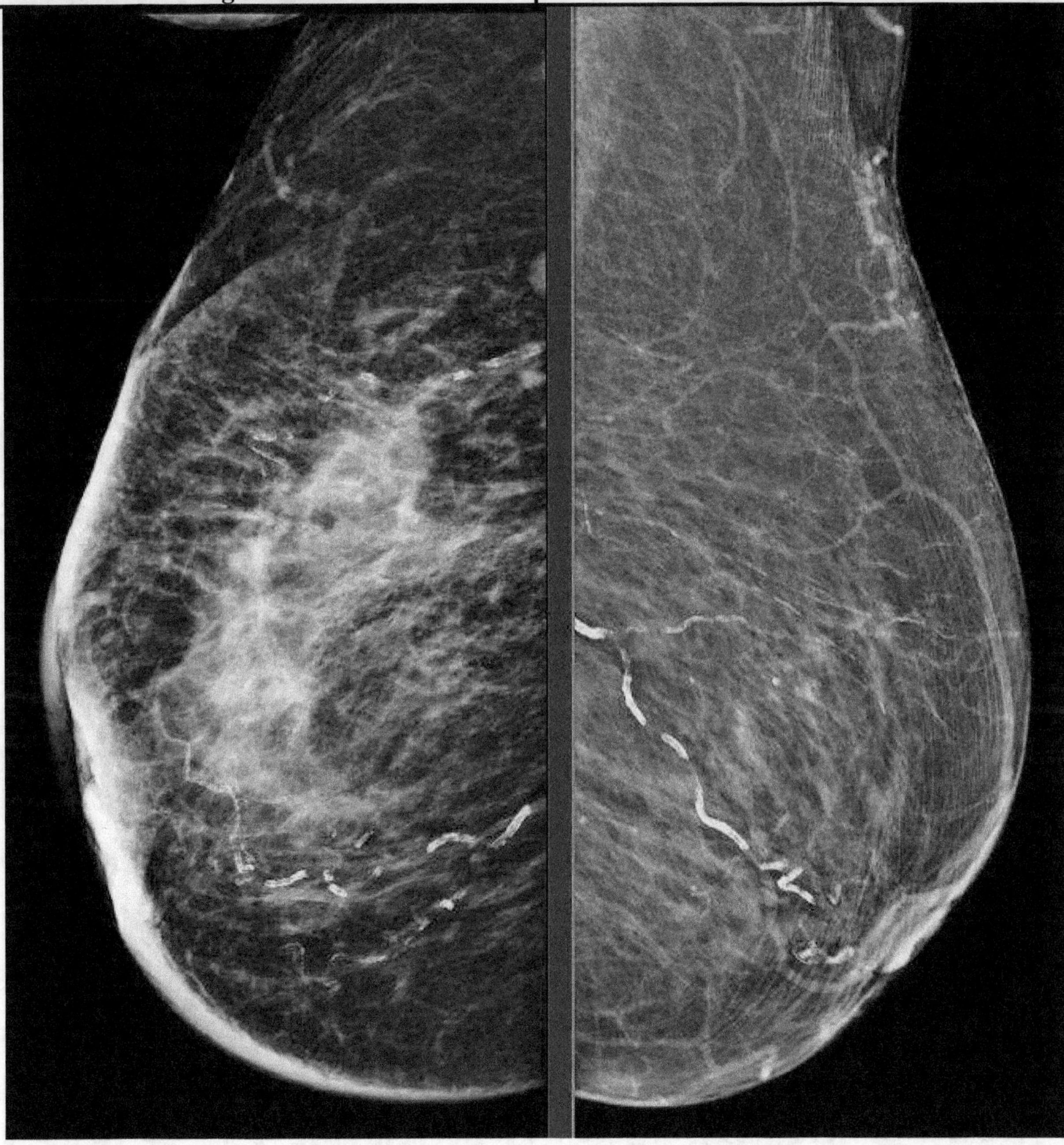

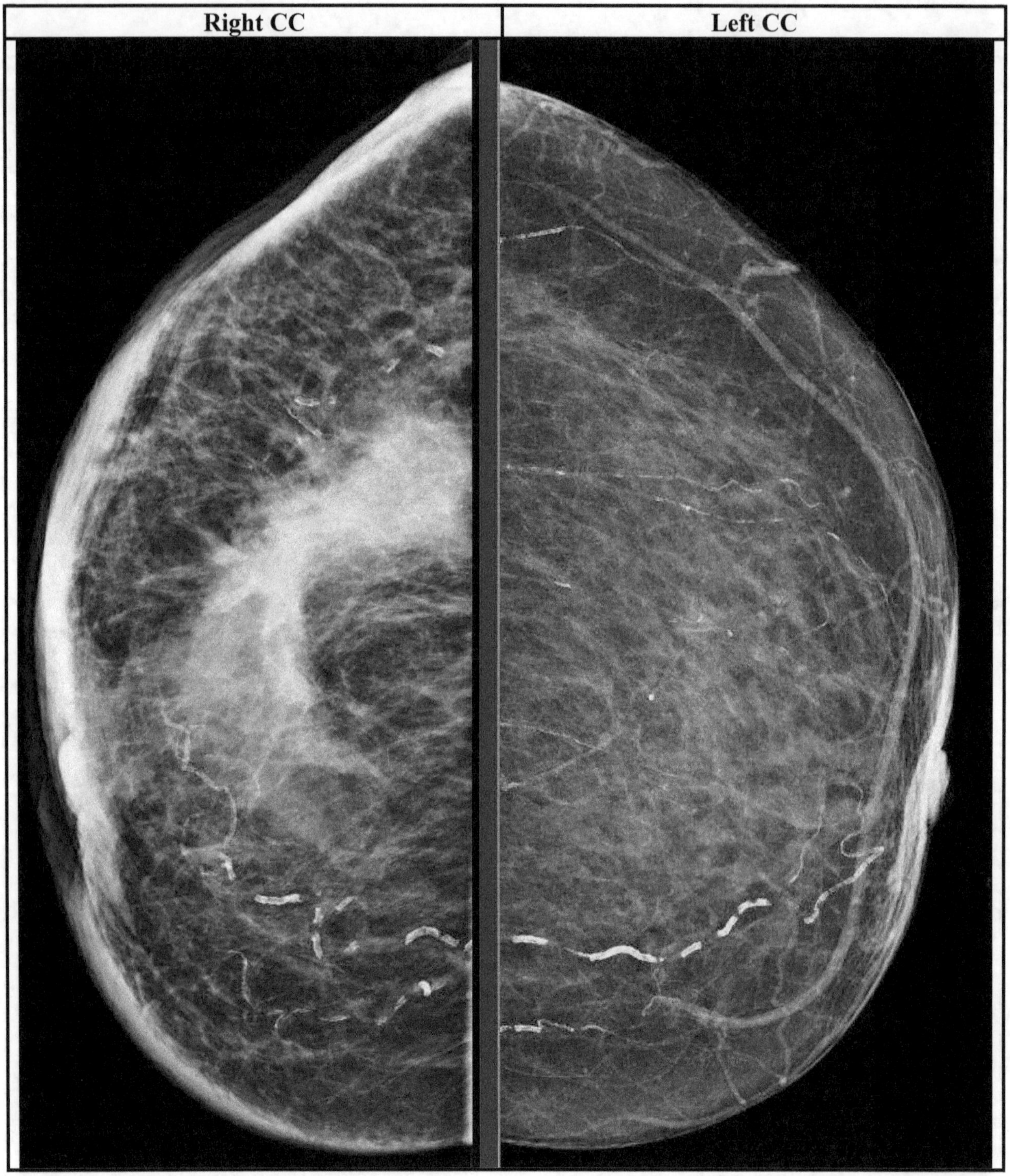
Right CC
Left CC

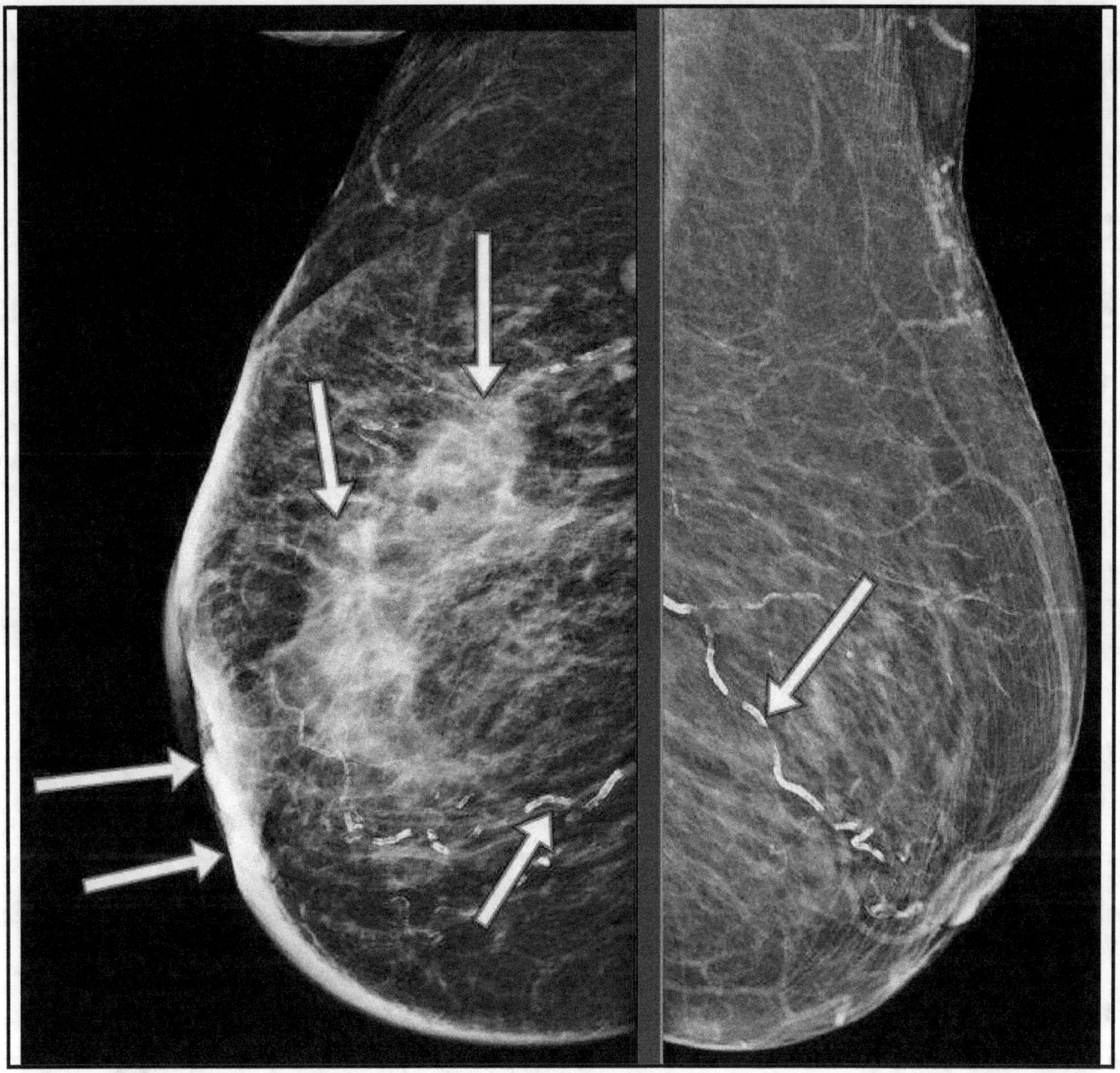

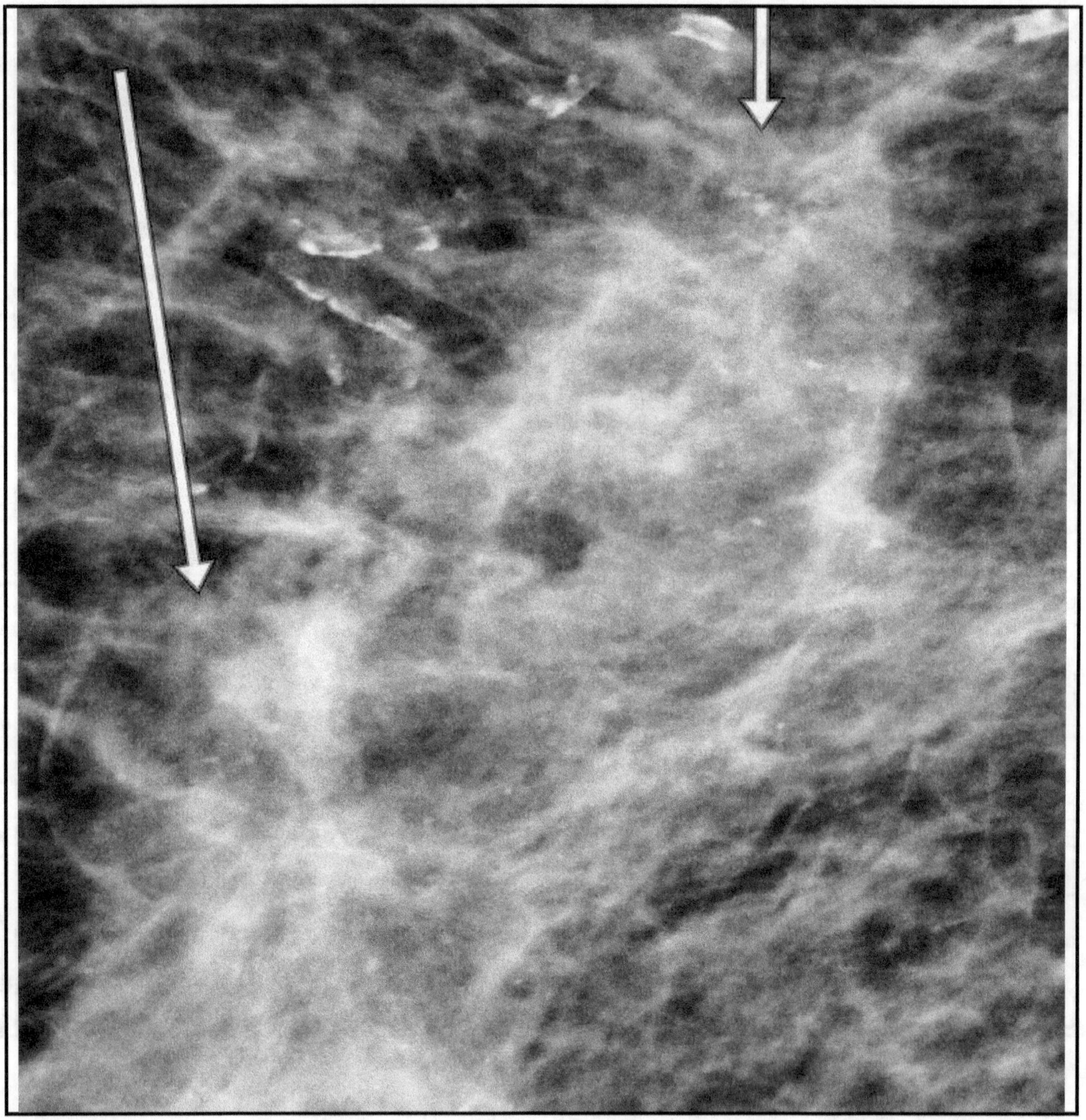

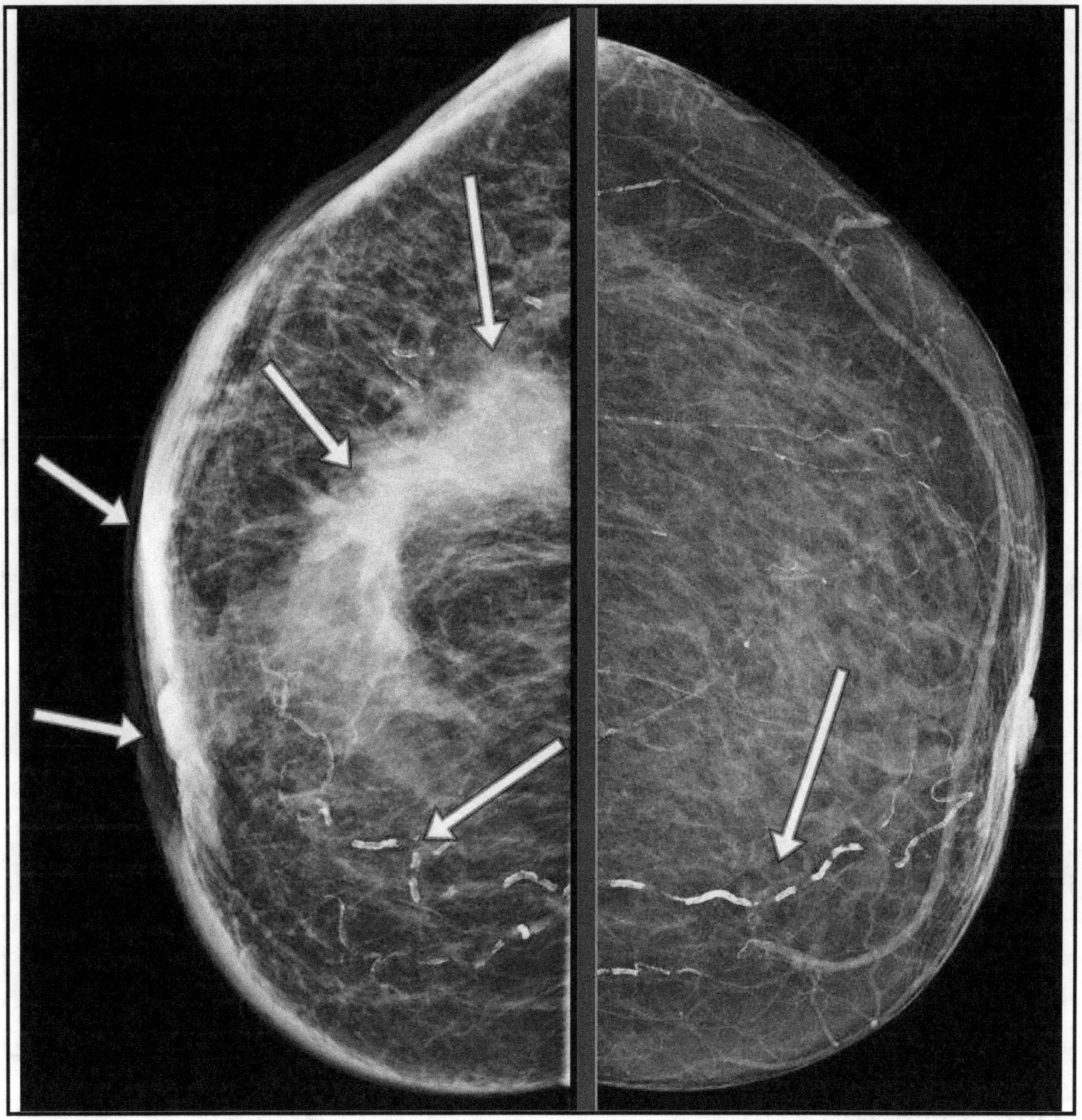

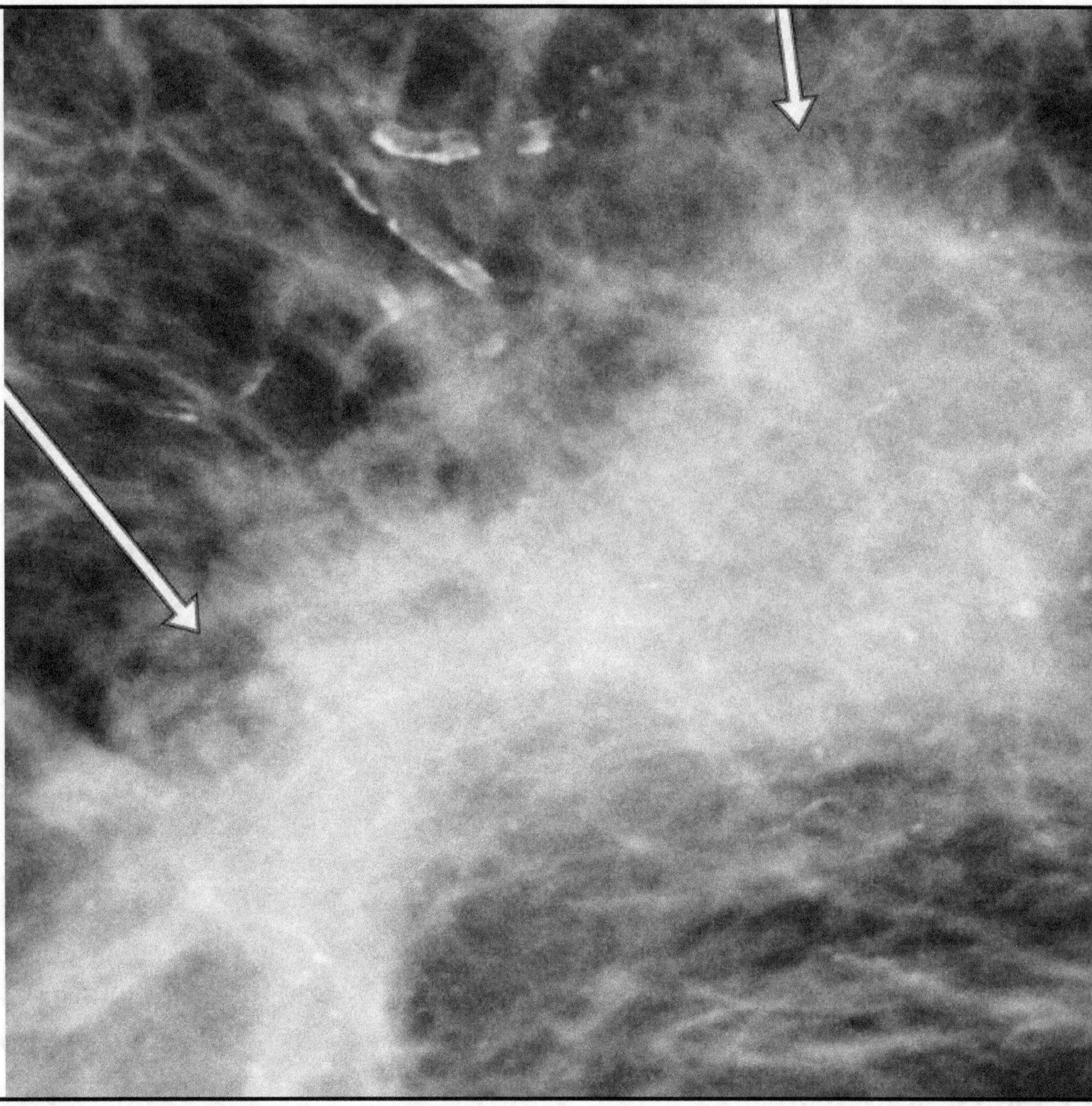

RIGHT BREAST	
Breast Parenchymal Density	***Scattered areas of fibroglandular density (ACR B)***
Focal Mass	None
Asymmetric Density	***UOQ focal asymmetry associated with suspicious amorphous micro-calcification***
Parenchymal Distortion	None
Calcification	***UOQ regional area of amorphous micro-calcification / Vascular Calcification***
Skin Thickening	***Positive /Nipple Retraction***
Axillary Nodes	None

LEFT BREAST	
Breast Parenchymal Density	***Almost entirely fatty (ACR A)***
Focal Mass	None
Asymmetric Density	None
Parenchymal Distortion	None
Calcification	***Vascular Calcification***
Skin Thickening	None
Axillary Nodes	None

IMPRESSION:

RIGHT BREAST: (BI-RADS 5)
LEFT BREAST: (BI-RADS 2)

RECOMMENDATION: Histopathological Correlation

CASE 83: 44-year-old female / diagnostic	
Right MLO	Left MLO

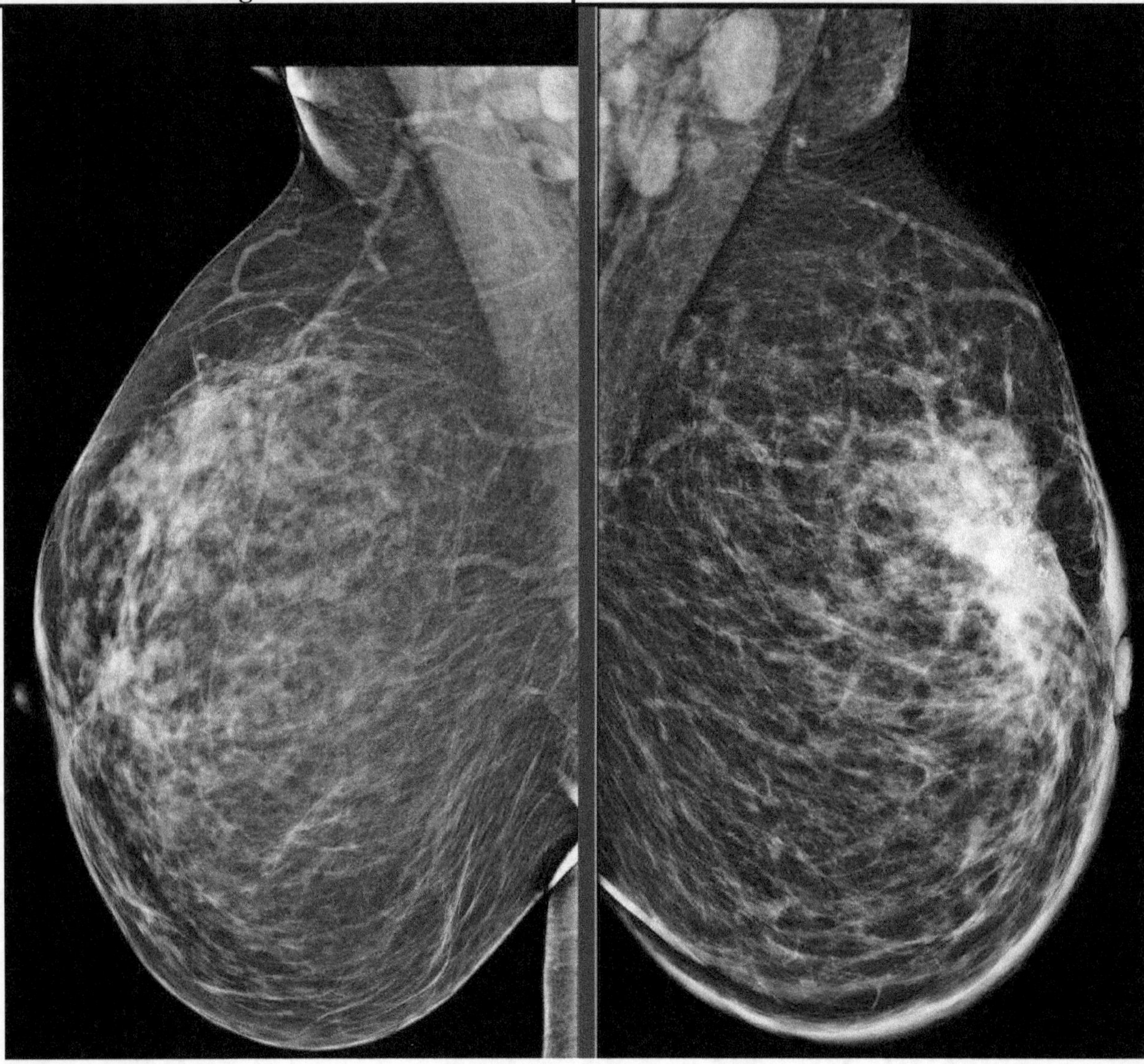

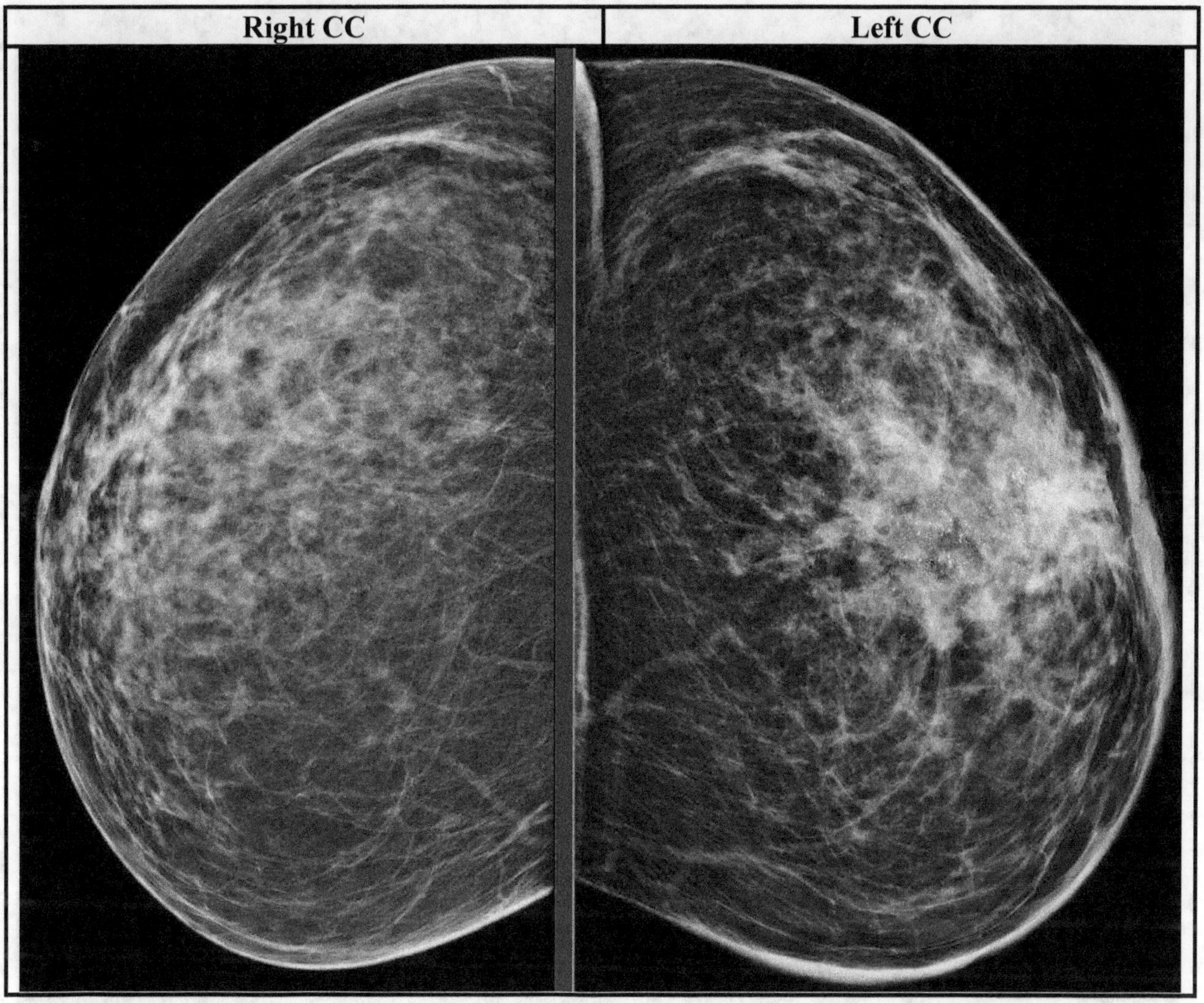
Right CC
Left CC

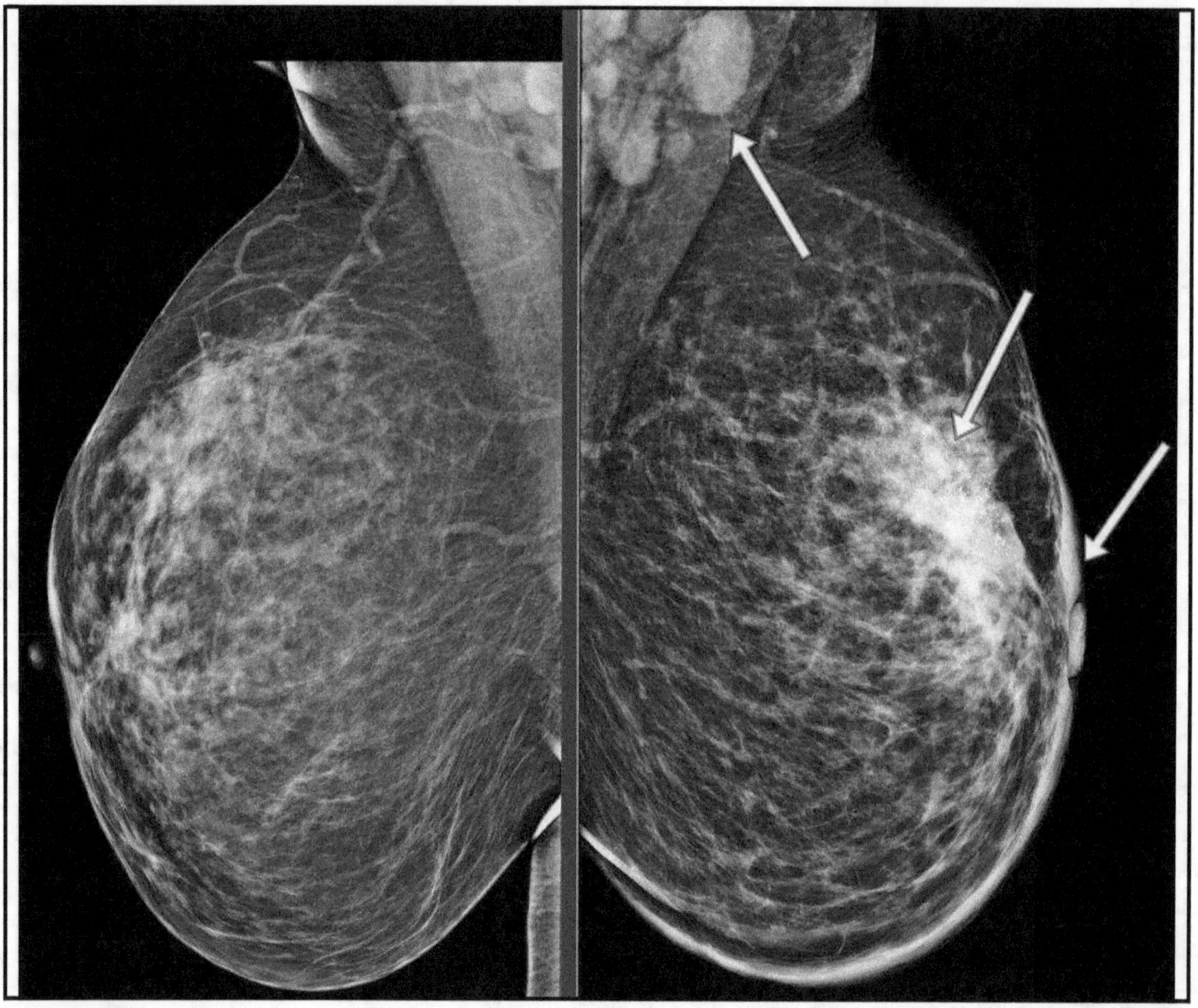

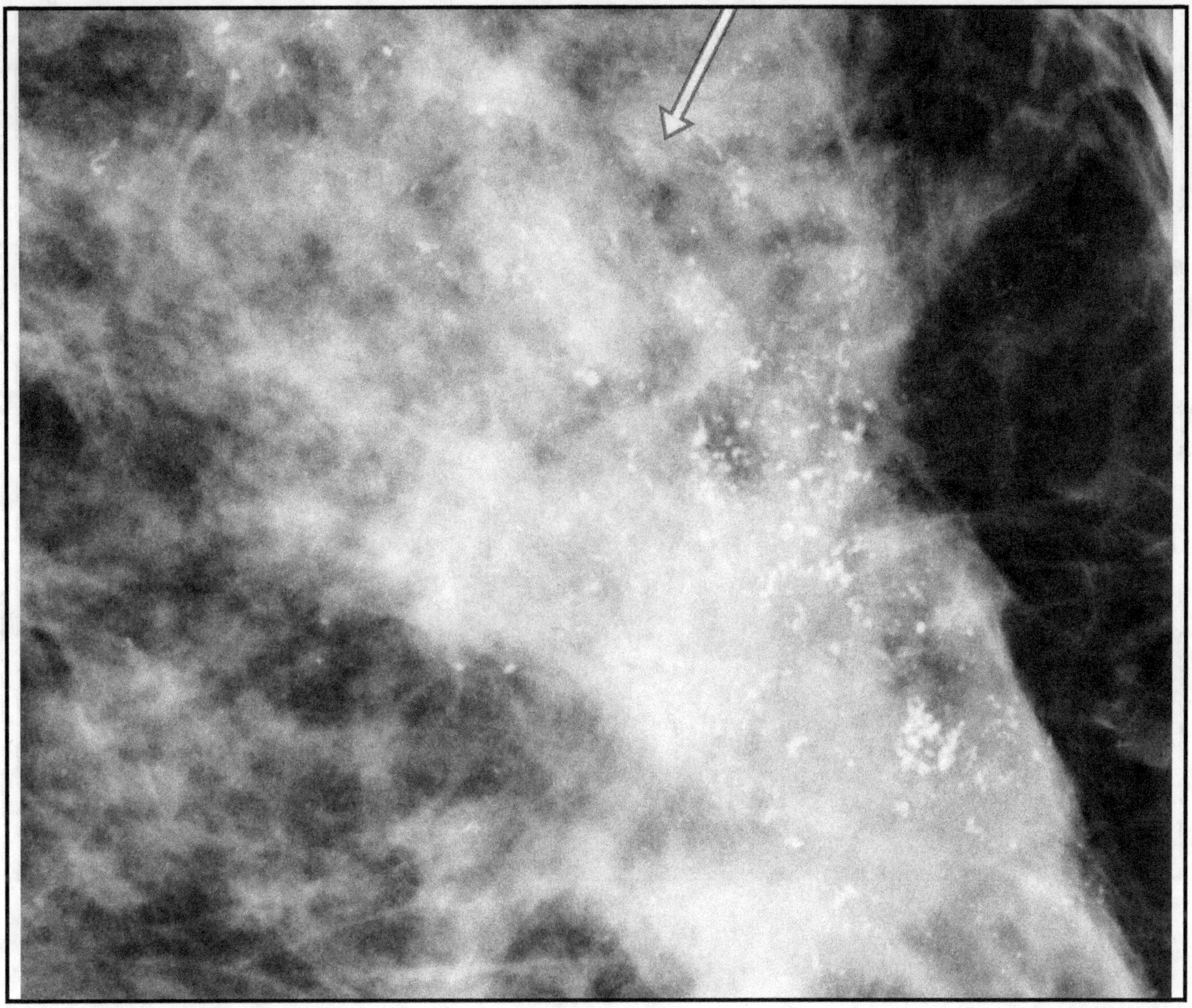

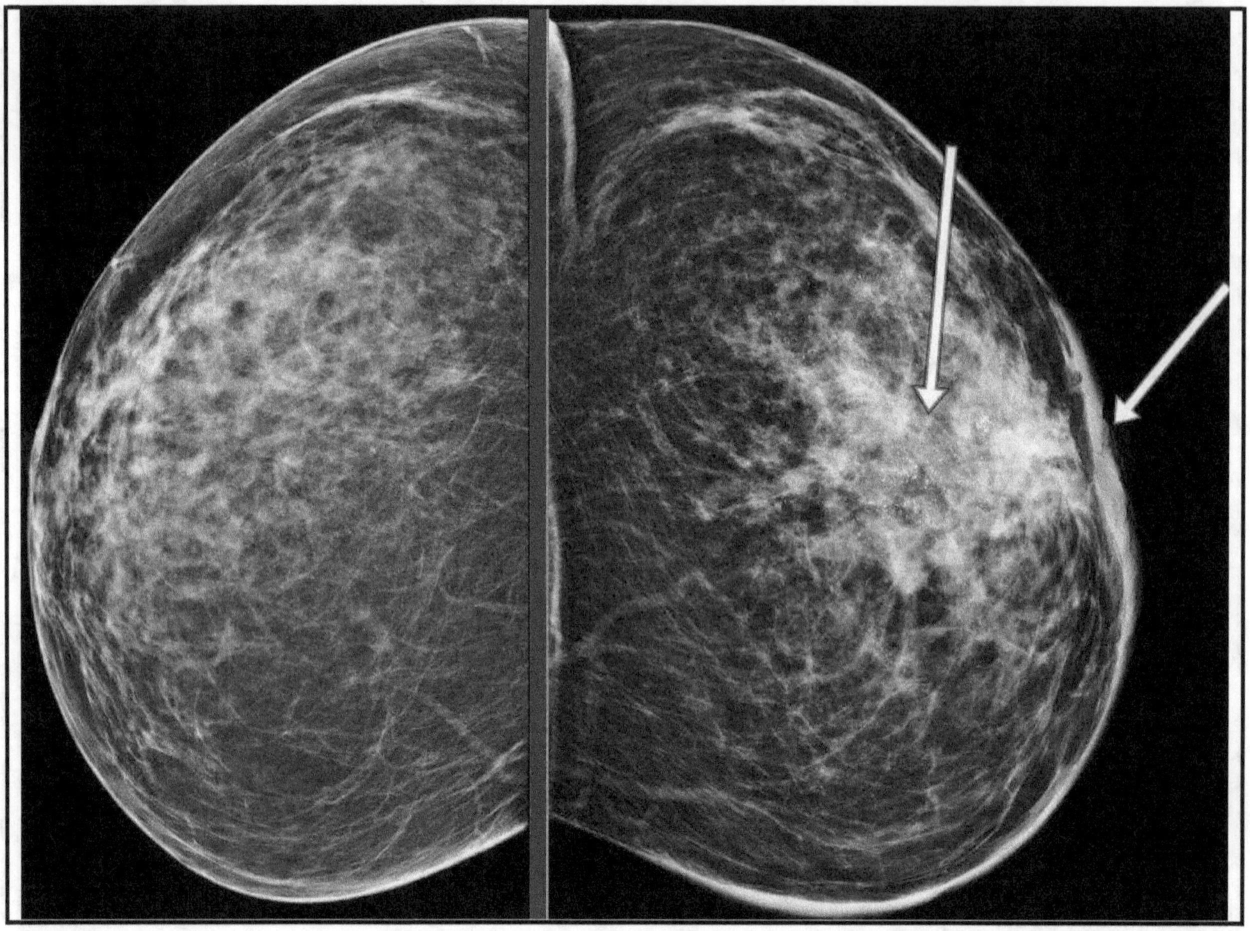

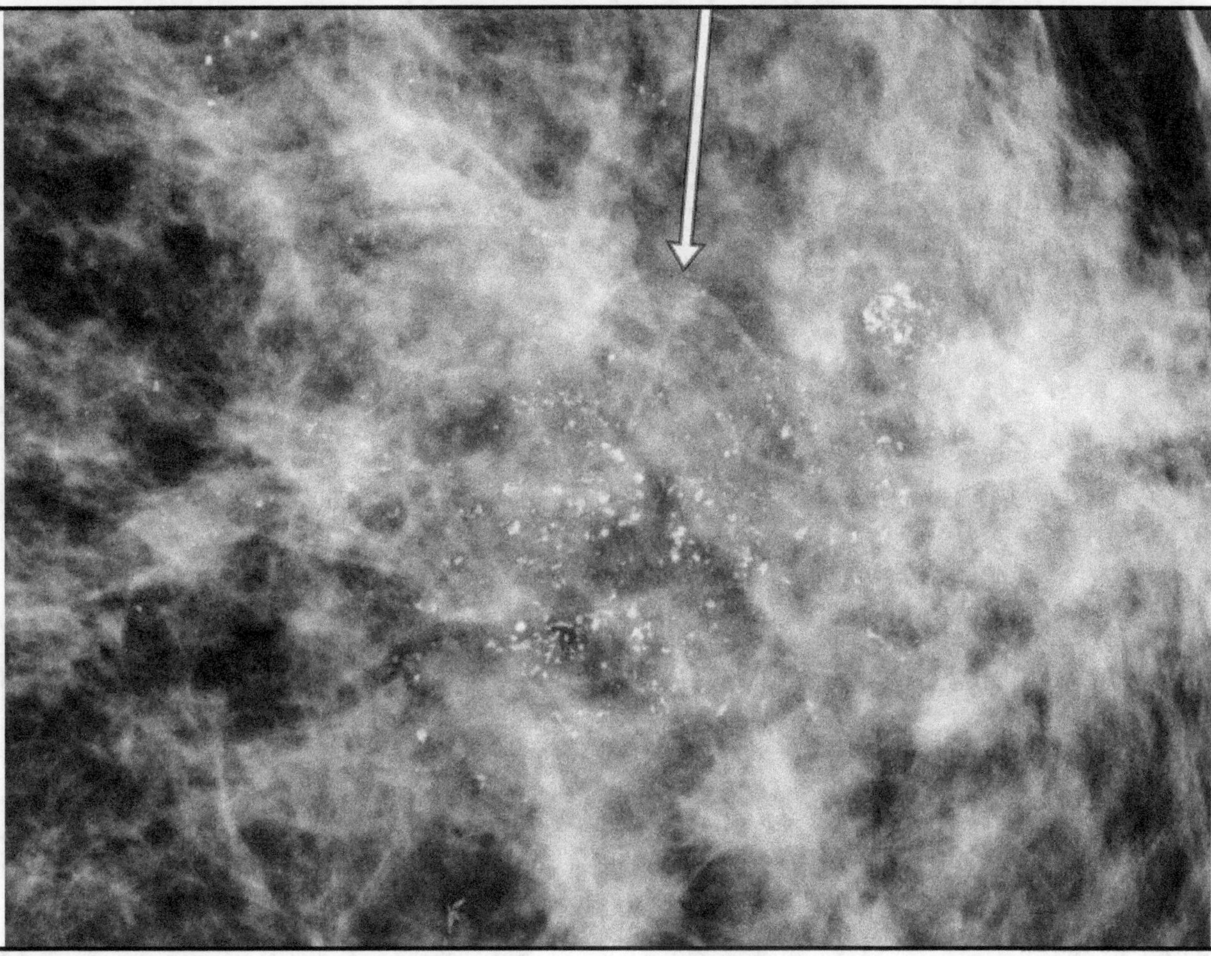

RIGHT BREAST	
Breast Parenchymal Density	***Scattered areas of fibroglandular density (ACR B)***
Focal Mass	None
Asymmetric Density	None
Parenchymal Distortion	None
Calcification	None
Skin Thickening	None
Axillary Nodes	None

LEFT BREAST	
Breast Parenchymal Density	***Scattered areas of fibroglandular density (ACR B)***
Focal Mass	None
Asymmetric Density	***UOQ focal asymmetry***
Parenchymal Distortion	None
Calcification	***UOQ segmental area of fine pleomorphic micro-calcification***
Skin Thickening	***Positive***
Axillary Nodes	***Lymphadenopathy***

IMPRESSION:

RIGHT BREAST: (BI-RADS 1
LEFT BREAST: (BI-RADS 4C)
RECOMMENDATION: Histopathological Correlation

CASE 84: 44-year-old female/ Diagnostic

Right MLO	Left MLO

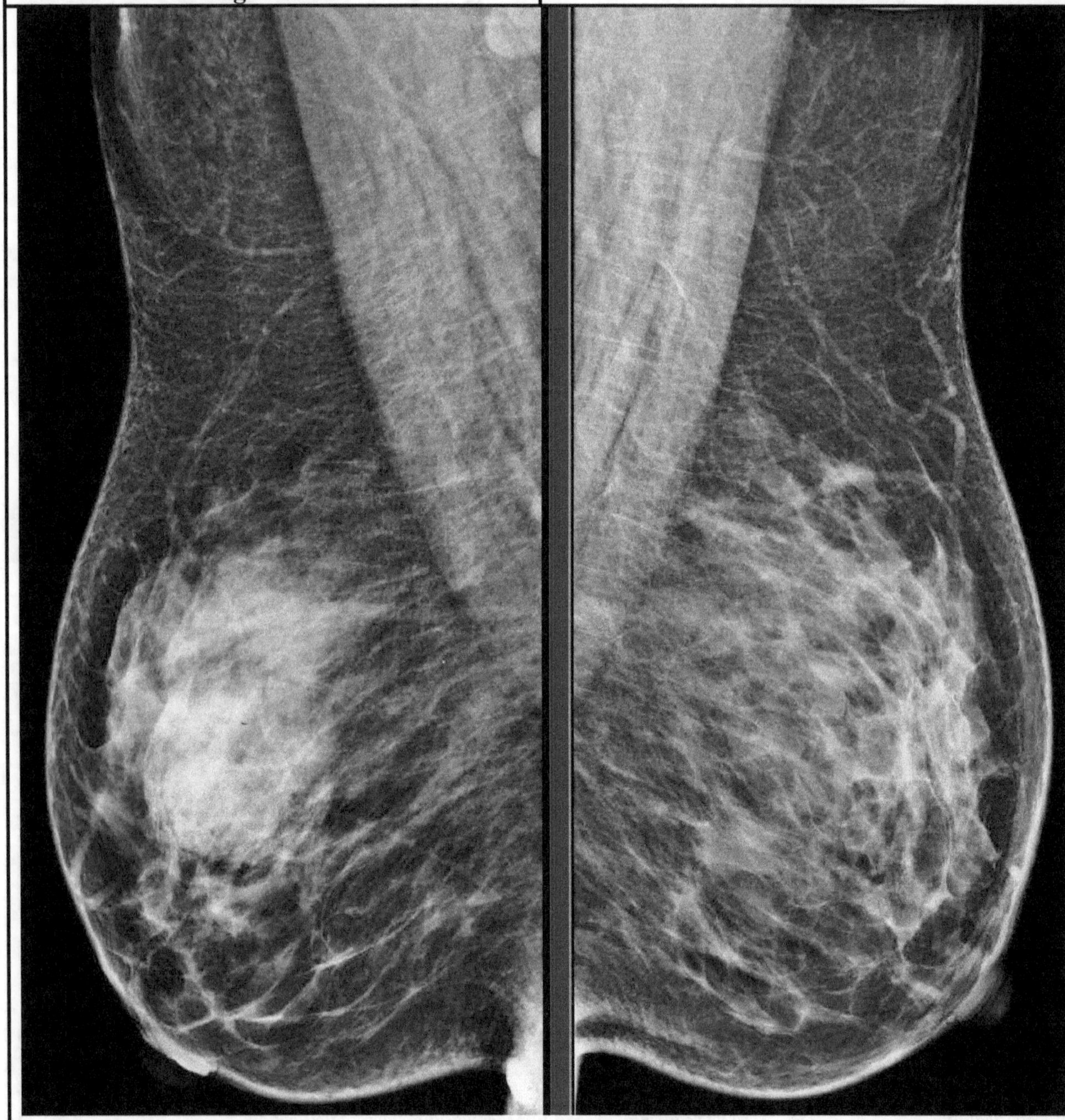

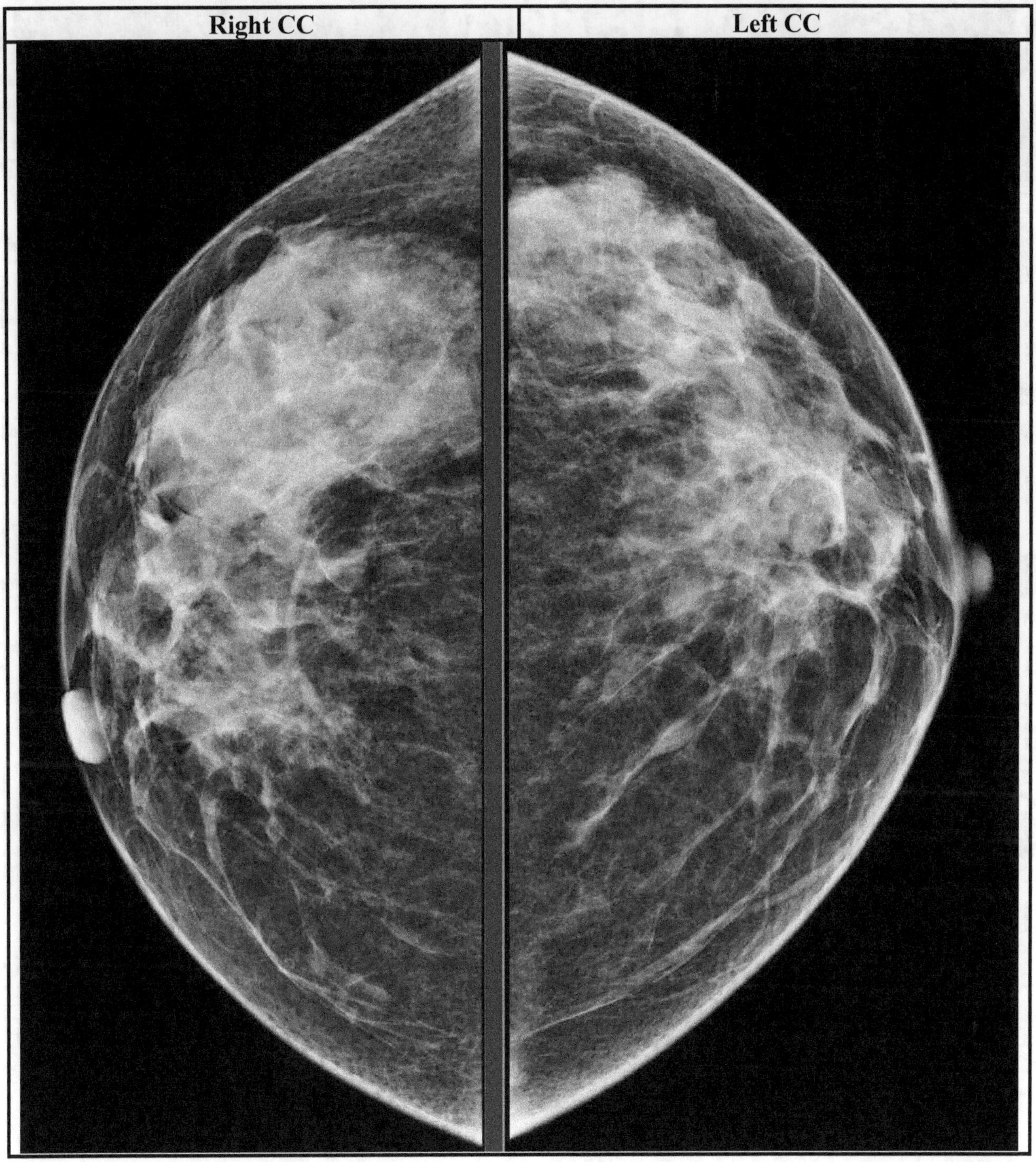
Right CC
Left CC

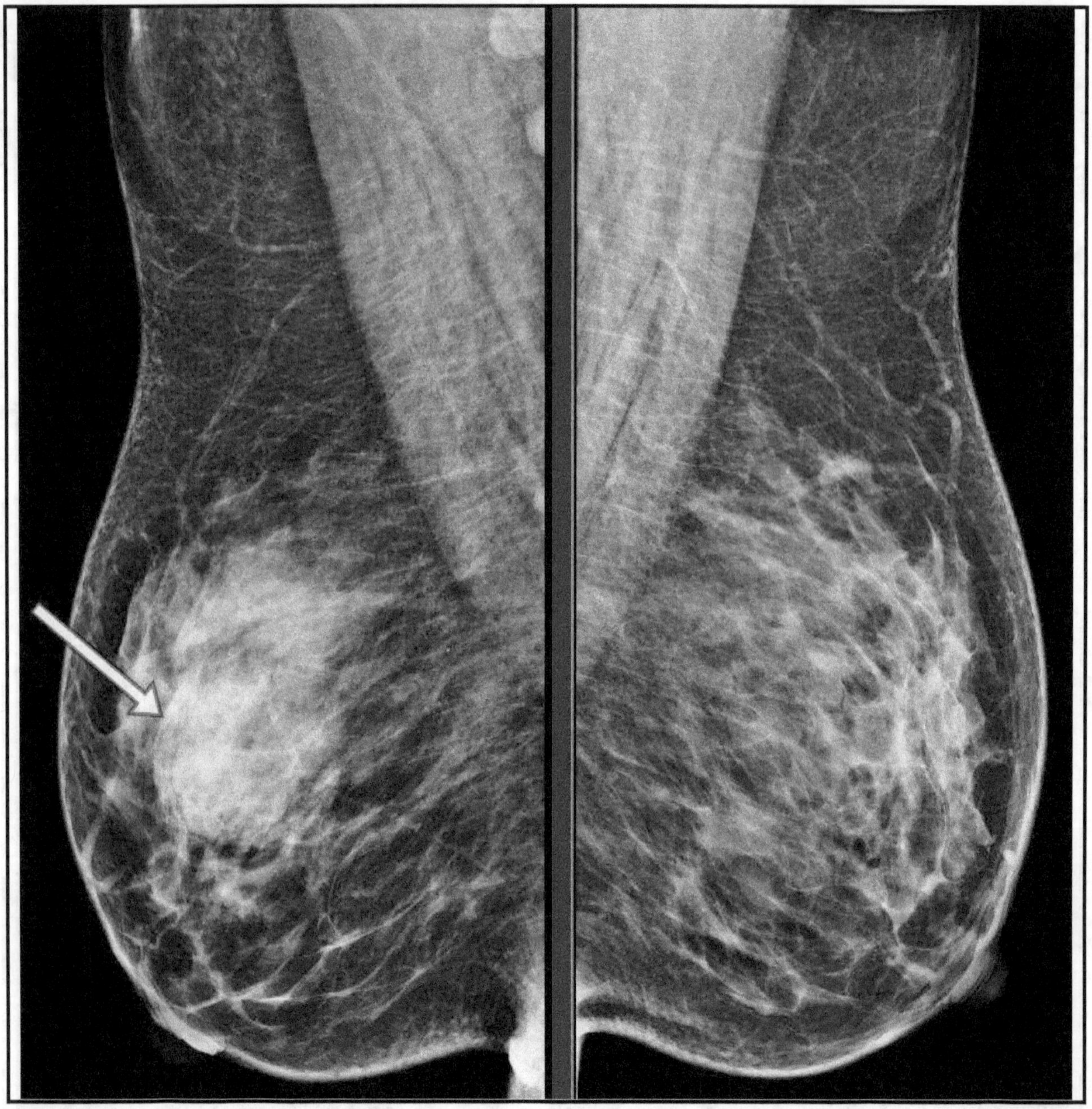

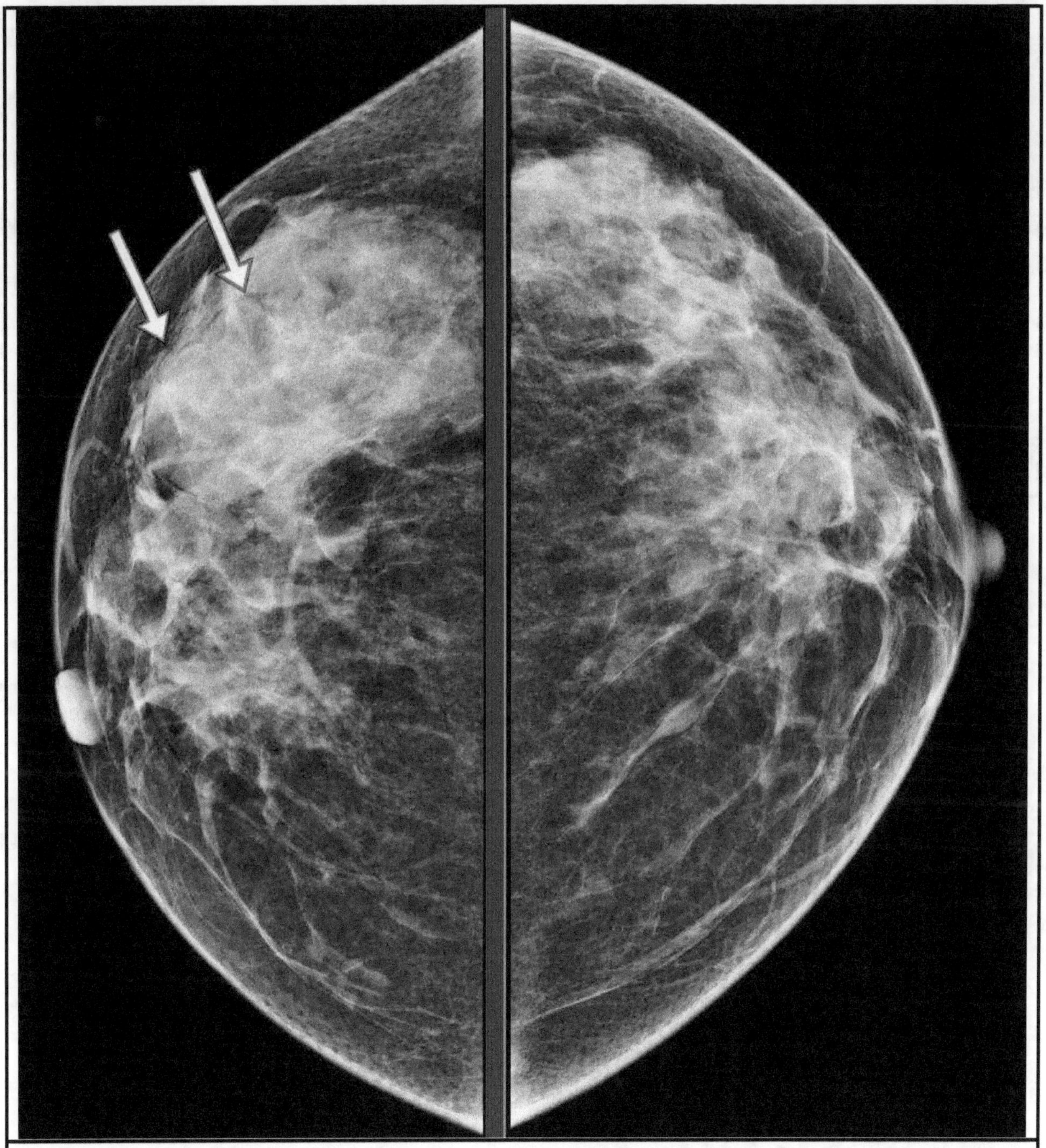

RIGHT BREAST	
Breast Parenchymal Density	***Heterogeneously dense, may obscure small masses (ACR C)***
Focal Mass	***UOQ multifocal round /oval circumscribed mass lesions***
Asymmetric Density	None
Parenchymal Distortion	None
Calcification	None
Skin Thickening	None
Axillary Nodes	None

LEFT BREAST	
Breast Parenchymal Density	***Heterogeneously dense, may obscure small masses (ACR C)***
Focal Mass	None
Asymmetric Density	None
Parenchymal Distortion	None
Calcification	None
Skin Thickening	None
Axillary Nodes	None

IMPRESSION:

RIGHT BREAST: (BI-RADS 0)
LEFT BREAST: (BI-RADS 1)

RECOMMENDATION: US Correlation

US demonstrate simple cysts

CASE 85: 40 -year-old female/ Diagnostic

Right MLO	Left MLO

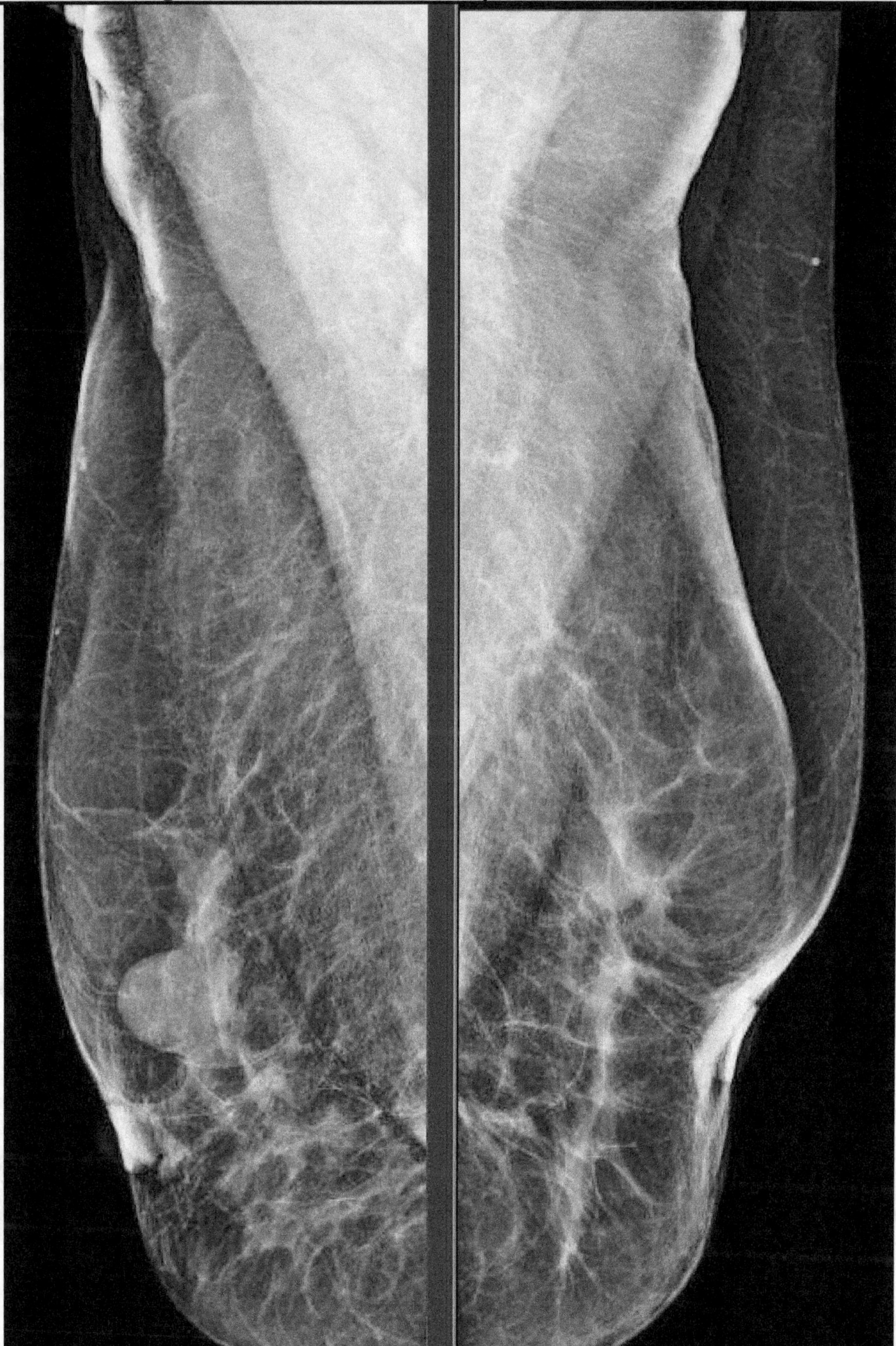

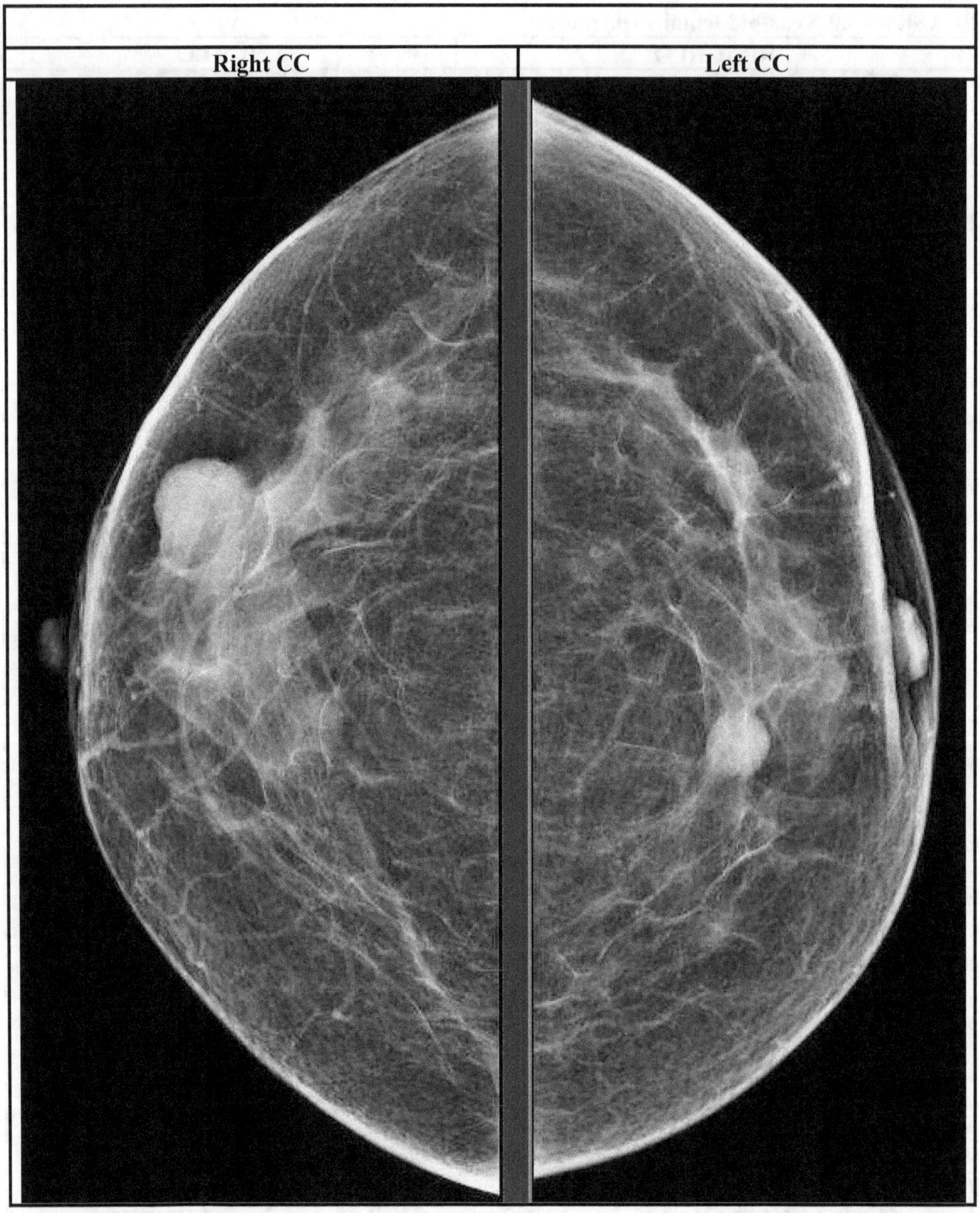
Right CC
Left CC

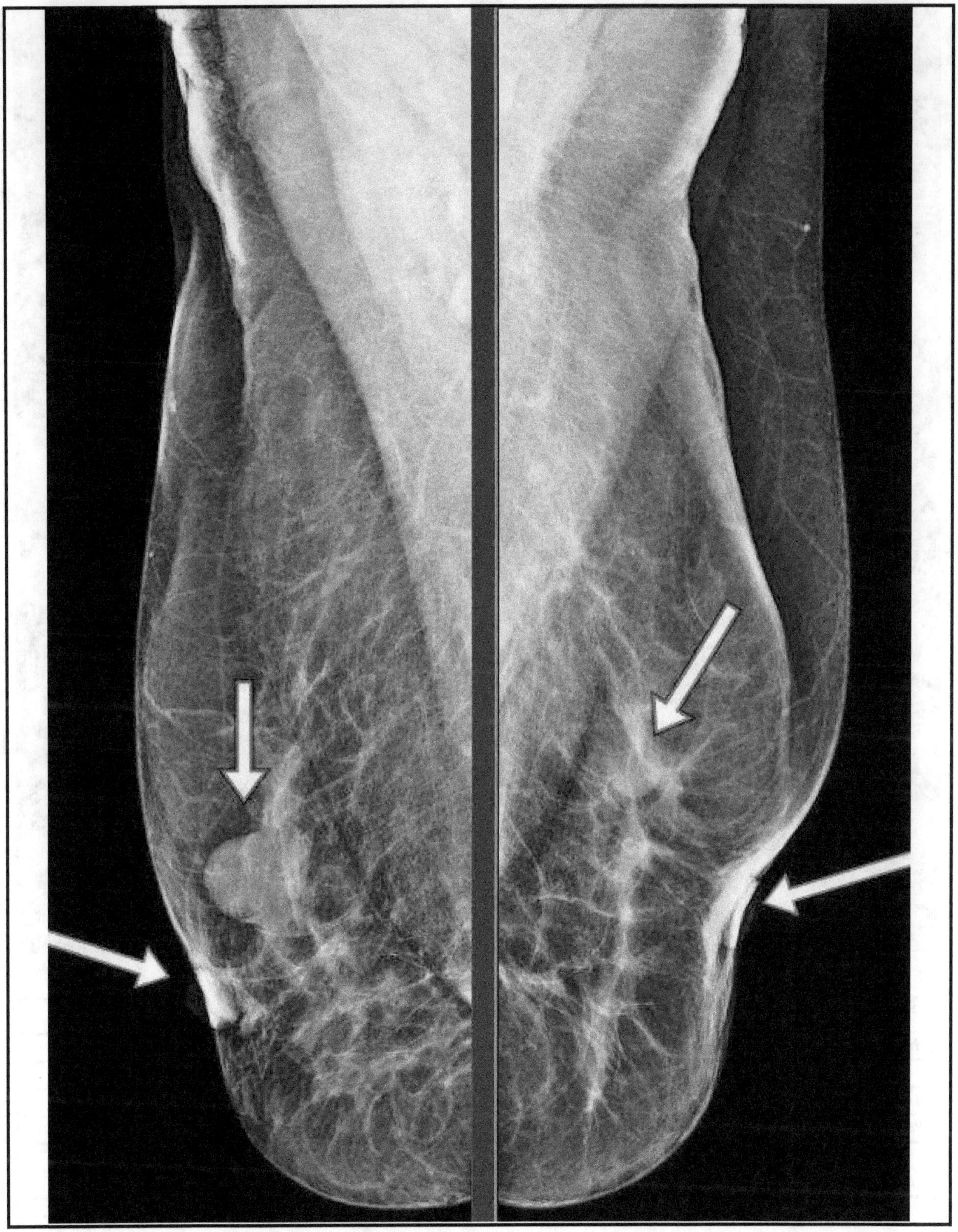

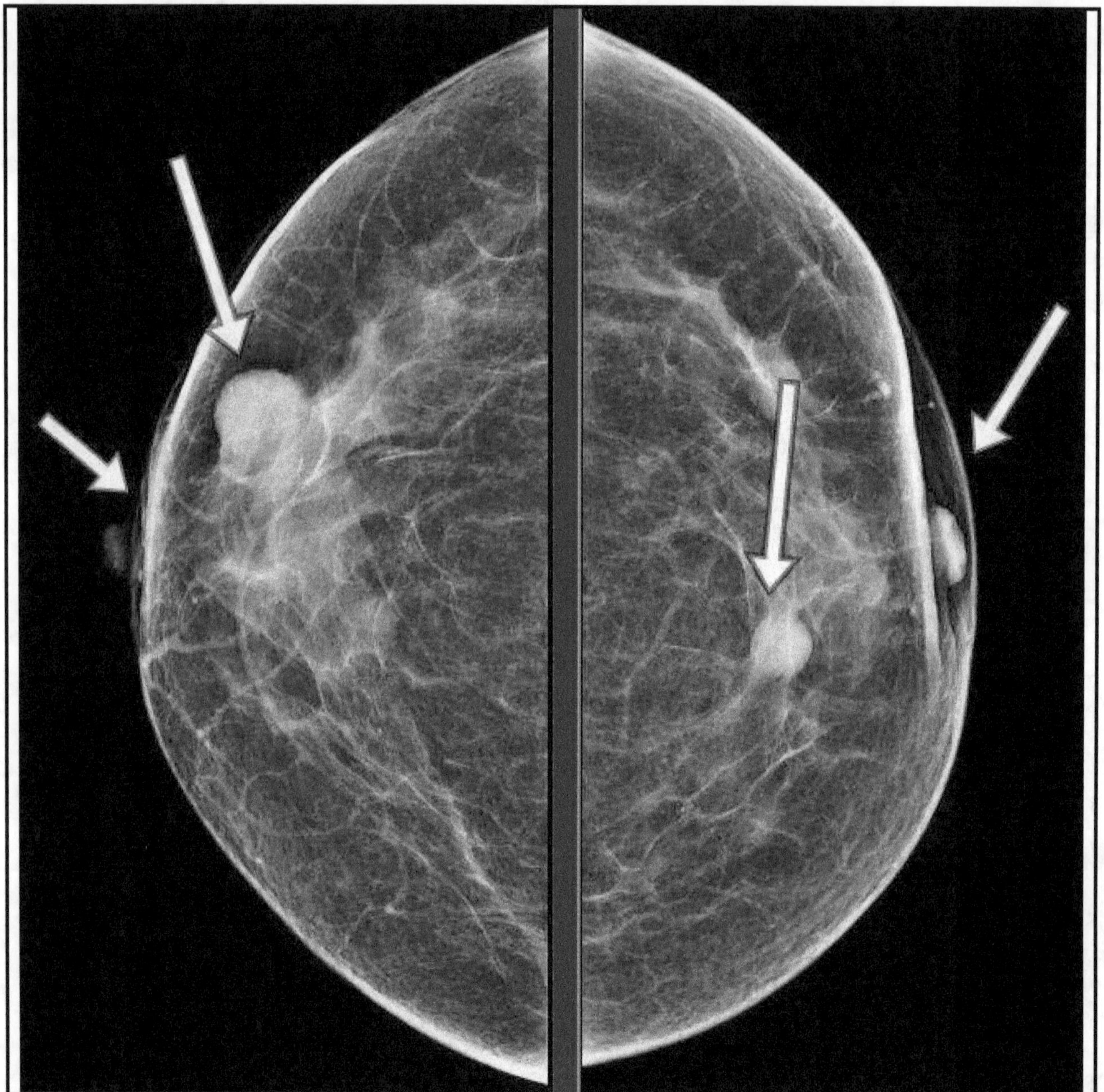

RIGHT BREAST	
Breast Parenchymal Density	***Scattered areas of fibroglandular density (ACR B)***
Focal Mass	***UOQ round obscured mass lesion***
Asymmetric Density	None
Parenchymal Distortion	None
Calcification	None
Skin Thickening	None / ***Nipple Retraction***
Axillary Nodes	None

LEFT BREAST	
Breast Parenchymal Density	***Scattered areas of fibroglandular density (ACR B)***
Focal Mass	***UIQ round circumscribed mass lesion***
Asymmetric Density	None
Parenchymal Distortion	None
Calcification	None
Skin Thickening	None/ ***Nipple Retraction***
Axillary Nodes	None

IMPRESSION:

RIGHT BREAST: (BI-RADS 0)
LEFT BREAST: (BI-RADS 0)

RECOMMENDATION: US Correlation

SUGGESTED READINGS

- The ACR BI-RADS® v2025 Manual the 5th Edition.
- ACR-AAPM-SIIM Practice parameter for determinants of image quality in digital mammography. Reston, VA: American College of Radiology; Amended 2014 (Resolution 39).
- American College of Radiology. ACR Practice parameters for the performance of screening and diagnostic mammography.
- Reston, VA: American College of Radiology; Amended 2014 (Resolution 39).
- Bahl M, Baker JA, Kinsey EN, Ghate SV. Architectural distortion on mammography: correlation with pathologic outcomes and predictors of malignancy. AJR Am J Roentgenol. 2015;205:1339–1345.
- Bassett LW, Hirbawi IA, DeBruhl N, Hayes MK. Mammographic positioning: evaluation from the view box. Radiology.1993;188:803–806.
- Bassett LW. Quality determinants of mammography: clinical image evaluation. RSNA Categorical Course in Breast Imaging Syllabus. 1995;57–67.
- Bird RE. Screening mammography: approach to interpretation and value of double reading. RSNA Categorical Course in Breast Imaging Syllabus. 1995;73–76.
- Cardenosa G, Eklund GW. Screening mammography in women 40 to 49 years old. AJR Am J Roentgenol.1995;164:1104–1106.
- Linver MN, Paster SB, Rosenberg RD, Key CR, Stidley CA, King WV. Improvement in mammography interpretation skills in a community radiology practice after dedicated teaching courses: 2-year medical audit of 38,633 cases. Radiology. 1992;184:39–43.
- Oeųnger KC, Fontham ET, Etzioni R, et al. Breast cancer screening for women at average risk. 2015 guideline update from the American Cancer Society. JAMA. 2015;314:1599–1614.
- Partyka L, Lourenco AP, Mainiero MB. Detection of mammographically occult architectural distortion on digital breast tomosynthesis screening: initial clinical experience. AJR Am J Roentgenol. 2014;203:216–222.

www.ingramcontent.com/pod-product-compliance
Lightning Source LLC
LaVergne TN
LVHW080013210926
848481LV00011B/3008
9798215708064